OKU

4

Orthopaedic Knowledge Update:

Foot and Ankle

AAOS
AMERICAN ACAD
ORTHOPAEDIC SU

OKU

4

Orthopaedic Knowledge Update:

Foot and Ankle

EDITOR:

Michael S. Pinzur, MD
Professor of Orthopaedic Surgery
Loyola University Medical School
Department of Orthopaedic Surgery
Loyola University Health System
Maywood, Illinois

Developed by the
American Orthopaedic Foot and Ankle Society

AMERICAN ORTHOPAEDIC
FOOT & ANKLE SOCIETY

AAOS
AMERICAN ACADEMY OF
ORTHOPAEDIC SURGEON

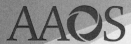

AMERICAN ACADEMY OF ORTHOPAEDIC SURGEONS

The material presented in **Orthopaedic Knowledge Update: Foot and Ankle 4** has been made available by the American Academy of Orthopaedic Surgeons for educational purposes only. This material is not intended to present the only, or necessarily best, methods or procedures for the medical situations discussed, but rather is intended to represent an approach, view, statement, or opinion of the author(s) or producer(s), which may be helpful to others who face similar situations.

Some drugs or medical devices demonstrated in Academy courses or described in Academy print or electronic publications have not been cleared by the Food and Drug Administration (FDA) or have been cleared for specific uses only. The FDA has stated that it is the responsibility of the physician to determine the FDA clearance status of each drug or device he or she wishes to use in clinical practice.

Furthermore, any statements about commercial products are solely the opinion(s) of the author(s) and do not represent an Academy endorsement or evaluation of these products. These statements may not be used in advertising or for any commercial purpose.

Some of the authors or the departments with which they are affiliated have received something of value from a commercial or other party related directly or indirectly to the subject of their chapter.

Published 2008 by the
American Academy of Orthopaedic Surgeons
6300 North River Road
Rosemont, IL 60018

Fourth Edition
Copyright 2008
by the American Academy of Orthopaedic Surgeons

ISBN 10: 0-89203-574-9
ISBN 13: 978-0-89203-574-8
Printed in the USA
Library of Congress Cataloging-in-Publication Data

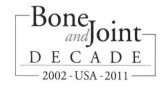

Acknowledgments

Editorial Board, Orthopaedic Knowledge Update: Foot and Ankle 4

Michael S. Pinzur, MD
Professor of Orthopaedic Surgery
Loyola University Medical School
Department of Orthopaedic Surgery
Loyola University Health System
Maywood, Illinois

Gregory C. Berlet, MD, FRCSC
Chief, Foot and Ankle Surgery
Orthopedic Foot and Ankle Center
Ohio State University
Columbus, Ohio

John T. Campbell, MD
Orthopaedic Surgeon
Institute for Foot and Ankle Reconstruction
Mercy Medical Center
Baltimore, Maryland

John S. Early, MD
Clinical Professor of Orthopedics
Southwestern Medical Center
Texas Orthopaedic Associates
Dallas, Texas

Stanley C. Graves, MD
Private Practice
Phoenix, Arizona

Sheldon S. Lin, MD
Associate Professor
Department of Orthopedics
University of Medicine and Dentistry of
  New Jersey
Newark, New Jersey

Stuart D. Miller, MD
Department of Orthopaedic Surgery
Union Memorial Hospital
Baltimore, Maryland

Ruth L. Thomas, MD
Professor
Department of Orthopaedics
University of Arkansas Medical Sciences
Little Rock, Arkansas

American Orthopaedic Foot and Ankle Society Board of Directors, 2008-2009

Robert B. Anderson, MD
President

Charles L. Saltzman, MD
President-Elect

Keith L. Wapner, MD
Vice-President

Judith F. Baumhauer, MD
Secretary

Lew C. Schon, MD
Treasurer

Steven D.K. Ross, MD
Immediate Past President

Lowell H. Gill, MD
Past President

Brian G. Donley, MD
Member-at-Large

Jeffrey E. Johnson, MD
Member-at-Large

Terrence M. Philbin, DO
Member-at-Large

Naomi N. Shields, MD
Member-at-Large

Contributors

Nicholas A. Abidi, MD
Santa Cruz Orthopaedic Institute
Dominican Santa Cruz Hospital
Santa Cruz, California

Richard G. Alvarez, MD
Director of Foot and Ankle Services
Department of Orthopaedic Surgery
University of Tennessee, Chattanooga
Chattanooga, Tennessee

LTC Romney C. Andersen, MD, MC, USA
Assistant Chief, Orthopaedic Surgery
Walter Reed National Military Medical Center
Washington, DC

James Aronson, MD
Professor and Chief
Department of Pediatric Orthopaedics
Arkansas Children's Hospital
University of Arkansas for Medical Sciences
Little Rock, Arkansas

Timothy M. Badwey, MD
Clinical Professor and Associate Program
  Director
Department of Orthopaedic Surgery
University of Missouri, Kansas City
Kansas City, Missouri

Wayne S. Berberian, MD, MBA
Associate Professor
Department of Orthopaedics
New Jersey Medical School
Newark, New Jersey

Eric M. Bluman, MD, PhD
Attending Orthopaedic Surgeon
Department of Orthopaedics
Brigham and Women's Hospital
Boston, Massachusetts

Michael E. Brage, MD
Associate Clinical Professor
Department of Orthopaedic Surgery
University of California, Irvine
South County Orthopaedic Specialists
Laguna Woods, California

Michael D. Castro, DO
Foot and Ankle Specialist
The Center for Orthopaedic Research and
Education
Phoenix, Arizona

Christopher P. Chiodo, MD
Foot and Ankle Division Chief
Department of Orthopedic Surgery
Brigham and Women's Hospital
Harvard Medical School
Boston, Massachusetts

Loretta B. Chou, MD
Associate Professor
Department of Orthopaedic Surgery
Stanford University
Stanford, California

Michael P. Clare, MD
Director of Fellowship Education
Foot and Ankle Fellowship
Florida Orthopaedic Institute
Tampa, Florida

J. Chris Coetzee, MD, FRCSC
Minnesota Sports Medicine and
  Twin Cities Orthopedics
Minneapolis, Minnesota

Henry DeGroot III, MD
Clinical Associate Professor
Newton Wellesley Hospital
Newton, Massachusetts

Alexis A. Dieter, MD
Columbia University College of
  Physicians and Surgeons
New York, New York

Thomas Dreher, MD
Section of Cerebral Palsy and Foot Deformities
Department of Orthopaedic Surgery
University of Heidelberg
Heidelberg, Germany

Patrick Ebeling, MD
Twin Cities Orthopaedics
Burnsville, Minnesota

Daniel C. Farber, MD
Assistant Professor of Orthopaedics
Department of Orthopaedics
University of Maryland School of Medicine
Department of Orthopaedics
Baltimore, Maryland

Jeff Feinblatt, MD
Oregon Orthopedics and Sports Medicine,
LLC
Oregon City, Oregon

James R. Ficke, MD
Chairman
Department of Orthopaedics and
Rehabilitation
Orthopaedic Consultant, US Army Surgeon
General
Brooke Army Medical Center
Fort Sam Houston, Texas

Adolph S. Flemister Jr, MD
Associate Professor
Department of Orthopedics
University of Rochester School of Medicine
Rochester, New York

Lorenzo Gamez, MD
Associate Professor
Department of Orthopaedic Surgery
University of Massachusetts Memorial
Medical Center
Worcester, Massachusetts

Stanley C. Graves, MD
Private Practice
Phoenix, Arizona

Gregory P. Guyton, MD
Faculty, Foot and Ankle Fellowship
Union Memorial Hospital
Baltimore, Maryland

Sharon Henry, MD
Associate Professor of Surgery
University of Maryland School of Medicine
Baltimore, Maryland

Keith J. Hill, MD
Team Physician, Lamar University Athletic
Program
Beaumont Bone and Joint Institute
Beaumont, Texas

Susan N. Ishikawa, MD
Assistant Professor
University of Tennessee
Campbell Clinic
Memphis, Tennessee

Clifford L. Jeng, MD
Attending Surgeon
Institute for Foot and Ankle Reconstruction
Mercy Medical Center
Baltimore, Maryland

CDR John J. Keeling, MD, MC, USN
Director, Orthopaedic Trauma and Foot and
Ankle Division
National Naval Medical Center
Walter Reed National Military Medical Center
Bethesda, Maryland

Derek M. Kelly, MD
Department of Pediatric Orthopaedic Surgery
University of Arkansas for Medical Sciences
Little Rock, Arkansas

Harold B. Kitaoka, MD
Consultant
Department of Orthopaedics
Mayo Clinic
Rochester, Minnesota

Alan C. League, MD
Clinical Instructor of Orthopaedic Surgery
Department of Orthopaedic Surgery
Loyola University Medical Center
Maywood, Illinois

John Logue, CPO
Prosthetist/Orthotist
D & J Medical
Baltimore, Maryland

Andrew Marini, DPT, ATC, MS
Owner/Physical Therapist
North River Physical Therapy
Chattanooga, Tennessee

James P. Maurer, DO
Department of Orthopedics
Philadelphia College of Osteopathic Medicine
Philadelphia, Pennsylvania

Robert G. Najarian, MD
Sports Medicine Fellow
Department of Orthopaedic Surgery
Cleveland Clinic Foundation
Cleveland, Ohio

John A. Nassar, MD
Private Practice
Scottsdale, Arizona

Steven K. Neufeld, MD
Director
Orthopaedic Foot and Ankle Center
   of Washington
Arlington, Virginia

Dror Paley, MD, FRCSC
Director
Rubin Institute for Advanced Orthopedics
Sinai Hospital of Baltimore
Baltimore, Maryland

Terrence M. Philbin, DO
Assistant Clinical Professor
Orthopedic Foot and Ankle Center
Ohio State University
Columbus, Ohio

Jason H. Pleimann, MD
Director, Foot and Ankle Service
Ozark Orthopaedic Clinic
Fayetteville, Arkansas

Julian Price, MD, ATC
Department of Orthopaedic Surgery
University of Tennessee, Chattanooga
Chattanooga, Tennessee

Amy Jo Ptaszek, MD
Clinical Associate
Northwestern University Medical School
Illinois Bone and Joint Institute
Glenview, Illinois

Steven M. Raikin, MD
Associate Professor of Orthopaedic Surgery
Director of Foot and Ankle Service
Rothman Institute
Philadelphia, Pennsylvania

Keri A. Reese, MD
Department of Orthopaedic Surgery
University of California, Irvine
Orange, California

Sanjeev Sabharwal, MD
Associate Professor
Department of Orthopaedics and Pediatrics
University of Medicine and Dentistry
   of New Jersey
New Jersey Medical School
Newark, New Jersey

Melanie Sanders, MD
Leesburg, Virginia

LTC Scott B. Shawen, MD, MC, USA
Director, Orthopaedic Foot and Ankle Surgery
Chief Consultant, Amputation Service
Department of Orthopaedics and
   Rehabilitation
Walter Reed Army Medical Center
Washington, DC

Naomi N. Shields, MD
Clinical Associate Professor
Department of Orthopaedic Surgery
University of Kansas School of Medicine
Wichita, Kansas

Paul S. Shurnas, MD
Director, Orthopaedic Foot and Ankle Surgery
Columbia Orthopaedic Group
Columbia, Missouri

Raymond J. Sullivan, MD
Associate Clinical Professor
University of Connecticut
Orthopaedic Associates of Hartford
Hartford, Connecticut

Norman S. Turner, MD
Assistant Professor of Orthopedics
Department of Orthopedic Surgery
Mayo Clinic
Rochester, Minnesota

Steven B. Weinfeld, MD
Associate Professor of Orthopaedic Surgery
Department of Orthopaedic Surgery
Mount Sinai School of Medicine
New York, New York

Wolfram Wenz, MD
Section of Cerebral Palsy and Foot Deformities
Department of Orthopaedic Surgery
University of Heidelberg
Heidelberg, Germany

Preface

The fourth edition of *Orthopaedic Knowledge Update: Foot and Ankle* reflects the expanded body of knowledge that has developed over the past several years in this relatively new subspecialty of orthopaedic surgery. As our discipline has matured, the contributors to this volume have attempted to provide a foundation of "state of the art" knowledge for both practicing orthopaedic surgeons and residents in training. We also have attempted to provide cutting-edge and controversial information for those with more sophisticated expertise in this rapidly evolving area of musculoskeletal medicine. It is our desire that the reader will be instilled with our enthusiasm for this subspecialty and that their patients will reap the benefits of the newest approaches to solving difficult problems of the foot and ankle.

I would especially like to express my gratitude to the authors and section editors for their willingness to share their knowledge with the readership. Their enthusiasm and efficiency allowed timely publication of this important orthopaedic text. I also want to thank the Academy publications staff: Marilyn L. Fox, PhD, Department Director; Lisa Claxton Moore, Managing Editor; and all the members of the production staff who contributed their time and efforts to this work. A very special thank you is given to Kathleen Anderson, Senior Editor, who translated "foot and ankle-ese" into a coherent and timely scientific resource.

I hope that the readership will find this work instructive and gain as much knowledge as I have obtained from the contributors during its preparation.

Michael S. Pinzur, MD
Editor

Table of Contents

Section 4: The Forefoot

Section 5: Neuromuscular Disease

Section 6: Special Problems of the Foot and Ankle

General Foot and Ankle Topics

SECTION EDITOR:

JOHN T. CAMPBELL, MD

Chapter 1

Biomechanics of the Foot and Ankle

Christopher P. Chiodo, MD   Eric M. Bluman, MD, PhD

Introduction

The lower extremity is a sophisticated and complex musculoskeletal unit that is essential to normal human function. Its evolution has allowed humans to stand upright, walk, and run. Describing the foot and ankle as a "pedestal" is inaccurate. Although the foot and ankle are stable and rigid structures that support weight and allow locomotion, they are also supple and flexible structures that absorb shock and adapt to movement over uneven ground.

Little was understood about the biomechanics of the foot and ankle until the 20th century. With the development of advanced imaging, videography, and modern electronics, knowledge in this field has grown exponentially.[1-4] Clinically, such knowledge has resulted in a better understanding of the biomechanical basis of normal function and has allowed insight into disorders of the foot and ankle, which often manifest in a disruption of normal biomechanical function.

A thorough understanding of the biomechanics of the foot and ankle is a prerequisite to treating patients with foot and ankle disorders and is essential for developing and advancing new procedures to treat such disorders.

Structural Anatomy and Kinematics

Kinetics is the branch of physics and mechanics concerned with the effect of forces on the motion of bodies and should not be confused with kinematics, which relates to the characteristics of motion without regard to the effects of force or mass.

At the most basic level, the foot can be conceptualized as a tripod that supports the ankle and body. With neutral alignment, ground pressure is almost evenly distributed between the heel, first metatarsal head, and the lesser metatarsal heads (**Figure 1**). Malalignment and deformity disrupt this balance. For example, a cavus deformity may cause increased pressure under the first metatarsal head and along the lateral border of the foot. In hallux valgus and other disorders that compromise the medial ray, there will be increased loading of the lesser metatarsals, which may result in the development of transfer metatarsalgia.

The foot has three arches: the medial longitudinal arch, the transverse metatarsal arch, and the lateral longitudinal arch. These arches are stabilized statically by bony anatomy and ligamentous constraints. For example, the transverse metatarsal and lateral longitudinal arches are stabilized by the cross-sectional wedge and keystone shapes of the cuboid, cuneiforms, and metatarsal bases.

The concept of dynamic stabilization is pertinent with regard to the sagittal plane and the medial longitudinal arch. This arch is a dynamic structure that allows shock absorption at heel strike and propulsion at toe-off. Two biomechanical models have been used to describe the medial longitudinal arch.[5] In one model, the arch is conceptualized as a curved, segmented beam

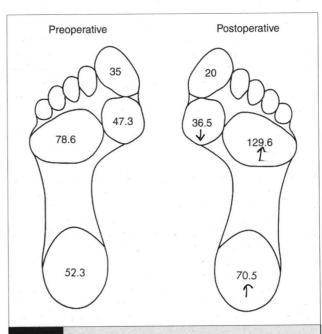

Figure 1	Peak forces, in Newtons, measured on the plantar foot before and after silicone arthroplasty of the first metatarsophalangeal joint. (*Reproduced with permission from Beverly MC, Horan FT, Hutton WC: Load cell analysis following silastic arthroplasty of the hallux. Int Orthop 1985;9:101-104.*)

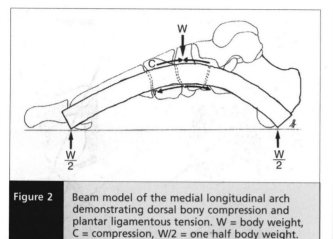

Figure 2 Beam model of the medial longitudinal arch demonstrating dorsal bony compression and plantar ligamentous tension. W = body weight, C = compression, W/2 = one half body weight. *(Reproduced with permission from Sarrafian SK: Anatomy of the Foot and Ankle: Descriptive, Topographic, Functional, ed 2. Philadelphia, PA, Lippincott, Williams and Wilkins, 1993, p 560.)*

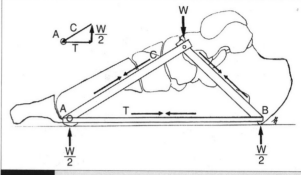

Figure 3 Truss model of the medial longitudinal arch. The bony architecture of the foot is conceptualized as two beams connected by the plantar fascia, which functions as a tie-rod. A and B = attachment points of the plantar fascia (or the rod) in the truss model, C = compression, T = tension, W = body weight, W/2 = one half body weight. *(Reproduced with permission from Sarrafian SK: Anatomy of the Foot and Ankle: Descriptive, Topographic, Functional, ed 2. Philadelphia, PA, Lippincott, Williams and Wilkins, 1993, p 559.)*

(**Figure 2**). The beam is made up of the calcaneus, talus, navicular, cuneiforms, and the first through third metatarsals. These segments are stabilized by ligamentous connections. With weight bearing, compression forces develop on the dorsal aspect of the beam whereas tensile forces are generated on the plantar aspect.[6] The dorsal compression forces are absorbed and resisted by the bony architecture of the arch whereas plantar tensile forces are resisted by the dense plantar ligaments.

The beam model of the medial longitudinal arch does not consider the role of the plantar fascia. This structure is incorporated in the truss model of the arch (**Figure 3**). In the truss model, the arch is conceptualized as a triangular structure composed of two oblique beams with a dorsal pivot connected plantarly by a tie-rod. Anatomically, the plantar fascia functions as the tie-rod, originating from the posterior calcaneal tuberosity and inserting onto the sesamoids and the bases of the proximal phalanges of the lesser toes. With loading, the plantar fascia resists the plantarly generated tensile forces.[7] A recent finite element analysis showed that surgical fasciotomy poses a risk to arch stability.[8]

The role of the plantar fascia in resisting plantar tensile forces and stabilizing the arch of the foot is sometimes referred to as the windlass mechanism. A windlass is a device used for transporting or lifting an object and is made up of a horizontal cylinder that is turned by a crank such that a cable or rope attached to the object is wound around the cylinder. The plantar fascia has been described as a windlass that stabilizes the arch by plantar flexion of the first metatarsal. Beginning at midstance, the hallux begins to dorsiflex. Because the plantar fascia inserts onto the hallux, this motion results in increased tension in the plantar fascia, thereby plantar flexion of the first metatarsal and stabilizing the medial arch. The forces involved are enhanced by the metatarsal head, which serves as the horizontal cylinder or pulley of the windlass.

Both the beam and truss models illustrate the biome-

chanical complexity of the medial longitudinal arch. This structure is critical to force dissipation during the early portions of stance and for effective propulsion later toward push-off.[6] A further understanding of the axes and articulations of the ankle and hindfoot is integral to this concept.

At heel strike, the subtalar and transverse tarsal (talonavicular and calcaneocuboid) joints are supple, allowing the foot and medial arch to absorb the ground reactive forces. In addition to the elasticity of the plantar fascia, absorption of forces is made possible by the unique articulations and axes of the three joints of the hindfoot. The subtalar joint has been classically conceptualized as a mitered hinge.[9] Its axis passes obliquely from plantar laterally to dorsomedially, deviating from the horizontal plane by approximately 42° and from the sagittal plane by approximately 16°.[10,11] Such obliquity allows the axial rotation of the tibia to be translated into inversion and eversion of the subtalar joint and allows pronation and supination of the midfoot and forefoot (**Figure 4**).

Because of their unique orientation, the axes of the talonavicular and calcaneocuboid joints are parallel and are therefore supple with subtalar eversion.[12] With subtalar inversion, the axes of these joints are convergent and locked (**Figure 5**). The teleology of the mitered hinge concept is apparent. At heel strike and initial stance, internal rotation of the tibia causes eversion of the subtalar joint. This, in turn, unlocks the transverse tarsal joint and allows shock absorption and accommodation during ambulation over uneven ground. Later during stance, external tibial rotation causes the subtalar joint to invert and lock the transverse tarsal joint. This allows the foot to become a rigid lever for more effective propulsion at push-off.

The unique anatomy of the ankle joint is important

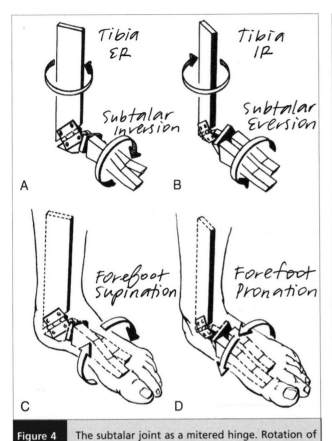

Tibia ER — *Subtalar Inversion*

Tibia IR — *Subtalar Eversion*

Forefoot Supination

Forefoot Pronation

A

B

C

D

Figure 4 The subtalar joint as a mitered hinge. Rotation of the tibia causes inversion (**A**) and eversion (**B**) of the subtalar joint, and supination (**C**) and pronation (**D**) of the forefoot. *(Reproduced with permission from Mann RA: Biomechanics of the foot and ankle, in Mann RA, Coughlin MJ (eds): Surgery of the Foot and Ankle, ed 6. St. Louis, MO, Mosby-Year Book, 1993, p 21.)*

of subtalar joint

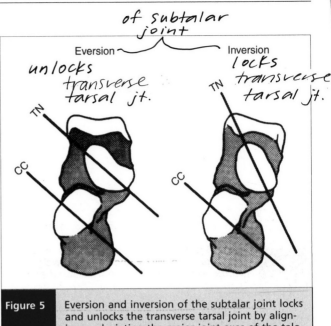

Eversion — *unlocks transverse tarsal jt.*

Inversion — *locks transverse tarsal jt.*

Figure 5 Eversion and inversion of the subtalar joint locks and unlocks the transverse tarsal joint by aligning or deviating the major joint axes of the talonavicular (TN) and calcaneocuboid (CC) joints. *(Reproduced with permission from Mann RA: Biomechanics of the foot and ankle, in Mann RA, Coughlin MJ (eds): Surgery of the Foot and Ankle, ed 6. St. Louis, MO, Mosby-Year Book, 1993, p 23.)*

to foot and ankle biomechanics. Composed of the talus and distal tibia and fibula, the ankle joint includes three articulations: tibiotalar, tibiofibular, and talofibular. The tibiofibular joint represents the inferior extent of the distal lower extremity syndesmosis. It is stabilized by the interosseous ligament, the inferior transverse tibiofibular ligament, and the anterior and posterior tibiofibular ligaments.[13,14] This articulation allows slight axial rotation of the foot about the vertical axis of the leg (> 15° in one recent study).[15] Specifically, there is a coupled motion with external rotation of the fibula linked to dorsiflexion of the ankle. The tibiofibular joint also plays a role in load sharing. Together, the tibiofibular and talofibular articulations allow the fibula to support approximately 15% to 20% of the load transmitted across the ankle.

The tibiotalar joint is one of the most remarkable joints of the body. Despite its small surface area and the relatively decreased thickness of its cartilage, this joint withstands up to four times body weight with normal ambulation. The empirical axis of the ankle joint is approximated by palpating the tips of the malleoli and does not correspond to the articular surface of the talus

(**Figure 6**). This axis is oriented obliquely at 82° from the midline of the tibia, running plantar laterally to dorsomedially.[12] The clinical significance of such obliquity allows concomitant horizontal rotation to occur in the foot or leg as the ankle moves in the sagittal plane. Specifically, when the foot is free (for example, during the swing phase of gait) the foot deviates outward with dorsiflexion and inward with plantar flexion. When the foot is stabilized by the ground, ankle dorsiflexion during early stance produces internal rotation of the leg. This coupled motion unlocks the transverse tarsal joint and allows both the hindfoot and leg to absorb the energy of heel strike. Later, as the foot pushes off, ankle plantar flexion results in external rotation of the leg. Such lower extremity external rotation is instrumental in forward progression of the trunk and body.

Because the empirical axis of the tibiotalar joint is oriented obliquely to the articular surface of the joint, the trochlear articular surface of the talus has been traditionally described as a truncated cone. This cone has a smaller medial and larger lateral radius. The articular surface of the talus is also narrower posteriorly than anteriorly. These relationships have substantial implications for ankle stability.[16,17] Because of the broader radius laterally, the supporting ligaments are more distinct and are divided into three components: the anterior talofibular ligament, the posterior talofibular ligament, and the calcaneofibular ligament. These ligaments have particular orientations.[18] The calcaneofibular ligament, which is always perpendicular to and stabilizes the subtalar joint, is perpendicular to the ankle joint in dorsiflexion. With ankle dorsiflexion, ligamen-

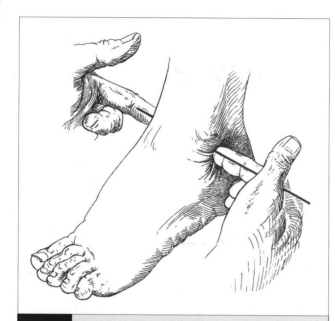

Figure 6 Estimation of the empirical axis of the ankle by palpation of the tips of the malleoli. *(Reproduced with permission from Mann RA: Biomechanics of the foot and ankle, in Coughlin MJ, Mann RA (eds): Surgery of the Foot and Ankle, ed 7. St. Louis, MO, Mosby-Year Book, 1999, p 15.)*

tous stability is a function of the calcaneofibular ligament. The anterior talofibular ligament is perpendicular to and stabilizes the ankle joint when the joint is plantar flexed. With ankle plantar flexion, the narrower posterior diameter of the talus also decreases the bony contribution to joint stability.[17]

Human Locomotion and Gait

Human locomotion is the activity by which an individual moves from one geographic location to another. Human gait is defined as that pattern or method by which the lower limbs are used for forward locomotion with the body held erect. During ambulation, the body progresses forward by means of a repetitive cycle during which alternating limbs are loaded and unloaded. At least one foot is always in contact with the ground. Walking also is characterized by a period of "double-limb support" during which both feet are in contact with the ground. This characteristic is in contrast to running, which is characterized by a period during which both feet are off the ground and there is no double-limb support.

Normal human gait is highly coordinated and efficient with regard to energy and oxygen consumption.[19] Stride length is defined as the distance covered between two consecutive heel strikes of the ipsilateral foot. Step length is the distance between the heel strike of one foot and heel strike of the other foot. Walking velocity is calculated from stride length and cadence (for exam-

ple, steps per second or minute). With gait dysfunction, alterations in these parameters lead to increased energy and oxygen consumption. In amputees, more proximal amputation levels correlate with higher rates of oxygen consumption. In patients who have been treated with ankle fusion, stride length is decreased.[20]

Gait analysis, the study of human locomotion, may be conducted in the clinic or more formally in a gait analysis laboratory. The latter option often involves a multidisciplinary team and the use of such tools as video analysis, pedobarographs, force plates, electromyography, and computerized gait assessment. Although most orthopaedic surgeons do not have direct access to such a facility, a complete orthopaedic physical examination should include visual observation of a patient's gait.

The gait cycle is defined as that period and activity encompassing one human stride, beginning at the heel strike of one limb and ending with the next heel strike of the same limb. There are two major phases of the gait cycle: stance and swing. The stance phase comprises approximately 60% of the gait cycle and represents the period during which one limb is loaded and in contact with the ground (**Figure 7**). Descriptive terms subdividing stance include heel strike, midstance (foot flat), and push-off (toe-off). The swing phase comprises the remaining 40% of the gait cycle and represents the period during which the limb advances forward and is not in contact with the ground.

The stance phase has been further divided into three intervals. The first interval extends from heel strike to foot flat. It is characterized by weight acceptance and rapid ankle plantar flexion, the latter controlled by eccentric contraction of the anterior compartment musculature. The second interval extends from foot flat through and past midstance. During this interval, the center of gravity of the body passes over the planted foot. Progressive ankle dorsiflexion is controlled by eccentric posterior compartment contraction, resulting in maximal loading across the ankle at more than four times body weight. The third interval extends from the second interval through toe-off. During this interval, the ankle rapidly plantar flexes (by means of concentric contraction of the posterior compartment musculature) in preparation for push-off and limb advancement during swing. During the third interval, the hindfoot is rigid and best suited for toe-off.

Many disorders of the foot and ankle lead to discernible and characteristic patterns of human gait. An antalgic gait results from pain and is defined by the shortened stance phase of the affected limb. A steppage gait results from footdrop or weakness of the anterior musculature of the leg. It is characterized by lifting the affected limb higher during the swing phase so that the foot adequately clears the ground. A calcaneal gait is characterized by exaggerated heel weight bearing and results from weakness or paralysis of the posterior compartment musculature. A waddling gait is the result of proximal myopathy and is characterized by a broad-

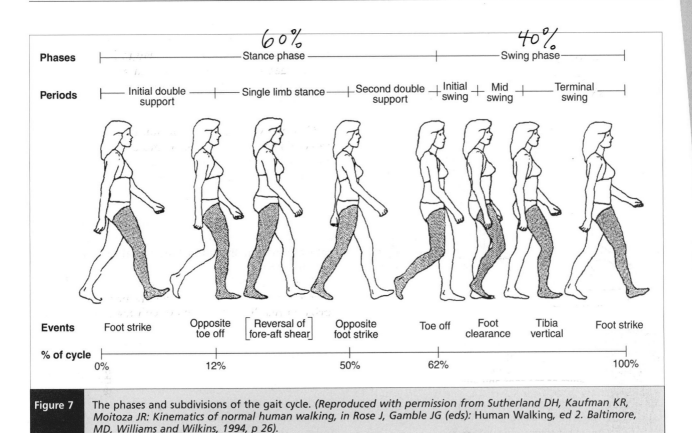

		60%			40%	
Phases	├─────── Stance phase ───────┤			├────── Swing phase ──────┤		
Periods	├─ Initial double support ─┤	├─ Single limb stance ─┤	├─ Second double support ─┤	├─ Initial swing ─┤	├─ Mid swing ─┤	├─ Terminal swing ─┤
Events	Foot strike	Opposite toe off	Reversal of fore-aft shear	Opposite foot strike	Toe off	Foot clearance	Tibia vertical	Foot strike
% of cycle	0%	12%		50%	62%			100%

Figure 7   The phases and subdivisions of the gait cycle. *(Reproduced with permission from Sutherland DH, Kaufman KR, Moitoza JR: Kinematics of normal human walking, in Rose J, Gamble JG (eds): Human Walking, ed 2. Baltimore, MD, Williams and Wilkins, 1994, p 26).*

based stance with the pelvis dropping toward the leg being raised during the swing phase. This gait abnormality is in contrast to a Trendelenburg gait, which is caused by weakness of the hip abductors and results in a compensatory lurching of the trunk toward the weakened side during stance.

Surgical Treatment

Advances in understanding foot and ankle biomechanics have led to the development of surgical procedures designed to correct and alter the abnormal biomechanics of certain foot and ankle disorders. These procedures often are used in conjunction with other procedures to tailor the surgical plan to the diagnosis and pattern of deformity of the individual patient.

Tendon Transfer

Successful tendon transfer requires consideration of multiple factors in planning and execution of the selected procedure. Failure to consider the strength, excursion, site of insertion, and phasic activity of the transferred muscle will risk insufficiency or failure of the procedure. In general, the strength of the musculotendinous unit to be transferred should be adequate to allow loss of one motor grade from that present in its native position. Muscle strength is proportional to the cross-sectional area of the muscle belly. Excursion also must be matched to the extent possible to ensure that

articular motion is returned to the physiologic range. The site of insertion will determine the moment arm of the portion of the extremity distal to the transfer. The moment arm is defined as the distance at which force is applied from a center of rotation. This distance also has a direct effect on the arc the joint can traverse. The contraction of the muscle to be transferred should occur during the same portion of gait as contraction of the motor unit it will replace or augment. Adherence to this concept maintains the principle of in-phase tendon transfer. Failure to achieve an in-phase transfer can lead to antagonistic activity of the transferred motor unit, which may prevent proper functioning of joints during the gait cycle. Location of the muscle relative to joint axes will determine the function it performs. Muscles that lie anterior and posterior to the axis of tibiotalar rotation will dorsiflex and plantar flex, respectively, the ankle during contraction. Those that lie medial and lateral to the axis of the subtalar joint will invert and evert the hindfoot, respectively.

Flexor digitorum longus (FDL) transfer with a calcaneal osteotomy for patients with adult acquired flatfoot deformity (AAFD) illustrates the application of these principles. The FDL is in phase with the posterior tibial tendon. Harvest of the FDL and transfer to the plantar and medial aspects of the navicular re-creates the moment arm of the dysfunctional posterior tibial tendon. The FDL has approximately 30% of the strength of the posterior tibial tendon and relatively less excursion, making isolated transfer prone to failure. Realignment

     7

of the hindfoot and/or forefoot can improve functional results by diminishing the loads required during weight bearing. A medial displacement calcaneal osteotomy reduces the antagonistic force of the Achilles tendon and decreases the strain on the medial supporting structures. Efficiency of the transferred tendon can be improved by medializing the insertion point of the transferred tendon. The navicular and transferred tendon can be further medialized in relationship to the subtalar axes by correcting the lateral subluxation of the talonavicular joint through spring ligament reefing and/or lateral column lengthening.

Gastrocnemius Recession and Achilles Tendon Lengthening

The triceps surae, composed of the gastrocnemius and soleus muscles, contributes to the pathology of many disorders affecting the foot and ankle. For example, Achilles tendon rupture results in decreased peak forefoot pressures.[21] Contracture of this musculoskeletal unit is especially problematic because it causes decreased ankle dorsiflexion, resulting in sagittal plane bending moments that are abnormally transmitted distally into the foot during late stance and push-off. This can lead to multiple pathologies, including joint instability (for example, peritalar subluxation) and bony overload (for example, metatarsalgia).

The tension and force generated by these muscles can be surgically decreased by gastrocnemius recession or Achilles tendon lengthening. These are not equivalent procedures and have different indications. Both the gastrocnemius and the soleus muscles insert on the calcaneus via the Achilles tendon. The soleus originates on the posterior tibia and crosses both the ankle and the subtalar joints. In contrast, the gastrocnemius originates on the distal femur and crosses the knee, the ankle, and the subtalar joints. Although both the gastrocnemius and soleus plantar flex the foot, differential amounts of pathologic contracture can be present. The Silfverskiöld test is used to differentiate Achilles tendon contracture from isolated gastrocnemius contracture. This test is performed by comparing the amount of passive ankle dorsiflexion obtainable when the knee is extended with the amount of passive ankle dorsiflexion when the knee is flexed. Flexion at the knee releases the gastrocnemius and allows testing of the soleus alone. Increased ankle dorsiflexion with the knee flexed indicates the presence of some degree of a gastrocnemius contracture. Limited ankle dorsiflexion, with and without knee flexion, indicates contracture of both the gastrocnemius and soleus muscles (the triceps surae).

An isolated gastrocnemius contracture can be corrected by recession of its aponeurosis above the level of the soleus tendon. Combined contracture of both the soleus and the gastrocnemius is treated with Achilles tendon lengthening. In one recent clinical study, the average improvement in ankle dorsiflexion following a Strayer procedure was 16°.[22] Another recent study investigated Achilles tendon lengthening with the Strayer procedure

in children with cerebral palsy.[23] The procedure was selected based on the Silfverskiöld test. Both groups showed significant improvement in static and dynamic dorsiflexion and in clinical outcomes. It was concluded that both procedures are effective in appropriately selected patients; however, overcorrection or undercorrection also was demonstrated with both procedures.

Medializing Calcaneal Osteotomy

The mild valgus present in the normal hindfoot becomes more pronounced in those with AAFD. A cornerstone of reconstructive surgery for this deformity is to restore the hindfoot to a more anatomic position and reestablish a more anatomic weight-bearing axis. Medial displacement calcaneal osteotomy is a joint-sparing procedure commonly used to accomplish this goal. The procedure translates the insertion of the Achilles tendon and triceps surae medially. As a result, the vector of pull promotes a varus moment at the subtalar joint and the ground reaction force is moved closer to the mechanical axis of the leg, decreasing torque at the subtalar joint. Another beneficial effect of medializing the calcaneal tuberosity is decreased tensile forces on the medial ligamentous structures, including the deltoid and spring ligament complexes.[24] Although there is theoretic concern that a medializing calcaneal osteotomy can affect tibiotalar contact and loading, it has been shown that large magnitudes of translation minimally shift the tibiotalar center of pressure. Although calcaneal osteotomies should have minimal effects in initiating joint degradation, they may have only a token effect in off-loading portions of the ankle joint that is demonstrating arthritic changes.

Lateral Column Lengthening

In some forms of AAFD, abduction of the midfoot exacerbates existing hindfoot valgus. Lateral column lengthening, either through calcaneal osteotomy or calcaneocuboid arthrodesis, is a potent surgical procedure commonly used for patients with more advanced stages of AAFD associated with substantial foot abduction. The procedure swings the midfoot and forefoot into a more adducted position through the talonavicular joint. Navicular coverage of the talar head, which is commonly subluxated medially, is an approximate gauge of the degree of correction obtained. In addition to correction of forefoot abduction, arch height is improved. It must be noted, however, that lateral column lengthening used for patients with AAFD often results in a midfoot and forefoot with residual varus that necessitates additional medial column procedures (for example, metatarsocuneiform arthrodesis or cuneiform osteotomy) to establish a plantigrade foot.

Technically, lateral column lengthening is performed using one of two methods. When performing calcaneocuboid distraction arthrodesis, the joint is sacrificed in the process of obtaining length. Typically, a 1.0- to 1.5-cm structural bone graft is placed between the anterior process of the calcaneus and the proximal cuboid. Alternatively, the graft can be placed in an osteotomy site created through the anterior calcaneus 1 cm proximal to the calcaneocuboid joint, thus sparing the calcaneocuboid joint.

In contrast with the effects of a medial translation calcaneal osteotomy, the tension in the spring ligament in intact feet is not decreased with lateral column lengthening. Recent studies show that these procedures decrease the load borne by the medial column while increasing the pressure in the lateral column.[25-27] Initial concerns that lengthening through the anterior calcaneus would increase calcaneocuboid pressure prompted some investigators to recommend bone block arthrodesis rather than a joint-sparing procedure. However, findings in a cadaver flatfoot model demonstrated increased lateral forefoot loading with arthrodesis when compared with osteotomy.[28]

Medial Cuneiform Osteotomy

The medial cuneiform (Cotton) osteotomy was described by Cotton in 1936.[29] This procedure consists of a dorsal opening wedge osteotomy through the medial cuneiform. It plantar flexes the first ray and is useful in realigning the distal portion of the medial column to a plantigrade position, essentially restoring the tripod configuration of the foot. This procedure typically is used when treating fixed forefoot varus (supination) associated with flatfoot deformities.

The Cotton osteotomy may play a role in reducing the increased lateral forefoot pressures associated with lateral common lengthening, although further research is needed. In one biomechanical study, the addition of a Cotton osteotomy to a lateral column lengthening procedure resulted in normalization of lateral forefoot pressures; however, high medial forefoot pressures were noted.[30] These results are inconsistent with those of another cadaver study in which the Cotton osteotomy, while increasing medial forefoot pressures, did not significantly decrease lateral pressures.[27]

Weil Osteotomy

The use of a shortening osteotomy of a distal lesser metatarsal was initially described by Barouk and further popularized by Weil.[31] This procedure is commonly performed using a long oblique osteotomy through the distal aspect of the metatarsal. It is primarily used to shorten the lesser metatarsals (by translation of the distal segment) to treat metatarsalgia and metatarsophalangeal joint instability. Fixation is obtained with Kirschner wires or 2.0-mm screws. In addition to shortening the metatarsal head through translation, the osteotomy also may incorporate bony wedge resection to elevate the metatarsal head.

An analysis of this procedure in a cadaver model found significant unloading of the head of the second metatarsal and remaining lesser metatarsals.[32] An increase in first metatarsal pressure also occurred. These results are similar to previous clinical data obtained using pedobarographs following Weil osteotomies.[33] The

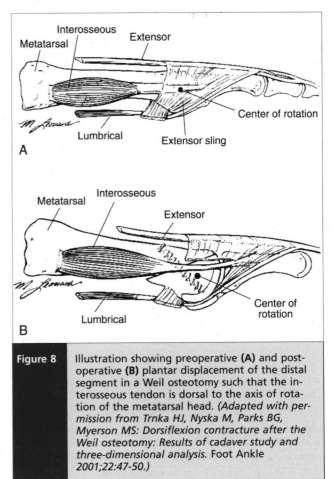

Figure 8 Illustration showing preoperative **(A)** and postoperative **(B)** plantar displacement of the distal segment in a Weil osteotomy such that the interosseous tendon is dorsal to the axis of rotation of the metatarsal head. *(Adapted with permission from Trnka HJ, Nyska M, Parks BG, Myerson MS: Dorsiflexion contracture after the Weil osteotomy: Results of cadaver study and three-dimensional analysis. Foot Ankle 2001;22:47-50.)*

authors of a 2005 study reported no decrease in pressure under the metatarsal head following a Weil osteotomy in a cadaver model, but noted that normal cadaver feet were assessed with a static model that did not examine peak pressures throughout the gait cycle.[34] Continued research is necessary to fully understand the biomechanical changes associated with a shortening osteotomy of a distal lesser metatarsal.

A biomechanical concern regarding the Weil osteotomy is that it displaces the center of rotation of the metatarsal head plantar to the axis of the intrinsic muscles (Figure 8). Clinically, this displacement may result in stiffness and/or a dorsiflexion contracture of the metatarsophalangeal joint. Possible surgical solutions include resecting a wedge of bone or using stacked saw blades to elevate the metatarsal head. Lengthening of the extensor tendon may lessen clinical dorsiflexion.

Subtalar Arthroereisis

Subtalar arthroereisis is a surgical procedure that uses an implant inserted into the sinus tarsi to stabilize the subtalar joint.[35] This procedure has been primarily used for treating flexible planovalgus deformities in children, but has recently been used in adults. The implant restricts subtalar and hindfoot eversion, corrects deformity, and probably functions as an "internal splint" to protect correction obtained with other surgical procedures. In patients with AAFD, arthroereisis is used as a surgical adjunct to other procedures, primarily medializing calcaneal osteotomy and FDL tendon transfer.

In one recent biomechanical study, arthroereisis performed in conjunction with calcaneal osteotomy and FDL transfer restored the talonavicular angle and medial cuneiform height in a severe flatfoot model.[36] In this model, the calcaneal osteotomy and FDL transfer alone did not restore these parameters.

Orthotics

Custom shoe orthoses are commonly prescribed by orthopaedic surgeons, podiatrists, and physical therapists to treat many types of foot and ankle disorders; however, these devices may be prescribed too often. Custom orthoses can be accommodative devices that unload a prominence or corrective devices that attempt to change the structure of the foot and correct a deformity. One recent study reported a beneficial effect on ankle and subtalar stability.[37] Hindfoot posting, in which the posterior aspect of the device is eccentrically augmented, is one technique by which an orthosis can correct a deformity. Medial hindfoot posting inverts the hindfoot and is useful in treating an acquired flatfoot deformity. Lateral hindfoot posting everts the hindfoot and is useful in treating pes cavus and ankle instability associated with hindfoot varus. More information on orthoses is available in chapter 2.

A 2005 study compared the effects of a University of California Biomechanics Laboratory (UCBL) orthosis to a medializing calcaneal osteotomy in a cadaver AAFD model.[38] Both conditions significantly decreased the global mean contact pressures at the tibiotalar joints. The UCBL orthosis had a significantly greater effect on pressure normalization than the osteotomy. Reduction in peak contact pressure also was significantly reduced from that observed in the flatfoot model when the UCBL orthosis was used.

Summary

The foot and ankle are complex structures that allow locomotion and enable us to stand erect. An understanding of their biomechanical basis is central to orthopaedics, for understanding disorders that affect the foot and ankle, and for optimal selection of surgical interventions to treat these disorders. Although knowledge of foot and ankle biomechanics has grown considerably, insight and knowledge of this academic field will continue to expand.

Annotated References

1. Arndt A, Westblad P, Winson I, Hashimoto T, Lundberg A: Ankle and subtalar kinematics measured with intracortical pins during the stance phase of walking. *Foot Ankle* 2004;25:357-364.

   In this study, cortical pins were inserted in the tibia, talus, and calcaneus of three patients. Video motion analysis was used to collect kinematic walking data. Large differences were seen in both ankle and subtalar axes of orientation. Most eversion and inversion occurred at the subtalar joint. Subtalar abduction and adduction was high, indicating that this motion is not purely attributable to the ankle joint.

2. Sheehan FT, Seisler AR, Siegel KL: In vivo talocrural and subtalar kinematics: A non-invasive 3D dynamic MRI study. *Foot Ankle* 2007;28:323-335.

   The authors of this study demonstrated that in vivo fast-phase contrast MRI had excellent precision and accuracy for tracking calcaneal, talar, and tibial movement. Three-dimensional subtalar kinematics showed that the talus and calcaneus do not move as a single unit and that most calcaneotibial supination occurred at the talocrural joint. A Stieda process markedly altered kinematics.

3. Kitaoka HB, Crevoisier XM, Hansen D, Katajarvi B, Harbst K, Kaufman KR: Foot and ankle kinematics and ground reaction forces during ambulation. *Foot Ankle Int* 2006;27:808-813.

   This study describes a three segment gait analysis model used to determine in vivo three-dimensional motion in the sagittal, coronal, and transverse planes. This model enabled the determination of calcaneotibial and metatarsocalcaneal movement in three planes. Ground reaction forces, temporal force factors, cadence, stance time, swing time, and the percentage of stance time were determined.

4. Segal A, Rohr E, Orendurff M, Shofer J, O'Brien M, Sangeorzan B: The effect of walking speed on peak plantar pressure. *Foot Ankle* 2004;25:926-933.

   The authors demonstrated that walking speed had an effect on peak plantar pressure and that this effect varied by plantar region. The authors recommended that walking speed be controlled in future measurement studies of plantar pressure. The pressure-speed relationships presented can be used as normative data for future evaluation of clinical interventions for pressure reduction.

5. Sarrafian SK: Functional anatomy of the foot and ankle, in Sarafian SK (ed): *Anatomy of the Foot and Ankle: Descriptive, Topographic, Functional*, ed 2. Philadelphia, PA, Lippincott-Williams & Wilkins, 1993.

6. Erdemir A, Hamel AJ, Fauth AR, Piazza SJ, Sharkey NA: Dynamic loading of the plantar aponeurosis in walking. *J Bone Joint Surg Am* 2004;86:546-552.

   In a cadaver model, the plantar aponeurosis forces gradually increased during stance and peaked in late stance. There was a strong correlation between aponeurosis tension and Achilles tendon force. It was concluded that the plantar aponeurosis transmits large forces between the hindfoot and forefoot during the stance phase. Surgical procedures that release this structure may disturb this mechanism and compromise efficient propulsion.

7. Hicks JH: The mechanics of the foot: II. The plantar aponeurosis and the arch. *J Anat* 1954;88:25-30.

8. Cheung JT, An KN, Zhang M: Consequences of partial and total plantar fascia release: A finite element study. *Foot Ankle* 2006;27:125-132.

   Using finite element analysis, the authors determined that partial and total plantar fascia release may decrease arch height but not necessarily cause total collapse. These procedures resulted in increased plantar strain and intensified midfoot and metatarsal stress. The authors concluded that plantar fasciotomy may pose a risk to arch stability and recommended that it be limited to less than 40% of the fascia.

9. Close JR, Inman VT, Poor PM, Todd FN: The function of the subtalar joint. *Clin Orthop Relat Res* 1967;50:159-179.

10. Inman VT: *The Joints of the Ankle.* Baltimore, MD, Williams & Wilkins, 1976.

11. Inman VT: *Human Walking.* Baltimore, MD, Williams & Wilkins, 1981.

12. Mann RA: Biomechanics of the foot and ankle, in Mann RA, Coughlin MJ (eds): *Surgery of the Foot and Ankle,* ed 6. St. Louis, MO, Mosby-Year Book, 1993, pp 3-43.

13. Beumer A, van Hemert WL, Swierstra BA, Jasper LE, Belkoff SM: A biomechanical evaluation of the tibiofibular and tibiotalar ligaments of the ankle. *Foot Ankle* 2003;24:426-429.

   The authors of this cadaver study investigated the strength and stiffness of the anterior and posterior syndesmotic tibiofibular ligaments and the posterior tibiotalar component of the deltoid ligament. The posterior tibiofibular ligaments exhibited the greatest strength; however, this was not significant. There was no difference in stiffness between the ligaments. It was confirmed that tibiofibular ligaments have greater strength than the lateral collateral and deltoid ligaments.

14. Hoefnagels EM, Waites MD, Wing ID, Belkoff SM, Swierstra BA: Biomechanical comparison of the interosseous tibiofibular ligament and the anterior tibiofibular ligament. *Foot Ankle* 2007;28:602-604.

   This biomechanical cadaver study compared the stiffness and strength of the interosseous tibiofibular ligament to the anterior tibiofibular ligament. The authors found that the interosseous ligament was significantly stiffer and also had a higher mean failure load. It was concluded that this ligament plays an important role in ankle stability.

15. Nester CJ, Findlow AF, Bowker P, Bowden PD: Transverse plane motion at the ankle joint. *Foot Ankle* 2003;24:164-168.

   The data from this dynamic noninvasive in vivo study suggest that the ankle is capable of considerable movement in the transverse plane (generally greater than 15°). It was concluded that both the ankle and subtalar joints play a role in allowing the foot to remain fixed on the floor while the leg above rotates in the transverse plane.

16. Fujii T, Kitaoka HB, Luo ZP, Kura H, An KN: Analysis of ankle-hindfoot stability in multiple planes: An in vitro study. *Foot Ankle* 2005;26:633-637.

   The authors devised a testing apparatus to critically determine ankle stability in all planes with a constant rotational force applied throughout the sagittal arc of motion. Cadaver data confirmed that ankle laxity varied depending on the plantar flexion-dorsiflexion position and the direction of the applied force. Specifically, the ankle was less stable in plantar flexion when inversion and internal rotation forces were applied.

17. Tochigi Y, Rudert MJ, Saltzman CL, Amendola A, Brown TD: Contribution of articular surface geometry to ankle stabilization. *J Bone Joint Surg Am* 2006;88:2704-2713.

   This combined cadaver and computer-modeling study illustrated the major role of articular geometry in passive ankle stabilization. The calculated contributions of the articular surface to joint stability were consistent with those previously reported in the literature. The data support the conceptual mechanism of ankle stabilization by redistribution of articular contact stress.

18. Ozeki S, Kitaoka H, Uchiyama E, Luo ZP, Kaufman K, An KN: Ankle ligament tensile forces at the end points of passive circumferential rotating motion of the ankle and subtalar joint complex. *Foot Ankle* 2006;27:965-969.

   The authors of this cadaver study measured tensile forces of the ankle ligaments at the end points of passive circumferential rotating motion of the ankle and subtalar joint complex in various foot positions. High tensile forces were observed, and peak forces were related to the anatomic position of individual ligaments. The anterior talofibular ligament played an important role in the supination position in plantar flexion, the calcaneofibular and tibiocalcaneal ligaments were important for pronation in plantar flexion, and the posterior talofibular ligament was an important stabilizer in dorsiflexion.

19. Saunders JB, Inman VT, Eberhart HD: The major determinants in normal and pathological gait. *J Bone Joint Surg Am* 1953;35:543-558.

20. Thomas R, Daniels T, Parker K: Gait analysis and functional outcomes following ankle arthrodesis for isolated ankle arthritis. *J Bone Joint Surg Am* 2006;88:526-535.

   Gait analysis was performed on patients in whom an ankle arthrodesis had been performed using modern surgical techniques. Compared with healthy controls, significant differences with regard to cadence and stride length were noted. The arthrodesis group showed decreased hindfoot and midfoot motion during the stance and swing phases of gait.

21. Costa ML, Kay D, Donell ST: Gait abnormalities following rupture of the tendo Achilles: A pedobarographic assessment. *J Bone Joint Surg Br* 2005;87:1085-1088.

Using plantar pressure measurements, patients with Achilles tendon ruptures were compared with normal controls. The authors reported a significant reduction in peak forefoot pressures in the early rehabilitation period and also at 6 months postoperatively. Pedobarographs confirmed gait abnormalities in the rupture group. Rehabilitation programs to treat these abnormalities were suggested.

22. Pinney SJ, Sangeorzan BJ, Hansen ST: The effect on ankle dorsiflexion of the gastrocnemius recession (Strayer procedure). *Foot Ankle* 2004;25:247-250.

This study assessed clinical ankle dorsiflexion achieved with gastrocnemius recession. An isolated gastrocnemius release was performed on 26 legs. Preoperative and postoperative ankle dorsiflexion was measured by an electrogoniometer. The average correction immediately following surgery was 18°. This correction was maintained at short-term follow-up.

23. Kay RM, Rethlefsen SA, Ryan JA, Wren TA: Outcome of gastrocnemius recession and tendo-achilles lengthening in ambulatory children with cerebral palsy. *J Pediatr Orthop B* 2004;13:92-98.

Gait analysis data were studied for children with cerebral palsy who underwent gastrocnemius recession or Achilles tendon lengthening based on the Silfverskiöld test. The group treated with Achilles tendon lengthening had greater preoperative equinus. Both groups showed improvement in static and dynamic dorsiflexion and outcome. Calf spasticity decreased and push-off power increased after gastrocnemius recession. Both procedures were effective in appropriately selected patients. However, both procedures also had the potential for overcorrection and undercorrection.

24. Arangio GA, Salathe EP: Medial displacement calcaneal osteotomy reduces the excess forces in the medial longitudinal arch of the flat foot. *Clin Biomech (Bristol, Avon)* 2001;16:535-539.

25. Arangio GA, Chopra V, Voloshin A, Salathe EP: A biomechanical analysis of the effect of lateral column lengthening calcaneal osteotomy on the flatfoot. *Clin Biomech (Bristol, Avon)* 2007;22:472-477.

A three-dimensional biomechanical model was used to analyze anatomic data from a normal foot, a flatfoot, and a foot corrected with a lateral column-lengthening calcaneal osteotomy. Lateral column lengthening reduced the excess force on the medial arch in an adult flatfoot, providing biomechanical rationale for this clinical procedure.

26. Logel KJ, Parks BG, Schon LC: Calcaneocuboid distraction arthrodesis and first metatarsocuneiform arthrodesis for correction of acquired flatfoot deformity in a cadaver model. *Foot Ankle* 2007;28:435-440.

The authors of this study evaluated radiographic and pressure changes in a cadaver flatfoot model with lateral column lengthening followed by first metatarsocuneiform arthrodesis. Lateral forefoot pressures increased after lateral column lengthening; however, the addition of a metatarsocuneiform arthrodesis reduced these pressures to normal.

27. Scott AT, Hendry TM, Iaquinto JM, Owen JR, Wanye JS, Adelaar RS: Plantar pressure analysis in cadaver feet after bony procedures commonly used in the treatment of stage II posterior tibial tendon insufficiency. *Foot Ankle* 2007;28:1143-1153.

This biomechanical cadaver study examined plantar pressures after various osteotomies performed for AAFD. Lateral column lengthening through both the calcaneocuboid joint and anterior calcaneus resulted in increased lateral forefoot pressures, although no significant differences between the two were noted. The addition of a medializing calcaneal osteotomy did not alter measurements of plantar pressures. The addition of a Cotton osteotomy resulted in increased medial forefoot pressures; a compensatory decrease in lateral forefoot pressures was not observed.

28. Tien TR, Parks BG, Guyton GP: Plantar pressures in the forefoot after lateral column lengthening: A cadaver study comparing the Evans osteotomy and calcaneocuboid fusion. *Foot Ankle* 2005;26:520-525.

The authors investigated differences between the Evans osteotomy and calcaneocuboid distraction arthrodesis with respect to lateral forefoot loading. A cadaver model showed that both procedures produced increased loading of the lateral forefoot. The increase was greater with the calcaneocuboid distraction arthrodesis than with the Evans osteotomy, leading the authors to conclude that lateral column overload may be more likely with calcaneocuboid distraction arthrodesis.

29. Cotton FJ: Foot statics and surgery. *N Engl J Med* 1936;214:353-362.

30. Benthien RA, Parks BG, Guyton GP, Schon LC: Lateral column calcaneal lengthening, flexor digitorum longus transfer, and opening wedge medial cuneiform osteotomy for flexible flatfoot: A biomechanical study. *Foot Ankle* 2007;28:70-77.

Using a cadaver flatfoot model, the authors confirmed that lateral column lengthening significantly corrects deformity but causes increased lateral forefoot pressures. Adding a medial cuneiform osteotomy normalized these lateral pressures; however, medial forefoot pressure was overcorrected. The cuneiform osteotomy also provided increased deformity correction.

31. Barouk LS: Weil's metatarsal osteotomy in the treatment of metatarsalgia. *Orthopade* 1996;25:338-344.

32. Khalafi A, Landsman AS, Lautenschlager EP, Kelikian AS: Plantar forefoot pressure changes after second metatarsal neck osteotomy. *Foot Ankle* 2005;26:550-555.

This cadaver study evaluated plantar pressure after a second metatarsal Weil osteotomy. Statistically significant decreases in pressure beneath the second metatarsal were noted both in neutral and at heel rise. However, a significant pressure increase occurred beneath the first metatarsal.

33. Vandeputte G, Dereymaeker G, Steenwerckx A, Peeraer L: The Weil osteotomy of the lesser metatarsals: A clinical and pedobarographic follow-up study. *Foot Ankle Int* 2000;21:370-374.

34. Snyder J, Owen J, Wayne J, Adelaar R: Plantar pressure and load in cadaver feet after a Weil or chevron osteotomy. *Foot Ankle Int* 2005;26:158-165.

This study used a cadaver forefoot model to evaluate resulting biomechanical changes from Weil and chevron osteotomies, which are often used to relieve central metatarsalgia.

35. Arangio GA, Reinert KL, Salathe EP: A biomechanical model of the effect of subtalar arthroereisis on the adult flexible flatfoot. *Clin Biomech (Bristol, Avon)* 2004;19:847-852.

The responses to applied load of a normal foot, a flatfoot, and a flatfoot treated with arthroereisis were analyzed with a three-dimensional biomechanical model. The flatfoot demonstrated an increase in first metatarsal load and in the moment about the talonavicular joint. Arthroereisis shifted load back toward the lateral column and decreased the moment about the talonavicular joint.

36. Vora AM, Tien TR, Parks BG, Schon LC: Correction of moderate and severe acquired flexible flatfoot with medializing calcaneal osteotomy and flexor digitorum longus transfer. *J Bone Joint Surg Am* 2006;88:1726-1734.

This study demonstrated that in a mild flatfoot model, medializing calcaneal osteotomy and tendon transfer corrected the talar-first metatarsal angle and talonavicular angle. In a severe flatfoot model, however, all radiographic parameters remained undercorrected following osteotomy and tendon transfer. After arthroereisis, the talonavicular angle and medial cuneiform height normalized.

37. Tochigi Y: Effect of arch supports on ankle-subtalar complex instability: A biomechanical experimental study. *Foot Ankle* 2003;24:634-639.

The authors examined the role of orthotics in simulated cadaver ankle-subtalar instability and found that insoles supporting the medial longitudinal and transverse arches decreased maximum ankle internal rotation but had no effect on subtalar rotation. It was concluded that such insoles improved abnormal joint kinematics in ankle-subtalar instability and that the observed changes were likely caused by improved arch configuration and stability.

38. Havenhill TG, Toolan BC, Draganich LF: Effects of a UCBL orthosis and a calcaneal osteotomy on tibiotalar contact characteristics in a cadaver flatfoot model. *Foot Ankle* 2005;26:607-613.

This study showed that both a UCBL orthosis and calcaneal osteotomy improve the altered tibiotalar contact characteristics of a cadaver flatfoot. For global and peak contact pressures, the orthosis demonstrated greater correction. Clinically, this finding supports the argument that management of pes planovalgus with a UCBL orthosis or calcaneal osteotomy may avert pantalar disease associated with chronic flatfoot.

1: General Foot and Ankle Topics

Chapter 2
Shoes and Orthotics

Clifford L. Jeng, MD   John Logue, CPO

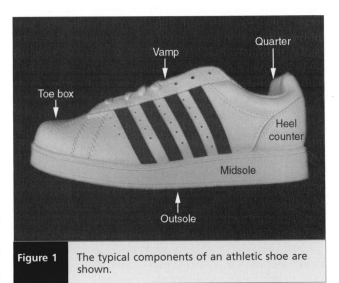

Introduction

The orthopaedic surgeon is responsible for both the surgical and nonsurgical care of musculoskeletal disorders, including the use of external mechanical devices. This chapter considers the role of shoes and orthoses in the care of foot and ankle disorders and discusses their roles in contemporary practice. Orthoses can be further subdivided into foot orthoses (in-shoe inserts or orthoses) and ankle-foot orthoses (AFOs). Most current knowledge in this area is based on the observations of AFO experts; efficacy is supported with only limited scientific data.[1] More biomechanical and clinical studies are needed to validate recent design developments and to establish standards to guide decision making.[2,3]

Shoes

Shoes play an important role in interacting with the environment because they interface with the ground. Shoes are critical in protecting the foot from injury and can enhance performance both in work and sports activites when certain features are incorporated into the shoe design. It is important to understand the basic elements of shoe construction and to be aware of the dramatic advances in technology that have occurred in athletic footwear. Different methods of modifying shoes to treat specific foot and ankle pathologies also are available.

Upper

The upper is the part of the shoe that encloses the foot (**Figure 1**). Everything above the insole of the shoe is considered the upper. The upper keeps the foot in place within the shoe and protects the top part of the foot from injury. It typically is made from either leather or a synthetic material and is composed of three elements: the toe box, the vamp, and the quarter.

Toe Box

The toe box is the front part of the upper that provides space for the toes. Its horizontal and vertical dimensions are determined by the last (a three-dimensional model of the foot), which is used to construct the shoe. Narrow toe boxes are common in fashion shoes for

women and have been widely implicated in the development of hallux valgus and hammer toe deformities. A study evaluating 255 women showed that 86% of women wore shoes that were too small for their feet; women with a greater shoe-foot size discrepancy were more likely to have foot pain.[1] Another study demonstrated that women who wore shoes that were too narrow were prone to hallux valgus and corns.[4] Women who wore shoes that were too short were more prone to lesser toe deformities. Patients with neuropathy secondary to diabetes mellitus are encouraged to wear shoes with a high, wide toe box to prevent ulcerations.

Vamp

The vamp is the middle section of the upper that covers the dorsum of the foot. The vamp is the part of the shoe with the greatest variability. It can be basically absent, such as in a sandal or a pump where almost the entire instep is exposed. It also can be complex, such as the vamp of a boot or running shoe with a tongue and lacing incorporated into the design. The vamp is usually the most decorated or stylized part of the shoe and is designed to appeal to the consumer.

Quarter

The quarter is the part of the shoe behind the vamp that covers the sides and back of the foot. The quarter can be absent in sandals or open-heeled shoes, or it can

Figure 1 The typical components of an athletic shoe are shown.

be built up to control hindfoot motion during gait (typically done with a heel counter). A heel counter is a reinforced material (usually fiberboard or molded plastic) that is built into the quarter that wraps around the back and sides of the heel. Its rigidity can vary and it can control excessive pronation when extended medially along the heel. The quarter also can control motion by extending the upper proximally, as is the case with a high-top sneaker or boot. One study showed that wearing a basketball shoe with a three fourths top resulted in a 20% to 30% increase in resistance to an inversion moment in healthy individuals.[5] This effect presumably results from the additional proprioceptive input and ability to limit extremes of motion provided by high-top shoes.

Lower

The lower refers to the part of the shoe located under the foot. It is made up of the insole, the midsole, and the outsole.

Insole

The insole is inside the shoe and is the part of the lower that comes in direct contact with the foot. It often is made of compressible foam that can mold to the contours of the foot and is frequently removable to allow room for a prescription or custom-made insole. More advanced insoles use nitrogen-impregnated ethylene vinyl acetate (EVA) or rubber to help absorb shock. Well-padded insoles can absorb a significant amount of shock when there is limited midsole cushioning, especially under low-impact energy conditions. One study showed that the conformity of the insole to the bottom of the foot was more important than the thickness of the insole or the material used in decreasing peak pressures; fully conforming insoles provided a 44% decrease in peak pressures versus only a 24% decrease with flat insoles.[6]

Midsole

The midsole is located between the insole and outsole. It provides cushioning from the impact forces associated with walking and running. Most of the design advances in athletic shoes have focused on midsole construction. The most common materials used for the midsole include EVA, dual-density EVA, and polyurethane foam. EVA is a lightweight foam that provides greater cushioning but less durability than polyurethane. Shock absorption results from the flow of air through interconnected air cells during shoe deformation under the pressure of body weight. Dual-density EVA often is used in certain sections of the lower to provide additional stability (for example, along the medial side of the shoe to limit pronation). Polyurethane foam is a durable material used for midsoles, but it is stiffer and heavier than EVA.

Much of the research and development in the multibillion-dollar athletic shoe industry is directed toward developing new materials to absorb shock. These materials include viscoelastic polymers, pressurized air bladders, encapsulated silicon gel or liquid inserts, urethane pillars, and matrices of synthetic strands to dissipate the impact of weight bearing. Other strategies include altering the manufacturing process of traditional EVA to improve its physical characteristics or combining EVA with polyurethane in different configurations to use the best attributes of each material.

Recent research has evaluated the durability of EVA in athletic shoes. With prolonged overuse of an athletic shoe, the air cells within the EVA collapse, resulting in a decrease in thickness and shock absorption of the midsole. One investigation demonstrated that a 50% loss of EVA thickness resulted in a 19% increase in peak heel pad stresses.[7] A second study evaluating EVA durability reported that the peak plantar pressures increased by 100% after a simulated 500-km run.[3] This finding corresponds well with the general recommendation that running shoes should be replaced after 300 to 500 miles of use.

Outsole

The outsole is the portion of the shoe that comes in contact with the ground and provides traction. It must be durable and protect the midsole from wear. In athletic shoes, the outsole is commonly made from solid, carbon, or blown rubber. Solid rubber is a blend of synthetic and natural rubber and is the most common material used in athletic shoes. It provides excellent traction and durability on indoor surfaces. Carbon rubber is a synthetic rubber with added carbon. It is the same material used in automobile tires and is extremely durable. Blown rubber is a synthetic rubber with injected air; it is lighter, more flexible, and provides more cushioning but is less durable than carbon rubber. Polyurethane is another material that often is used in the outsole of athletic shoes. It is flexible and provides high shock absorption with minimal thickness. The outsole pattern and composition may vary according to the demands of the sport or activity. For example, a herringbone outsole pattern is popular in basketball shoes because it provides increased traction for lateral motion.

Fashion Shoes

Fashion shoes are selected for different characteristics than athletic shoes and are constructed according to different principles. Cosmesis may be a greater priority than functionality and comfort, which affects the materials chosen and can prove detrimental to shoe construction. The entire lower is often made from a thin layer of leather with little cushioning or traction ability. The toe box is often narrow or tapered, which can make the foot appear more slender, but crowds the toes. The insole is often very thin and provides limited support to the foot. Shoes that have little or no vamp, such as loafers or pumps, must grasp the forefoot tightly to prevent the shoe from falling off. This alteration can lead to further overcrowding of the toes and subsequent deformity. The heels in fashion shoe wear can be of variable heights. Research has shown that shoes with high heels have the effect of decreasing the load on the hindfoot and increasing the load on the forefoot, especially on the medial forefoot and hallux. Over the past decade, the shoe industry has increasingly recognized the value of cushioning in dress shoes and has developed hybrid shoes with a fashionable upper combined with a lower similar to that found in athletic shoes.

Last

The last is a three-dimensional model of the foot that is the form on which shoes are fabricated. Shoe dimensions are statistically modeled to accommodate the average foot; however, the last usually does not provide an exact replica of the foot. Dimensions are typically modified in certain areas to provide specific functions or to give a certain appearance. Lasts can be made from metal, plastic, or wood and are made in one of three shapes: straight, semicurved, or curved. Straight lasts are generally a good choice for people with flat feet who have a straight foot shape and require stability. A semicurved last has a gentle arc that is best for the average or normal foot, whereas a curved last is best suited for use by individuals with high arches who typically have a curved foot shape.

Shoe Modifications

Off-the-shelf shoes generally are designed for the average foot with no consideration for pathologic conditions. For severely deformed or neuropathic feet, custom-made shoes may be necessary to protect against ulceration or trauma. Shoe modifications offer an alternative to standard, off-the-shelf shoe wear and more expensive custom-made shoes. Uppers, especially in the area of the toe box, can be stretched to accommodate bunions, hammer toes, or other toe deformities. Such stretching is limited by the material composition of the upper and/or by stitching in the local area where stretching is needed. The desired direction of stretching also is important. More stretching is possible in a mediolateral or vertical direction, with minimal stretching possible to lengthen the shoe.

More significant alterations can be made to the midsole or outsole of a shoe, which can alter the alignment or mechanics of the lower limb. Shoe lifts are the most common modification used in off-the-shelf shoes. These lifts add thickness to the midsole between the outsole and upper. External shoe lifts are prescribed for patients with limb-length discrepancies of greater than 0.5 inch because in-shoe orthoses thicker than 0.5 inch would raise the heel out of the quarter and cause the shoe to slip off. Dress shoes can incorporate even less of an internal heel lift than athletic shoes because they typically have a lower heel counter.

Medial or lateral wedges can be inserted into the midsole to correct the alignment of a flexible hindfoot deformity or to resist excessive pronation or supination. These wedges can be placed under only the heel or over the entire length of the shoe. A medial heel wedge inverts the heel and is helpful for pes planus or posterior tibial tendon dysfunction. A lateral heel wedge everts the heel and can improve lateral ankle instability and relax the peroneal tendons. Medial or lateral wedges also can be used in the front of the shoe to accommodate a fixed forefoot varus or valgus deformity, helping the floor to meet the foot.

A flare is a triangular-shaped extension (either medially or laterally) of the lower, causing the bottom edge of the sole in contact with the ground to be wider than the top of the sole. This increase in the base of support improves stability and resists excessive ankle inversion or eversion. A medial flare increases the varus moment of the ground reaction force and a lateral flare increases the valgus moment of the ground reaction force. A lateral flare is especially beneficial in patients with recurrent ankle instability, acting as an outrigger to prevent inversion sprains.

A solid ankle cushion heel modification involves removing a triangular-shaped wedge from the heel midsole posteriorly and replacing it with a material with a lower durometer (hardness). This allows the heel of the shoe to compress at heel strike and absorb more energy and then immediately rebound for the next heel strike. When prescribed for patients treated with ankle fusion, the solid ankle cushion heel modification can mimic ankle plantar flexion following heel strike.

A rocker bottom sole adds material to the midsole, which is then beveled anteriorly or posteriorly (or both). The apex or thickest part of the rocker can be positioned more proximally or distally to treat different conditions. The modification may reduce the energy expended during gait by propelling the body forward after the center of gravity passes over the apex. Rocker bottom soles also can significantly assist ambulation in patients who have decreased ankle or forefoot motion and can improve the gait of patients who have lost motion following ankle fusion. Rocker bottom soles also help to decrease the need for metatarsophalangeal dorsiflexion in patients with hallux rigidus, metatarsophalangeal pathology, and first metatarsophalangeal joint fusions. They can offload the metatarsal heads in patients with metatarsalgia or diabetic neuropathic ulcerations.

A metatarsal bar consists of material added transversely across the bottom of the outsole just proximal to the metatarsal heads. This modification relieves pressure under the metatarsal heads by transferring pressure from the metatarsal shafts directly to the toes, effectively bypassing the metatarsal heads. It also decreases the need for metatarsophalangeal joint motion. This modification, however, requires greater ankle dorsiflexion than is normally required. A metatarsal bar should be prescribed for patients with metatarsalgia or metatarsophalangeal joint pathology.

A stiffener is a rigid addition to the midsole that limits flexion primarily at the midfoot and forefoot. It is

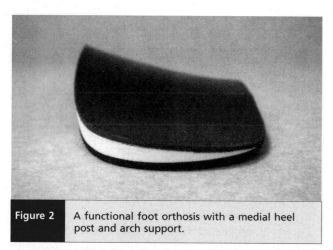

Figure 2   A functional foot orthosis with a medial heel post and arch support.

usually made from a steel shank or carbon fiber plate that extends from the heel to the toe. This modification is beneficial in patients with midfoot or forefoot arthritis, stress fractures, and metatarsophalangeal joint pathology.

Orthoses

In-shoe orthoses can serve multiple purposes if prescribed and fabricated properly. The two main types of orthoses are accommodative and functional. Accomodative orthoses are the least intrusive and usually are made of materials with a lower durometer and are shaped to closely match the sole of the foot. These devices function to distribute body weight along the entire plantar surface of the foot, providing cushioning and support. Orthoses are useful in accommodating foot deformities that are rigid and cannot be corrected. Functional orthoses, on the other hand, intentionally alter the alignment or mechanics of the foot and ankle to treat flexible pathologic conditions (**Figure 2**).

A complete orthotic prescription requires several components, including the diagnosed condition of the patients. Many manufacturers of orthoses have algorithms or formulas for constructing shoe inserts based almost entirely on the diagnosis provided by the orthopaedic surgeon. The prescription should specify whether the insert should be accommodative or functional. The desired length of the orthotic device should be specified as full length, sulcus (terminating at the metatarsophalangeal joints), or behind the metatarsal heads. The durometer (rigid, semirigid) of the orthotic device should be included. A rigid orthosis should be prescribed for taller patients or patients weighing more than 200 pounds because these patients would easily "bottom out" a softer orthosis. Semirigid orthoses are good choices for patients of average size. Any specific modifications to the insert should be specified. A list of commonly prescribed modifications and applicable diagnoses are shown in **Table 1**.

Foot and Ankle Bracing

Introduction
The orthotist uses external mechanical devices to oppose the mechanical abnormalities caused by various medical conditions. The orthopaedic surgeon should have a sound understanding of the principles and devices used by the orthotist to appropriately supervise the provision of orthotic services. An understanding of the terminology used to classify braces will facilitate communication between the surgeon and orthotist.

Terminology
The terminology used to specify and characterize orthotic devices has changed from a narrow set of colloquial terms, primarily consisting of the phrases "short leg brace" and "long leg brace," to a nomenclature system based on the joints crossed by a given device. This scheme uses two- or three-letter acronyms to identify the joints crossed. For example, foot orthosis (FO) refers to the entire group of devices that cross the joints of the foot but do not extend above the ankle. Ankle-foot orthosis (AFO) refers to the entire category of devices that cross the joints of the ankle and the foot. A particular device is defined by the above acronyms to identify its general category and an additional descriptive term is used to identify the particular device. Recently, several commercially manufactured products have been introduced that do not fit within these standard category definitions. As a result, product brand names have replaced the more generic terminology in communications between the orthopaedic surgeon and the orthotist. Familiarity with such devices may assist the surgeon in prescribing braces until generic nomenclature is established for these new devices.

Materials Used for Fabricating Orthoses
The materials used to apply therapeutic forces to the foot and ankle have evolved from metal uprights and leather cuffs to molded plastics. Metal and leather braces still are used for patients with variable edema, high-risk skin conditions, and for those requiring low contact about the ankle. Molded plastics are the most commonly used material for custom-made orthoses. More recently, composites of different materials have been used to fabricate certain specialized orthoses. These composite constructions, which are manufactured over custom molds, are continuing to gain market share as improved product designs appear.

Custom-Molded Plastic
Custom-molded orthoses usually are formed with thermoplastics derived from the olefin (alkene) family. These compounds are composed of a series of monomer hydrocarbons with the basic formula C_nH_{2n}. The most common examples are ethylene (C_2H_4) and propylene (C_3H_6). They may be polymerized by various

Table 1

Orthotic Modifications

Prescribed Orthosis	Description	Indication
Arch support	Material added under orthosis in arch area to elevate and support arch	Flatfoot, overpronation, heavy patients
Forefoot post	Wedge under medial or lateral forefoot to elevate floor to foot	Fixed forefoot varus/valgus
Forefoot well/depression	Cutout or depression to unload specific area	Metatarsalgia (multiple etiologies), sesamoiditis, plantar callus
Heel cushion	Soft foam cushion on top of heel module of orthosis	Plantar fasciitis, heel fat pad atrophy
Heel lift	Rigid neutral wedge under the heel module to elevate heel and relax Achilles tendon	Limb-length discrepancy, Achilles tendinitis, Haglund deformity, retrocalcaneal bursitis
Heel post	Rigid wedge under medial or lateral aspect of heel to tilt hindfoot	Valgus heel = medial post; varus heel = lateral post
Heel spur cutout	Central cutout in heel module to relieve pressure	Plantar fasciitis, heel fat pad atrophy
Horseshoe accommodation	U-shaped cushion applied to top of heel module to relieve pressure	Plantar fasciitis, heel fat pad atrophy
Medial flange	Semirigid "ramp" built up along medial side of arch to elevate arch	Severe flatfoot deformity
Metatarsal bars	Padding placed behind metatarsal heads to offload them	Metatarsalgia (multiple etiologies), Morton neuroma
Midfoot/arch cutout	Cutout or depression to unload specific area	Plantar bony prominences, plantar fibroma
Morton extension	Plastic or carbon fiber extension that extends under the hallux to limit first metatarsophalangeal motion	Hallux rigidus, sesamoiditis, turf toe
Rigid forefoot extension	Rigid plastic/carbon fiber that extends out to tip of all toes to restrict metatarsophalangeal motion	Hallux rigidus, lesser metatarsophalangeal synovitis, Morton neuroma, midfoot arthritis
Sesamoid cutout	Area under sesamoids that is cut out or depressed to relieve pressure	Sesamoiditis, plantar-flexed first ray

methods into polyethylene, polypropylene, or copolymers that contain both ethylene and propylene monomers. Stiffness is the most important characteristic that distinguishes these materials. Thermoplastics all mold well, machine well, and are biologically inert, chemically stable, and inexpensive. The density and stiffness of polyethylene can vary across a wide range. High-density polyethylene is commonly used for in-shoe orthotic supports. Low-density polyethylene is commonly used for the inner shells in certain two-layer constructions. Polypropylene is the most common plastic used in molded braces for the foot and ankle; it is less tough and less brittle than high-density polyethylene and less flexible than low-density polyethylene. In addition to its desirable level of stiffness, polypropylene is particularly resistant to fatigue from repetitive loading. This characteristic makes it the ideal plastic for AFOs because ambulation involves much repetitive loading.

To understand the recent advances in foot and ankle bracing, it is important to understand the difference between elasticity and stiffness. Elasticity is a material property that refers to resistance of deformation under load. Stiffness refers to the resistance of a solid body to deformation under load and is determined by the elasticity of the constituent material in addition to the size, shape, and thickness of the body. The stiffness of the brace is controlled by the material choice in combination with its wall thickness, trimlines, and whether it has a conventional or composite construction.

Composite Constructions

Composite orthoses produce a set of desirable characteristics from the combined effects of two or more materials with different physical characteristics. The two different materials can be assembled in a geometry that influences the net effect. Because these devices are more complex to construct, they are generally manufactured on an industrial assembly line rather than in a craftsman's workshop. The role of the orthotist is to provide expert guidance on the various centrally fabricated devices available. The orthotist makes a plaster or fiberglass cast of the foot and ankle in the best available position by considering the patient's pathology and anatomic alignment as well as the mechanical capabilities of the chosen orthotic device. The cast is then sent to the central facility for manufacturing of the final orthosis.

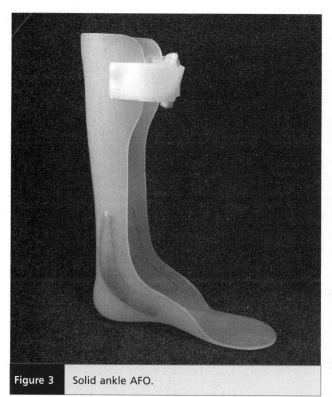

Figure 3 Solid ankle AFO.

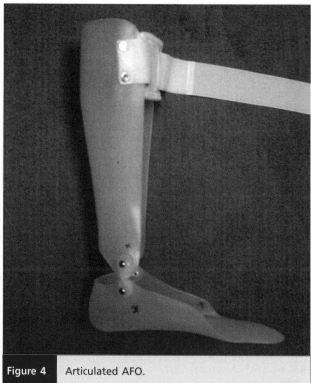

Figure 4 Articulated AFO.

Mechanisms of Orthotic Treatment

All orthotic treatment is mechanical in nature and the mechanisms used depend on pressure applied to the skin. Five outcomes can be achieved with orthoses: protection of the skin from mechanically induced breakdown, control of anatomic alignment, mitigation of bending forces acting on the anatomy as a result of weight bearing, support of muscular weakness, and mitigation of gait deviations. To achieve these outcomes, the materials through which the mechanisms act must be formed to match the best available anatomic position for the patient. Orthotic devices also must provide adequate stiffness to transmit therapeutic forces to the anatomy.[8-11]

The concept of skin protection is critical because all orthotic devices rely on pressure applied to the skin. The protection of skin from mechanically-induced breakdown is a separate concern because if the skin is compromised, the orthosis will not be tolerated by the patient. Skin protection involves control of pressure distribution and friction and is primarily achieved by the skill of the treating orthotist. Pressure and friction are controlled by means of brace contours and material selection. Brace contours may be depressed to reduce pressure concentration in high-risk areas and elevated to increase pressure concentration in more tolerant areas. Materials of different durometers also may be positioned over strategic areas of the anatomy to alter pressure distribution. Friction is controlled by keeping the involved anatomy immobile inside the orthotic enclosure and by an appropriate selection of materials based on their coefficient of friction.

Selected Orthotic Devices

The following devices illustrate the materials and mechanisms previously described but are by no means a comprehensive list. Few rigorous data are available regarding brace design or clinical outcomes, and there are no validated guidelines to assist the orthopaedic surgeon in choosing an orthosis. It is imperative that the orthopaedic surgeon consult with a competent orthotist to collaborate about patient care.

Standard AFOs

A standard AFO is made of molded thermoplastic in one of four versions: solid ankle (**Figure 3**), semisolid, posterior leaf spring, or articulated (**Figure 4**). These orthoses usually are made by the treating orthotist. Their molded, three-dimensional design facilitates the application of three-point pressure systems to the foot and ankle to control the alignment of articulating body segments including the ankle, subtalar joint, and midfoot complex. Inclined planes or wedges also may be included under the plantar surface of the foot. Such additions can affect anatomic alignment through the mechanism of force couples. Force couples and three-point pressure systems are the primary tools used by the orthotist to treat the alignment of the foot and ankle.

In a standard solid ankle AFO, the trimlines fully enclose the malleoli. Such a brace is intended to fully immobilize the foot and ankle complex. In a standard semisolid AFO, the trimlines wrap around the sides of the ankle anatomy but do not extend to fully enclose the malleoli. This configuration allows some ankle mo-

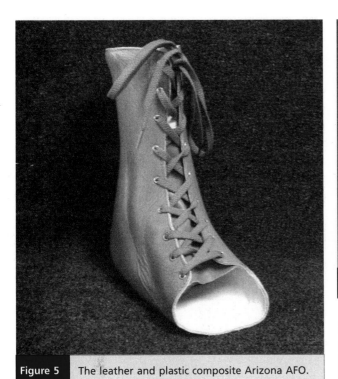

Figure 5 The leather and plastic composite Arizona AFO.

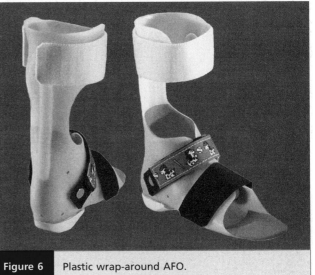

Figure 6 Plastic wrap-around AFO.

tion during weight bearing, but only against resistance. The resistance dampens or reduces the effect of the ground reaction forces that otherwise would act on the anatomic structures. In this sense, semisolid AFOs may be referred to as torque-absorbing AFOs. Diseased anatomy, such as an attenuated tendon, can be spared stress through this torque-absorbing mechanism. The amount of stiffness built into the brace determines the amount of torque energy absorbed and determines the amount of motion that is blocked. Generally, a semisolid AFO is intended to protect anatomic structures and allow enough motion for normal walking. No standards currently exist to guide the amount of stiffness built into such braces. The skill and judgement of the orthotist will determine the optimal stiffness of an AFO for a given patient.

The posterior leaf spring version of the standard AFO is used to support weakened dorsiflexor muscles. The leaf spring part of the brace is supple enough to allow normal ankle motion during weight bearing but stiff enough to maintain dorsiflexion during the swing phase of gait and to ensure toe clearance.

The articulated AFO consists of two moving segments joined by a mechanism that allows motion, such as a simple hinge. The articulating mechanism aligns with the anatomic ankle. Many such mechanisms exist and they may be classified by the ankle motion that they block. For example, if no pathology is present around the ankle, a free-motion device may be appropriate. If Achilles tendon pathology is present, a joint that blocks dorsiflexion may be needed. Joints exist to block or allow motion in any subset of the ankle's normal range. In instances of ankle weakness, a joint may

be used that provides assistance to the user's motor power, such as dorsiflexion assistance during the swing phase of gait. Joints in articulated AFOs also vary in bulk and weight. It is always necessary to consider how the AFO will fit into the patient's shoe. An articulated AFO often requires more room in the shoe than other types of AFOs.

Plastic and Leather Composite Orthoses
The original plastic and leather orthosis, the Arizona AFO (Arizona AFO Inc, Mesa, AZ), is a design that does not fit into the standard nomenclature system (**Figure 5**). It uses thin polypropylene as a reinforcing material between two layers of molded leather, which completely surrounds the lower leg, ankle, hindfoot, and midfoot. Because numerous braces with a similar design made by competing manufacturers are now available, there may be some confusion when ordering this type of brace.

Some manufacturers have expanded on the original design by exploring other material choices or geometric configurations. Most manufacturers of this type of full-enclosure, composite orthosis will provide customized configurations based on specifications of the treating orthotist. No evidence-based data exist to assist in specifying a particular configuration for a particular diagnosis.

Other variations of this type of AFO include a woven polymer fabric that conforms to compound curves, instead of molded leather as an enclosing material or an AFO that uses a laminated composite for a stiffening material. These variations are lighter in weight.

Plastic Wrap-Around AFOs
Another form of full-enclosure AFO with a composite construction is the plastic wrap-around AFO (**Figure 6**). These AFOs are most commonly used for pediatric patients. The manufacture and design of these devices is sophisticated. Numerous models are available

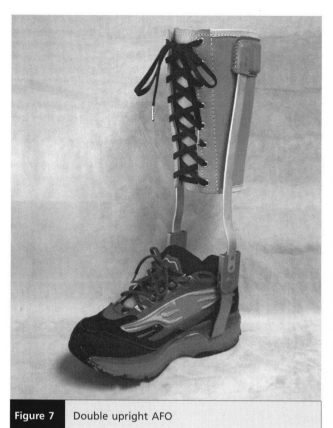

Figure 7   Double upright AFO

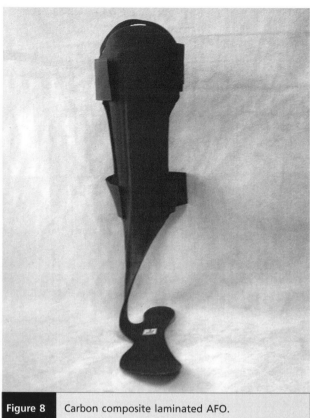

Figure 8   Carbon composite laminated AFO.

that can be matched to a wide variety of biomechanical presentations. In the same manner as leather and plastic composite braces, plastic wrap-around braces completely enclose the midfoot, hindfoot, ankle, and lower leg. They effectively immobilize the anatomy inside the orthotic enclosure and maximize the area of surface contact with the skin; therefore, they are often more comfortable and more effective at maintaining the desired anatomic alignment.

Double Upright AFOs

Double upright AFOs are the best devices for certain patients (**Figure 7**). When edema varies too much to be accommodated by any enclosing device, double upright devices can control ankle motion without skin contact in the ankle and lower leg areas. The exact controls exerted on the ankle can range from free motion to assisted motion, resisted motion, or completely blocked motion. This type of brace also obviates difficulties with shoe fittings because it attaches to the exterior of the patient's regular shoes.

Carbon Fiber AFOs

Modern resilient materials, particularly carbon fiber composite laminations, have made energy storage and return available as a new mechanism for treating orthopaedic foot and ankle conditions[12] (**Figure 8**). The achievement of world records in running competitions by amputees is evidence of the power of this mechanism. New marathon and other running competition

records have been set since the introduction of carbon fiber leaf springs to the design of prosthetic feet and ankles. At least 11 orthotic devices with integrated carbon leaf springs are now available in marketed manufactured products. Some individual orthotic facilities also fabricate custom-laminated devices for their patients. There are three key differences between these resilient leaf spring devices and the simpler torque-absorbing plastic AFOs previously described: (1) the resilient leaf spring operates in both plantar flexion and dorsiflexion; (2) in addition to allowing limited motion against resistance, the carbon leaf spring recoils with force; and (3) the rhythm of resistance and recoil matches the energy sequence exerted by eccentric and concentric muscle activity during normal gait. Wearing such a brace may diminish the muscle action crossing the foot and ankle. The diminished muscle activity may then be expected to diminish the compressive forces acting within the involved joints and diminish the tensile forces acting through the involved tendons. Diminished pain has been observed in patients with arthritis and tendon pathology.

The thin cross-sectional area necessary for these braces to fit around the foot and ankle limits the magnitude of energy storage and return that the orthotic device can achieve compared with bulkier prosthetic devices for amputees. The limits of what can be achieved with these new materials are still being explored as new products with innovative new approaches continue to emerge.

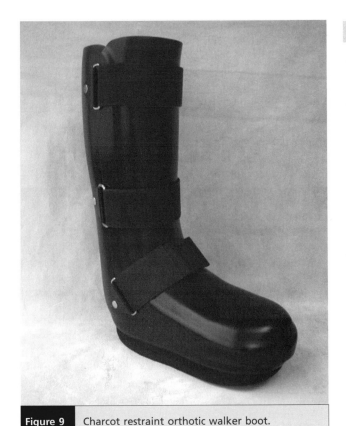

| Figure 9 | Charcot restraint orthotic walker boot. |

Charcot Restraint Orthotic Walker Boot

The Charcot restraint orthotic walker is a custom molded, clam-shell orthosis that attempts to completely immobilize the foot and ankle anatomy (**Figure 9**). It is essentially a removable version of a total contact cast with a rocker bottom shoe sole to facilitate walking. The contours of the molded plastic shells are supplemented with a molded foam lining to protect the skin. A removable closed-cell, expanded, polyethylene foam insert is typically included under the plantar surface of the foot. This device is intended for use in patients with severe foot and ankle deformity, severe instability, and/or skin at high risk for ulceration.

Summary

Because shoes are important for protecting the foot from injury, manufacturers are using specific design characteristics for the upper, insole, midsole, and outsole to maximize protection, performance, and comfort during work and sporting activities. When standard shoe wear does not provide adequate cushioning, support, or stability, shoe modifications and orthoses are available to treat foot and ankle pathology. Orthoses (both in-shoe and AFOs) work by one or a combination of different mechanisms including protection of skin, controlling anatomic alignment, mitigating bending forces caused by weight bearing, supporting muscular weakness, or correcting deviations in gait.

Annotated References

1. Frey C, Thompson F, Smith J: Update on women's footware. *Foot Ankle Int* 1995;16:328-331.

2. Alvarez RG, Marini A, Schmitt C, Saltzman CL: Stage I and II posterior tibial tendon dysfunction treated by a structured nonoperative management protocol: An orthosis and exercise program. *Foot Ankle Int* 2006;27: 2-8.

   Stage I and II posterior tibial tendon dysfunction can be effectively treated in 89% of patients with a short, articulated AFO or foot orthosis and a physical therapy program.

3. Verdejo R, Mills NJ: Heel-shoe interaction and the durability of EVA foam running-shoe midsoles. *J Biomech* 2004;37:1379-1386.

   After a 500 km run, peak plantar pressures in running shoes increase by 100% because of fatigue of the EVA foam in the midsole. Failure of the EVA foam results in less heel cushioning, which may lead to injury.

4. Menz HB, Morris ME: Footwear characteristics and foot problems in older people. *Gerontology* 2005;51: 346-351.

   Hallux valgus deformities and corns developed in individuals who wore shoes that were too narrow. Shoes that were too short were associated with the development of hammer toes. High heeled shoe wear was associated with hallux valgus and plantar callosities.

5. Ottaviani RA, Ashton-Miller JA, Kothari SU, Wojtys EM: Basketball shoe height and the maximal muscular resistance to applied ankle inversion and eversion moments. *Am J Sports Med* 1995;23:418-423.

6. Goske S, Erdemir A, Petre M, Budhabhatti S, Cavanagh PR: Reduction of plantar heel pressures: Insole design using finite element analysis. *J Biomech* 2006;39:2363-2370.

   Conformity of an insole to the foot is more important than the thickness of the insole or the material used in reducing peak plantar pressures.

7. Even-Tzur N, Weisz E, Hirsch-Falk Y, Gefen A: Role of EVA viscoelastic properties in the protective performance of a sport shoe: Computational studies. *Biomed Mater Eng* 2006;16:289-299.

   Midsole EVA wear in athletic shoes increases heel pad stresses. A 50% reduction in EVA thickness resulted in an increase in peak heel pad stress by 19%.

8. Crincoli MG, Trepman E: Immobilization with removable walking brace for treatment of chronic foot and ankle pain. *Foot Ankle Int* 2001;22:725-730.

9. Imhauser CW, Abidi NA, Frankel DZ, Gavin K, Siegler S: Biomechanical evaluation of the efficacy of external stabilizers in the conservative treatment of acquired flatfoot deformity. *Foot Ankle Int* 2002;23:727-737.

10. Nagaya M: Shoehorn-type ankle foot orthoses: Prediction of flexibility. *Arch Phys Med Rehabil* 1997;78:82-84.

11. Raikin SM, Parks BG, Noll KH, Schon LC: Biomechanical evaluation of the ability of casts and braces to immobilize the ankle and hindfoot. *Foot Ankle Int* 2001;22:214-219.

12. Alimusaj M, Knie I, Wolf S, Fuchs A, Braatz F, Doderlein L: Functional impact of carbon fiber springs in ankle-foot orthoses. *Orthopade* 2007;36:752-756.

Carbon fiber leaf springs in AFOs provide support throughout the stance phase of gait and increase the energy of push-off.

Chapter 3

Imaging

Steven M. Raikin, MD

Introduction

Following a careful history and clinical examination of a patient, radiographic imaging is the next step in formulating a diagnosis and establishing a treatment plan for patients with conditions affecting the foot and ankle. Numerous imaging modalities are available to the physician. Appropriate indications and current applications of many of these modalities will be discussed in this chapter.

Plain Radiographs

Plain radiographs are the foundation of imaging for most foot and ankle pathologies. Bony anatomy, integrity, and alignment along with joint congruency can be assessed using routine radiographs, which can usually be obtained in the office at the time of the patient's initial visit. Weight-bearing radiographs should be obtained whenever possible for the best images of the foot and ankle. Non–weight-bearing techniques to assess structural anatomy and rule out fractures may be better tolerated in patients with acute traumatic injuries; however, non–weight-bearing views do not show the physiologic position of the foot and ankle and may hinder detection of malalignment or some pathologic conditions.

Digital radiology is gaining in popularity. There are two methods to capture radiographs digitally. Computed radiography is affordable, offers excellent image quality, and uses existing x-ray systems. Digital radiography technology is more expensive, but offers increased efficiency and the capacity for higher image quality or lower dose radiation. Images are archived in a picture archiving and communication system that replaces hard-copy films.[1] Medical images are most commonly stored in Digital Imaging and Communication in Medicine (DICOM) format, which allows safe, high-quality, off-site viewing and analysis of radiographs. Other potential advantages include computer-assisted measurements of distances or angles used in diagnosing various foot and ankle pathologies.[2]

Radiographs of the Foot

Routine radiographs of the foot include lateral, AP, and oblique views. The internal (medial) oblique view is usually obtained as part of the routine three-view set and is useful in viewing the lateral tarsometatarsal joints and for assessing possible calcaneonavicular tarsal coalitions. The external (lateral) oblique view is used if clearer visualization of the perinavicular joints is required or for identifying the presence of an accessory navicular bone.

In specific circumstances, special views can be helpful in obtaining information about the bony anatomy. The sesamoid axial projection may show sesamoid-metatarsal arthritis, fractures or osteonecrosis of the hallux sesamoids, and sesamoid alignment relative to the crista on the plantar aspect of the metatarsal head. The calcaneal axial view (Harris-Beath view) is taken at a 45° angle from a posteriorly proximal direction. This view allows analysis of the posterior and middle facet of the subtalar joint for arthritis or a tarsal coalition. Broden views are a sequence of angled radiographs centered over the sinus tarsi and taken between 10° and 40° of cephalic tilt. These views provide reliable imaging of the posterior facet of the subtalar joint in calcaneal fracture management and subtalar fusions. The talar neck view provides a true AP view of the talar neck that is useful in assessing talar neck fractures. This view is taken with the foot internally rotated 15°, and the x-ray beam angled 15° cephalad while centered over the talar neck.

Radiographs of the Ankle

As is the case with radiographs of the foot, a three-view weight-bearing set is routinely recommended for analysis of the ankle. Anatomic AP, lateral, and mortise views are obtained. In the anatomic AP view, the ankle mortise is anatomically aligned 20° externally rotated to the sagittal plane; a true AP radiograph is taken with the beam 20° medially (internally) directed. A mortise view provides the best assessment of mortise congruity and the talar dome.[3]

Special views also may be needed to evaluate the ankle joint. The 50° external rotation view is used for optimal visualization of posterior malleolar fracture fragments. The hindfoot alignment view is obtained with the patient standing on a raised platform with the x-ray beam directed from the posterior and angled 20° caudally.[4] The cassette is placed perpendicular to the beam.

Stress views of the ankle are used in assessing ankle instability. While a lateral radiograph is taken, an anterior drawer test is performed manually (with the evaluator's hands protected by lead gloves) or with the use of

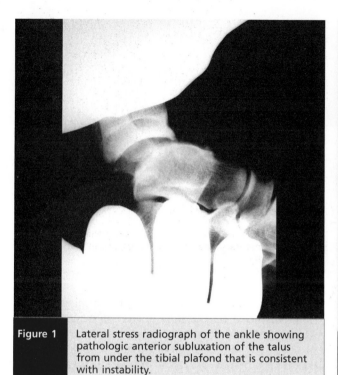

Figure 1 Lateral stress radiograph of the ankle showing pathologic anterior subluxation of the talus from under the tibial plafond that is consistent with instability.

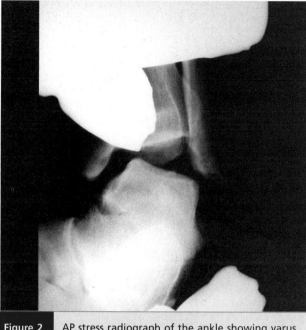

Figure 2 AP stress radiograph of the ankle showing varus ankle instability secondary to lateral ankle ligament complex dysfunction.

a mechanical jig. Anterior displacement of the talus of more than 10 mm (or 5 mm more than displacement caused by stressing the uninvolved ankle) is consistent with lateral ankle ligament dysfunction (**Figure 1**). Similarly, varus and valgus stress radiographs are used to assess the lateral ligament complex and deltoid ligament integrity, respectively. A 10° difference in the talar tilt between the normal and injured extremity is considered pathologic (**Figure 2**). However, the reliability and reproducibility of stress testing is questionable because of the wide variation in findings in healthy patients with normal ankles, the variations in the tester-dependent forces applied against the ankle, and variations in force resistance from the patient. The results of stress testing alone should not dictate the ultimate treatment of ankle instability.

Intraoperative fluoroscopic evaluation has become a vital tool in assessing joint or bone alignment and for positioning internal hardware. Technical advances have allowed significant improvements in the quality of fluoroscopy units in terms of image quality, machine size, and ease of handling. Mini C-arm fluoroscopy is used by many foot and ankle surgeons and exposes the surgical team to minimal radiation during routine use, unless they are in the direct path of the beam.[5]

Radiographic Measurements

Various radiographic measurements have been described to evaluate the alignment of the foot and ankle. All of the measurements are more accurate when radiographs are taken under weight-bearing conditions. The hallux valgus angle and the first-second intermetatarsal angles are the mainstay for assessing severity of hallux valgus deformities. These measurements have good intraobserver and interobserver reliability when standardized methods are used.[6] The first and second metatarsal axes are each drawn by connecting the midpoint of the shaft of the metatarsal 2 cm from the proximal and distal articular surfaces. The axis of the phalanx is drawn through the shaft midpoints 0.5 cm from each of its articulations. A third angle, the hallux valgus interphalangeus angle, is drawn between the phalangeal axis of the proximal and distal phalanx of the hallux (**Figure 3**). Using the distal metatarsal articular angle for determining joint congruency does not have the same degree of reliability and reproducibility.[7] Measurements can be enhanced with computer assistance, but this is usually unnecessary.[8]

The talus-first metatarsal angle (Meary angle) is drawn through the long axes of the talus and the first metatarsal on a lateral radiograph. This angle is useful in determining planus or cavus of the arch with a normal angle of −4° to 4°[9] (**Figure 4**).

The talonavicular coverage angle is useful for evaluating pes planovalgus deformities to determine the degree of forefoot abduction as determined by the degree of lateral subluxation of the navicular at the talar head or the amount of uncovered talar head. The angle is measured on a weight-bearing AP radiograph of the foot by measuring the angle created by a line joining the two ends of the articular surface of the talar head and a line joining the matching two ends of the joint surface of the navicular. The angle created between the perpendicular lines drawn off the midpoints of each of these two lines represents the talonavicular coverage angle; a normal value is less than 7°.

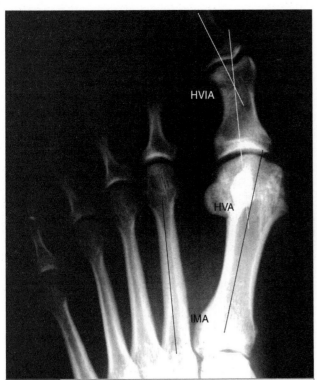

Figure 3 AP radiograph showing the angles measured for determining hallux valgus deformity. HVIA = hallux valgus interphalangeus angle, HVA = hallux valgus angle, IMA = first-second intermetatarsal angle.

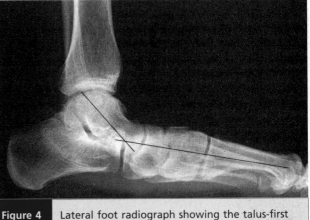

Figure 4 Lateral foot radiograph showing the talus-first metatarsal angle for diagnosing pes planovalgus deformity.

Tenography

Plain radiographs are used to view secondary changes caused by tendon dysfunction, but are not used to evaluate the tendons. Tenography involves the injection of contrast material (under fluoroscopy) into the tendon sheath (often followed by a therapeutic steroid injection) to allow tendon evaluation. This is a cost-effective but invasive technique and may cause tendon rupture. Tenography can show tenosynovitis, stenosing tenosynovitis, or tendon tears or rupture.[10] In the absence of tendon tears, intrasheath steroid injection associated with tenography can relieve symptoms in up to 46% of patients with tenosynovitis around the foot and ankle. With the advent of MRI, tenography is used less often for diagnostic purposes.[11]

Ultrasound

Ultrasound evaluation of tendons around the foot and ankle offers numerous advantages compared with other modalities.[12] It is a cost-effective, safe, noninvasive modality that is nonradiation-based and offers real-time assessment of the structures being evaluated. A major advantage of ultrasound is that it permits dynamic evaluation of the tendons, allowing conditions such as subluxation of the peroneal tendons to be viewed di-

rectly during the actual subluxation. Another advantage is that the transducer can be manipulated to avoid interference from metallic implants within the ankle. This modality is useful in determining associated tendon injuries following surgical fixation of prior foot or ankle disorders in which interference from the implanted hardware makes MRI suboptimal. MRI evaluations of tendons passing around the ankle also are susceptible to the "magic ankle phenomenon" (artifact seen within tendons orientated at 54.7° to the magnetic field), which may suggest intratendinous pathology. This drawback is not associated with ultrasound evaluation. According to recent studies, ultrasound was slightly less sensitive in diagnosing posterior tibial tendon (PTT) pathology compared with MRI, but no discrepancies resulted in altered clinical management.[13,14] Ultrasound also has 100% sensitivity and 90% specificity in detecting peroneal tendon tears, and a 100% positive predictive value in detecting peroneal subluxation when correlated with intraoperative findings.[15,16]

Ultrasound can be used to evaluate lateral ankle ligament tears, with a sensitivity and specificity comparable with MRI. Interdigital (Morton) neuromas and recurrent interdigital neuroma can be detected on ultrasound if clinical evaluation is equivocal; other soft-tissue masses or cysts also can be detected. Ultrasound can assist with guided aspiration, biopsy, or directed therapeutic injections in specific pathologies. Foreign bodies (such as wooden splinters) that are not radiopaque can be detected and localized with ultrasound guidance to facilitate removal.

The major disadvantage of ultrasound is that it is a technician-dependent modality and many medical centers do not have a trained radiologist experienced in interpreting the results of musculoskeletal ultrasound studies. Other disadvantages include the inability to perform the study through a cast or splint (direct skin contact via gel is required), and poor visualization of bone.

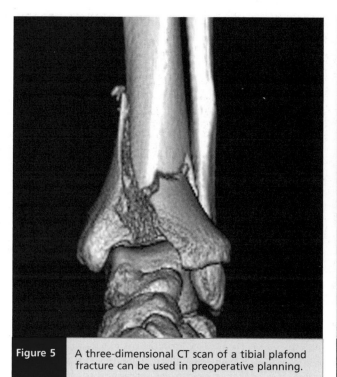

Figure 5 A three-dimensional CT scan of a tibial plafond fracture can be used in preoperative planning.

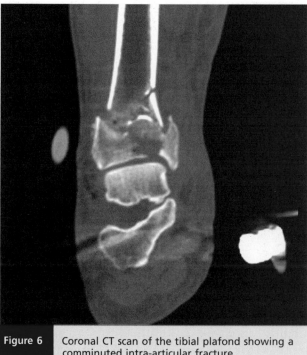

Figure 6 Coronal CT scan of the tibial plafond showing a comminuted intra-articular fracture.

CT Scanning

CT scanning offers high-resolution, thin-slice scanning of the foot and ankle. Over the past 10 years, CT imaging of osseous structures has evolved significantly with the development and implementation of multidetector-row slip-ring technology. Source images can be acquired in the axial, coronal, or sagittal planes, allowing three-dimensional views of the bony anatomy for diagnostic and therapeutic planning. Newer computer software allows reconstruction in additional planes without added exposure to ionizing radiation (such as coronal images reconstructed from axial images). Three-dimensional reconstruction models also can be created from the initial source images for preoperative planning (**Figure 5**). A disadvantage of CT is that imaging cannot be performed with the patient in a physiologic weight-bearing stance; however, simulated weight-bearing scans are being investigated. Around the foot and ankle, scanning with 3-mm or thinner slices is routinely recommended. Foot position in the scanner is important, with the source image planes obtained parallel to the osseous structures of the foot in each plane using a tomographic scout localizer image. Cast or splinting material around the region does not interfere with CT imaging, but may make positioning of the foot more difficult during the study. With the advent of multidetector-row systems, rapid image acquisition and improved three-dimensional reconstruction can be achieved with lower radiation doses.

CT scanning can be used for diagnosing fractures, infections, osteochondral injuries, arthritis, osteonecro-

sis, and tumors or congenital abnormalities affecting bones or joints of the foot and ankle. CT is particularly useful in providing fine osseous detail not obtainable with plain radiographs. Subtle fractures, joint diastasis, or articular incongruity (including Lisfranc and syndesmotic injuries and tibial plafond fractures) not detectable on plain radiographs frequently are seen on CT scans. CT scans can be used to assess the degree of joint comminution in calcaneal or plafond fractures to assist in preoperative planning (**Figure 6**).

CT scanning also is useful in detecting fracture nonunions, showing an accuracy of 90% and a sensitivity of 100%.[17] CT is more reliable in determining the degree of union after surgical arthrodesis than serial radiographic studies[18] (**Figure 7**). This accuracy may be enhanced in the future with new microCT and nanoCT technology, which is currently being studied in small animals.[19]

Nuclear Medicine

Nuclear medicine studies involve the intravenous administration of a radioactive tracer followed by subsequent scanning with a gamma camera, which can detect concentration of the tracer in a given area of study. Conventional nuclear medicine studies of the musculoskeletal system (bone scans) involve the administration of technetium Tc 99m methylene diphosphonate (^{99m}Tc MDP), which binds to hydroxyapatite crystals during bone formation. This technique can identify bone turnover caused by occult fractures, stress fractures, tumors, infections, and metabolic disorders.

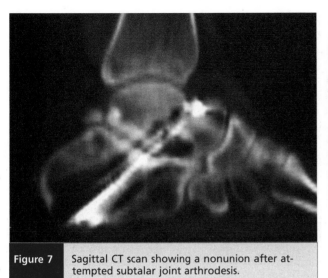

Figure 7 | Sagittal CT scan showing a nonunion after attempted subtalar joint arthrodesis.

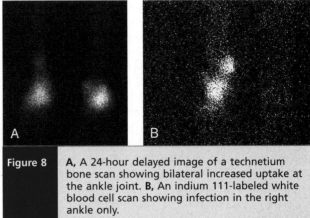

Figure 8 | **A,** A 24-hour delayed image of a technetium bone scan showing bilateral increased uptake at the ankle joint. **B,** An indium 111-labeled white blood cell scan showing infection in the right ankle only.

Scanning is performed at three different phases. The first scan is performed within 1 minute of tracer administration and is termed the blood flow phase; this scan identifies increased blood flow to the studied area caused by inflammation. The second phase, which detects blood pooling, is obtained after 5 minutes. The third phase (the delayed phase) is performed 4 hours after injection of the tracer and specifically detects bone turnover. The scan can be performed over the entire body or by obtaining pinhole views of the area of interest.[20] Because many conditions affect blood flow and bone turnover, bone scanning is very sensitive but has poor specificity. Some conditions, such as sympathetically mediated complex regional pain syndrome, may show increased tracer in the affected area in all three phases of the study. Following a fracture, the earliest that a bone scan will return to normal levels is after 6 months, with 10% of uncomplicated fractures still demonstrating increased local tracer uptake after 2 years.[20]

Leukocyte-labeled scanning can increase the specificity for diagnosing bone infections. Peripheral blood is aspirated from the patient and the white blood cells are labeled with radioactive tracer. Common labels include Tc 99m hexamethylpropyleneamineoxide (^{99m}Tc HMPAO) or indium 111 oxime. It is advantageous to use ^{99m}Tc HMPAO because of the lower radiation dose and quicker scanning time (scan performed after 4 hours instead of 24 hours for indium 111). Delayed scanning will localize areas of increased leukocyte uptake, signifying inflammation or infection. When combined with a standard three-phase bone scan, synchronous uptake in the same area on both scans indicates bone activity caused by infection, thus improving specificity[21] (**Figure 8**).

[99m]Tc sulfur colloid scanning is a technique for identifying marrow infection. This technique can be used in combination with a leukocyte-labeled study to further improve the specificity of the study.

Positron emission tomography (PET) is the newest generation of nuclear medicine scanning. PET usually involved the intravenous injection of fluorodeoxyglucose (FDG) with scanning for positron emission decay in the area of study 1 hour after administration. FDG-PET has been shown to exclude bone or soft-tissue infection in a Charcot foot in the presence of a foot ulcer, with an overall sensitivity and accuracy of 100% and 93.8%, respectively. FDG-PET scanning is more accurate in diagnosing active chronic osteomyelitis than indium 111-labeled scanning.[22]

Nuclear medicine imaging has been advocated as a method for assessing arterial limb perfusion, particularly in the presence of calcified vessels in which the ankle-brachial index may be spuriously elevated. Thallium 210 scanning can detect perfusion abnormalities and deficiencies in muscle perfusion reserves in asymptomatic diabetic patients with clinically normal perfusion, whereas FDG-PET scanning is accurate in determining the degree of atherosclerosis within the extremities of diabetic patients.[23]

Magnetic Resonance Imaging

After conventional radiography, MRI is the most frequently used modality for imaging foot and ankle pathology. MRI can be used to evaluate osseous, ligamentous, tendon, and muscular injuries about the foot and ankle using a standard, noncontrast protocol. MRI also can be used to characterize an injury based on known patterns of abnormal signal indicating stress along a specific biomechanical axis. Advantages of MRI compared with other imaging modalities include its multiplanar capabilities, its sensitivity for both osseous and soft-tissue edema, and its use of a magnetic field to generate diagnostic images without exposing tissue to ionizing radiation. Potential disadvantages include cost and imaging time. Some patients with implanted ferromagnetic devices, including some cardiac pacemakers, cerebral aneurysm clips, automatic defibrillators, biostimulators, implanted infusion devices, internal hearing aids, and any metallic foreign bodies about the orbits, are not candidates for MRI. Many implanted medical devices and fixation hardware are nonferromagnetic and are MRI compatible. Although the number of MRI studies dedicated to the foot and ankle has increased dramatically over the past 10 years, it is still not typically used as a first-line modality in imaging foot and ankle pathology. Most commonly, MRI of the foot and ankle is indicated when radiographic or CT findings are inconclusive or inconsistent with clinical symptomatology, when pain persists atypically during a treatment course, or when a primary soft-tissue process, such as tendon or ligament dysfunction, is suspected.

An MRI of the foot or ankle should include both fluid-sensitive (T2-weighted) and anatomy-specific (T1-weighted) sequences. Optimally, an MRI of the foot or ankle should include at least two fat-suppressed sequences to maximize fluid sensitivity. MRI examinations of the ankle should be distinct from those dedicated to the foot. Ankle MRI scans should image from proximal to the tibiotalar joint down to the midfoot level, including posterior tibial and peroneus brevis insertions. In contrast, an MRI of the foot should image areas from the talar head through the toes. All MRI protocols for imaging the ankle or foot should include three anatomic planes. At the ankle, recommended protocols use two sagittal, one fluid-sensitive with fat suppression, and one anatomy-specific (T1-weighted spin-echo) sequences, as well as two axial sequences with similar parameters. A coronal, fluid-sensitive sequence should be tailored to evaluate potential osteochondral lesions at the tibiotalar joint. Acquisition of these five sequences on most MRI systems can be accomplished in approximately 22 minutes. For MRI dedicated to the foot, optimal plane selection can be difficult because of varying perceptions on the definition of terms such as coronal and axial. For this reason, descriptive terms including short axis, long axis, and sagittal are recommended for plane selection. Both fluid-sensitive and anatomy-specific short axis (or bread slice) sequences should be acquired for detecting metatarsal and intermetatarsal pathology. Inversion recovery sequences often provide the most homogeneous fat suppression in the sagittal plane, and a long axis, fluid-sensitive sequence should be acquired along the metatarsals, simulating an AP radiograph.

Intravenous gadolinium contrast is occasionally indicated when imaging the foot and ankle with MRI. Evaluation of a soft-tissue mass or osteomyelitis are indications for precontrast and postcontrast imaging. Other relative indications for intravenous contrast with foot and ankle MRI include inflammatory arthropathies, stenosing tenosynovitis, postoperative scar evaluation, and intermetatarsal neuromas. Severe renal insufficiency is a relative contraindication for gadolinium-based contrast agents because of their suspected association with the development of nephrogenic systemic fibrosis. With specific indications, including assessment of the integrity of the lateral ankle ligaments and the stability

of osteochondral lesions, intra-articular contrast injection with a dedicated arthrographic MRI protocol may ultimately prove useful.[24]

Circumferential receiver coil designs, such as a head or extremity coil, can be used effectively to generate adequate signal throughout the ankle or foot. With the exception of specific indications such as reflex sympathetic dystrophy, attempting to image both the foot and the ankle using one protocol and acquisitions in large fields of views is strongly discouraged. Based on the clinical examination and patient history, indications for MRI of the ankle should generally be discernible from indications for MRI of the foot. If there is concern for injury involving the ankle and the forefoot, two separate MRI studies are recommended.

Although numerous MRI system designs and field strengths are widely available, limitations encountered with some patients including claustrophobia and obese body habitus are rarely an issue when imaging the foot and ankle. To allow adequate resolution of ligaments, tendons, and articular surfaces in the distal lower extremity, MRI studies acquired at standard- or high-field strengths (1.0 tesla (T) and above) are recommended. In rare instances in which patients cannot tolerate a standard, closed, 1.5-T MRI unit, a high-field strength, dedicated, extremity system has potential benefits compared with low-field strength (0.2 and 0.3 T) open systems. Although little scientific evidence exists to mandate imaging the foot and ankle at 3.0-T strength, early applications with these high-field strength systems have shown promise for improving current MRI protocols dedicated to articular cartilage lesions, and tendinopathies. Regardless of field strength, MRI will be limited by the quality and efficiency of the receiver coil; therefore, dedicated extremity coils or ankle coils are preferable for adequate imaging of the foot and ankle.[25]

Osseous Injury

Displaced fractures usually are diagnosed with plain radiographs or CT scans; in contrast, nondisplaced fractures and contusions about the foot and ankle can be identified on MRI scans. Nondisplaced fractures and contusions will manifest on fluid-sensitive, fat-suppressed MRI sequences as hyperintense T2-weighted signal. In the setting of a fracture, the T2-weighted hyperintense signal is more focal, more intense, and may exhibit a linear morphology compared with an osseous contusion in which the T2-weighted hyperintense signal is less intense and more diffuse. Another tool for distinguishing a fracture from a contusion is abnormal signal on T1-weighted sequences. Linear, hypointense, T1-weighted signal in the location of T2-weighted hyperintensity in patients with known trauma can be interpreted as a fracture with some degree of certainty. When abnormal T2-weighted hyperintense and T1-weighted hypointense signal extends in a sunburst pattern from an articular surface, the term osteochondral impaction injury is preferred. This is a relatively nonspecific term because a discrete

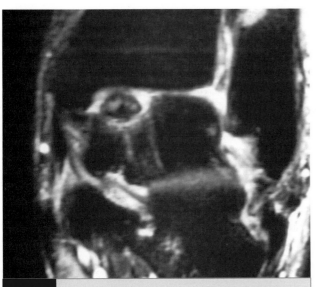

Figure 9	Coronal MRI scan of the ankle joint showing an osteochondral lesion with an underlying fluid level consistent with an unstable lesion.

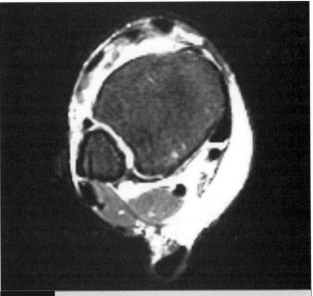

Figure 10	Axial MRI scan taken 1 cm above the ankle joint level showing a complete rupture of the anterior distal tibiofibular syndesmotic ligament and avulsion of the posterior ligament.

osteochondral lesion can be difficult to distinguish from an osteochondral contusion in the setting of acute trauma. MRI is routinely used for diagnosing osteochondral defects. Typical signal characteristics include a subchondral osseous T1-weighted hypointense crescent (or T2-weighted hyperintense signal), signifying fluid undercutting the bone fragment and implying instability of the fragment (**Figure 9**). On the talar dome, osteochondral defect lesions are located medially at the anterior to posterior equator by a ratio of nearly 2:1 compared with lateral lesions.[26] Medial talar dome osteochondral defect lesions also involve a larger surface area and tend to be deeper in craniocaudal dimensions than lateral lesions. Less common locations for osteochondral lesions about the foot and ankle include the talar head, the tibial plafond, the calcaneocuboid joint, and the metatarsal heads. Lesions at these locations also can be effectively diagnosed with MRI.

Traumatic ankle and foot injuries often cause reproducible patterns of bony contusion that can be seen on MRI scans. Knowledge of these patterns can result in a better understanding of injury mechanisms and can aid in diagnosing associated soft-tissue injuries. With inversion ankle injuries, common locations for T2-weighted hyperintense osseous contusions include the tip of the fibula, the entire medial malleolus, the anterior process and anterolateral body of the calcaneus, the talar neck or anteromedial talus extending to the middle subtalar joint, and the proximal cuboid at the calcaneocuboid articulation. An eversion injury is characterized by bony contusion of the proximal aspect of the cuboid at the calcaneocuboid joint and malleoli. Marrow edema in the distal fibula tends to be diffuse and ill-defined whereas bone marrow edema in the medial malleolus tends to be isolated to its tip (suggestive of an avulsion injury). MRI of the foot also is useful in assessing sub-

tle bony injuries that can be difficult to assess with plain radiographs alone. Bony contusions and osteochondral injuries involving the distal articular surfaces of the cuneiforms and the proximal articular surfaces of the metatarsals should raise suspicion for Lisfranc ligament injury. MRI is extremely sensitive for detecting acute nondisplaced or stress fractures of the metatarsals, which are easily identified on short axis sequences through the forefoot in injuries characterized by diffuse, abnormal, medullary T2-weighted hyperintensity. Plantar plate injury can be diagnosed by MRI by identifying T2-weighted hyperintensity within the metatarsal head and a breach in the soft-tissue structures intimate to the plantar aspect of each metatarsal head. Osseous injuries of the first metatarsophalangeal sesamoids can be identified with MRI and are characterized as fractures, contusions, or osteonecrosis.

Ligament Injuries

Normal ligaments should appear hypointense or dark on all MRI sequences. The appearance of a ligament with an acute sprain includes poor definition along with periligamentous fluid signal. Diffuse enlargement, attenuation, or complete disruption can indicate either a subacute or chronic high-grade injury. It is difficult to establish the clinical competence of a sprained ligament with the use of MRI alone.

Acute injury of the distal tibiofibular syndesmosis generally presents on axial MRI sequences as focal enlargement and edema of ligamentous structures (**Figure 10**). Although the anterior inferior tibiofibular ligament is often disrupted, the posterior syndesmosis rarely shows abnormality on non–weight-bearing images. Syndesmotic structures often ossify over time af-

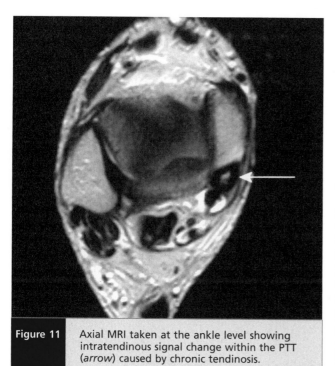

Figure 11 | Axial MRI taken at the ankle level showing intratendinous signal change within the PTT (*arrow*) caused by chronic tendinosis.

ter injury and appear diffusely dark, thickened, and heterogenous on axial MRIs. MRI also can be useful in diagnosing injuries of the lateral ligaments of the ankle. Given the frequency of inversion injury and subsequent trauma to the anterior talofibular ligament (ATFL), this structure rarely appears normal on MRI scans. In patients with an acute or subacute ATFL sprain, the ill-defined or enlarged ligament is accompanied by bony contusions in or by edema within the lateral soft tissues. Chronic ATFL injuries appear as diffuse ligament hypertrophy with scar tissue (as may be seen in antero-lateral impingement) or as complete absence of the ligament (suggesting lateral instability). Less frequently, the calcaneofibular ligament appears abnormal on MRI scans. The calcaneofibular ligament should appear as a thin, hypointense, linear structure that runs deep to the peroneal tendons in the subfibular region. It is best assessed on sequential coronal images; a normal insertion on the lateral calcaneus should be documented on every ankle MRI. Acute injury often manifests as disruption of the ligament from the calcaneal periosteum with surrounding soft-tissue edema, whereas chronic injury can appear as diffuse ligamentous enlargement. The sensitivity of MRI in diagnosing medial deltoid ligament injury is suboptimal, but an osseous contusion pattern indicating eversion injury may correlate with a deltoid sprain. With a high-grade deltoid injury, the ligament can be entirely disrupted from its medial malleolus origin on coronal MRI scans.

MRI can be useful in diagnosing ligament sprains in the foot, particularly sprains that are subtle or clinically confusing. With suspicion of a Lisfranc ligament injury, long axis sequences should be acquired in the plane of the medial cuneiform–second metatarsal (Lisfranc) lig-

ament for assessing morphology and signal pattern.[27] With these sequences, the Lisfranc ligament can be assessed in a similar manner by directly identifying intraligamentous edema, partial tears, or complete disruption. In the forefoot, sprains or tears of the plantar plate of the first metatarsophalangeal joint (turf toe) are recognizable on T2-weighted MRI scans. MRI can be used to differentiate ligamentous and osseous injuries and can aid in differentiating complete tears from partial sprains.

Tendon Injuries

As is the case with other soft-tissue conditions, MRI is an ideal modality for assessing tendon structures of the foot and ankle. Tendons are imaged in cross-sectional axial views or with sagittal views. Tendons should appear hypointense with homogenous signal and smooth contours. Tenosynovitis is characterized by peritendinous high signal intensity consistent with fluid. Abnormal tendons appear heterogenous with intratendinous medium signal intensity, along with abnormal morphology such as hypertrophy, thickening, marked attenuation, or even complete absence in instances of rupture. MRI can confirm a clinical diagnosis of tendon pathology and quantify the severity of disease.

MRI can play a role in assessing patients with a degenerative PTT.[28] Conventional non–weight-bearing MRI can show abnormal valgus alignment of the hindfoot on coronal images at the level of the midsubtalar joint. MRI also is useful in identifying midfoot sag on sagittal images (the analogue of an abnormal Meary angle) and uncovering of the talar head by the navicular on axial images. This triad of malalignments along with PTT pathology will confirm PTT dysfunction. Earlier in the course of PTT tendinopathy, MRI is less sensitive for tendon degeneration. The normal MRI appearance of the distal PTT insertion on axial MRI scans is similar to that of an inverted "Hershey's Kiss." The navicular insertion of the PTT blends with the medial bundle of the spring ligament, creating a broad footprint. More proximally, the spring ligament is directed medially, and the PTT tapers quickly on axial images to an ovoid configuration, appearing slightly larger than the adjacent flexor hallucis longus tendon. The absence of this rapid tapering and a broader PTT proximal to the navicular with more of a "Tootsie Roll" configuration can be the earliest clue to insertional PTT tendinopathy. Posterior tibial tendinopathy also can present more proximally behind the medial malleolus. Enlargement and intratendinous heterogeneity of the PTT along with subcortical malleolar marrow edema are hallmarks of advanced PTT degeneration (**Figure 11**). Common patterns of PTT pathology include hypertrophic appearance or marked attenuation of the tendon; less commonly, a complete rupture appears with absence of the tendon within its sheath.

At the lateral ankle, numerous peroneal tendon pathologies can be reliably diagnosed with MRI. In the retrofibular or subfibular regions, a peroneus brevis

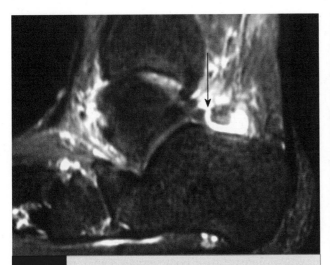

| Figure 12 | Sagittal MRI scan of the ankle showing a fractured os trigonum process (*arrow*) with associated edema. |

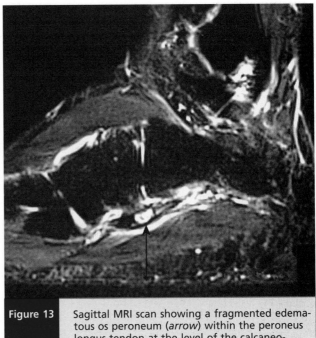

| Figure 13 | Sagittal MRI scan showing a fragmented edematous os peroneum (*arrow*) within the peroneus longus tendon at the level of the calcaneocuboid joint. |

split tear can appear as a wishbone-shaped tendon or as two separate tendon bellies on axial images. At the level of the lateral malleolus, peroneal instability can manifest as redundancy or tear of the superior peroneal retinaculum, stripping of the retinaculum off the periosteum of the malleolus, or frank dislocation of the peroneus longus out of the groove and adjacent to the lateral malleolus itself.[29] With degenerative peroneal tendon conditions, either tendon may show diffuse enlargement (tendinosis) or longitudinal, intratendinous high signal on T2-weighted sequences (interstitial tearing). With dorsiflexion injury, it is important to follow the peroneus longus under the calcaneocuboid joint and the midfoot to its insertion on the plantar surface of the first metatarsal, because distal peroneus longus tears can mimic other plantar soft-tissue injuries. Accessory ossicles around the foot and ankle area also are prone to injuries that may not be discernible on plain radiographs, such as injuries to the os trigonum posterior to the talus in which MRI may show increased signal intensity within the synchondrosis, or injury indicated by fluid collection around the os on T2-weighted sequences (**Figure 12**). In ballet dancers using the en pointe or demi pointe position, posterior ankle impingement also can be caused by flexor hallucis longus tendinitis or tenosynovitis, which can be differentiated from an os trigonum on MRI evaluation. Similarly, painful os peroneum syndromes can be diagnosed on MRI scans by signal change within the os (located within the peroneus longus tendon at the level of the calcaneocuboid joint) demonstrating inflammatory changes, a stress fracture, or osteonecrosis of the ossicle (**Figure 13**).

Ankle MRI is an accurate diagnostic modality for traumatic and degenerative pathologies involving other ankle tendons including the Achilles tendon and anterior tibial tendon. Achilles tendon injury can occur at the critical zone or the insertion, including enthesopa-

thies such as retrocalcaneal bursitis, and bone marrow edema of the dorsal calcaneus associated with a Haglund exostosis and insertional spurring. Tendinosis is characterized on MRI scans as morphologic thickening of the tendon, signal change within the substance of the tendon itself, and linear splits within the tendon suggestive of degenerative tears (**Figure 14**). In addition to providing diagnostic assistance, MRI studies also can guide the management of insertional Achilles tendinitis. A recent study showed that the absence of acute inflammatory changes associated with confluent areas of intrasubstance signal change in the distal Achilles tendon is a poor prognostic indicator of the potential success of nonsurgical treatment of the condition.[30] The identification of the location of intrasubstance tears and mucinous changes within the tendon on MRI scans can guide the surgeon in determining the amount of tendon involved and in débriding the involved areas of the tendon at the time of surgery. Although usually diagnosable by clinical evaluation alone, MRI can be beneficial in confirming a rupture within the tendon and quantifying any retraction gaping between the tendon ends.

Other Indications

MRI can be used to identify sources of ankle pain related to impingement of soft-tissue structures including infiltration of the sinus tarsi, the effect of a mass within the tarsal tunnel causing nerve compression, and intra-articular anterolateral or anteromedial ankle impingement. It can be useful in identifying atraumatic osseous pathologies including os trigonum syndrome and patchy bone marrow edema related to altered biomechanics or stress response. MRI plays an essential role in the work-up of symptomatic midfoot or hindfoot co-

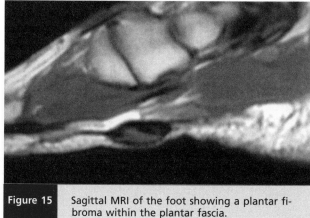

Sagittal MRI of the foot showing a plantar fibroma within the plantar fascia.

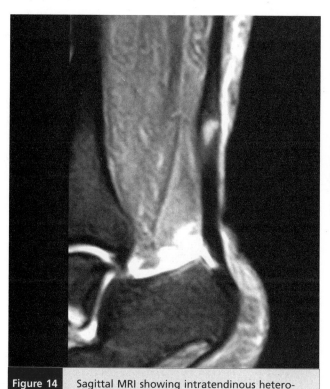

Figure 14 | Sagittal MRI showing intratendinous heterogeneity within the Achilles tendon at the vascular watershed area 7 cm above the calcaneal insertion.

alition because it can show osseous morphology and the sequelae of abnormal weight distribution.

MRI of the foot is a useful tool for evaluating both soft-tissue and osseous pathologies in acute injuries and degenerative conditions.[31] It is useful in evaluating refractory plantar fasciitis and can identify fascial tears and reactive marrow edema at the plantar calcaneus. MRI is the imaging modality of choice for various common soft-tissue conditions of the foot, including plantar fibromatosis (**Figure 15**), intermetatarsal neuromas, ganglion cysts of tendon sheaths or joint capsules, and synovial chondromatosis of the ankle. With inflammatory arthropathies, MRI delineates the extent of osseous erosions and periarticular synovitis. MRI has evolved into the modality of choice for imaging osteomyelitis caused by foot infections because it can accurately identify the presence and extent of osseous involvement and soft-tissue abscesses or phlegmon.[32-34]

Summary

Appropriate imaging of the foot and ankle is essential to the orthopaedic surgeon for diagnosing and guiding treatment of many lower extremity pathologies. An understanding of the available imaging modalities and their advantages and shortfalls will contribute to optimal outcomes for patients with foot and ankle disorders.

Annotated References

1. Gallet J, Titus H: CR/DR systems: What each technology offers today. What is expected for the future. *Radiol Manage* 2005;27:30-36.

   Computed radiography is affordable, offers excellent image quality and exposure latitude, and uses existing x-ray systems. Computed radiographic systems are indicated in lower volume areas. Digital radiography is more expensive but has the capacity for higher efficiency, better image quality, and lower-dose radiation.

2. Raikin SM, Bley LA, Leb RB: Emerging technology: Remote analysis of traumatic musculoskeletal radiographs transmitted by electronic mail. *J Orthop Trauma* 1999;13:516-519.

3. Brage ME, Bennett CR, Whitehurst LB, Getty PJ, Toledano A: Observer reliability in ankle radiographic measurements. *Foot Ankle Int* 1977;18:324-329.

4. Cobey JC: Posterior roentgenogram of the foot. *Clin Orthop Relat Res* 1976;118:202-207.

5. Giordano BD, Ryder S, Baumhauer JF, DiGiovanni BF: Exposure to direct and scatter radiation with use of mini-c-arm fluoroscopy. *J Bone Joint Surg Am* 2007;89:948-952.

   The authors assessed the safety of using mini C-arm radiographic imaging in the operating room without lead gown protection and concluded that the surgical team is exposed to minimal radiation, except when in the direct path of the radiation beam.

6. Coughlin MJ, Freund E: The reliability of angular measurements in hallux valgus deformities. *Foot Ankle Int* 2001;22:369-379.

7. Chi TD, Davitt J, Younger A, Holt S, Sangeorzan BJ: Intra- and inter-observer reliability of the distal metatarsal articular angle in adult hallux valgus. *Foot Ankle Int* 2002;23:722-726.

8. Piqué-Vidal C, Maled-García I, Arabi-Moreno J, Vila J:

Radiographic angles in hallux valgus: Differences between measurements made manually and with a computerized program. *Foot Ankle Int* 2006;27:175-180.

In patients with hallux valgus deformities, angular measurements made on computer-assisted weight-bearing radiographs were more reliable than those made with a goniometer. For large angles, such as the hallux valgus and distal metatarsal articular angles, results obtained with both techniques were similar. Manual measurements may underestimate the true values of the smaller intermetatarsal and proximal phalangeal articular angles.

9. Younger AS, Sawatzky B, Dryden P: Radiographic assessment of adult flatfoot. *Foot Ankle Int* 2005;26: 820-825.

The authors of this study concluded that the talar-first metatarsal angle is an accurate radiographic identifier of patients with symptomatic adult flatfoot.

10. Jaffee NW, Gilula LA, Wissman RD, Johnson JE: Diagnostic and therapeutic ankle tenography: Outcomes and complications. *AJR Am J Roentgenol* 2001;176:365-371.

11. Schreibman KL: Ankle tenography: What, how, and why. *Semin Roentgenol* 2004;39:95-113.

Tenography is an invasive yet effective method of evaluating tendon structure for rupture and tenosynovitis. A steroid injection can be added as a therapeutic adjuvant to the diagnostic injection.

12. Rockett MS, Waitches G, Sudakoff G, Brage M: Use of ultrasonography versus magnetic resonance imaging for tendon abnormalities around the ankle. *Foot Ankle Int* 1998;19:604-612.

13. Nallamshetty L, Nazarian LN, Schweitzer ME, et al: Evaluation of posterior tibial pathology: Comparison of sonography and MR imaging. *Skeletal Radiol* 2005;34: 375-380.

In this study, ultrasonography and MRI of the PTT were concordant in most patients. Ultrasonography was slightly less sensitive than MRI for PTT pathology, but these discrepancies did not affect clinical treatment.

14. Premkumar A, Perry MB, Dwyer AJ, et al: Sonography and MR imaging of posterior tibial tendinopathy. *AJR Am J Roentgenol* 2002;178:223-232.

15. Grant TH, Kelikian AS, Jereb SE, McCarthy RJ: Ultrasound diagnosis of peroneal tendon tears: A surgical correlation. *J Bone Joint Surg Am* 2005;87:1788-1794.

The authors of this study found that the sensitivity, specificity, and accuracy of ultrasonography in diagnosing peroneal tendon tears was 100%, 85%, and 90%, respectively. The use of dynamic ultrasound is effective for determining the presence or absence of a peroneal tendon tear and should be considered a first-line diagnostic tool.

16. Neustadter J, Raikin SM, Nazarian LN: Dynamic sonographic evaluation of peroneal tendon subluxation. *AJR Am J Roentgenol* 2004;183:985-988.

Dynamic sonography is an effective technique for diagnosing peroneal tendon subluxation and associated tears of the peroneal tendons. A high intraoperative correlation was demonstrated in this study.

17. Bhattacharyya T, Bouchard KA, Phadke A, Meigs JB, Kassarjian A, Salamipour H: The accuracy of computed tomography for the diagnosis of tibial nonunion. *J Bone Joint Surg Am* 2006;88:692-697.

CT shows good accuracy in the evaluation of tibial fracture healing. However, it is limited by low specificity and may sometimes cause a physician to misdiagnose a healed fracture as a nonunion.

18. Coughlin MJ, Grimes JS, Traughber PD, Jones CP: Comparison of radiographs and CT scans in the prospective evaluation of the fusion of hindfoot arthrodesis. *Foot Ankle Int* 2006;27:780-787.

This prospective study compared radiographs and CT scans for the quantitative evaluation of healing of hindfoot arthrodeses. Progress of the fusion cannot be determined accurately from standard radiographs. CT scanning appears to be significantly more reliable.

19. Schmidhammer R, Zandieh S, Mittermayr R, et al: Assessment of bone union/nonunion in an experimental model using microcomputed technology. *J Trauma* 2006;61:199-205.

Study results showed that microCT with three-dimensional reconstruction was the optimal diagnostic tool for assessing fracture healing, especially in instances of fracture nonunion.

20. Frater C, Emmett L, van Gaal W, Sungaran J, Devakumar D, Van der Wall H: A critical appraisal of pinhole scintigraphy of the ankle and foot. *Clin Nucl Med* 2002;27:707-710.

21. Poirier JY, Garin E, Derrien C, et al: Diagnosis of osteomyelitis in the diabetic foot with a 99mTc-HMPAO leucocyte scintigraphy combined with a 99mTc-MDP bone scintigraphy. *Diabetes Metab* 2002;28:485-490.

22. Basu S, Chryssikos T, Houseni M, et al: Potential role of FDG PET in the setting of diabetic neuro-osteoarthropathy: Can it differentiate uncomplicated Charcot's neuroarthropathy from osteomyelitis and soft-tissue infection? *Nucl Med Commun* 2007;28:465-472.

The results of this study support the valuable role of FDG-PET in treating Charcot neuroarthropathy by reliably differentiating it from osteomyelitis both in general and when a foot ulcer is present.

23. Lin CC, Ding HJ, Chen YW, Huang WT, Kao A: Usefulness of thallium-201 muscle perfusion scan to investigate perfusion reserve in the lower limbs of type 2 diabetic patients. *J Diabetes Complications* 2004;18:233-236.

The perfusion reserve in the lower limb muscles in patients with type 2 diabetes can be measured by a thallium-201 muscle perfusion scan.

24. Cerezal L, Abascal F, Garcia-Valtuille R, Canga A: An-

kle MR arthrography: How, why, when. *Radiol Clin North Am* 2005;43:693-707.

The authors of this study reviewed current indications and potential applications for both intravenous and intra-articular uses of gadolinium-based contrast agents in MRIs of the foot and ankle.

25. Calisir C, Murat Aynaci AI, Korkmaz C: The accuracy of magnetic resonance imaging of the hands and feet in the diagnosis of early rheumatoid arthritis. *Joint Bone Spine* 2007;74:362-367.

The authors reviewed MRI findings in both the hands and feet in 21 patients who fulfilled the 1987 American College of Rheumatology criteria for the diagnosis of rheumatoid arthritis to assess the prevalence of MRI findings early in the course of the disease.

26. Raikin SM, Elias I, Zoga AC, Morrison WB, Besser MP, Schweitzer ME: Osteochondral lesions of the talus: Localization and morphologic data from 424 patients using a novel anatomic grid scheme. *Foot Ankle Int* 2007; 28:154-161.

The authors established the true frequency of osteochondral lesions on the talar dome by location using a nine zone grid and compared the morphology of lesions at the medial dome to those at the lateral dome.

27. Potter HG, Deland JT, Gusmer PB, Carson E, Warren RF: Magnetic resonance imaging of the Lisfranc ligament of the foot. *Foot Ankle Int* 1998;19:438-446.

28. Lim PS, Schweitzer ME, Deely DM, et al : Posterior tibial tendon dysfunction: Secondary MR signs. *Foot Ankle Int* 1997;18:658-663.

29. Wang XT, Rosenberg ZS, Mechlin MB, Schweitzer ME: Normal variants and diseases of the peroneal tendons and superior peroneal retinaculum: MR imaging features. *Radiographics* 2005;25:587-602.

A review of the appearance of MRIs and several recent scientific articles regarding both traumatic and degenerative injuries to the peroneal tendons and the superior peroneal retinaculum are presented.

30. Nicholson CW, Berlet GC, Lee TH: Prediction of the success of nonoperative treatment of insertional Achilles tendinosis based on MRI. *Foot Ankle Int* 2007;28:472-477.

Patients with insertional Achilles tendinitis underwent MRI evaluation. Tendinosis was classified based on tendon size and degree of involvement (type I, II, or III). After failure of nonsurgical treatment, 12.5% of patients with type I, 90.8% with type II, and 70.4% with type III tendinosis required surgery. The authors concluded that early identification of these patients and surgical treatment may lead to earlier return to function.

31. Labovitz JM, Schweitzer ME: Occult osseous injuries after ankle sprains: Incidence, location, pattern, and age. *Foot Ankle Int* 1998;19:661-667.

32. Kapoor A, Page S, Lavalley M, Gale DR, Felson DT: Magnetic resonance imaging for diagnosing foot osteomyelitis: A meta-analysis. *Arch Intern Med* 2007;167: 125-132.

These authors performed a meta-analysis of clinical trials from 1980 through 2006 and compared MRI with scintigraphy for diagnosing foot infections. They concluded that MRI outperformed other imaging modalities for diagnosing osteomyelitis of the foot.

33. Lipman BT, Collier BD, Carrera GF, et al: Detection of osteomyelitis in the neuropathic foot: Nuclear medicine, MRI and conventional radiography. *Clin Nucl Med* 1998;23:77-82.

34. Morrison WB, Carrino JA, Schweitzer ME, Sanders TG, Raiken DP, Johnson CE: Subtendinous bone marrow edema patterns on MR images of the ankle: Association with symptoms and tendinopathy. *AJR Am J Roentgenol* 2001;176:1149-1154.

Chapter 4
Arthroscopy of the Foot and Ankle

Gregory P. Guyton, MD   Lorenzo Gamez, MD

Introduction

An increasing array of techniques has expanded the indications for arthroscopic procedures about the foot and ankle in recent years. These minimally invasive approaches hold promise for significantly reducing patient morbidity and decreasing recovery times compared with open procedures. In addition to a better understanding of the appropriate indications for routine anterior ankle arthroscopy, recent attention has focused on alternative uses of the arthroscope in posterior ankle arthroscopy, subtalar arthroscopy, Haglund débridement, and first metatarsophalangeal (MTP) joint arthroscopy. As in all arthroscopic procedures on small joints, the special demands on the hindfoot arthroscopist to avoid iatrogenic injury to the surrounding nerves or joint structures remain unchanged.

Anterior Ankle Arthroscopy

Approach, Positioning, and Equipment

Anterior ankle arthroscopy is the most routine of the foot and ankle arthroscopic procedures. The patient is typically positioned supine with the operative leg in a well-leg holder or on a bolster. A variety of noninvasive joint distraction devices are available that use a foot strap and jackscrew to provide gentle ankle distraction while allowing access to both the anterior and posterior aspects of the ankle. Invasive distraction with the use of an external fixator is of historic interest only.

The availability of pressure and flow-regulated arthroscopic pumps makes it unnecessary to routinely use a separate posterolateral portal for outflow. Most procedures can be performed through standard anteromedial and anterolateral portals with appropriate pump settings and intermittent use of a shaver and suction to clear the joint. If outflow is required for unique situations, it can easily be accomplished with an 18-gauge spinal needle through a posterolateral approach.

Most procedures are appropriately accomplished with a short 30°, medium-sized arthroscope, typically 2.9 mm in diameter. The equipment is the same as that used in many institutions for elbow arthroscopy. Smaller arthroscopes (2.0 mm or smaller) used in wrist arthroscopy are prone to bending and do not afford sufficient inflow. Larger instruments, such as those used in knee arthroscopy, are prone to causing iatrogenic gouging or scuffing of the cartilage. Large arthroscopes have a role in situations in which high flow or a powerful large-diameter shaver or burr is required, such as débridement of large anterior osteophytes, extensive arthrofibrosis, or arthroscopic arthrodesis.

The anteromedial portal is established at the level of the joint line immediately adjacent to the anterior tibial tendon. Although no major nerve structures are at risk at this location, care must be taken to hug the tendon closely; establishing this portal too medially will allow access to the anterior aspect of the joint but will limit visualization of the medial gutter of the ankle. Immediately prior to making the portal, the joint can be injected through the same approach with a local anesthetic containing epinephrine using a 20-gauge needle; this allows an appropriate check of the position.

The anterolateral portal is established only after the arthroscope has been inserted medially. The primary risk of anterior ankle arthroscopy is injury to the superficial peroneal nerve or, more commonly, its intermediate dividing branch. This risk can be minimized with several techniques but cannot be completely eliminated because of the anatomic variability of the nerve. Several studies have reported the risk of nerve injury as approximately 1%.[1,2] Several methods should be routinely used to avoid this type of nerve injury. (1) The nerve can be marked preoperatively. If the patient is thin or fair-skinned, the nerve can often be palpated or directly visualized subcutaneously. Marking is often best accomplished in the preoperative holding area where the nerve can be marked with a permanent marker. Passive flexion of the fourth toe places the nerve under tension and may make it more prominent and easier to visualize near the ankle. (2) Anatomic landmarks can be used to locate the nerve. The location of the superficial peroneal nerve branches with regard to the portals used for ankle arthroscopy has been described. The literature generally advises locating the portal at least 2 to 4 mm lateral to the peroneus tertius tendon.[1] (3) Transillumination can be used to visualize the nerve. The medial portal is routinely established first and the arthroscope is used to transilluminate the joint, potentially revealing larger nerve branches or veins that should be avoided during the procedure. (4) The nerve may be located by a gentle spreading technique. The portal itself should be made with a skin-only incision followed by a vertical spreading motion

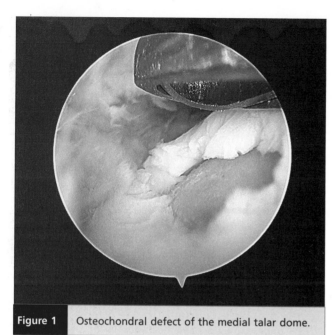

Figure 1 Osteochondral defect of the medial talar dome.

with a hemostat to go through the subcutaneous tissues.

Other portals are not routinely used. The anterocentral portal that was once described for ankle arthroscopy was associated with an unacceptably high rate of neurovascular injury to the deep peroneal nerve. If a posterolateral portal is required, it can be established immediately adjacent to the Achilles tendon, 1 cm above the level of the tip of the fibula.

After the joint is entered, the ankle is examined using a systematic approach that includes the medial and lateral gutters, medial and lateral talar dome, central talar dome, tibial plafond, syndesmosis, and anterior aspect of the talus at the capsular reflection. A small probe should be used to check the integrity of the cartilage with special attention paid to the anterolateral and posteromedial talar dome, which are the most common locations of osteochondral injury.

Osteochondral Lesions

Osteochondral lesions of the talus are among the most common indications for ankle arthroscopy (**Figure 1**). They are typically located either anterolaterally or posteromedially on the shoulder of the talar dome. Arthroscopic treatment is typically aimed at débridement and microfracture of the lesion; in rare circumstances an acute traumatic lesion may be amenable to arthroscopically assisted fixation.

Posteromedial and anterolateral lesions have different characteristics that must be appreciated by the arthroscopist. Posteromedial lesions are often deeper and cup shaped, yet may be more confined in the area of the talar dome they occupy. Anterolateral lesions tend to be shallower and shaped like a wafer. In the setting of the multiply injured ankle with chronic instability, the anterolateral lesion may be surrounded by an area

of chondromalacia, making it difficult to determine the precise boundaries of the lesion.

Patient presentation and history may differ depending on the type of lesion present. Although all osteochondral lesions probably have a traumatic origin, a specific known incident is more commonly determined in patients with anterolateral lesions. Posteromedial lesions may be noted as incidental findings in patients with other ankle pathologies, such as ankle instability or peroneal pathology.

Microfracture techniques are used most commonly for osteochondral lesions (Figure 2). Modern microfracture awls are available in a variety of angles and allow ready access to essentially all anatomic locations within the ankle. Older techniques, such as transmalleolar drilling, cause trauma to the tibial chondral surface and are no longer recommended.

There is continued debate regarding the surface dimension and depth of osteochondral lesions that are suitable for microfracture. The literature provides guidance on the types of lesions that will have poor outcomes and those that are likely to fill with stable fibrocartilage following the procedure. The current alternate technologies for cartilage replacement include autologous osteochondral grafting, allograft osteochondral grafting, reimplantation of cultured chondrocytes, and synthetic replacements. These techniques usually require arthrotomy; in patients with posteromedial lesions, a medial malleolar osteotomy may be necessary. There is no evidence that an attempt at arthroscopy and microfracture will diminish the possibility of ultimate salvage if the initial procedure fails. As a general guideline, arthroscopy should be used as the primary method to treat all lesions smaller than 1 cm. There are strong indications that arthroscopic microfracture can be used to treat larger lesions without cystic change.[3,4]

Determining the size of an osteochondral lesion preoperatively can present a significant challenge. MRI is routinely used to screen for the pathology; however, the dramatic reactive marrow edema surrounding the true lesion may result in a significant overestimation of the size of the pathologic bone volume. CT is often a useful adjunct if the size of the lesion is considered borderline or if a large cystic component is suspected that may require an alternative technique to fill the void.

The technical aspects of a microfracture procedure are usually straightforward. It is most critical to remove all loose bone and cartilage debris and to obtain a stable cartilage margin around the entire lesion. A series of passes is made with the microfracture awl into the deeper bone to ensure free backbleeding from the lesion; this bleeding should be confirmed by observing the lesion with the pump occluded and/or the shaver suction running over the site. It is usually best to use a twisting hand motion to pass the awl through the bone rather than striking it with a mallet. This technique provides greatly improved control in the small space of the ankle joint.

Access to anterolateral lesions is not complicated; however, access to posteromedial lesions may present

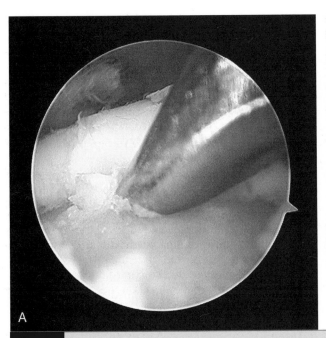 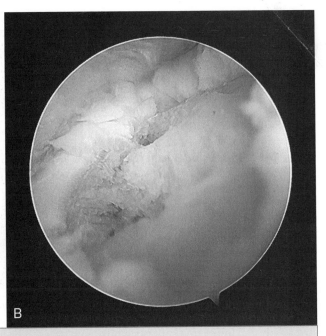

Figure 2 A, Microfracture of a talar osteochondral lesion. B, The lesion after microfracture.

special challenges. Despite their location, these lesions can often be approached via a purely anterior technique if the medial portal is used as the working portal for passing the curettes, shaver, and awls. A 30° arthroscope often fails to provide adequate visualization of a posteromedial lesion when placed through the anterolateral portal, and a 70° arthroscope is often required in this situation. If adequate débridement cannot be accomplished through an anterior approach, an additional posterolateral portal can serve as an additional working portal.

The success rates for microfracture of osteochondral lesions of the talus have been reported at 75% to 85%.[3-7] A number of factors that can influence outcome include size of the lesion, concurrent ankle arthritis or instability, and age of the patient. No specific data are available to guide the appropriate postoperative protocol, but 1 month of non–weight-bearing restrictions is typically advised to allow a suitable mechanical environment for fibrocartilage ingrowth. After microfracture, continued improvement may occur for several months following the procedure. In the absence of mechanical symptoms, an interval of 6 months or more is usually recommended before using a secondary procedure for patients who are unsatisfied with their outcomes. Repeat arthroscopic débridement and microfracture achieves essentially the same rate of success as the primary procedure in patients with recurrent symptoms and should be strongly considered.[8]

Soft-Tissue Impingement Lesions

Anterolateral soft-tissue impingement of the ankle following an inversion ankle sprain was first described in a 1990 study.[9] The authors described a distal and often

separate fascicle of the anteroinferior tibiofibular ligament that is part of the syndesmotic ligament complex. This fascicle runs obliquely for a course between 17 and 22 mm in length from the anterior aspect of the distal tibia to the anterior aspect of the fibula, crossing just over the lateral corner of the talar dome. Following major inversion ankle injuries, hypertrophy of the ligament and accompanying synovitis can lead to persistent pain in the area regardless of whether the ankle has regained stability following the original sprain. Resection of this low-lying band, now commonly called Bassett's ligament, usually results in pain relief.

Bassett's ligament is not a pathologic structure. It is present in most ankles and is seen routinely at the time of arthroscopy. This ligament is often responsible for symptoms following injury. In severe injuries, the hypertrophic response of the ligament can lead to direct erosion of the lateral dome of the talus (a kissing lesion).

Anterolateral soft-tissue impingement is mainly a clinical diagnosis.[10,11] MRI studies suggest that thickening of the ligament or fluid outlining may occur in some patients who are later believed to have clinically significant anterolateral soft-tissue impingement; however, findings are subtle.[12,13] Changes in the talar dome that can be identified arthroscopically often are not seen on conventional MRI scans, likely because they are largely restricted to the cartilage without accompanying marrow changes.

Patients with persistent pain localized over the anterolateral corner of the joint 4 to 6 months after a major inversion ankle sprain are appropriate candidates for arthroscopy. Resection of Bassett's ligament alone does not appear to have mechanical sequelae. The surgeon should recognize the possibility of subtle ankle instability as an alternate cause of the symptoms. The patient should be questioned concerning any history of ankle instability. The anesthetized patient should be examined for anterior talofibular ligament laxity at the time of arthroscopy.

Anterior Bony Decompression

The formation of anterior ankle osteophytes is a common early presentation of ankle arthritis and often occurs while central joint space is maintained. This condition is particularly common in patients who participate in sports requiring cutting motions, and has been termed footballers' ankle. Anterior osteophytes may form off the tibia (typically in an anterolateral location) and off the talus (typically anteromedially). Because the tibial spur and talar spur may not match the sagittal plane, a lateral radiograph often overestimates the severity of the disorder; kissing spurs may simply be overlapping. The patient should be carefully assessed for ankle instability that may require concurrent correction; there is a high incidence of significant chondral injury.

Arthroscopic resection of anterior bony osteophytes is usually associated with a high degree of patient satisfaction, although the potential for recurrence and progression of arthritic changes is significant. Most athletes can resume participation in sports activities, and weight bearing is usually restricted for only a few days. Aggressive rehabilitation and therapeutic exercises are then used to regain motion.

Arthroscopic resection of larger spurs can be challenging. Standard portals are used but the usual type of ankle arthroscope may not provide adequate flow or visualization to accomplish extensive débridement of bone. A standard large-joint arthroscope can be used if care is taken to avoid gouging the cartilage surface and the instruments are confined to the anterior capsule of the joint. A 4.5-mm shaver is typically used to outline the spur and a shielded 4.0- to 5.0-mm burr, such as those used for subacromial decompression, allows resection of the spur while protecting the anterior soft tissues. Lateral fluoroscopic imaging is recommended to achieve the desired degree of resection.

The tibial osteophyte is located within the capsular reflection of the ankle joint whereas the talar osteophyte is typically located on the anteromedial talar neck and is embedded in the capsular insertion.[14] The talar osteophyte is typically resected with a burr placed through the medial portal with the arthroscope placed laterally. Because the capsule is partially taken down in the process, anterior decompression may result in significant extravasation. Pump pressures should be kept as low as feasible (50 mm Hg) and a tourniquet should be considered to facilitate visualization with these low pressures.

Concurrent Arthroscopy With Ligament Stabilization

The incidence of significant concurrent ankle pathology in the presence of chronic ankle instability is believed to be approximately 20%.[15] Talar chondral injury and peroneal tendon tears are among the most common comorbidities, but occasional loose bodies or unusually located chondral lesions on the tibia or fibula also occur. Because conventional MRI scans often cannot detect subtle chondral injury that does not lead to marrow changes, a strong case can be made for routine concurrent ankle arthroscopy at the time of lateral ankle ligament reconstruction. Arthroscopy can provide prognostic information, such as early arthritic changes or unrecognized chondral erosions, and also allows treatment of cartilage flap tears of the talar dome or removal of synovitis, fibrosis, or loose bodies. Arthroscopic examination also may provide improved visualization of the medial and posterior ankle than that allowed by open anterolateral arthrotomy.

It is not necessary to alter the arthroscopic technique when the procedure is performed in conjunction with lateral ankle ligament reconstruction, but excessive fluid extravasation should be avoided when possible by limiting pump pressures and efficiently executing the procedure.

Arthroscopic Ankle Fusion

The use of arthroscopic débridement of the ankle in conjunction with percutaneous screw fixation has been advocated for more than 25 years. The purported advantages of this procedure include diminished pain for the patient and more rapid healing. The literature on ankle fusions reports a wide range of fusion rates, which is likely a result of varying initial pathologies and the possibility that fusion is not well assessed by plain radiography used in most studies.[16-18] No prospective, randomized studies exist that directly compare open and arthroscopic ankle fusion, nor have any studies used more rigorous CT-based criteria to evaluate the speed and ultimate success of arthroscopic fusion. One retrospective review comparing open versus arthroscopic ankle arthrodesis has shown comparable fusion rates between groups.[19] Patients treated with arthroscopic fusion had shorter surgical times, shorter tourniquet times, and a decreased number of in-hospital days. The range of reported fusion rates based on the limited number of existing studies appears to show results that are at least as good as those achieved with open techniques.

Arthroscopic ankle fusion is accomplished through two anterior portals; a large arthroscope is used if adequate distraction can be achieved. Curettes, osteotomes, and motorized burrs can be used for decortication. Backbleeding from the subchondral bone should be observed prior to fixation. Two or three antegrade

6.5- to 8.0-mm lag screws are typically placed in antegrade fashion across the joint.

Arthroscopic ankle fusion also has influenced surgeons who advocate open procedures. A small miniarthrotomy technique uses short anterolateral and anteromedial incisions that mimic the arthroscopic portals. This method easily accomplishes ankle fusion without extensive soft-tissue stripping and preserves the blood supply. Miniarthrotomy is suitable for patients with limited deformity and represents a significant departure from more extensive traditional techniques that involved larger lateral incisions and fibular resection.

Posterior Ankle Arthroscopy

Approach, Positioning, and Equipment

Posterior ankle arthroscopy is performed with the patient prone. A bump is placed under the distal tibia to elevate the foot. For posterior impingement, distraction is not usually necessary. The dense ligamentous structures about the posterior ankle and subtalar joint usually require establishment of a working area just outside the capsule, particularly if an os trigonum must be resected. A large-bore arthroscope is helpful when working outside the joint capsule because it provides the flow necessary for using a larger 4.5-mm shaver. Pump pressures should be kept as low as feasible (approximately 50 mm Hg) to avoid excessive extravasation; tourniquet use should be considered.

The standard portals for posterior ankle arthroscopy are established immediately adjacent to the Achilles tendon (**Figure 3**). The portals usually are established approximately 1 cm proximal to the level of the distal tip of the fibula. It is safe to use posterior portals if absolutely no deviation away from the medial and lateral margins of the Achilles tendon is tolerated. Anatomic analysis of posterior portal placement has established clearance guidelines of approximately 6 to 7 mm from the tibial nerve and 3 to 4 mm from the sural nerve.[20]

After creating an initial central working space using triangulation between the shaver and the arthroscope, the anatomic key to posterior ankle arthroscopy is the flexor hallucis longus (FHL) tendon. Manipulating the hallux during the early stages of the procedure may help establish the location of the FHL tendon. The neurovascular bundle will be medial and immediately adjacent to the FHL; all work should be carried out lateral to this tendon.

Posterior Impingement and Os Trigonum Resection

The most common indication for posterior ankle arthroscopy is posterior impingement or a painful os tri-

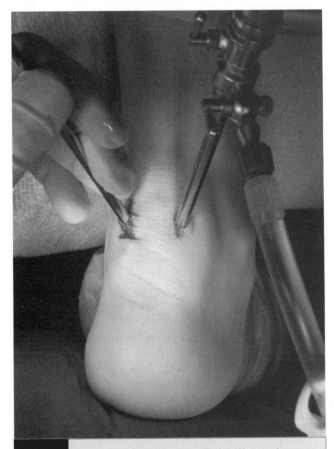

Figure 3   Posterior ankle arthroscopic portals are shown.

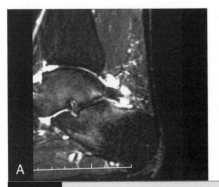 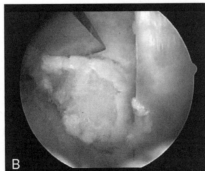 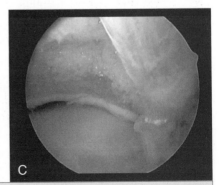

Figure 4   **A,** T2-weighted MRI showing symptomatic os trigonum. **B,** Arthroscopic resection of os trigonum. **C,** Arthroscopic image after ossicle excision.

1: General Foot and Ankle Topics

gonum (**Figure 4**). Patients will present with pain with forced plantar flexion in the posterior ankle that is often initially confused with Achilles tendon pathology. The incidence of a fully separate os trigonum is reported in 2.7% to 7.7% of skeletally mature adults.[21] The ossicle is usually bilateral but other variations are possible. Incomplete separation of the ossification center has been reported in 11% of adults.[21] A large but fused separate process of bone may be present that is called the trigonal process.

Any of these anatomic variants can occur with posterior impingement symptoms. Bone scans may show increased activity in the posterior talus and MRI may demonstrate a frank fracture or excessive marrow edema of the ossicle. Impingement also can be indicated by edema in adjacent areas of the posterior tibia and calcaneus. Resection is indicated if immobilization fails to relieve symptoms.

No studies are available that directly compare open and arthroscopic os trigonum resection, but the arthroscopic technique allows remarkably rapid mobilization and return to activity. Most patients achieve unprotected weight bearing within days of the procedure. The depth of exposure required for the open technique appears to have risks related to the required soft-tissue retraction. The largest study of open posterolateral resections reported 8 of 41 patients had sural nerve injury; four of these injuries were permanent.[22] In theory, the arthroscopic technique avoids these concerns.

Pathology of the FHL

Triggering of the FHL is a relatively common pathology in dancers who perform en pointe; however, it can occur even without a history of activities that require extreme plantar flexion. The pathology is akin to triggering of the A1 pulley in the hand; tenosynovitis and thickening of the tendon cause entrapment as the tendon passes through a restrictive band. In the FHL, this location is the tight sheath just above the sustentaculum tali.

FHL triggering should be considered in patients with posterior ankle pain; it can be relatively subtle to diagnose because no associated findings appear on imaging studies. Clinically, it is usually demonstrated by active plantar flexion of the toe with the ankle plantar flexed. Triggering of the FHL can occur with or without concurrent posterior impingement symptoms. If an os trigonum or large trigonal process is present, it should be treated concurrently with release of the FHL sheath.

Nonsurgical treatment can be as simple as a short respite from the inciting activity, particularly dancing en pointe. If this treatment is not successful, immobilization with a removable boot can be considered. Steroid injection of the sheath also can be effective if used sparingly. Fill of the FHL sheath can be shown on a concurrent live fluoroscopic tenogram to ensure proper placement of the needle and is recommended when possible.

Typically, 4 to 6 mL of a mixture of equal parts of steroid, local anesthetic, and radiographic contrast agent are injected using a 25-gauge needle along the same path as would be used for a posteromedial arthroscopy portal.

Arthroscopic release of the FHL sheath has been suggested and reported as an aspect of larger studies. The tibial nerve and the medial calcaneal sensory branch (in particular) lie directly on the FHL sheath and are vulnerable to injury.[23] One study that attempted FHL release under laboratory conditions reported that release down to the level of the sustentaculum was not possible even with the addition of a separate superomedial portal to provide a more acute angle for the arthroscopic instruments.[23] It is unclear exactly how far inferiorly the FHL sheath must be released to relieve symptoms. Because of these uncertainties and concerns about proximal neurologic structures, it is recommended that FHL release be performed through an open medial approach unless data supporting an all-arthroscopic technique become available.

Other Indications

The entire range of arthroscopic procedures performed from the anterior aspect of the ankle also can be performed from a posterior approach. Far posteromedial osteochondral lesions that are present well over the apex of the dome may be accessible only from the back of the ankle. If broader access to the talocrural joint is required, the arthroscopic portals can be located somewhat more inferiorly to allow access up the posterior slope of the talus. If the posterior subtalar joint is the primary focus of the examination, a standard location 1 cm above the level of the tip of the fibula usually provides excellent visualization.

Subtalar Arthroscopy

Approach, Positioning, and Equipment

Arthroscopy of the subtalar joint is usually focused on the interosseous ligament located within the sinus tarsi and the posterior facet of the joint. A lateral decubitus position with a small bump under the distal tibia is used to allow the foot to fall into slight inversion, opening up the sinus tarsi. For débridement of the sinus tarsi, distraction is not routinely necessary but may facilitate access to the posterior facet of the joint.

A number of different landmarks have been suggested to help locate the lateral portals that are used to introduce the arthroscope into the sinus tarsi, but simple palpation of the anterior process of the calcaneus and the angle of Gissane is usually the most straightforward approach. One portal is placed at the anterior aspect of the angle of Gissane and a second portal is placed at its posterior aspect. These locations are free of major neurovascular structures. If simultaneous access to the posterior aspect of the subtalar joint is necessary or the lateral recess of the joint must be explored, an additional posterolateral portal placed immediately adjacent to the Achilles tendon can be made. The location is identical to that used for the posterolateral portal in ankle arthroscopy. It is important to avoid the sural nerve.

Arthroscopy equipment that is appropriate for small joints is typically used. Because the two lateral portals are located very close together, a 70° arthroscope may occasionally be helpful to avoid impingement of the arthroscope, shaver, or other instruments.

Sinus Tarsi Pain

Pain localized to the sinus tarsi well after an inversion hindfoot sprain remains one of the most common indications for subtalar arthroscopy. The nonspecific term sinus tarsi syndrome is used to describe persistent localized pain in that area. Attempts to better define the nature of the disorder have generally followed either mechanical or neurologic approaches.

Tears of the interosseous ligament, diffuse arthrofibrosis, or subtle degenerative changes in patients with posttraumatic sinus tarsi pain undergoing arthroscopy have been documented.[24] Many authors have recommended preoperative sinus tarsi injection both as a potential therapeutic and diagnostic procedure. At the time of arthroscopic examination, débridement of the torn segment of the interosseous ligament is performed using the shaver and other hand tools as necessary. Only case series evidence (level 4) is available, but good or excellent results in more than 80% of patients have been reported.[24]

Recently, other researchers have focused attention on the innervation of the subtalar joint, suggesting that chronic sinus tarsi syndrome often represents a traction injury to the series of two to four small branches of the deep peroneal nerve that pass to the lateral aspect of the subtalar joint. Only case study evidence exists to support the contention, but a significant proportion of good to excellent results have been reported.[25] Whether the neurologic approach to sinus tarsi pain represents a separate and distinct entity from mechanical pathology or simply represents an alternative surgical method of masking pain from an injured structure remains to be determined.

Subtalar Fusion

The use of the arthroscope to perform subtalar fusion involving the posterior facet in select patients without deformity has been studied. The patient must be prone when posterior arthroscopic subtalar arthrodesis (called the PASTA approach) is used to facilitate access to the posterior facet. A small number of available case studies indicate an acceptable fusion rate.[20,26] The procedure is likely to have only limited application because of issues related to prone positioning of the patient and the reality that the combined incision length of the arthroscopic portals approaches that of an open technique via the sinus tarsi. This procedure may be most useful in patients with extensive soft-tissue damage, such as occurs after calcaneal fractures.

Endoscopic Calcaneal Exostectomy

Retrocalcaneal pain from a prominent posterior prominence of the calcaneus, or Haglund deformity, has been traditionally treated using an open surgical incision. Even when débridement of the Achilles tendon is not needed, the procedure can be associated with postoperative pain of significant longevity. During the past decade, there has been a focus on the development of endoscopic techniques to prevent this complication.

The arthroscopic technique is appropriate for patients who require a simple bony resection. If a symptomatic insertional calcaneal spur is present or degenerative MRI signal changes are evident within the Achilles tendon, an open technique should be used. Patients who are candidates for a simple bony removal are usually younger and athletic. Two portals are established on either side of the Achilles tendon and a shielded burr is used to resect the posterior margin of the calcaneus. The Achilles tendon insertion itself is avoided and the degree of bony resection is verified using intraoperative fluoroscopy.

Only evidence from level 4 case studies is available to support the technique, and most data are anecdotal. In a recent study of 32 patients, two complications were reported—one early postoperative Achilles tendon rupture and one patient with persistent pain requiring resurgery with an open procedure.[27] Anatomic studies of the portals have emphasized the proximity of the sural nerve and its lateral calcaneal branch, but neuritic complications have not been prominent in clinical reports.[1]

First MTP Joint Arthroscopy

Arthroscopy of the first MTP joint has been advocated for suspected chondral pathology in appropriate joints with little or no deformity (**Figure 5**). A small joint arthroscope, such as that typically used in the wrist (2.0 mm), is used with dorsolateral and dorsomedial portals. A direct medial portal also can be used if necessary. The joint usually can be easily distracted with a soft finger trap.

No comparative data exist comparing open débridement of chondral lesions of the metatarsal head with arthroscopic techniques. The open procedures can usually be accomplished with remarkably little morbidity and allow immediate weight bearing. Only a small case series supports use of the arthroscopic technique.[28] Arthroscopic débridement of early hallux rigidus has been advocated, but no comparison to traditional open methods is available. First MTP joint arthroscopy is best viewed as a technique with some potential advan-

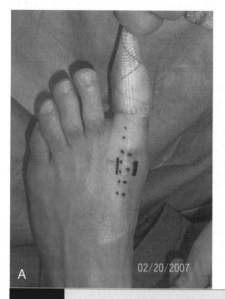
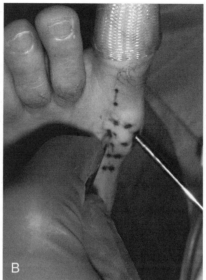
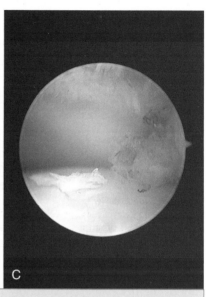

02/20/2007

A

B

C

Figure 5   **A,** Hallux MTP arthroscopic portals. The extensor hallucis longus tendon is marked by dotted lines. **B,** Arthroscopy of the hallux MTP joint is performed with a sterile finger trap for distraction. **C,** Arthroscopic view of the hallux MTP joint. The metatarsal head is inferior, the phalangeal base is superior, and synovitis is seen on the right side.

tages over traditional methods that remain to be proven.

Summary

Arthroscopy of the foot and ankle continues to evolve. New techniques of cartilage regeneration will likely allow ever greater flexibility in the arthroscopic treatment of chondral injury. In addition, as greater follow-up is documented, other arthroscopic procedures may prove to have significant benefits in recovery time or morbidity compared with open procedures.

Annotated References

1. Feiwell LA, Frey C: Anatomic study of arthroscopic portal sites of the ankle. *Foot Ankle* 1993;14:142-147.

2. Ferkel RD, Heath DD, Guhl JF: Neurological complications of ankle arthroscopy. *Arthroscopy* 1996;12:200-208.

3. Chuckpaiwong B, Berkson EM, Theodore GH: Microfracture for osteochondral lesions of the ankle: Outcome analysis and outcome predictors of 105 cases. *Arthroscopy* 2008;24:106-112.

   This study showed a correlation between the size of the osteochondral lesion and success of treatment. Treatment of lesions smaller than 15 mm had excellent results regardless of location. Increasing patient age, a higher body-mass index, trauma, and the presence of osteophytes negatively affected outcome.

4. Han SH, Lee JW, Lee DY, Kang ES: Radiographic

changes and clinical results of osteochondral defects of the talus with and without subchondral cysts. *Foot Ankle Int* 2006;27:1109-1114.

   The authors evaluated 38 patients (20 patients with subchondral cysts and 18 patients with an osteochondral defect without cysts). At follow-up, there was no difference in American Orthopaedic Foot and Ankle Society scores or radiographic results between the groups. The authors concluded that arthroscopic microfracture can be used to treat small cystic lesions and that the existence of a small cyst may not affect the prognosis.

5. Mologne TS, Ferkel RD: Arthroscopic treatment of osteochondral lesions of the distal tibia. *Foot Ankle Int* 2007;28:865-872.

   The authors concluded that arthroscopic treatment of osteochondral lesions of the tibia by curettage, abrasion arthroplasty, microfracture, or iliac crest bone grafting resulted in excellent and good results in 14 of 17 patients at medium-term follow-up.

6. Saxena A, Fakin C: Articular talar injuries in athletes: Results of microfracture and autogenous bone graft. *Am J Sports Med* 2007;35:1680-1687.

   The use of either talar bone grafting or microfracture allowed athletes to return to sports activities. The use of talar bone graft was associated with a longer time to return to activity in high-demand patients.

7. Takao M, Uchio Y, Kakimaru H, Kumahashi N, Ochi M: Arthroscopic drilling with debridement of remaining cartilage for osteochondral lesions of the talar dome in unstable ankles. *Am J Sports Med* 2004;32:332-336.

   In 69 patients, arthroscopic drilling of osteochondral lesions left remaining cartilage at the lesion in 39 patients and removed all cartilage at the lesion in 30 patients. At 1-year follow-up, the group in whom all cartilage was removed showed significantly more improvement than the other group. Removal of all cartilage at the time of arthroscopic drilling may be beneficial.

8. Savva N, Jabur M, Davies M, Saxby T: Osteochondral lesions of the talus: Results of repeat arthroscopic debridement. *Foot Ankle Int* 2007;28:669-673.

   Twelve patients underwent revision arthroscopic microfracture treatment for symptomatic talar osteochondral lesions. With an average follow-up of 6 years, eight patients returned to their preinjury level of activity and sports, whereas three returned to sports at a lower level. One patient with poor results required cartilage transplantation surgery. The authors concluded that in selected patients, revision microfracture surgery may yield acceptable outcomes and avoid more extensive salvage surgery, such as cartilage transplantation or grafting.

9. Bassett FH, Gates HS, Billys JB, Morris HB, Nikolaou PK: Talar impingement by the anteroinferior tibiofibular ligament: A cause of chronic pain in the ankle after inversion sprain. *J Bone Joint Surg Am* 1990;72:55-59.

10. Baums MH, Kahl E, Schultz W, Klinger HM: Clinical outcome of the arthroscopic management of sports related "anterior ankle pain": A prospective study. *Knee Surg Sports Traumatol Arthrosc* 2006;14:482-486.

    Anterior ankle arthroscopy for the treatment of both bony and soft-tissue impingement was reviewed in active athletes. At a mean follow-up of 31 months, 25 of 26 athletes were very satisfied with the procedure. No differences in outcome for bony and soft-tissue impingement were reported, indicating the efficacy of arthroscopic débridement for soft tissues.

11. Gulish HA, Sullivan RJ, Aronow M: Arthroscopic treatment of soft-tissue impingement lesions of the ankle in adolescents. *Foot Ankle Int* 2005;26:204-207.

    The authors evaluated 11 adolescent patients at an average follow-up of 25 months after arthroscopic débridement for soft-tissue ankle impingement. They reported improvement in American Orthopaedic Foot and Ankle Society scores and a high level of patient satisfaction. Ten of 11 patients had good to excellent results.

12. Duncan D, Mologne T, Hildebrand H, Stanley M, Schreckengaust R, Sitler D: The usefulness of magnetic resonance imaging in the diagnosis of anterolateral impingement of the ankle. *J Foot Ankle Surg* 2006;45:304-307.

    MRI findings were compared with surgical findings in patients with anterolateral ankle impingement. Sensitivity for the diagnosis ranged from 75% to 83%. The axial image was most useful in demonstrating the presence of anterolateral scar tissue.

13. Lee JW, Suh JS, Huh YM, Moon ES, Kim SJ: Soft tissue impingement syndrome of the ankle: Diagnostic efficacy of MRI and clinical results after arthroscopic treatment. *Foot Ankle Int* 2004;25:896-902.

    A specific MRI sequence, contrast-enhanced, fat-suppressed, three-dimensional, fast-gradient–recalled acquisition in the steady state with radiofrequency-spoiling MRI was used in the diagnosis of patients with suspected anterolateral ankle impingement. When compared with surgical findings, the sensitivity was 91.9% and the specificity was 84.4%.

14. Tol JL, van Dijk CN: Etiology of the anterior ankle impingement syndrome: A descriptive anatomical study. *Foot Ankle Int* 2004;25:382-386.

    The attachment point of the anterior ankle capsule was noted to be well proximal to the typical location of origin of anterior tibial osteophytes. The authors interpreted this finding as evidence against the traditional theory that anterior tibial osteophytes represent traction spurs from the capsular origin.

15. DiGiovanni BF, Fraga CJ, Cohen BE, Shereff MJ: Associated injuries found in chronic lateral ankle instability. *Foot Ankle Int* 2000;21:809-815.

16. Collman DR, Kaas MH, Schuberth JM: Arthroscopic ankle arthrodesis: Factors influencing union in 39 consecutive patients. *Foot Ankle Int* 2006;27:1079-1085.

    This retrospective study assessed 39 consecutive patients treated with arthroscopic ankle arthrodesis. Thirty-four of 39 patients achieved radiographic and clinical union. Poor bone quality and ankle deformity were identified as risk factors for nonunion. Smoking, diabetes mellitus, peripheral neuropathy, and other medical comorbidities or use of demineralized bone matrix or platelet-rich plasma during surgery did not influence union rates.

17. Ferkel RD, Hewitt M: Long-term results of arthroscopic ankle arthrodesis. *Foot Ankle Int* 2005;26:275-280.

    The authors report on 35 patients with end-stage ankle arthritis treated with arthroscopic ankle arthrodesis (average follow-up, 72 months). The overall fusion rate was 97% (34 of 35 patients). Average time to fusion was 11.8 weeks. No infections or neurovascular injuries were reported. Postoperative grading showed 74% and 83% good to excellent results using the Mazur and Morgan outcome scales, respectively. In three patients with delayed union, nonunion occurred in one patient.

18. Gougoulias NE, Agathangelidis FG, Parsons SW: Arthroscopic ankle arthrodesis. *Foot Ankle Int* 2007;28:695-706.

    A retrospective review of 78 consecutive in situ arthroscopic ankle fusions in 74 patients is presented. Forty-eight ankles had minor deformity (group A) whereas 30 ankles had varus/valgus deformities of greater that 15° (group B). Results show a fusion rate of 97.9% in group A versus 96.7% in group B. Acceptable ankle alignment in the frontal and sagittal plane was reported in both groups. Symptomatic arthritis from the adjacent joint developed in six ankles (7.7%). The outcome was graded as very good in 79.2% (38 feet) in group A and 80% (24 feet) in group B, fair in 18.8% (9 feet) in group A and 16.7% (5 feet) in group B, and poor in 1 ankle in each group ($P = 0.68$).

19. O'Brien TS, Hart TS, Shereff MJ, Stone J, Johnson J: Open versus arthroscopic ankle arthrodesis: A comparative study. *Foot Ankle Int* 1999;20:368-374.

20. Amendola A, Lee KB, Saltzman CL, Suh JS: Technique and early experience with posterior arthroscopic subtalar arthrodesis. *Foot Ankle Int* 2007;28:298-302.

Retrospective review of 10 patients (11 feet) treated with posterior arthroscopic subtalar arthrodesis. Patients were evaluated on level of satisfaction, American Orthopaedic Foot and Ankle Society scores, union rate, time to union, and postoperative complications. Eight patients were very satisfied with the procedure. American Orthopaedic Foot and Ankle Society scores improved from an average of 36 points preoperatively to 86 points on follow-up evaluation. Ten of 11 joints successfully fused and no postoperative complications were reported. The authors concluded that posterior arthroscopic subtalar arthrodesis provides excellent results with low rates of morbidity.

21. Willits K, Sonneveld H, Amendola A, Giffin JR, Griffin S, Fowler PJ: Outcome of posterior ankle arthroscopy for hindfoot impingement. *Arthroscopy* 2008;24:196-202.

Twenty-four posterior ankle arthroscopies for hindfoot impingement in 23 patients were evaluated at a mean follow-up of 32 months. Return to work occurred at a mean of 1 month and return to sports at a mean of 5.8 months. No permanent neurovascular complications occurred, although temporary numbness around the scar was evident in five patients.

22. Abramowitz Y, Wollstein R, Barzilay Y, et al: Outcome of resection of a symptomatic os trigonum. *J Bone Joint Surg Am* 2003;85:1051-1057.

Forty-one patients were treated with an open posterolateral approach for resection of a painful os trigonum. Complications developed in some patients including sural nerve sensory loss in eight patients, which proved permanent in four of these patients. Reflex sympathetic dystrophy occurred in another patient. The length of recovery was not documented.

23. Keeling JJ, Guyton GP: Endoscopic flexor hallucis longus decompression: A cadaver study. *Foot Ankle Int* 2007;28:810-814.

This cadaveric study evaluated the use of endoscopic FHL decompression. Three of eight FHL tendons were injured during attempted release. No FHL sheath was completely released. Posterolateral portal placement was, on average, only 6.1 mm from the lateral calcaneal branch of the sural nerve. In all instances, the medial calcaneal nerve and the first branch of the lateral plantar nerve were in close proximity to the FHL sheath. The authors concluded that endoscopic FHL release is technically demanding and has significant risks to local neurovascular structures.

24. Frey C, Feder KS, DiGiovanni C: Arthroscopic evaluation of the subtalar joint: Does sinus tarsi syndrome exist? *Foot Ankle Int* 1999;20:185-191.

25. Dellon AL, Barrett SL: Sinus tarsi denervation: Clinical results. *J Am Podiatr Med Assoc* 2005;95:108-113.

Thirteen patients with sinus tarsi syndrome were treated with sinus tarsi denervation. No arthroscopies were performed. Ten of 13 patients had complete relief of pain in this retrospective review. This small study represents the largest evaluation of denervation as an alternative approach to mechanical débridement of the sinus tarsi in patients with recalcitrant pain.

26. Phisitkul P, Tochigi Y, Saltzman CL, Amendola A: Arthroscopic visualization of the posterior subtalar joint in the prone position: A cadaver study. *Arthroscopy* 2006;22:511-515.

The authors performed a cadaver study of the available working area of the posterior facet of the subtalar joint. A nearly 50% increase in the available working area was achieved by adding the posteromedial portal to dorsal and ventral posterolateral portals. The authors advocated the use of the prone position because it allows easy use of the posteromedial portal.

27. Ortmann FW, McBryde AM: Endoscopic bony and soft-tissue decompression of the retrocalcaneal space for the treatment of Haglund deformity and retrocalcaneal bursitis. *Foot Ankle Int* 2007;28:149-153.

Thirty-two endoscopic retrocalcaneal débridements in 30 patients were reviewed at a mean follow-up of 35 months. The authors reported 1 poor, 3 good, and 26 excellent results. One Achilles tendon rupture occurred postoperatively and one procedure was treated with resurgery using an open procedure. The authors advocate the use of the procedure because it spares greater morbidity. This was the only study that reported Achilles rupture as a complication.

28. Davies MS, Saxby TS: Arthroscopy of the first metatarsophalangeal joint. *J Bone Joint Surg Br* 1999;81:203-206.

Chapter 5

Adolescent Foot and Ankle Conditions

Raymond J. Sullivan, MD

Accessory Navicular

Accessory navicular or os naviculae is present in 10% to 14% of normal feet and is usually asymptomatic. There are three types of accessory navicular.[1-3] Type I is present in approximately 30% of patients and is a small, oval ossicle that is separate from the navicular body and lies completely within the substance of the posterior tibial tendon. A type II accessory navicular is larger and has a distinct synchondrosis at the junction of the navicular tuberosity. The navicular insertion of the posterior tibial tendon attaches directly to the ossicle. Type III is fused directly to the navicular and the tuberosity is enlarged at the medial border.

Presentation

Children usually present with medial navicular tuberosity pain or irritation secondary to shoe wear. Most patients with type II accessory navicular are symptomatic secondary to chronic injury at the synchondrosis.[4,5] This condition is more common in girls than in boys (ratio, 5:1).[5,6] Patients usually become symptomatic in early adolescence, and approximately 50% have a pes planovalgus deformity at the time of presentation; however, an accessory navicular is not associated with the development of a flexible flatfoot.[7] Symptoms often increase secondary to activity and worsen over time. Patients with type II and III accessory navicular ossicles often have tenderness directly over the navicular synchondrosis or tuberosity and frequently have associated symptoms of insertional posterior tibial tendinitis.

Radiographic Evaluation

Radiographic evaluation consists of standing AP, external oblique, and lateral views (Figure 1). The addition of an internal oblique view can be helpful to visualize the accessory ossicle. Global alignment of the foot is assessed, including the presence of pes planus. Three-phase radionuclide bone scanning and MRI can be useful but usually are unnecessary. Bone scans typically show intense signal increase at the site of the accessory bone. MRI offers excellent imaging of the ossicle, synchondrosis interface, and posterior tibialis tendon. In most patients, the tendon appears normal whereas the

accessory ossicle may show intraosseous edema. Injury to the synchondrosis is indicated by fluid in the fibrous interface between the navicular and the ossicle.[8]

Nonsurgical Treatment

Initial treatment of a painful accessory navicular includes rest and the use of an over-the-counter orthotic arch support. Nonsteroidal anti-inflammatory medications also can be helpful. Patients with associated pes planovalgus deformity often have an associated gastrocnemius-soleus complex contracture. The initiation of a heel cord and gastrocnemius stretching program should be started when the patient is placed in orthotic arch supports so that excessive pronation and medial arch strain are avoided during weight bearing. If the patient remains symptomatic, the use of a walking cast or removable fracture boot for 4 to 6 weeks is indicated. Long-term treatment with over-the-counter arch supports and an Achilles tendon stretching program have shown success rates ranging from 20% to 50%.[1,4]

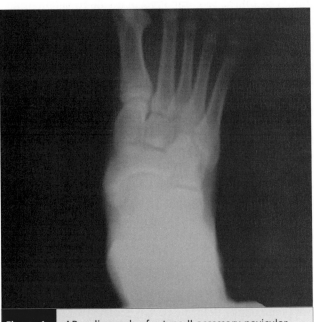

Figure 1   AP radiograph of a type II accessory navicular.

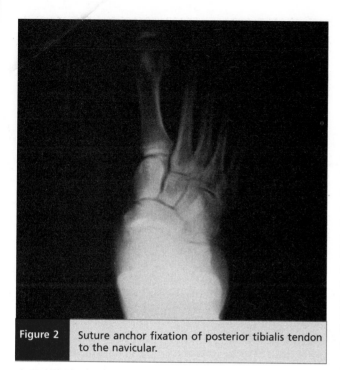

Figure 2 | Suture anchor fixation of posterior tibialis tendon to the navicular.

Surgical Treatment

If nonsurgical treatment is unsuccessful, the accessory navicular can be excised. The classic Kidner procedure consisted of excision of the accessory ossicle and advancement of the posterior tibial tendon to the medial cuneiform.[9] More recent literature has shown that the classic Kidner procedure offers no additional benefit compared with simple excision.[3,4,10,11] Most surgeons now prefer to use a modification of the original Kidner procedure.

Type I accessory navicular ossicles are excised through a longitudinal split in the posterior tibial tendon. The split is then repaired in a side-to-side manner with nonabsorbable sutures. Type II or III accessory navicular ossicles should be subperiosteally dissected from the posterior tibial tendon insertion. Additional excision of the remaining navicular tuberosity will ensure adequate decompression of the medial prominence. The talonavicular capsule must be preserved during the bony resection. The posterior tibial tendon insertion can be reattached to the residual navicular tuberosity using a suture anchor with nonabsorbable sutures (Figure 2).

Significant Achilles tendon contracture or gastrocnemius contracture should be treated at the time of surgery. Most patients have an isolated gastrocnemius contracture that can be released with a gastrocnemius recession through a posterior or medial longitudinal incision at the musculotendinous junction. Controversy exists regarding whether concomitant bony procedures, such as osteotomies, should be added to improve overall alignment of the foot. Patients with an associated pes planovalgus deformity may benefit from a medializing calcaneal osteotomy, lengthening osteotomy of the

anterior calcaneus, or implantation of a subtalar arthroereisis device. To date, there is no substantial evidence of improved outcomes in these patients compared with those treated by ossicle excision and tendon reattachment alone.

Tarsal Coalition

Tarsal coalition is an abnormal connection between the bones of the hindfoot or midfoot and is believed to result from failure of mesenchymal segmentation.[12] These connections can be fibrous, cartilaginous, or bony. An association between rigid pes planus in the presence of tarsal coalition has been described.[13] Classic studies have linked peroneal spastic flatfoot with talocalcaneal coalitions.[12,14] Calcaneonavicular and talocalcaneal coalitions, especially of the middle facet, are the most common types, with coalitions between other tarsal bones occurring less commonly. Fifty percent of coalitions are bilateral. Tarsal coalitions are autosomal dominant with variable penetrance.[15]

Presentation: Calcaneonavicular Coalition

Calcaneonavicular coalitions usually occur in children from 8 to 12 years of age and often are noted after acute ankle sprains. Patients report persistent lateral hindfoot pain and tenderness in the sinus tarsi. Hindfoot range of motion is usually limited, especially in patients with complete bony coalitions. Pes planovalgus deformity is typical and can have an associated contracture of the Achilles tendon or gastrocnemius muscle. On single-limb heel rise testing, the foot shows poor restoration of the medial longitudinal arch and persistence of hindfoot eversion. Patients often present with peroneal muscle spasms secondary to the pain.

Presentation: Talocalcaneal Coalition

Talocalcaneal coalitions usually occur in children age 12 to 16 years. Patients often present for treatment following minor trauma. Hindfoot range of motion is often more limited than in children with calcaneonavicular coalitions, and hindfoot valgus is often more severe. Patients rarely present with cavovarus deformity. Patients with talocalcaneal coalitions are more likely to have the classic finding of peroneal muscle spasms. The evaluation of a patient with peroneal spasms includes injection of an anesthetic agent into the sinus tarsi or common peroneal nerve for both diagnostic and potentially therapeutic purposes. Other causes of peroneal spastic flatfoot, including osteochondral lesions of the talus, inflammatory arthritis, infection, fracture, and tumor, must be ruled out.

Radiographic Evaluation

Initial radiographic evaluation includes standing AP, lateral, 45° internal oblique, and axial (Harris) views of the hindfoot. Talar beaking (dorsal osteophyte) at the talonavicular joint is often seen in either talocalcaneal

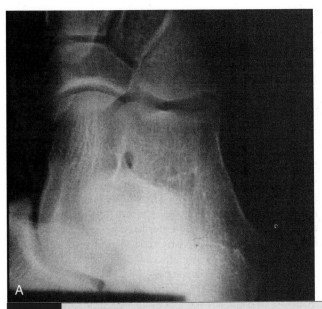

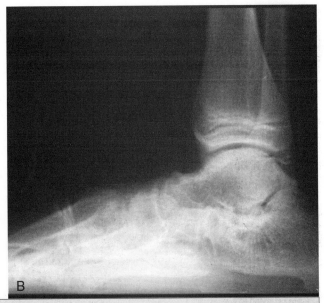

Figure 3 Oblique (**A**) and lateral (**B**) radiographs showing calcaneonavicular coalition and anteater's nose sign.

or calcaneonavicular coalitions and is not associated with true talonavicular arthritis.[16] A calcaneonavicular coalition is best seen on the 45° lateral oblique view. The lateral radiographic view also may indicate prominence of the anterior process of the calcaneus toward the navicular, the so-called anteater's nose sign (**Figure 3**). The talocalcaneal coalition is best seen on the axial view and less consistently on the lateral view. The axial (Harris) view shows irregularity and oblique orientation of the middle facet, whereas visualization of the subtalar joint is poorly defined on the lateral view because of valgus obliquity of the joint.

CT and MRI Evaluation
The difficulty in diagnosing tarsal coalitions, especially talocalcaneal coalitions, with plain radiographs has led to the increased use of CT and MRI. CT scans can be used to identify the presence and extent of the coalition, can differentiate between bony and fibrous coalitions, and are useful for evaluating the presence of arthritis or additional coalitions within other parts of the foot (**Figure 4**). MRI is the preferred modality for evaluating younger patients who are more likely to have fibrous coalitions because of incomplete ossification.[17]

Nonsurgical Treatment
Nonsurgical treatment is recommended for patients with any type of tarsal coalition. The presence of symptomatic peroneal spasms requires the use of casting and often anesthetic injections for spasm relief. Subsequent treatment with a University of California at Berkeley Laboratories orthotic arch support and an Achilles tendon stretching program can be initiated only after resolution of painful peroneal spasms. In the absence of peroneal spasms, a University of California at Berkeley Laboratories orthotic device rather than

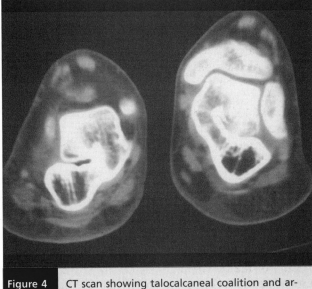

Figure 4 CT scan showing talocalcaneal coalition and arthrosis of the subtalar joint.

over-the-counter orthotic arch supports are often necessary to adequately control hindfoot eversion and achieve successful long-term results. Patients who present with severe symptoms should be treated with rest, restriction from sports activities, and temporary cast or boot brace immobilization. After symptoms subside, the patient can advance to the use of an orthotic device and slowly resume activities. An Achilles tendon and gastrocnemius stretching program is needed for patients with gastrocnemius-soleus complex contracture. Surgery for tarsal coalition is indicated when nonsurgical treatments fail, which typically occurs when symptoms are not relieved by initial treat-

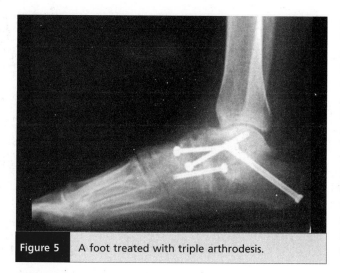

Figure 5   A foot treated with triple arthrodesis.

ment or when they recur as the patient ages and hindfoot stiffness worsens.

Surgical Treatment

Calcaneonavicular Coalition

Calcaneonavicular coalitions are excised through a longitudinal incision over the sinus tarsi. Adequacy of the excision is assessed both clinically and radiographically; the return of full hindfoot motion should be obtained intraoperatively. The extensor digitorum brevis (EDB) muscle belly and fascia can be advanced and interposed into the excision site. The use of suture anchors into the lateral aspect of the navicular makes the interposition easier and quite stable. Care must be taken not to injure the talonavicular joint and the talar head (specifically) during resection. Associated Achilles tendon contracture or gastrocnemius contracture should be treated at the time of surgical resection. Many authors have reported good to excellent results with calcaneonavicular coalition excision and EDB interposition.[16,18,19] Excision with EDB interposition has improved outcomes compared with excision alone. An increased recurrence of the coalition was reported when the EDB was not interposed.[20] Long-term results are somewhat less encouraging, with up to 25% of patients requiring subsequent surgical intervention.[21] Isolated gastrocnemius contractures can be treated with a gastrocnemius recession, whereas combined gastrocnemius and soleus contracture should be treated with percutaneous Achilles lengthening.[22,23]

Talocalcaneal Coalition

Talocalcaneal coalitions are excised through a medial approach between the flexor digitorum longus and flexor hallucis longus tendons. Care must be taken to avoid the medial plantar neurovascular bundle. It is crucial that the surgeon adequately resect the coalition, particularly from anterior to posterior. Good visualization of the posterior subtalar facet is necessary after removal of the coalition. Most surgeons interpose bone wax and local fat in the resected coalition site. Local fat

graft can be obtained anterior to the Achilles tendon. Good results have been reported.[24,25] Good short-term coalition resection results were reported at 5-year follow-up with resection of the sustentaculum and use of a flexor hallucis longus graft.[26] Similar results were reported in another study using flexor hallucis longus interposition without resection of the sustentaculum.[27] A 2003 study reported excellent results in 14 of 14 patients (100%) on short-term follow-up with the addition of an arthroereisis screw in the subtalar joint.[28] Many authors have reported poorer outcomes in talocalcaneal coalition excisions when more than 50% of the posterior facet is involved, which may require revision with subtalar or triple arthrodesis.[29-33] These finding do not seem to apply to anterior and middle facet coalitions.

Failed Tarsal Coalition Excisions

Patients who do not improve after tarsal coalition excision ideally should not be treated again until skeletal maturity is reached. A decision on surgical reconstruction with subtalar fusion or triple arthrodesis should be made based on the arthritic changes, hindfoot rigidity, and severity of planovalgus deformity. Triple arthrodesis is a more reliable salvage procedure than isolated subtalar arthrodesis[16,21,31-34] (Figure 5).

Flexible Pes Planovalgus Deformity

Pes planovalgus deformity (pediatric flexible flatfoot) is usually asymptomatic. By definition, the deformity is reducible at the level of the midfoot and hindfoot into neutral position. Children with this deformity often have an associated Achilles tendon or gastrocnemius contracture. Pes planus is present in approximately 10% to 20% of the adult population, whereas up to 80% of the pediatric population has a flexible flatfoot. Pes planus has been shown to decrease with age.[35] Flexible flatfoot is more common in patients with a tight Achilles tendon. In 1948, the differences among patients with flexible flatfoot with or without an Achilles tendon contracture were described.[36] Several authors have shown that muscle activity has minimal influence in the development or persistence of flexible flatfoot deformity.[37,38]

Presentation

Children with flexible flatfoot are often asymptomatic. They present for treatment with a supple deformity, with loss of the normal medial longitudinal arch and hindfoot valgus. The talar head is often palpable medially, secondary to navicular uncovering. Symptomatic children usually have an associated Achilles tendon or gastrocnemius contracture. On examination, the deformity is easily reducible at the midfoot and hindfoot. On heel rise, the arch is restored and the hindfoot inverts. The arch also is well restored on "Jack testing" by passive dorsiflexion of the first metatarsophalangeal

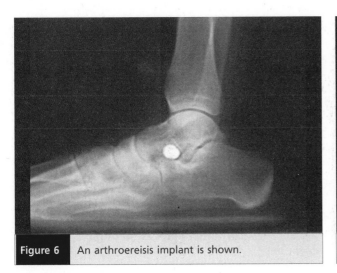

Figure 6   An arthroereisis implant is shown.

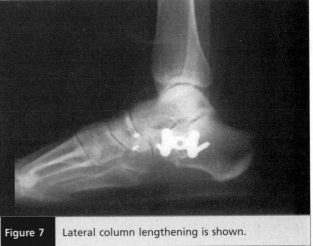

Figure 7   Lateral column lengthening is shown.

joint.[39] Symptomatic patients present with tenderness along the talonavicular joint or medial longitudinal arch in the region of the midsubstance of the plantar fascia. Younger patients often report night pain along the muscle groups of the medial compartment of the lower leg. In patients with more severe deformity, sinus tarsi pain can develop secondary to calcaneofibular abutment.

Radiographic Evaluation

Radiographic evaluation of patients with a flexible flatfoot deformity includes standing AP, 45° internal oblique, and lateral radiographs. Most other pathologies can be ruled out with standing AP ankle and axial hindfoot views. Patients with pes planovalgus will have an increased Meary (talar-first metatarsal) angle on the lateral radiograph. The weight-bearing AP view will show uncovering of the talar head by the navicular, which is subluxated laterally. Patients with an Achilles tendon or gastrocnemius contracture have a decreased calcaneal pitch.

Nonsurgical Treatment

Treatment of asymptomatic patients with flexible flatfoot deformity is not necessary. Counseling and educating the patient and parents on the benign nature of the condition is warranted. If the patient presents with an Achilles tendon or gastrocnemius contracture, initiation of an Achilles tendon stretching program may be useful; however, no long-term studies have proven such programs to be beneficial. The use of orthotic arch supports, braces, or corrective shoes in asymptomatic patients has not been shown to prevent pes planovalgus or assist in the development of a normal arch.[40-44]

A prescription orthotic arch support or scaphoid pad can be used for patients with a painful flexible flatfoot. Long-term studies have not shown clear benefits of using custom orthotics for this condition. Patients should be started on an Achilles tendon and gastrocnemius stretching program. Many patients will respond to nonsurgical treatment; however, no long-

term studies exist regarding outcomes of nonsurgical treatment.[45]

Surgical Treatment

Surgery should be considered for patients with persistent pain who had unsuccessful nonsurgical treatment. Historically, insertion of a polymeric silicone arthroereisis into the sinus tarsi was used with some initial short-term success.[46] Unfortunately, this procedure was complicated by significant foreign body reaction in the sinus tarsi.[47] This complication led to the development of metallic implants (**Figure 6**). Published results have shown improved short-term success with decreased foreign body reaction and sinus tarsi pain.[48,49] Complications, including the need for subsequent hardware removal, remain an issue. A 2007 study described a calcaneal-stop method with similar short-term results using a bone screw.[50] Complications included a high incidence of screw breakage. The surgeon also must assess the need for a concomitant gastrocnemius or Achilles tendon lengthening because patients often have an associated contracture. No long-term results have been published on either of these techniques. Patients who do not improve with subtalar arthroereisis can undergo revision with a lateral column calcaneal lengthening osteotomy after hardware removal.

Many authors have reported on a variety of procedures that include a variation of a limited naviculocuneiform Hoke fusion.[22,39,51] This procedure was further modified to include the talonavicular joint.[52] One long-term follow-up study on this procedure showed good results.[53] The drawbacks associated with permanent hindfoot fusion in a growing child has caused most surgeons to limit the use of these procedures.

As an alternative procedure, calcaneal osteotomy can avoid fusion in the growing child. A lateral column lengthening osteotomy (**Figure 7**) can be performed through a sinus tarsi incision from the tip of the fibula to the base of the metatarsals. Care must be taken to protect the peroneal tendons during the lateral dissection of the calcaneal wall. Using fluoroscopic guidance, a saw or osteotome is used to perform a lateral to medial calcaneal osteotomy starting in the Gissane angle and angling medially between the anterior and middle facets of the subtalar joint. The medial wall can be left intact and a laminar spreader is used to distract the osteotomy. An 8-mm to 10-mm wedge-shaped bone graft is then inserted, using autologous or allograft bone. Graft placement and foot positioning is crucial to correct both midfoot abduction and any residual supination. Compression screws or lateral plating are used for fixation. Excessive dorsal graft within the sinus tarsi must be trimmed to prevent impingement. No studies are available to show a clear superiority of autograft over allograft. One study reported very good results in 45 patients using isolated lateral column lengthening.[45] Although there are many reports on these procedures for adult patients, no long-term results are available for the pediatric population. In patients with severe deformity and weak inversion, a talonavicular capsulotomy, spring ligament repair, and flexor digitorum longus transfer can be added to improve deformity correction and inversion strength.

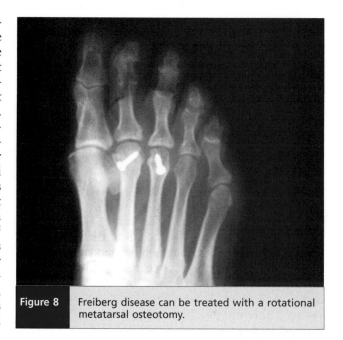

Figure 8 Freiberg disease can be treated with a rotational metatarsal osteotomy.

Osteochondrosis

Sever Disease

Sever disease (calcaneal apophysitis) occurs in children age 9 to 12 years. It was first described by Sever in 1912, who noted radiographic changes and pain at the calcaneal apophysis in children.[54] Symptomatic children usually report pain during activities and often have an associated Achilles tendon or gastrocnemius contracture. Patients have isolated tenderness at the calcaneal apophysis that is believed to be caused by tension from the heel cord. There is some evidence that Sever symptoms may represent a stress fracture at the calcaneal apophysis. Evaluation with plain radiographs usually shows no abnormalities.[55] Imaging with radionuclide bone scanning or MRI are usually unnecessary.

Symptomatic children are treated with activity modifications, including relative rest and restricted participation in sports activities. Other treatment modalities include the use of felt or silicone heel wedges, icing, nonsteroidal anti-inflammatory medications at an appropriate dosage, and an Achilles tendon stretching program.[56] Patients with severe or recalcitrant symptoms may require a brief period of immobilization in a cast or fracture boot. Sever disease is a self-limiting condition and surgery is rarely indicated. Patients will have resolution of symptoms when the calcaneal apophysis fuses, which relieves tension on the apophysis. Successful treatment includes education of the patient and parents to provide realistic expectations on the course of this benign but frustrating condition.

Köhler Disease

Köhler[57] first described the radiographic findings of navicular osteonecrosis in symptomatic children in 1908. The etiology remains unclear. The condition is more common in boys than girls. Patients have tenderness and swelling over the navicular and walk with an antalgic gait. Treatment is based on the severity of symptoms. In patients with mild symptoms, the use of soft arch supports, rest, and activity modifications is an effective treatment. Many patients require the use of a walking cast for 6 to 8 weeks for full resolution of symptoms, with all patients showing radiographic resolution by 8 months.[58]

Freiberg Infraction

In 1924, Freiberg[59] described the radiographic changes seen in the second metatarsal head in symptomatic young women. These changes include sclerosis, metatarsal head flattening, and enlargement of the second metatarsal head. Any of the metatarsal heads can be involved, but the second metatarsal head is the most commonly affected. Freiberg infraction occurs more commonly in athletic adolescent girls than in boys. Various etiologies have been described, including trauma, vascular insult to the metatarsal head, and stress fractures. Patients present with swelling and tenderness over the affected joint.

Initial treatment consists of activity modification, nonsteroidal anti-inflammatory medications, and off-loading with soft shoe inserts. Patients with severe symptoms may benefit from a short period of cast immobilization. Spontaneous repair and reconstitution of the metatarsal head may take up to 2 years. If nonsurgical treatment fails, surgical débridement of the metatarsophalangeal joint may be necessary. Synovitis, loose bodies, and osteophytes should be excised and necrotic bone débrided. In patients with significant metatarsal head enlargement, resurfacing of the metatarsophalangeal joint improves motion and relieves impingement. A dorsal wedge osteotomy of the metatarsal neck has been described to bring the normal plantar cartilaginous surface into an articulating position[60] (Figure 8). Better outcomes have been reported with improved fixation of metatarsal osteotomies.[61,62] Complete metatarsal head resection should be avoided because of resultant joint instability, continued pain, and transfer metatarsalgia. More information on Freiberg infraction is available in chapter 21.

Summary

Adolescent foot and ankle conditions are often self limiting and respond well to nonsurgical treatment. Arch supports, heel wedges, and Achilles tendon stretching programs are often the keys to successful nonsurgical management. Surgical treatment for selected conditions can be challenging. Fixed deformity and arthritis can be salvaged after the child's growth plates have been fused with arthrodesis.

Annotated References

1. Geist E: The accessory scaphoid bone. *J Bone Joint Surg* 1925;7:570-574.

2. Chen YJ, Hsu RW, Liang SC: Degeneration of the accessory navicular synchondrosis presenting as rupture of the posterior tibial tendon. *J Bone Joint Surg Am* 1997;79:1791-1798.

3. Sella EJ, Lawson JP, Ogden JA: The accessory navicular synchondrosis. *Clin Orthop Relat Res* 1986;209:280-285.

4. Grogan DP, Gasser SI, Ogden JA: The painful accessory navicular: A clinical and histopathological study. *Foot Ankle* 1989;10:164-169.

5. Lawson JP, Ogden JA, Sella E, Barwick KW: The painful accessory navicular. *Skeletal Radiol* 1984;12:250-262.

6. Mygind HB: The accessory tarsal scaphoid: Clinical features and treatment. *Acta Orthop Scand* 1953;23:142-151.

7. Sullivan JA, Miller WA: The relationship of the accessory navicular to the development of the flat foot. *Clin Orthop Relat Res* 1979;144:233-237.

8. Sizensky JA, Marks RM: Imaging of the navicular. *Foot Ankle Clin* 2004;9:181-209.

   A concise review of the use of different imaging techniques in the diagnosis of navicular abnormalities is presented. The authors discuss specific signal changes seen on MRI scans in patients with symptomatic accessory navicular.

9. Kidner FC: The pre-hallux (accessory scaphoid) in its relation to flat-foot. *J Bone Joint Surg* 1929;11:831-837.

10. Sullivan JA, Miller WA: The relationship of the accessory navicular to the development of the flat foot. *Clin Orthop Relat Res* 1979;144:233-237.

11. Macnicol MF, Voutsinas S: Surgical treatment of the symptomatic accessory navicular. *J Bone Joint Surg Br* 1984;66:218-226.

12. Harris B: Anomalous structure in the developing human foot. *Anat Rec* 1995;121:399.

13. Slomann HC: On coalition calcaneo-navicularis. *J Orthop Surg (Hong Kong)* 1921;3:586-602.

14. Harris RI, Beath T: Etiology of peroneal spastic flat foot. *J Bone Joint Surg Br* 1948;30:624-634.

15. Leonard MA: The inheritance of tarsal coalition and its relationship to spastic flat foot. *J Bone Joint Surg Br* 1974;56:520-526.

16. Swiontkowski MF, Scranton PE, Hansen S: Tarsal coalitions: Long-term results of surgical treatment. *J Pediatr Orthop* 1983;3:287-292.

17. Thometz J: Tarsal coalition. *Foot Ankle Clin* 2000;5:103-118.

18. Andreasen E: Calcaneo-navicular coalition: Late results of resection. *Acta Orthop Scand* 1968;39:424-432.

19. Gonzalez P, Kumar SJ: Calcaneonavicular coalition treated by resection and interposition of the extensor digitorum brevis muscle. *J Bone Joint Surg Am* 1990;72:71-77.

20. Moyes ST, Crawfurd E, Aichroth PM: The interposition of extensor digitorum brevis in the resection of calcaneonavicular bars. *J Pediatr Orthop* 1994;14:387-388.

21. Inglis G, Buxton RA, Macnicol MF: Symptomatic calcaneonavicular bars, the results 20 years after surgical excision. *J Bone Joint Surg Br* 1986;68:128-131.

22. Hoke M: An operation for the correction of extremely relaxed flatfeet. *J Bone Joint Surg* 1931;13:773-783.

23. DiGiovanni CW, Langer P: The role of isolated gastrocnemius and combined Achilles contractures in the flat foot. *Foot Ankle Clin* 2007;12:363-379.

   The authors review the association between gastrocnemius or Achilles contractures and the development of pes planus. The authors stress the importance of addressing the contracture surgically at the time of the flatfoot reconstruction procedure. The authors outline their procedure of choice.

24. McCormack TJ, Olney B, Asher M: Talocalcaneal coalition resection: A 10-year follow-up. *J Pediatr Orthop* 1997;17:13-15.

25. Olney BW, Asher MA: Excision of symptomatic coalition of the middle facet of the talocalcaneal joint. *J Bone Joint Surg Am* 1987;69:539-544.

26. Westberry DE, Davids JR, Oros W: Surgical management of symptomatic talocalcaneal coalition by resection of the sustentaculum tali. *J Pediatr Orthop* 2003; 23:493-497.

    Good to excellent results were reported in 11 of 12 patients after resection of the talocalcaneal coalition with additional resection of the sustentaculum tali. The mean patient age was 13 years at the time of the resection and the mean follow-up period was 5 years.

27. Raikin S, Cooperman DR, Thompson GH: Interposition of the split flexor hallucis longus tendon after resection of a coalition of the middle facet of the talocalcaneal joint. *J Bone Joint Surg Am* 1999;81:11-19.

28. Giannini S, Ceccarelli F, Vannini F, Baldi E: Operative treatment of flatfoot with talocalcaneal coalition. *Clin Orthop Relat Res* 2003;411:178-187.

    The authors present 2- to 4-year follow-up results for 14 patients treated with tarsal coalition excision and the addition of a subtalar arthroereisis implant. All patients showed significant clinical improvement.

29. Comfort TK, Johnson LO: Resection for symptomatic talocalcaneal coalition. *J Pediatr Orthop* 1998;18:283-288.

30. Ehrlich MG, Elmer EB: Tarsal coalition, in Jahs M (ed): *Disorders of the Foot and Ankle*, ed 2. Philadelphia, PA, WB Saunders, 1991, pp 921-928.

31. Luhmann SJ, Schoenecker PL: Symptomatic talocalcaneal coalition resection: Indications and results. *J Pediatr Orthop* 1998;18:748-754.

32. Wilde PH, Torode IP, Dickens DR, Cole WG: Resection for symptomatic talocalcaneal coalition. *J Bone Joint Surg Br* 1994;76:797-801.

33. Cohen BE, Davis WH, Anderson RB: Success of calcaneonavicular coalition resection in the adult population. *Foot Ankle Int* 1996;17:569-572.

34. Mosier KM, Asher M: Tarsal coalitions and peroneal spastic flatfoot: A review. *J Bone Joint Surg Am* 1984; 66:976-984.

35. Staheli LT, Chew DE, Corbett M: The longitudinal arch: A survey of eight hundred and eighty-two feet in normal children and adults. *J Bone Joint Surg Am* 1987; 69:426-428.

36. Harris RI, Beath T: Hypermobile flat-foot with short tendo Achillis. *J Bone Joint Surg Am* 1948;30:116-138.

37. Basmajian JV, Stecko G: The role of muscles in arch supports of the foot. *J Bone Joint Surg Am* 1963;45: 1184-1190.

38. Mann R, Inman VT: Phasic activity of intrinsic muscles of the foot. *J Bone Joint Surg Am* 1964;46:469-481.

39. Jack EA: Naviculo-cuneiform fusion in the treatment of flat foot. *J Bone Joint Surg Br* 1953;35:75-82.

40. Sim-Fook L, Hodgson AR: A comparison of foot forms among the non-shoe and shoe wearing Chinese population. *J Bone Joint Surg Am* 1958;40:1058-1062.

41. Staheli LT, Griffin L: Corrective shoes for children: A survey of current practice. *Pediatrics* 1980;65:13-17.

42. Wenger DR, Mauldin D, Speck G, Morgan D, Lieber RL: Corrective shoes and inserts as treatment for flexible flatfoot in infants and children. *J Bone Joint Surg Am* 1989;71:800-810.

43. Gould N, Moreland M, Alvarez R, Trevino S, Fenwick J: Development of the child's arch. *Foot Ankle* 1989;9: 241-245.

44. Penneau K, Lutter LD, Winter RD: Pes planus: Radiographic changes with foot orthoses and shoes. *Foot Ankle* 1982;2:299-303.

45. Mosca VS: Flexible flatfoot and skewfoot, in Drennan JC (ed): *The Child's Foot and Ankle*. New York, NY, Raven Press, 1992, pp 335-376.

46. Viladot A: Surgical treatment of the child's flat foot. *Clin Orthop Relat Res* 1992;283:34-38.

47. Smith SD, Millar EA: Arthrorisis by means of a subtalar polyethylene peg implant for correction of hindfoot pronation in children. *Clin Orthop Relat Res* 1983;181:15-23.

48. Giannini BS, Ceccarelli F, Benedetti MG, Catani F, Faldini C: Surgical treatment of flexible flatfoot in children: A four-year follow-up study. *J Bone Joint Surg Am* 2001;83(suppl 2):73-79.

49. Needleman RL: A surgical approach for flexible flatfeet in adults including a subtalar arthroereisis with the MBA sinus tarsi implant. *Foot Ankle Int* 2006;27:9-18.

    The author reports on 23 patients with flexible flatfoot who had correction with subtalar arthroereisis and were followed for a mean of 44 months. The average American Orthopaedic Foot and Ankle Society score improved from 52 to 87. Radiographic correction was significant in all patients and persisted after implant removal. Forty-six percent of patients reported sinus tarsi pain, but most had symptom improvement after implant removal.

50. Roth S, Sestan B, Tudor A, Ostojic A, Sasso A, Durbesic A: Minimally invasive calcaneo-stop method for idio-

pathic, flexible pes planovalgus in children. *Foot Ankle Int* 2007;28:991-995.

Ninety-four minimally invasive calcaneo-stop procedures were performed in 48 children (age, 8 to 14 years). Significant radiographic improvements occurred in all the children. Hardware was removed in all patients. At 5-year follow-up, 91 feet maintained the correction.

51. Butte FL: Navicular-cuneiform arthrodesis for flatfoot: An end-result study. *J Bone Joint Surg* 1937;19:496-502.

52. Miller GR: The operative treatment of hypermobile flatfeet in the young child. *Clin Orthop Relat Res* 1977;122:95-101.

53. Giannestrus NJ: Flexible valgus flatfoot resulting from naviculocuneiform and talonavicular sag: Surgical correction in the adolescent, in Bateman JE (ed): *Foot Science*. Philadelphia, PA, WB Saunders, 1976, pp 67-105.

54. Sever JW: Apophysitis of the os calsis. *NY Med J* 1912;95:1025.

55. Volpon JB, de Carvalo Filho G: Calcaneal apophysitis: A quantitative radiographic evaluation of the secondary ossification center. *Arch Orthop Trauma Surg* 2002;122:338-341.

56. Micheli LJ, Ireland ML: Prevention and management of calcaneal apophysitis in children: An overuse syndrome. *J Pediatr Orthop* 1987;7:34-38.

57. Kohler A: Ueber eine haufige bisher anscheinend unbekannte Erkrankung einzelner Kinklicherkernochen . *Munchen Med Wochnscbr* 1908;55:1923.

58. Ippolito E, Ricciardi Pollini PT, Falez F: Kohler's disease of the tarsal navicular: Long-term follow up of 12 cases. *J Pediatr Orthop* 1984;4:416-417.

59. Freiberg AH: Infraction of the second metatarsal bone: A typical injury . *Surg Gynecol Obstet* 1914;19:191.

60. Gauthier G, Elbaz R: Freiberg's infraction: A subchondral bone fatigue fracture. A new surgical treatment. *Clin Orthop Relat Res* 1979;142:93-95.

61. Katcherian DA: Treatment of Freiberg's disease. *Orthop Clin North Am* 1994;25:69-81.

62. Chao KH, Lee CH, Lin LC: Surgery for symptomatic Freiberg's disease: Extraarticular dorsal closing-wedge osteotomy in 13 patients followed for 2-4 years. *Acta Orthop Scand* 1999;70:483-486.

1: General Foot and Ankle Topics

Foot and Ankle Trauma

SECTION EDITORS:

JOHN S. EARLY, MD

STANLEY C. GRAVES, MD

Chapter 6

Fractures of the Ankle

Michael D. Castro, DO   James P. Maurer, DO

Introduction

Fractures of the ankle are among the most common orthopaedic injuries and can occur as a result of the application of a purely rotational force or a milieu of rotational, translational, and axial forces. Ankle fractures resulting from low-energy, twisting injuries have few or no long-term sequelae. High-energy ankle injuries, such as those caused by a fall from a height or a motor vehicle crash, commonly cause debilitating injuries and frequently are associated with the need for revision surgery. The goal of treatment is to optimize the patient's short- and long-term functional outcomes. This goal is most consistently achieved by anatomic reduction of articular surfaces, restoring metaphyseal stability, preserving the blood supply, and allowing early motion. The treatment strategy requires a complete understanding of the extent of injury to both the bone and soft tissue and is achieved by obtaining a thorough patient history, performing a careful physical examination, and obtaining appropriate imaging studies. The age, physical condition, demands, and lifestyle of the patient should be evaluated in terms of the risks and benefits of the proposed treatment.

Biomechanics

The ankle is a complex joint made up of the talus set in a mortise composed of the distal tibia and fibula. The sagittal plane motion consists of rotation and translation about a transient axis. The joint is stabilized by the tibiofibular, deltoid, and collateral ligaments, which primarily function to regulate coupled motion occurring among the mortise, talus, hindfoot, and midfoot. The talus is classically referred to as a truncated cone. The tibia rotates and translates anteriorly and posteriorly over the talus during dorsiflexion and plantar flexion, respectively. The articular surfaces of the distal tibia and talus are not completely congruent and the contact area, location, and size change with ankle joint position. The medial and lateral margins differ in their radii of curvature, with the medial side made up of two different radii, whereas the lateral side is constant and larger than the medial side. This unique architecture allows internal rotation of the tibia from plantar flexion through dorsiflexion. The tibiotalar articular surface is widened anteriorly

and tapers posteriorly. As the wider portion of the talus engages the ankle mortise, external rotation of the fibula occurs, tensioning the anterior talofibular ligament. This action, along with the deltoid ligament, allows stable, consistent tracking of the talus within the mortise.

The ankle joint is efficient at withstanding axial and shear forces. It appears to be resistant to primary osteoarthritis. Injury resulting from impact and/or displacement of the articular surface and compromise of the regulating soft tissues leads to alteration in mechanics and degeneration of the articular surfaces.[1,2] Given the complexity of the hindfoot joints, the goals of surgical treatment should focus on restoration of the articular surfaces and overall alignment.

Malleoli Fractures

Infrasyndesmotic Fractures

Infrasyndesmotic injuries generally occur with the forefoot in supination, causing an avulsion fracture of the distal fibula. Isolated lateral malleolar fractures at this level are stable and can be treated with a stirrup and early functional rehabilitation.

The overall stability of this fracture pattern is based on injury to the medial side of the joint. Medial displacement of the talus causes an oblique or vertical fracture of the medial malleolus. In a retrospective review, 42% of the vertical medial malleolar fracture patterns involved marginal impaction of the plafond.[3] Anatomic reduction can be performed through an anteromedial approach. If marginal impaction is present, the cartilage must be elevated to restore the joint surface; bone grafting is performed if the defect is sufficiently large. Fixation of the medial malleolus can be performed with two screws placed through the fragment that is oriented perpendicular to the joint or by using a one third tubular plate as a buttress.

Transsyndesmotic Fractures

Transsyndesmotic fractures account for 40% to 75% of malleolar fractures. These injuries involve a fracture of the fibula starting at the level of the plafond and propagating from an anteroinferior to a posterosuperior direction along the fibular shaft. This type of injury occurs when the forefoot is in supination and there is a subsequent external rotation (SER) force.

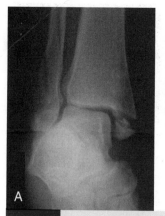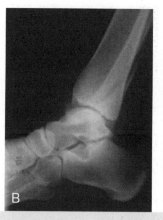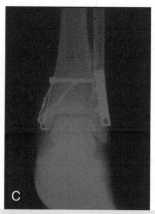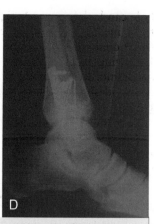

Figure 1 Mortise **(A)** and lateral **(B)** radiographic views showing an AO/OTA 44-B2 fracture. Postoperative AP **(C)** and lateral **(D)** radiographs show antiglide fixation of the fibula and tension band fixation medially. The inherent stability of this construct allows early range of motion.

Treatment of these fractures is based on the stability of the talus within the ankle mortise. Lateral shift of the talus causes a decrease in the tibiotalar contact area and a subsequent increase in contact pressure at the talar dome. One study showed that 1 mm of lateral displacement of the talus caused a 42% decrease in contact area of the tibiotalar joint.[4]

Closed treatment of isolated lateral malleolus fractures (AO/Orthopaedic Trauma Association [OTA] classification 44-B1, SER-II with cast or brace immobilization and early weight bearing has traditionally produced acceptable results in low-demand patients or those who are poor candidates for surgery. Acceptable fibular shortening of up to 5 mm and a talocrural angle within 2° to 5° of the opposite side is considered acceptable displacement for the isolated lateral malleolus fractures. However, these injuries often result in rotation of the distal fragment and loss of fibular length. Because of the potential for degenerative changes and low morbidity, surgical treatment of these fractures should be considered.

Medial malleolus fracture or deltoid ligament incompetence make SER fractures unstable and are best treated with surgery (**Figure 1**). Determination of whether an injury is an AO/OTA 44-B1 fracture or whether medial injury is involved (AO/OTA 44-B2 or 44-B3 fracture) is key to selecting the appropriate treatment. In radiographs showing an apparent isolated lateral malleolus fracture, determination of the competence of the deltoid ligament is necessary to appropriately treat SER ankle fractures. Recently, the tenet of medial-sided ecchymosis and pain on examination as evidence of deep deltoid ligament rupture has been questioned. Medial-sided tenderness is a poor indicator of deep deltoid ligament rupture as proven by external rotation stressing of a transsyndesmotic fracture.[5] Medial-sided tenderness was found to be 57% specific and 59% sensitive for deep deltoid ligament rupture. Manual and gravity external rotation testing are good indicators of deltoid ligament competence. Both tests are generally well tolerated by the patient.

Medial widening of clear space of greater than 4 mm is considered a positive test.[6,7]

Management of AO/OTA 44-B1 Fractures

Multiple options exist for the treatment of AO/OTA type B lateral malleolus fractures. The goal of treatment is anatomic reduction with restoration of fibular length. Traditional fixation uses an anterior to posterior lag screw followed by a lateral neutralization plate. Drawbacks to this technique include prominent hardware, dependence on distal unicortical screws for fixation, and the possibility of intra-articular hardware.

In one study of patients younger than 50 years of age, fixation of oblique lateral malleolus fractures using only lag screws was shown to be efficacious when used for the proper fracture.[8] Fractures amenable to this fixation have no comminution and are long enough to accept two lag screws placed 1 cm apart. There was no loss of reduction, prominent hardware, or nonunions in the study.

Fixation with antiglide plating offers advantages over traditional plating. The soft-tissue coverage avoids skin irritation and sensitivity to cold and there is little risk of the screws violating the tibiofibular joint. The anterior cortex is denser, offering better screw purchase and a stronger biomechanical construct. The main drawback of this technique is the possibility of peroneal tendinitis. This complication can be avoided if proper technique is used. The distal end of the implant should extend no farther distally than the apex of the posterior tubercle. A five-hole, one-third, tubular plate fixator (Synthes, Paoli, PA) provides versatile placement because of the screw hole spacing (**Figure 2**). The first screw can be placed in the proximal fragment as close to the fracture line as possible. This placement decreases the moment arm, reduces the chance of plate deformation, and provides a more rigid construct. A second screw can be placed in the most proximal hole. A posterior to anterior lag screw can be placed through the plate in the third screw hole. The most distal screw hole can be left open. Antiglide plating has been shown to be mechanically stronger than lateral plating with a traditional or locking plate and lag screw construct.[9,10] Following fixation of the fibula, the integrity of the syndesmotic constraints should be tested. Disruption of the syndesmosis is not uncommon with this fracture pattern.[11] If necessary, the syndesmosis is stabilized with screw fixation through a neutralization plate or anterior to an antiglide plate. When fixing the syndesmosis in conjunction with an antiglide plate, the syndesmosis screws should be placed through the proximal fragment or both the proximal and distal fragments (Figure 3). Displacement of the fracture may occur when attempting to stabilize the syndesmosis through the distal fragment alone.

Management of AO/OTA 44-B2 Fractures

The deltoid ligament has a superficial and deep portion. The superficial portion of the ligament arises from the anterior colliculus of the medial malleolus and has a broad attachment on the talus and navicular. The deep portion of the ligament arises from the posterior colliculus of the medial malleolus and inserts onto the talus. The deep portion of the ligament provides the greatest resistance to external rotation of the talus. It was demonstrated that fractures of the anterior colliculus could be associated with deep deltoid ligament avulsions off the posterior colliculus.[12] Medial-sided incompetence can persist despite fracture fixation, secondary to the complex anatomy of the deltoid ligament.

In bimalleolar equivalent fractures, the medial injury is a tear or avulsion of the deltoid ligament. Repair of the lateral malleolus alone should provide adequate stability for deltoid ligament healing, provided that the syndesmosis is intact. The medial side of the joint should only be approached if part of the deltoid ligament is blocking anatomic reduction of the joint. Acute repair of the deltoid ligament is unnecessary; however, initial postoperative immobilization in neutral to slight dorsiflexion (a position of inherent stability) will maintain reduction of the talus in the mortise. This will close down the medial gutter and preclude thickening of the scarring ligament.

Fractures of the medial malleolus should be repaired by anatomic reduction and internal fixation and can be approached through an anteromedial approach. Large fracture fragments can be fixed with two cancellous screws. A partially threaded screw must be of sufficient length that all screw threads pass the fracture line, yet short enough that the threads purchase the denser metaphyseal bone surrounding the subchondral region. Lag fixation with fully threaded screws may avoid potential complications.

Tension-band fixation of a medial malleolar fracture has been shown to be efficacious. The technique may be most beneficial in small or comminuted medial malleolar fractures. The tension-band construct is four times stiffer than two cancellous screws.[13] This technique is beneficial when the subchondral bone is com-

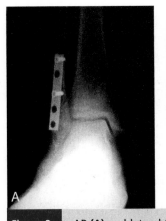
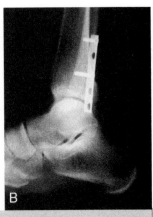

Figure 2 AP **(A)** and lateral **(B)** radiographic views of an AO/OTA 44-B1 fracture stabilized with a five-hole one-third tubular plate in antiglide fashion. The five-hole plate provides versatility because of the screw-hole spacing. The three regularly spaced holes allow for antiglide screw placement immediately proximal to the fracture line without the plate extending beyond the apex of the fibular tubercle. This placement reduces the risk of irritation of the peroneal tendons. In isolated lateral injuries, weight bearing begins 2 weeks after surgery in a stirrup support.

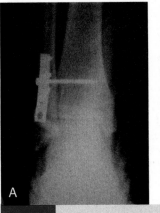
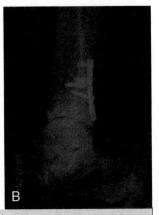

Figure 3 AP **(A)** and lateral **(B)** radiographic views of an AO/OTA 44-B2 fracture with involvement of the distal syndesmosis as demonstrated by intraoperative testing. The fracture was stabilized with antiglide fixation and the syndesmosis with a 3.5-mm fully threaded cortical screw placed anterior to the plate through the proximal fragment.

minuted. In such instances, lag screw fixation may cause a valgus deformity of the malleolus. Tension-band fixation allows anatomic alignment without compromising compression at the fracture.

Placement of hardware in the medial malleolus can injure the posterior tibial tendon. In a cadaver study, hardware placed at or posterior to the intracollicular groove placed the posterior tibial tendon at risk.[14] The anterior colliculus was a safe zone.

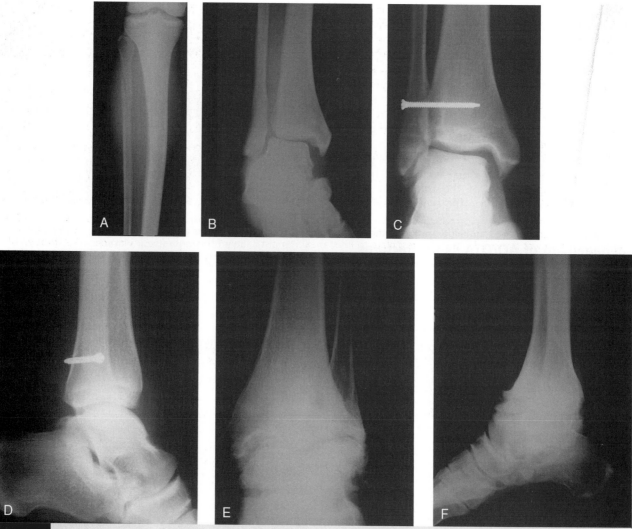

Figure 4 AP radiograph of a tibia/fibula injury showing an oblique fracture of the proximal fibula **(A)** associated with widening of the ankle mortise **(B)**. AP **(C)** and lateral **(D)** radiographic views of single screw fixation that left the syndesmosis malreduced. Weight bearing began after hardware was removed 5 weeks after placement. AP **(E)** and lateral **(F)** radiographic views obtained 18 years after the injury, showing end-stage degenerative changes to the ankle joint.

Injuries Involving the Syndesmosis

External rotation of the ankle joint with the foot in a pronated position will subject the fibula to external torque, which results in disruption of the tibiofibular (anteriorly and, depending on the impulse, posteriorly) and interosseous ligaments. This disruption is accompanied by a medial injury, either bony or ligamentous (AO/OTA 44-C fracture). The fibula may be fractured within 8 to 10 cm of the ankle joint or at the proximal neck. Transverse fractures of the medial malleolus or widening of the medial clear space that suggest a deltoid injury with an otherwise intact fibula should arouse suspicion of a fracture of the proximal fibula. These injuries require meticulous attention to the restoration of length and rotation of the fibula and stabilization of the syndesmosis.

A fracture involving the distal one third of the fibula should be reduced and stabilized with rigid internal fix-

ation using anterior to posterior interfragmentary compression and neutralization plating. The syndesmosis then can be stabilized by a screw or screws placed through the plate and directed along the transmalleolar axis. The benefit of using a lateral plate is the distribution of force distal to the screw, which is ideally placed proximal to the articular surfaces of the syndesmosis (1.5 to 2 cm proximal to the ankle mortise). More proximal fractures of the fibula associated with disruption of the distal syndesmosis (Maisonneuve fractures) may not require internal fixation of the fracture; however, care should be taken to restore length and rotation of the fibula before fixation of the syndesmosis. Loss of fibular length and lateral buttress of the talus can result in traumatic arthritis in much the same manner as a widened syndesmosis (**Figure 4**). A limited approach allowing reduction and provisional fixation

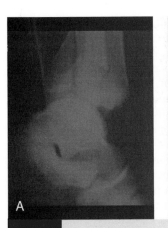 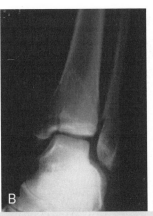 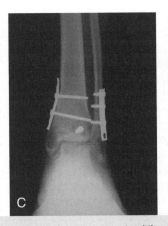 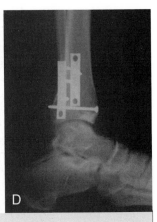

Figure 5 AP **(A)** and mortise **(B)** radiographic views of an AO/OTA 44-B3 fracture. Mortise **(C)** and lateral **(D)** postoperative radiographs show antiglide fixation of the fibula and lag screw fixation of the Volkmann fragment. The medial fracture was stabilized with a buttress plate to resist shear. No instability of the syndesmosis was seen after fixation of the fractures.

with bone-holding forceps may be necessary to restore length and correct rotation.

Techniques used to stabilize the syndesmosis vary widely. The number and size of the screws used, the number of cortices engaged, and whether the hardware is removed or allowed to break are some controversial issues regarding this procedure. The principle is to provide fixation adequate to maintain the fibula in a reduced position and restrict weight bearing until the soft tissues heal. If necessary, a reliable technique is to reduce the syndesmosis using fluoroscopic imaging to compare the contralateral side. If a neutralization plate is used to stabilize the fracture, a 4.0-mm solid screw is placed along the transmalleolar axis immediately proximal to the articular surface of the syndesmosis. The screw is used with a washer and is placed anterior to the lateral edge of the plate if used in conjunction with antiglide fixation. When stabilizing the syndesmosis without associated fracture fixation, two screws placed through a four-hole plate provide rigid fixation of the otherwise unstable distal fragment. Four cortices are engaged and the screw length is sufficient to allow the screw tip to be proud on the medial side so the shank can be removed if the screw breaks. Alternatively, a plate may be used to distribute the stress applied by the screws. Use of a plate will allow screw fixation slightly more proximal to the ideal position. This fixation may be beneficial in revision surgery or in injuries that compromise the fibular cortex. Weight bearing is determined by fracture healing (6 to 8 weeks). Fixation is removed at approximately 16 weeks, allowing the fibula to externally rotate during ankle dorsiflexion.

Outcomes after surgical fixation of ankle fractures are generally good. However, some subgroups of patients have a worse prognosis. In a 2007 study, the authors found functional outcomes at 1 year after surgery were worse in patients with bimalleolar ankle fracture when compared with outcomes in those with bimalle-

olar equivalent fractures.[15] In a prospective observational study, factors including the presence of a medial malleolar fracture, patient smoking, and those with a lower educational level were predictive of poor functional ability at 3 months after surgery.[16]

Posterior Malleolus Fractures (AO/OTA 44-B3 Fractures)

Fracture of the posterior malleolus can be caused by direct impact from the talus or more commonly as avulsion fracture caused by the posteroinferior tibiofibular ligament. A recent study used CT to examine the morphology of posterior malleolus fractures.[17] Most fractures consisted of a large posterolateral fragment. A subset of fractures extended from the posterior malleolus into the medial malleolus. The authors recommended preoperative CT to assist in surgical planning.

Fixation of posterior malleolus fractures is recommended when fragments are greater than 25% of the joint surface or there is persistent posterior subluxation of the talus. The fracture fragment generally is reduced by closed methods through ligamentotaxis after the fibula is reduced. Open treatment is required if the posterior malleolus remains malreduced despite lateral and medial malleoli reduction (**Figure 5**). The fracture can be approached through a posteromedial or posterolateral approach. CT scans may help in determining which approach will allow the easiest reduction and fixation.

If the fragment is reduced by closed means, a tenaculum or Kirschner wires can provide provisional fixation. Fixation can be performed with anterior-to-posterior screw fixation. If partially threaded screws are used, all threads must cross the fracture to ensure compression. Fully threaded screws placed in lag fashion may be a more efficient option. If open reduction is performed, the fragment can be held in place with posterior-to-anterior lag screws or an antiglide plate.

2: Foot and Ankle Trauma

Osteoporotic Fractures

As the population continues to age, the incidence of osteoporotic fractures will continue to increase. Previously, poor results have been reported for nonsurgically treated unstable ankle fractures in elderly patients.[18] Maintaining stable fixation in osteoporotic bone is challenging. Traditional lag screw fixation and lateral neutralization plating depend on two to three unicortical screws in the small distal fragment to maintain reduction. This fixation may be tenuous in many instances. Screw purchase can be enhanced by augmentation with polymethylmethacrylate, intramedullary Kirschner wire augmentation of the screw and plate construct, or intramedullary fibular fixation. New technology and techniques should be investigated to improve fixation methods.

Locking plates are advantageous in other osteoporotic fractures. A recent cadaver study using locking and conventional one third tubular plates placed as neutralization plates on the lateral fibula showed that locking plates function independently of bone mineral density. In severely osteoporotic bone, the locking one third tubular neutralization plates provided better torque-to-failure performance than conventional plates.[19]

Antiglide and lateral locking plate fixation was compared in a cadaver study of short oblique fractures of lateral malleoli in osteoporotic bone.[9] The antiglide plate had a higher torque to failure and construct stiffness than the lateral locking plate. The authors concluded that use of antiglide plate fixation can be advantageous in osteoporotic ankle fractures.

Augmentation of the construct with absorbable bone cement also is being investigated. In a cadaveric model, injectable tricalcium phosphate improved plate-screw fixation strength to cantilever bending by 3.6 times using conventional plating and by 5 times in locked-plate constructs.[20] A Norwegian study showed augmentation of "stripped screw holes" with synthetic bone filler to be safe and effective at gaining screw purchase in osteoporotic bone. At 2-year follow-up, the cohort showed no increase in clinically adverse effects.[21]

Currently, no clinical studies are available comparing locking and conventional plates in the treatment of ankle fractures. Additional clinical evaluation of these technologies is necessary to determine cost effectiveness and to improve clinical results compared with those achieved with traditional treatment protocols.

Fixation in the Neuropathic Patient

In addition to the systemic effects of diabetes mellitus, impaired circulation and decreased sensation predispose patients to complications involving both soft tissues and fracture healing and also increase the risk of infection. Management of unstable ankle fractures in patients with diabetic neuropathy, neuropathy arising from alcoholism, or other diseases of the peripheral nervous system demand an awareness of potential problems and should include a team approach to treating the patient. If surgical treatment is indicated and the patient is a candidate for surgery, the procedure should be performed after the soft tissues are stabilized. This may require a period of splinting or stabilization with an external fixator.

Methods of internal fixation should take into account the potential for poor bone quality, delayed healing, and some degree of patient noncompliance. Similar to fixation in osteoporotic bone, locked antiglide plating of the fibula may be beneficial. Screw purchase can be improved in the fibula by first placing multiple Kirschner wires within the medullary canal.[22] Tetracortical tibiofibular screws have shown improved stability and resistance to failure in neuropathic ankle fracture-dislocations in which bone quality of the fibula is poor.[23] A technique using a 4.5-mm dynamic compression plate and multiple 4.5-mm cortical screws has been described as a salvage for failed fixation.[24] The stability imparted by this construct has led to its use as primary fixation in neuropathic ankle fractures. The risks of altering ankle mechanics in these patients are not as severe as the risks associated with loss of reduction and the need for revision surgery.

It is important that patients with neuropathic conditions understand the risks and the need for compliance when undergoing fracture fixation. Postoperatively, the patient should be immobilized in a well-padded or total contact cast. Weight bearing should be restricted for 12 weeks, but can be tailored to the patient's progress. Follow-up radiographic studies are needed to evaluate healing, loss of reduction, and skin conditions.

Weight Bearing After Open Reduction and Internal Fixation of Unstable Ankle Fractures

Traditionally, surgically treated ankle fractures are placed in a cast or brace and the patient does not bear weight for 4 to 6 weeks. Recently, early weight bearing after ankle fractures in patients with stable fixation has been proposed. In a prospective study, patients with stable fixation of ankle fractures were allowed partial weight bearing in a stirrup brace in the immediate postoperative period. If radiographs showed fracture stability at 3-week follow-up, patients were allowed to progress to full weight bearing. In comparison with patients treated with immobilization and a non–weight-bearing protocol, the early weight-bearing group had a faster return to full weight bearing, earlier return to work, and similar pain scores.[25]

Fractures of the Weight-Bearing Surface

Fractures involving the weight-bearing surface of the distal tibial plafond or pilon occur from axial loading of the joint surface. The fracture pattern is dictated by the quality of the bone and the force absorbed. Lower energy injuries produce simpler fracture patterns whereas high-energy injuries, such as a fall from a height or a motor vehicle crash, tend to result in comminuted articular fractures with impaction of the metaphysis. The outcome of these injuries tends to be unpredictable and often disappointing. Although debilitating arthritis often occurs despite anatomic reduction; every attempt should be made to optimize function.[26] This goal is best achieved by accurate reduction of the articular surface and restoration of metaphyseal integrity and overall alignment.

History and Physical Examination

It is important to establish the mechanism of injury because this information is useful in determining the amount of energy imparted to the limb and the potential for associated injuries. Clinical assessment should include the condition of the skin, degree of swelling, motor and sensory status, and circulation. Obvious deformities that compromise circulation and/or nerve function should be corrected immediately. Particular attention should be given to the signs and symptoms of compartment syndrome.

Imaging

In addition to standard AP and lateral radiographs of the ankle, the entire tibia and fibula should be evaluated in the AP and lateral planes. CT is indicated in fractures involving the articular surface and helps in classifying the fracture pattern and planning the methods of surgical approach and fixation. CT scanning is best after application of external traction. By restoring length and rotation, information can be obtained regarding defects, impacted fragments, and the location of fracture lines, all of which are helpful in formulating the preoperative plan. MRI is of little use in the acute setting but may be useful later for identifying devitalized bone using intravenous contrast.

Classification

The AO/OTA fracture classification system for pilon fractures has been widely accepted as a descriptive schema for purposes of data collection and publication.[27] This system has been studied regarding its power to predict functional outcomes and intraobserver variations.[28] Interobserver and intraobserver agreement was better with the AO/OTA system than with the Rüedi and Allgöwer classification system.[29] However, although agreement among subtypes 43-A through 43-C was satisfactory, further subtyping (among types 43-C1 through 43-C3) did not produce satisfactory results. In attempting to correlate functional outcome with injury severity, type C fractures were associated with a worse functional outcome than type B injuries, but there was no significant difference in the functional outcome of type A fractures compared with type B or C fractures. Although descriptive, it is difficult to use validation as a predictive tool because of multiple variables, such as the degree of individual injury. A recent study showed that fracture of the fibula is more common in type C than type B fractures; however, there was no difference in the severity of injury in patients with type C fibula fractures compared with those with intact fibulae.[30]

A 2005 study provided a detailed description of fracture variation, describing 10 subtypes, primarily coronal or sagittal fracture patterns.[31] This principle is important in planning optimal fixation. The fibula is not considered in these systems.

Initial Management

The initial focus in the treatment of pilon fractures should be soft-tissue management. Length alignment and rotation should be treated urgently to avoid neurovascular compromise. The limb should be stabilized in a well-padded splint and plain radiographs should be obtained. Nonsurgical management may be an option in stable, less severe injuries (low-energy, nonarticular, or nondisplaced articular injuries) or in patients who are not candidates for surgery. Such injuries should be evaluated with serial radiographs to monitor alignment. Casting is applied after swelling has stabilized; the patient is regularly evaluated for skin breakdown.

If surgical treatment is indicated, several options should be considered. All treatments should include immediate stabilization with external fixation as a temporizing measure. The rationale for external fixation is to stabilize the limb, allow soft-tissue observation, and prevent dynamic soft-tissue contracture while unloading the joint surface. Typically, a less complex and inexpensive system is used for temporary stabilization. A transcalcaneal pin and two tibial pins spanned by supports on either side constitute a delta configuration. This construct stabilizes the fracture in the sagittal, coronal, and transverse planes and maintains the foot in an anatomic position relative to the tibial axis. Meticulous placement of the fixator and alignment of the limb precludes the need to stabilize the fibula by open means, which may compromise soft tissues or other surgical approaches. Bars can be added to support pins placed in the medial cuneiform (between the anterior and posterior tibial tendons) or the first metatarsal to avoid intrinsic contracture of the foot.

Grade 1 and 2 open injuries may be irrigated, débrided, and closed. Contaminated wounds should be evaluated and débrided every 48 hours until clean. Wound care consisting of synthetic or vacuum dressings may be used as needed. The focus then becomes edema control. In the absence of other concerns requiring continued hospitalization, the patient may be discharged. It is essential that the patient understand the severity and consequences of the injury and the importance of controlling swelling.

Internal Fixation

Open treatment with plate fixation can provide satisfactory results after soft tissues are stabilized.[32-34] Low-profile periarticular implants allowing compression, neutralization, and locking provide a variety of treatment options based on the fracture pattern and surgical approach.[35] Although implants and techniques have evolved, the fundamental treatment concepts are still the standard of care. Fibular length and rotation should

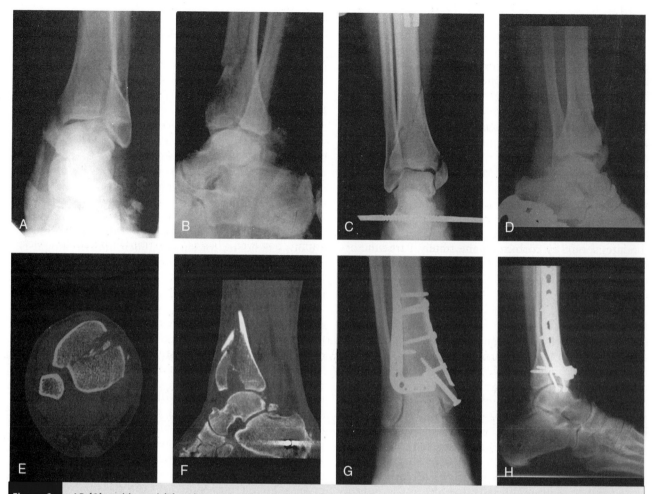

Figure 6 AP **(A)** and lateral **(B)** radiographs of a comminuted, intra-articular fracture of the tibial plafond (AO/OTA 43-B3.3) in a 57-year-old woman who fell from counter height. The fibula is intact, suggesting that most of the impact force was sustained by the tibia. AP **(C)** and lateral **(D)** radiographic views after external fixation. The deltoid ligament appears to be intact and the joint surfaces are unloaded. Posttraction CT axial **(E)** and sagittal **(F)** cuts showing comminuted articular fragments interposed within the primary coronal fracture line. Postoperative weight-bearing AP **(G)** and lateral **(H)** radiographic views. The fracture was stabilized with an anterolateral plate through a Böhler approach. In addition to the screw fixation medially, a buttress plate was used to stabilize the medial diaphysis.

be restored, serving as a reference for the tibia. The articular surface of the tibia is reconstructed and the metaphyseal void is filled with cancellous graft or bone graft substitute[29] (**Figure 6**). Corticocancellous structural graft may be needed, depending on the defect and need for cortical support. If bone grafting is contraindicated because of wound contamination, grafting may be done secondarily at approximately 6 weeks. The construct is supported with plate fixation as required by the fracture pattern.

The patient is positioned supine on a radiolucent table. A tourniquet is placed around the proximal thigh. The skin is prepared and the limb draped to the knee. The leg is elevated from the table with a cushioned bump. Elevation should be sufficient to allow a lateral fluoroscopic image to be unimpeded by the contralateral limb. This degree of knee flexion also relaxes the gastrocnemius, avoiding the potential for a deforming plantar flexion force.

The anteromedial approach had been the standard. However, the incision(s) chosen are based on the fracture pattern seen on the CT scan after traction. The approach must provide optimal visualization, allow reduction and implant placement, and should be extensile to avoid undue tension on the wound margins and further soft-tissue injury.[32,36-39] The need for additional incisions must be considered in the preoperative plan. Adequate skin bridges must be maintained to avoid devitalization and slough.

In fractures involving a coronal fracture line and anterolateral or valgus compression, if an anterolateral plate is preferred, the Böhler (anterolateral) approach provides broad visualization of the plafond and facilitates buttressing of the anterolateral column and Chaput fragment.[37] The incision is initiated 5 cm proximal to the ankle joint and 1.5 to 2 cm medial to the anterior margin of the fibula. The incision progresses distally in line with the third intermetatarsal space. The superficial peroneal nerve is visualized and protected. Both the superior and inferior extensor retinaculum is divided. The peroneus tertius, extensor digitorum longus, deep peroneal nerve, and dorsalis pedis are mobilized and retracted medially. If fractured, the fibula may be anteriorly stabilized by beginning the incision slightly more laterally, approximating the anterior margin of the fibula. If necessary, this approach may be combined with a medial or posteromedial approach, maintaining an adequate soft-tissue bridge to address a medial malleolar or posterior fragment, respectively.

A combined medial and lateral approach can provide visualization and reduction of the articular surface of the tibia. These objectives are accomplished from the medial side by reflecting the medial malleolus and from the lateral side by mobilizing the fibula if fractured.[38] The medial approach consists of an incision through the midline of the medial malleolus while maintaining full-thickness skin margins. The saphenous nerve and vein will lie in the anterior flap. The incision curves anteriorly distal to the tip of the malleolus. The ankle joint capsule, if intact, can be opened to expose the anteromedial portion of the joint. By releasing the posterior tibial retinaculum, a medial malleolar fragment can be hinged on the deltoid ligament and reflected distally. This approach can provide visualization of the articular surface to the tibia from anterior to posterior and allows manipulation of the posterior fragment.

The lateral approach follows the anterior margin of the fibula, progressing distally by paralleling the anterior talofibular ligament. The superficial peroneal nerve is identified and protected and the incision carried to bone at the tubercle of Chaput. The extensors and anterior neurovascular bundle are retracted medially. In addition to reduction and fixation of the fibula, the distal fragment can be retracted posteriorly, which affords access to the incisure of the fibula and/or a posterior fragment.

External Fixation

Pilon fractures associated with severe soft-tissue injury can be treated definitively with external fixation (**Figure 7**). This technique may be beneficial in decreasing the incidence of soft-tissue complications. Simple articular fractures can be satisfactorily reduced by indirect techniques and fixed with lag screws placed percutaneously or through limited incisions, or with tensioned olive wires using nonspanning ring or hybrid systems. More complex articular fractures that require direct reduction techniques should be staged.[40-42] Minimally invasive techniques can be used with external fixation as a means of stabilization. Initially, the fixator can span the ankle using ligamentotaxis to align larger fragments and unload the articular surface. Once the soft tissues stabilize, the fixator can be converted to a nonspanning construct after definitive articular reconstruction and metaphyseal bone grafting are performed.[43,44] In such instances, the frame is secured proximally with diaphyseal pins. Distally, tensioned fine wires and/or olive wires are used with strict adherence to anatomic safe

zones to avoid injury to neurovascular structures and tendons and intracapsular pin placement.[45,46]

Results

Researchers have achieved acceptable rates of soft-tissue complications with immediate external fixation and delayed definitive stabilization.[33] In 29 closed type 43-C injuries, superficial infections occurred in 17% and deep infection in 3.4%. Time from external fixation to definitive plate fixation was 12.7 days. In 17 open injuries, 2 superficial and 2 deep infections occurred; one required amputation. Higher rates of complications were found in type C fractures treated with initial external fixation and delayed internal fixation compared with those treated with primary internal fixation; however, better functional outcomes were achieved in patients treated with a staged protocol.[47] In a 2007 study, 43 patients (44 fractures; 8 type 43-B and 36 type 43-C fractures) were treated with open reduction and plate fixation after soft tissues were stabilized. The authors reported two superficial and two deep infections.[32] In another study, researchers compared open reduction and internal fixation with two methods of external fixation.[48] Twenty-four fractures (18 closed, 6 open) were treated with open reduction and internal fixation at an average of 2.2 days after injury. Two deep infections occurred, leading to below-knee amputation, and there were six minor wound complications. Comparing the groups treated with external fixation with the group treated with plate fixation, no significant difference was found in the rate of wound complications. However, a greater number of malunions occurred in the groups treated with external fixation. A similar study concluded that staged surgery results in better motion, better workability, and a lower incidence of end-stage degenerative joint disease.[49] Other authors reviewed 107 fractures initially stabilized with calcaneal traction and treated definitively with internal or limited internal or external fixation.[40] Regardless of treatment, satisfactory outcomes were achieved in patients with type 43-A and 43-B fractures. However, the authors reported higher rates of infection, nonunion, and malunion in patients with type C fractures treated with internal fixation compared with those treated with limited internal fixation with external fixation. Although several studies showed poorer outcomes in patients with type C fractures regardless of the treatment method, complication rates were higher in patients treated with external fixation.[41,50] Late infection resulted in amputation in five patients treated with external fixation.[51]

Two recent studies using validated outcome instruments have shown that pilon fractures have profound effects on the overall health and well being of patients.[51,52] Although one study showed continued improvement in pain and functional levels over a minimum follow-up of 5 years, both studies showed negative long-term effects. Significant numbers of patients were unable to return to work and some of those

2: Foot and Ankle Trauma

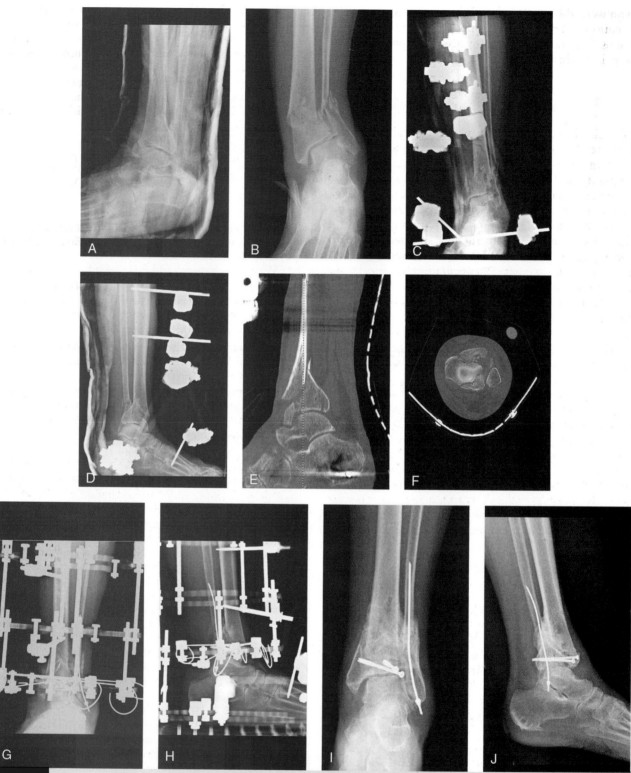

Figure 7 Lateral **(A)** and AP **(B)** radiographs of an intra-articular fracture of the tibial plafond and fibula fracture (AO/OTA 43-C2) in a 44-year-old man involved in a motor vehicle crash. AP **(C)** and lateral **(D)** radiographic views after spanning external fixation was applied. The anterior tibial fragment is posteriorly rotated. Sagittal **(E)** and axial **(F)** CT images are vital in planning the approach, reduction, and fixation of the articular surface. Because of the degree of soft-tissue compromise, the spanning fixator was converted to a hybrid ring. AP **(G)** and lateral **(H)** radiographic images show improvement of the axial alignment. The articular surface was reduced and stabilized with limited internal fixation consisting of two anterior to posterior screws. The fibula was stabilized with an olive wire. **I** and **J**, After removal of the frame, although the mortise is widened, the overall alignment is satisfactory and the soft tissues are intact. *(Courtesy of J. Tracy Watson, MD.)*

who were able to work found it necessary to change occupations. Return to recreational activity was nearly impossible and daily function was poor; prolonged use of pain medication was common.

Summary

Historically, surgical management of distal tibial pilon fractures has resulted in high rates of soft-tissue loss, deep infection, osteomyelitis, and not uncommonly, amputation. These complications have been attributed to surgery performed through swollen and otherwise compromised soft tissues. The most important advance in the treatment of severe pilon fractures has been the delay in definitive reconstruction sufficient to allow soft-tissue stabilization. This rationale should be explained to the patient to encourage compliance and promote comfort. The discrepancies in results regarding fracture type and treatment methods highlight the challenge of treating these injuries. The decision to treat this injury with internal or external fixation depends on several factors, such as the degree of bone and soft-tissue injury, the patient's expectations, and experience of the surgeon.

The goal of surgical management of ankle fractures is optimization of function by restoration of form. Although improved imaging methods and implants have enhanced the surgeon's armamentarium for treating these common injuries, the importance of having a thorough understanding of the anatomy and biomechanics of the ankle joint cannot be overemphasized. The surgeon also must have the skills and judgement needed to formulate and execute a treatment plan that will achieve anatomic reduction using an atraumatic technique.

Annotated References

1. McKinley TO, Rudert MJ, Tochigi Y, et al: Incongruity-dependent changes of contact stress rates in human cadaveric ankles. *J Orthop Trauma* 2006;20:732-738.

   The authors describe a cadaver study illustrating changes in contact pressure with displacement of the tibial plafond. Contact pressure was measured in 10 normal specimens subjected to physiologic load applied through a range of motion simulating the stance phase of gait. The anterolateral 25% of the tibial plafond was osteotomized. Measurements were made with the fragment fixed anatomically and after proximal displacement of 4 mm at 1 mm intervals. Changes in contact stress approximating 300% of that seen in controls were observed.

2. Fitzpatrick DC, Otto HK, McKinley TO, Marsh JL, Brown TK: Kinematic and contact stress analysis of posterior malleolus fractures of the ankle. *J Orthop Trauma* 2004;18:271-278.

   Using a cadaver model, contact stress was measured under physiologic load from 25° of plantar flexion to 15°

of dorsiflexion. Measurements were in four posterior malleolar fracture models (AO/OTA 44-B3) involving 50% of the plafond—no internal fixation, two malreduced configurations, and anatomic reduction with fixation. No increase in peak contact stress was seen; however, stress shifted anteromedially (a region where little load is applied in the intact ankle). The authors concluded that these findings did not explain the incidence of arthrosis seen after a fracture.

3. McConnell T, Tornetta P III: Marginal plafond impaction in association with supination-adduction ankle fractures: a report of eight cases. *J Orthop Trauma* 2001;15:447-449.

4. Ramsey PL, Hamilton W: Changes in tibiotalar area of contact caused by lateral talar shift. *J Bone Joint Surg Am* 1976;58:356-357.

5. DeAngelis NA, Eskander MS, French BG: Does medial tenderness predict deep deltoid ligament incompetence in supination-external rotation type ankle fractures? *J Orthop Trauma* 2007;21:244-247.

   In this study, patients with lateral malleolus fractures and normal medial clear space were examined to determine the presence of medial ankle tenderness. Stress radiographs were then obtained to determine the competence of the deep deltoid ligament. The study showed no statistically significant correlation between medial tenderness and deep deltoid incompetence.

6. Egol KA, Amirtharajah M, Tejwani NC, Capla EL, Koval KJ: Ankle stress test for predicting the need for surgical fixation of isolated fibular fractures. *J Bone Joint Surg Am* 2004;86:2393-2398.

   The authors evaluated the prevalence of medial ankle widening in patients with isolated fibula fracture and examined the outcomes of nonsurgical treatment. This study evaluated 101 patients with isolated fibula fractures and symmetric mortise on injury radiographs. Positive stress radiographs (≥ 4 mm of medial widening) were seen in 65% of patients. Medial tenderness, swelling, or ecchymosis was not predictive of medial widening. Symptomatic patients with medial widening were surgically treated. Asymptomatic patients with positive stress radiographs were treated nonsurgically and had good to excellent clinical results at an average follow-up of 7.4 months.

7. Gill JB, Risko T, Raducan V, Grimes JS, Schutt RC: Comparison of manual and gravity stress radiographs for the evaluation of supination-external rotation fibular fractures. *J Bone Joint Surg Am* 2007;89:994-999.

   Manual and gravity stress radiographs were obtained for 25 patients with isolated lateral malleolus fractures. The two methods were equivalent for determining deltoid ligament injury in isolated lateral malleolus fractures.

8. Tornetta P III, Creevy W: Lag screw only fixation of the lateral malleolus. *J Orthop Trauma* 2001;15:119-121.

9. Minihane KP, Lee C, Ahn C, Zhang L, Merk BR: Comparison of lateral locking plate and antiglide plate for fixation of distal fibular fractures in osteoporotic bone: A biomechanical study. *J Orthop Trauma* 2006;20:562-566.

    In this cadaver study, oblique distal fibula fractures were created in osteoporotic bone. The fractures were repaired with either a posterolateral antiglide plate with a lag screw or a lateral neutralization plate with independent lag screw. The posterolateral antiglide plate was found to have a higher torque to failure and construct stiffness in the osteoporotic bone.

10. Schaffer JJ, Manoli A: The antiglide plate for distal fibular fixation: A biomechanical comparison with fixation with a lateral plate. *J Bone Joint Surg Am* 1987;69:596-604.

11. Stark E, Tornetta P III, Creevy WR: Syndesmotic instability in Weber B fractures: A clinical evaluation. *J Orthop Trauma* 2007;21:643-646.

    The authors present the results of a retrospective study of syndesmosis instability in Weber B supination external rotation fracture patterns. Instability was found in 39% of ankles by external rotation stress examination under fluoroscopy after rigid fixation of the lateral malleolus fracture.

12. Tornetta P III: Competence of the deltoid ligament in bimalleolar ankle fractures after medial malleolar fixation. *J Bone Joint Surg Am* 2000;82:843-848.

13. Ostrum RF, Litsky AS: Tension band fixation of medial malleolus fractures. *J Orthop Trauma* 1992;6:464-468.

14. Femino JE, Gruber BF, Karunakar MA: Safe zone for the placement of medial malleolar screws. *J Bone Joint Surg Am* 2007;89:133-138.

    In this cadaveric study, screws were placed via fluoroscopic guidance into the medial malleolus. The proximity of the head of the screw to the posterior tibial tendon was then determined. The authors found that screws placed posterior to the anterior colliculus placed the posterior tibial tendon at risk for iatrogenic injury.

15. Tejwani NC, McLaurin TM, Walsh M, Bhadsavle S, Koval KJ, Egol KA: Are outcomes of bimalleolar fractures poorer than those of lateral malleolar fractures with medial ligamentous injury? *J Bone Joint Surg Am* 2007;89:1438-1441.

    The authors compare functional outcomes of patients with lateral malleolar fractures with deltoid injury and bimalleolar ankle fractures treated with stabilization. Patients were evaluated using Short Musculoskeletal Function Assessment and the American Orthopaedic Foot and Ankle Society scores. Although both groups had few restrictions and mild pain, patients with bimalleolar fractures had worse functional scores at 1 year.

16. Bhandari M, Sprague S, Hanson B, et al: Health-related quality of life following operative treatment of unstable ankle fractures. *J Orthop Trauma* 2004;18:338-345.

    The authors report on a prospective study correlating health-related quality of life to outcome in 30 patients with unstable type Weber B fractures. A history of smoking, the presence of a medial malleolar fracture, and a lower education level were predictive of decreased physical function at the 3-month postoperative follow-up.

17. Haraguchi N, Haruyama H, Toga H, Kato F: Pathoanatomy of posterior malleolar fractures of the ankle. *J Bone Joint Surg Am* 2006;88:1085-1092.

    The authors evaluated 57 consecutive ankle fractures with posterior malleolar involvement. They classified the fractures into three types: posterolateral-oblique, medial-extension, and small-shell. The posterior malleolus fracture extended into the medial malleolus 20% of the time. With the high variability in the posterior malleolus fragment, preoperative CT may aid in surgical planning for these fractures.

18. Ali MS, McLaren CA, Rouholamin E, O'Connor BT: Ankle fractures in the elderly: Nonoperative or operative treatment. *J Orthop Trauma* 1987;1:275-280.

19. Kim T, Ayturk UM, Haskell A, Miclau T, Puttlitz CM: Fixation of osteoporotic distal fibula fractures: A biomechanical comparison of locking versus conventional plates. *J Foot Ankle Surg* 2007;46:2-6.

    In this cadaveric study, a supination external rotation injury was simulated in osteoporotic specimens. The fibula was stabilized with either a construct consisting of a lag screw and conventional plate with three distal unicortical screws or a lag screw and a locking plate with two distal unicortical screws. The constructs were then mechanically stressed. The authors found the locking plate construct functioned independent of the bone mineral density of the specimen.

20. Collinge C, Merk B, Lautenschlager EP: Mechanical evaluation of fracture fixation augmented with tricalcium phosphate bone cement in a porous osteoporotic cancellous bone model. *J Orthop Trauma* 2007;21:124-128.

    This study used a bone model to test the pullout strength of 4.5-mm cortical screws with fixation augmented with tricalcium phosphate bone cement. The augmented screws had almost four times the pullout strength as nonaugmented screws in this model. The authors then tested a locked plate construct with screw fixation augmented with tricalcium phosphate cement and found the construct strength was five times greater than a nonlocked, nonaugmented construct.

21. Andreassen GS, Hoiness PR, Skraamm I, Granlund O, Engebretsen L: Use of synthetic bone void filler to augment screws in osteopenic ankle fracture fixation. *Arch Orthop Trauma Surg* 2004;124:161-165.

    A prospective study of 37 patients with type Weber B ankle fractures showed radiographic signs of osteopenia. Stripping of at least one screw occurred during internal fixation. Eighty-six screws were augmented with synthetic bone void filler. Two wound infections occurred. All fractures healed by 3-month follow-up. At 2 years postoperatively, all patients had resumed normal activity and no loosening was observed in the augmented screws.

22. Koval KJ, Petraco DM, Kummer FJ, Bharam S: A new technique for complex fibula fracture fixation in the elderly: A clinical and biomechanical evaluation. *J Orthop Trauma* 1997;11:28-33.

23. Schon LC, Marks RM: The management of neuroarthropathic fracture-dislocations in the diabetic patient. *Orthop Clin North Am* 1995;26:375-392.

24. Perry MD, Taranow WS, Manoli A II, Carr JB: Salvage of failed neuropathic ankle fractures: Use of large-fragment fibular plating and multiple syndesmotic screws. *J Surg Orthop Adv* 2005;14:85-90.

The authors describe a technique used in revision surgery for failed ankle fixation in six patients with neuropathy. Although wound complications were common, no amputations were needed. Fractures healed in all six patients and all were able to perform activities of daily living with the use of a brace.

25. Simanski CJ, Maegele MG, Lefering R, et al: Functional treatment and early weightbearing after an ankle fracture: A prospective study. *J Orthop Trauma* 2006;20: 108-114.

This prospective study compared early weight bearing and functional rehabilitation with a non–weight-bearing and immobilization protocol for patients with surgically treated ankle fractures. The authors found that patients with the early weight-bearing protocol returned to full weight bearing earlier with no increase in the rate of complications.

26. Furman BD, Olson SA, Guilak F: The development of posttraumatic arthritis after articular fracture. *J Orthop Trauma* 2006;20:719-725.

These authors discuss the potential roles of impact and altered biomechanics resulting from fracture. The spectrum of injury includes metabolic and inflammatory changes affecting joint cartilage and the possible role of genetic factors.

27. Marsh JL, Slongo TF, Agel J, et al : Fracture and dislocation classification compendium—2007: Orthopaedic Trauma Association classification, database and outcome committee. *J Orthop Trauma* 2007;21(suppl 10): S1-S133.

The compendium provides a comprehensive classification system for facilitating standardization of research and communication. A review of new scientific information on the classification of fractures published within the past 11 years is included.

28. Swiontkowski MF, Agel J, McAndrew MP, Burgess AR, MacKenzie EJ: Outcome validation of the AO/OTA fracture classification system. *J Orthop Trauma* 2000; 14:534-541.

29. Rüedi T, Matter P, Allgöwer M: Intra-articular fractures of the distal tibial end. *Helv Chir Acta* 1968;35: 556-582.

30. Barei DP, Nork SE, Bellabarba C, Sangeorzan BJ: Is the absence of an ipsilateral fibular fracture predictive of increased radiographic tibial pilon fracture severity? *J Orthop Trauma* 2006;20:6-10.

Twenty tibial pilon fractures without associated fibular fracture were compared with a cohort of 20 age- and gender-matched patients with pilon fractures with fractured fibulae. Three evaluators ranked the severity of the fractures. Fibula fracture was more commonly associated with type C fractures compared with type B fractures. However, there was no significant difference in severity between type C fractures with or without fibula fracture.

31. Topliss CJ, Jackson M, Atkins RM: Anatomy of pilon fractures of the distal tibia. *J Bone Joint Surg Br* 2005; 87:692-697.

The authors evaluated 126 tibial pilon fractures. Fractures were categorized as being primarily sagittal or coronal. The sagittal type was associated with a high-energy injury and a varus moment, whereas coronal injuries occurred with lower energy forces and in older patients. Five subtypes were identified in the coronal group and three in the sagittal group. Intraobserver agreement was superior to that of the Rüedi and Allgöwer or AO classification systems.

32. Grose A, Gardner MJ, Hettrich C, et al: Open reduction and internal fixation of tibial pilon fractures using a lateral approach. *J Orthop Trauma* 2007;21:530-537.

Forty-four tibial pilon fractures were treated with delayed open reduction and internal fixation using a lateral approach. Results were based on reduction of the articular surface and soft-tissue healing. Reduction was judged to be anatomic in 41 fractures; 13.6% of patients underwent secondary surgery for infection or nonunion. The authors observed that this approach preserves soft tissues and provides excellent visualization of the lateral distal tibia.

33. Sirkin M, Sanders R, DiPasquale T, Herscovici D: A staged protocol for soft tissue management in the treatment of complex pilon fractures. *J Orthop Trauma* 2004;18:S32-S38.

The authors present a retrospective evaluation of 56 AO 43-C fractures (34 closed injuries [group I] and 22 open injuries [group II]). Treatment consisted of open reduction and internal fixation of the fibula and application of a spanning external fixator within 24 hours. Average time to definitive treatment was 12.7 days and 14 days, respectively. In group I, five patients sustained partial thickness necrosis treated with local wound care. In group II, five Gustilo type IIIB injuries were treated with free-flap placement. Two patients were treated with local wound care for partial-thickness necrosis. Two patients were treated for deep infection including an amputation for osteomyelitis involving the calcaneus. The authors concluded that their relatively low complication rate was the result of allowing adequate time for soft-tissue stabilization before performing the definitive procedure.

34. Patterson MJ, Cole JD: Two-staged delayed open reduction and internal fixation of severe pilon fractures. *J Orthop Trauma* 1999;13:85-91.

2: Foot and Ankle Trauma

35. Hasenboehler E, Rikli D, Babst R: Locking compression plate with minimally invasive plate osteosynthesis in diaphyseal and distal tibial fracture: A retrospective study of 32 patients. *Injury* 2007;38:365-370.

   The authors present a retrospective review of diaphyseal and distal tibial shaft fractures treated with minimally invasive plate osteosynthesis. Fracture healing was evaluated radiographically at 3-month intervals. Healing was defined as bridging of one cortex and pain-free weight bearing; 27 of 32 patients met these criteria at 9 months. The authors reported favorable results in simple fracture patterns when bridging was indicated.

36. Bhattacharyya T, Crichlow R, Gobezie R, Kim E, Vrahas MS: Complications associated with the posterolateral approach for pilon fractures. *J Orthop Trauma* 2006;20:104-107.

   A retrospective review of 19 patients treated for tibial pilon fractures with initial external fixation and delayed open reduction and internal fixation is presented. The authors hypothesized that fewer wound complications would occur using a posterolateral approach. Average follow-up was 13 months. No benefit was found in terms of decreased complication rates. The authors recognized the benefit of this approach if needed because of soft-tissue compromise but did not recommend its routine use.

37. Herscovici D, Sanders RW, Infante A, DiPasquale T: Bohler incision: An extensile anterolateral approach to the foot and ankle. *J Orthop Trauma* 2000;14:429-432.

38. Chen L, O'Shea K, Early JS: The use of medial and lateral surgical approaches for the treatment of tibial plafond fractures. *J Orthop Trauma* 2007;21:207-211.

   The authors report on 65 patients with distal tibial plafond fractures treated with a medial and lateral approach. CT scans after reduction were routinely obtained to plan the approach. Surgery was delayed until the soft tissue was deemed stable. Follow-up ranged from 6 to 16 months. During the observation period, no amputations, deep infections, or need for flap placement occurred. This two-incision technique provided better visualization than a single incision and allowed accurate articular reduction and fixation placement.

39. Kao KF, Huang PJ, Chen YW, Cheng YM, Lin SY, Koh SH: Postero-medio-anterior approach of the ankle for the pilon fracture. *Injury* 2000;31:71-74.

40. Watson JT, Moed BR, Karges DE, Cramer KE: Pilon fractures: Treatment protocol based on severity of soft tissue injury. *Clin Orthop Relat Res* 2000;375:78-90.

41. Anglen JO: Early outcome of hybrid external fixation for fractures of the distal tibia. *J Orthop Trauma* 1999;13:92-97.

42. Manca M, Narchette S, Restuccia G, Faldini A, Faldini C, Giannini S: Combined percutaneous internal and external fixation of type-C tibial plafond fractures: A review of twenty-two cases. *J Bone Joint Surg Am* 2002;84(suppl 2):109-115.

43. El-Shazly M, Dalby-Ball J, Burton M, Saleh M: The use of trans-articular and extra-articular external fixation for management of distal tibial intra-articular fractures. *Injury* 2001;32(suppl 4):SD99-SD106.

44. French B, Tornetta P III: Hybrid external fixation of tibial pilon fractures. *Foot Ankle Clin* 2000;5:853-871.

45. Lee PT, Clarke MT: Bearcroft PW, Robinson AH: The proximal extent of the ankle capsule and safety for the insertion of percutaneous fine wires. *J Bone Joint Surg Br* 2005;87:668-671.

   Eighteen patients were evaluated with magnetic resonance arthrograms to assess the proximal extent of the ankle joint capsule. The mean extent of the capsule was 9.6 mm proximal to the anteroinferior tibial margin and 3.8 mm proximal to the dome of the tibial plafond. In the tibiofibular recess, the mean capsular extension was 19.2 mm proximal to the anteroinferior margin and 13.4 mm proximal to the dome of the tibial plafond. When applying external fixation, awareness of this anatomy should minimize intra-articular placement of fine wires and the risk of septic arthritis.

46. Vives MJ, Abidi MA, Ishikawa SM, Taliwal RV, Sharkey PF: Soft tissue injuries with the use of safe corridors for transfixion wire placement during external fixation of distal tibia fractures: An anatomic study. *J Orthop Trauma* 2001;15:555-559.

47. Kilian O, Bündner MS, Horas U, Heiss C, Schnettler R: Long-term results in the surgical treatment of pilon tibial fractures: A retrospective study. *Chirurg* 2002;73:65-72.

48. Pugh KJ, Wolinsky PR, McAndrew MP, Johnson K: Tibial pilon fractures: A comparison of treatment methods. *J Trauma* 1999;47:937-941.

49. Blauth M, Bastian L, Krettek C, Knop C, Evans S: Surgical options for the treatment of severe tibial pilon fractures: A study of three techniques. *J Orthop Trauma* 2001;15:153-160.

50. Harris AM, Patterson BM, Sontich JK: Results and outcomes after operative treatment of high-energy tibial plafond fractures. *Foot Ankle Int* 2006;27:256-265.

   The authors present a retrospective review of 79 fractures (OTA types B or C). Twenty-one fractures were open. Open reduction and internal fixation was used to treat 63 patients and 16 were treated with limited internal and external fixation. Fewer complications and less posttraumatic arthritis occurred in the group treated with open reduction and internal fixation. The authors hypothesized that there was a bias of treating more severe injuries with external fixation.

51. Pollak AN, McCarthy ML, Bess S, Agel J, Swiontkowski MF: Outcomes after treatment of high-energy tibial plafond fractures. *J Bone Joint Surg Am* 2003;85:1893-1900.

   Eighty patients were treated for distal tibial pilon fractures; most were closed type C fractures. Average follow-up was 3.2 years. The patients were evaluated regarding overall health and ankle function. Most patients had significant functional restrictions. Socioeconomic issues were correlated with outcomes; 43% of patients could not return to work. Physical and psychosocial health was negatively impacted. The authors detail the difficulty in comparing the outcome of these injuries as well as the limitations of the study.

52. Marsh JL, Weigel DP, Dirschl DR: Tibial plafond fractures: How do these ankles function over time? *J Bone Joint Surg Am* 2003;85-A(suppl 2):287-295.

The authors report on the intermediate outcomes of 40 tibial plafond fractures using validated outcome instruments. Between 5 and 12 years after injury there was an overall negative effect on general health, with ankle pain and functional restrictions. Fourteen patients changed occupations. Most patients had limitations in recreational activities. However, the authors observed continued improvement over a 2.4-year period in nine patients.

2: Foot and Ankle Trauma

Chapter 7

Calcaneal Fractures

Michael P. Clare, MD

Introduction

Fractures of the calcaneus are among the most challenging lower extremity fractures to effectively manage. Approximately 60% to 75% of all calcaneal fractures are displaced intra-articular fractures; 10% of patients with calcaneal fractures have associated spine fractures.[1,2]

Intra-articular Fractures

Displaced intra-articular calcaneal fractures generally result from high-energy trauma, such as a motor vehicle crash or fall from a height. The exact pattern of fracture lines and extent of comminution are influenced by the position of the foot at impact, the extent of force involved, and the overall bone quality of the patient.[3-6]

Pathoanatomy

In a displaced intra-articular calcaneal fracture, there is loss of height through the calcaneus resulting in a shortened and widened heel and classic varus malalignment of the tuberosity. This loss of height is reflected in a decreased tuber angle of Böhler, whereby the normal declination of the talus is diminished and the talus becomes relatively more horizontal, which, if not restored, leads to secondary loss of ankle dorsiflexion. As the superolateral fragment of the posterior facet is impacted plantarward, the thin lateral wall explodes laterally just posterior to the crucial angle of Gissane and can trap the peroneal tendons against the lateral malleolus. In some instances, a violent contracture of the peroneal tendons may avulse the tendon sheath from the fibula, resulting in an avulsion fracture of the lateral malleolus and dislocation of the peroneal tendons. The anterior process typically displaces superiorly, which directly limits subtalar joint motion by impinging against the lateral process of the talus.

Understanding fragment terminology is necessary to appreciate the relevant pathoanatomy. The anterolateral fragment encompasses the lateral wall of the anterior process and may include a portion of the calcaneocuboid articular surface; the anterior main fragment is the large fragment anterior to the primary fracture line. The superomedial fragment (also known as the sustentacular or constant fragment) is found posterior to the primary fracture line and almost always remains attached to the talus through the deltoid ligament complex and is therefore stable. The superolateral fragment is the lateral portion of the posterior facet that is sheared from the remaining posterior facet in joint depression fractures. The tongue fragment refers to the superolateral fragment that remains attached to a portion of the posterior tuberosity in tongue-type fractures; the posterior main fragment represents the posterior tuberosity.

Diagnosis and Evaluation

The severity of fracture displacement and extent of soft-tissue injury are directly related to the amount of energy absorbed by the limb at the time of injury. Higher energy injuries produce more severe soft-tissue disruption and may result in an open fracture. Bleeding into the tightly enveloped fascial planes surrounding the heel produces severe pain overlying the fracture and may result in compartment syndrome of the foot, which is discussed in this chapter. The normal skin creases typically disappear within several hours following the injury; in the event of extreme swelling, cleavage at the dermal-epidermal junction may produce fracture blisters.

Plain Radiography

Plain radiographic evaluation includes a lateral view of the hindfoot, an AP view of the foot, an axial view of the heel, and a mortise view of the ankle.[7] The lateral view of the hindfoot shows loss of height in the posterior facet in which the articular surface is impacted within the body of the calcaneus and usually rotated anteriorly relative to the remaining subtalar joint. A decreased tuber angle of Böhler and an increased crucial angle of Gissane are seen in fracture patterns in which the entire posterior facet is separated from the sustentaculum and depressed (**Figure 1, A**). If only the lateral portion of the posterior facet is involved, the split in the articular surface is manifest as a "double density"; in these instances, the tuber angle of Böhler and crucial angle of Gissane may remain normal[8] (**Figure 1, B**). The lateral view also allows delineation to determine if the fracture is a joint depression or tongue fracture.[5] The AP view of the foot shows anterolateral fragments and extension of fracture lines into the calcaneocuboid joint. The axial view of the heel shows loss of calcaneal length, increased width, and typically shows varus angulation of the tuberosity fragment. A mortise view of

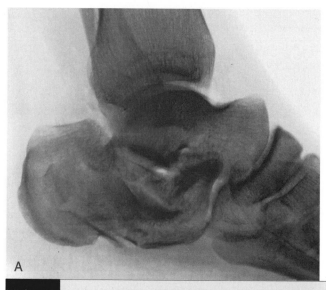

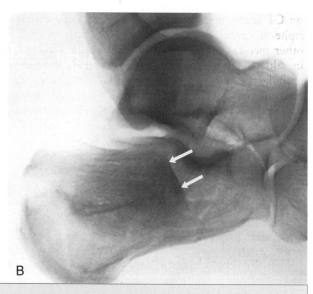

Figure 1 **A,** Lateral injury radiograph of the calcaneus with severe impaction of entire posterior facet; note decreased tuber angle of Böhler and increased crucial angle of Gissane from loss of calcaneal height. **B,** Lateral injury radiograph with impaction of superolateral fragment manifest as the "double density" sign (*arrows*).

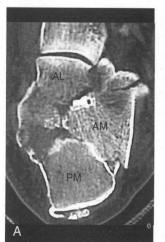

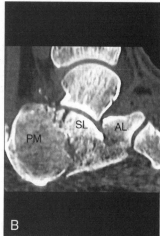

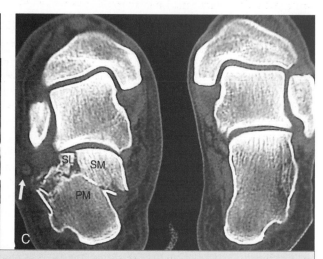

Figure 2 Axial **(A)**, sagittal **(B)**, and semicoronal **(C)** CT images delineating typical calcaneal fracture fragments. Note lateral wall expansion and peroneal tendon dislocation (*arrow*) on the semicoronal image. AL = anterolateral, AM = anterior main, PM = posterior main, SL = superolateral, SM = superomedial.

the ankle usually demonstrates involvement of the posterior facet.

Computed Tomography

CT is indicated if plain radiographs suggest intra-articular extension. Images are obtained in 2- to 3-mm intervals in the axial, sagittal, and 30° semicoronal planes. The axial cuts show extension of fracture lines into the anterior process and calcaneocuboid joint and the sustentaculum tali and anteroinferior margin of the posterior facet **(Figure 2, A)**. The sagittal reconstruction views show displacement of the tuberosity fragment, anterior process involvement including superior displacement of the anterolateral fragment, anterior rotational displacement of the superolateral posterior facet fragment, and delineation of the fracture as a joint depression or tongue-type pattern[5] **(Figure 2, B)**. The semicoronal images show displacement of articular fragments in the posterior facet, the sustentaculum tali, the extent of widening and shortening of the calcaneal body, expansion of the lateral calcaneal wall, and varus angulation of the tuberosity **(Figure 2, C)**. Fractures are then classified according to the Sanders classification system to assist in determining the optimal treatment method[9] **(Figure 3)**.

Treatment

Nonsurgical

Nonsurgical treatment is best reserved for truly nondisplaced (Sanders type I) intra-articular fractures as seen on CT scans, and fractures in patients with severe peripheral vascular disease, type I diabetes mellitus, or other medical comorbidities that prohibit surgery, and in elderly patients who are minimal (household) ambulators.[8-11] Chronologic age is not necessarily a contraindication to surgical treatment because many older patients are healthy and active well into their seventh decade.[12] Nonsurgical treatment also may be necessary because of injury severity, such as severe blistering, prolonged edema, large open wounds, or in patients with life-threatening injuries. In these instances, the patient may be later treated for calcaneal malunion.[13]

Nonsurgical treatment consists of initial splint immobilization followed by conversion to an elastic compression stocking and prefabricated fracture boot locked in neutral flexion to allow range-of-motion exercises. Weight bearing is not allowed for 10 to 12 weeks, until radiographic union is confirmed.

Surgical Treatment

Surgical treatment is generally indicated for displaced intra-articular fractures involving the posterior facet and is ideally performed within 3 weeks of injury before early fracture consolidation. Beyond 3 weeks, fragments become increasingly difficult to separate to obtain an adequate reduction and the articular cartilage may delaminate from the underlying subchondral bone. Surgery must be delayed, however, until the associated soft-tissue swelling has adequately dissipated. Splint immobilization and limb elevation are performed initially, with later conversion to a compression stocking and fracture boot. Full resolution of soft-tissue edema is verified by a positive wrinkle test, indicating that surgical intervention may be safely undertaken.[9]

Essex-Lopresti Technique for Tongue-Type (Sanders Type IIC) Fractures

The patient is placed in the lateral decubitus position; using fluoroscopic guidance in the lateral view, two terminally threaded guide pins are inserted in the superior edge of the posterior tuberosity and advanced parallel to the tongue fracture line (in the axial plane) toward the anteroinferior edge of the posterior facet[14] (Figure 4, *A*). With the dorsum of the foot held in the palm of one hand and the guide pins with the palm of the other hand, both thumbs are placed on the plantar foot at the midportion of the calcaneus. The guide pins are levered plantarward while simultaneously plantar flexing the midfoot. The reduction of the tongue fragment is confirmed fluoroscopically with the midfoot still held in plantar flexion, and the guide pins are advanced into the anterior process region (Figure 4, *B*). A Broden view is obtained to assess the reduction of the articular surface; the position of the guide pin is confirmed with lateral, axial, and AP views.[15] Definitive fixation is achieved with either two large cannulated screws or multiple small fragment lag screws (Figure 4, *C* and *D*).

If the tongue fragment fails to disimpact, a small periosteal elevator may be used through a small stab inci-

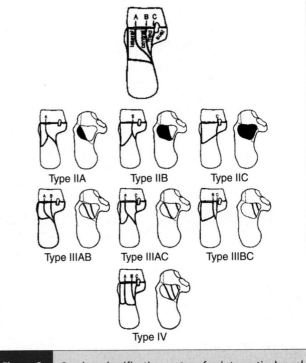

Type IIA	Type IIB	Type IIC
Type IIIAB	Type IIIAC	Type IIIBC
	Type IV	

Figure 3   Sanders classification system for intra-articular calcaneal fractures. This system uses the semi-coronal image with the widest undersurface of the posterior facet of the talus and is based on the number and location of articular fracture fragments. (*Reproduced with permission from Sanders R: Intra-articular fractures of the calcaneus: Present state of the art.* J Orthop Trauma 1992;6:252-265.)

sion to disimpact the fragment and assist with reduction. If widening remains between the sustentaculum and the articular portion of the tongue fragment in the coronal plane, a small fragment lag screw may be placed in the sustentaculum to narrow the posterior facet. If the tongue fragment is irreducible, the reduction is converted to a formal open reduction using a standard extensile lateral approach.

The percutaneous incisions are closed and a supportive splint is placed, with later conversion to a compression stocking and fracture boot to allow range-of-motion exercises; postoperative weight bearing is not permitted for 10 to 12 weeks.

Extensile Lateral Approach for Joint Depression-Type Fractures

The patient is placed in the lateral decubitus position on a beanbag. Attention to detail with respect to placement of the incision and gentle soft-tissue handling is of paramount importance because soft-tissue complications are a major cause of morbidity with these injuries.[16-19] A full-thickness, subperiosteal flap is raised and 1.6-mm Kirschner wires (K-wires) are placed in the fibula, talar neck, and cuboid, for retraction of the subperiosteal flap.

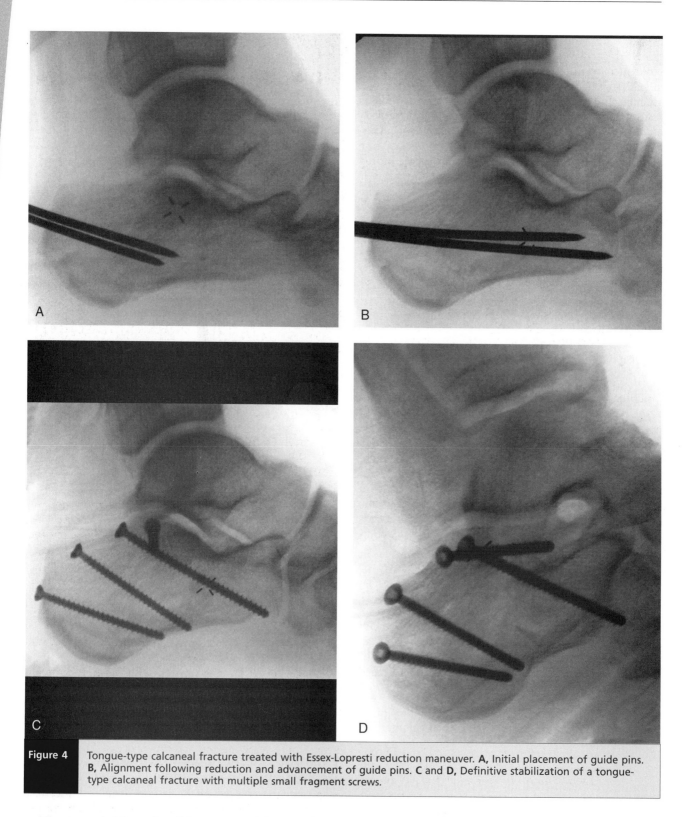

Figure 4 Tongue-type calcaneal fracture treated with Essex-Lopresti reduction maneuver. **A,** Initial placement of guide pins. **B,** Alignment following reduction and advancement of guide pins. **C** and **D,** Definitive stabilization of a tongue-type calcaneal fracture with multiple small fragment screws.

The expanded lateral wall fragment and impacted superolateral articular fragment are carefully mobilized and preserved in saline on the back table, which affords exposure of the superomedial fragment and the obliquely oriented primary fracture line (**Figure 5**). A blunt periosteal elevator is introduced into the primary fracture line and levered plantarward, thereby disimpacting the posterior main fragment from the superomedial fragment and restoring calcaneal height and length along the medial calcaneal wall[20] (**Figure 5**). A 4.5-mm Schanz pin is placed in the posteroinferior corner of the calcaneal tuberosity for further manipulation.[21]

Next, the anterior process fragments are pulled inferiorly and provisionally secured with 1.6-mm K-wires.

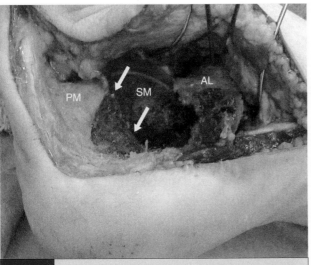

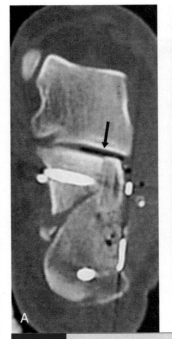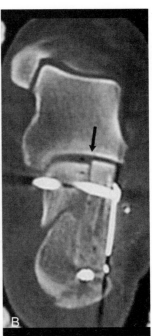

| **Figure 5** | Intraoperative view following excision of a lateral wall fragment and superolateral fragment. Mobilization through the primary fracture line (*arrows*). AL = anterolateral; SM = superomedial; PM = posterior main. |

| **Figure 6** | **A** and **B,** Sagittal plane rotational malalignment of superolateral fragment from inadequate "window visualization." **A,** Semicoronal image through the anterior portion of the posterior facet showing satisfactory intra-articular reduction (*arrow*). **B,** Semicoronal image through the posterior portion of the posterior facet showing intra-articular step-off (*arrow*). |

Variability in fracture lines through the anterior process is common, such that there may be three separate fragments and, as the anterolateral fragment is reduced, the central fragment may remain superiorly displaced. A lamina spreader then may be used to facilitate reduction of the central fragment. A transverse fracture line may be present through the crucial angle of Gissane, in essence rotating the superomedial fragment beneath the anterior main fragment. In this instance, before reduction of the superolateral articular fragment, the superomedial fragment must be derotated, reduced, and provisionally stabilized to the anterior main fragment to prevent malrotation of the entire posterior facet articular surface.

The superolateral fragment (Sanders type II fracture) is brought back into the wound and two parallel 1.6-mm K-wires are placed to facilitate reduction; in the event of two separate fragments (Sanders type III fracture), the central articular fragment is first reduced to the superomedial fragment and stabilized with 1.5-mm bioresorbable (poly-L-lactic acid) pins. The protruding ends of the bioresorbable pins are removed flush with the bony surface with a handheld electrocautery unit. The superolateral (lateral most articular) fragment is then reduced and provisionally stabilized with 1.6-mm K-wires to the central and superomedial fragments. The articular fragment(s) must be precisely reduced so that (superoinferior) height, (anteroposterior) rotation, and coronal plane (varus-valgus) alignment are correct. The articular reduction is verified through "window" visualization; the superolateral and superomedial fragments should align both anteriorly and posteriorly. Failure to visualize the posterior facet from both sides of the window may lead to malreduction of the fragment(s) in the sagittal plane (Figure 6).

At this point in the procedure, the posterior edge of the anterolateral fragment should "key" into the anteroinferior edge of the superolateral fragment, indicating restoration of the crucial angle of Gissane. The lateral wall and the body of the calcaneus should align with simple valgus manipulation of the Schanz pin and the previously excised lateral wall fragment should anatomically reduce, confirming (at the least) that the lateral column is anatomically restored. The reduction is then confirmed by intraoperative fluoroscopy, including lateral, Broden, and axial views.

The posterior facet is secured with 3.5-mm cortical lag screws placed just beneath the articular surface angling toward the sustentaculum. A low-profile lateral neutralization plate is then selected and secured with 4.0-mm cancellous screws, starting with the most distal screw holes overlying the anterior process. The oblique orientation of the calcaneocuboid articulation is accommodated by aiming slightly posteriorly. Screw placement on power will bring the plate to bone, restoring calcaneal width. Next, the calcaneal tuberosity is secured to the plate while maintaining a simultaneous lateral-to-medial force on the plate and a valgus-directed force on the tuberosity. The main components of the calcaneus (anterior process, posterior tuberosity, and articular surface) are further secured to the plate so that a minimum of two screws traverse each component (Figure 7).

2: Foot and Ankle Trauma

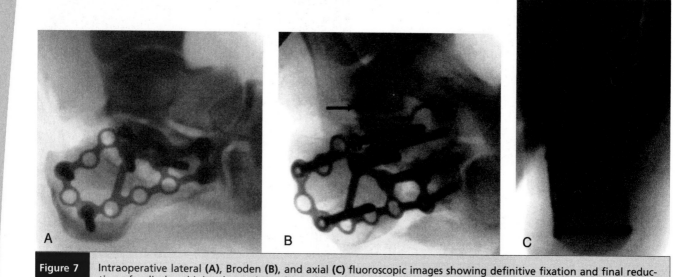

Figure 7 Intraoperative lateral **(A)**, Broden **(B)**, and axial **(C)** fluoroscopic images showing definitive fixation and final reduction of a displaced joint depression calcaneal fracture.

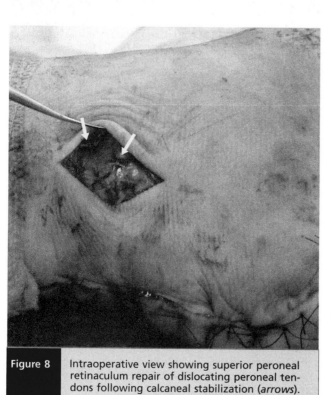

Figure 8 Intraoperative view showing superior peroneal retinaculum repair of dislocating peroneal tendons following calcaneal stabilization (*arrows*).

The peroneal tendons are assessed for stability by advancing a Freer elevator within the peroneal tendon sheath to the level of the lateral malleolus and levering forward. If the superior peroneal retinaculum and tendon sheath are unstable, the elevator will easily slide anterior to the fibula, in which case a tendon sheath repair is required (**Figure 8**). The full-thickness flap is closed over a deep drain with deep No. 0 absorbable sutures placed starting at the proximal and distal ends and progressing toward the apex of the incision. The sutures are hand tied sequentially in similar fashion to eliminate tension at the apex of the incision. The skin layer is closed with 3-0 monofilament sutures using the modified Allgöwer-Donati technique.

After splint immobilization, conversion to a compression stocking and fracture boot occurs at 3 weeks postoperatively and range-of-motion exercises are begun. The sutures are removed once the incision is fully sealed and dry, typically at 3 to 4 weeks; however, weight bearing is not initiated until 10 to 12 weeks postoperatively.

Combined (Open and Closed) Techniques for Split Tongue Fractures

Intra-articular tongue-type patterns (Sanders types IIA, IIB, and III) require an extensile lateral approach because of the pull of the Achilles tendon on the fragment, which often precludes reduction of the lateral articular tongue fragment in proper sagittal plane rotation. For such fractures, the Essex-Lopresti reduction technique is performed on the tongue fragment in an open fashion and a 4.5-mm Schanz pin is placed percutaneously into the tongue fragment, which neutralizes the deforming forces of the Achilles tendon and allows anatomic reduction of the articular surface in the sagittal plane (Figure 9). The remainder of the procedure is then completed as previously described.

Other Percutaneous Techniques

A recent study described minimally invasive reduction techniques combined with small fragment fixation for tongue-type fractures.[22] Small incisions are used for the placement of Schanz pins, small periosteal elevators assist with the reduction in combination with the Essex-Lopresti reduction maneuver, and multiple small fragment screws then are used axially and laterally. Although technically demanding, these applications can

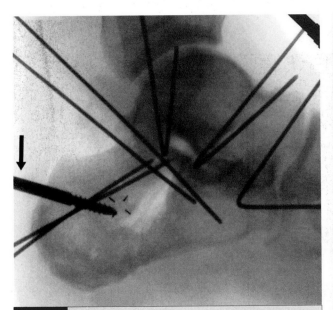

Figure 9 Radiograph showing the Essex-Lopresti technique for intra-articular, split tongue, fracture patterns. Note the Schanz pin (*arrow*) within the tongue fragment to neutralize the pull of the Achilles tendon.

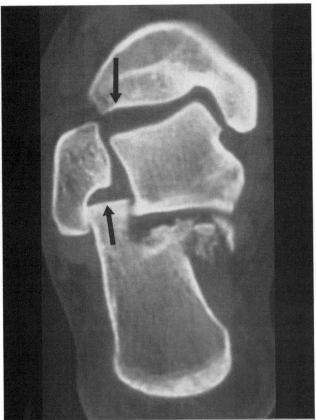

Figure 10 Coronal CT image showing a fracture-dislocation of the calcaneus. Note varus tilt within the ankle mortise and the posterolateral fragment wedged within the talofibular joint (*arrows*).

be expanded to include certain simple joint depression-type fractures (Sanders type IIA or IIB) by controlling the articular reduction with subtalar arthroscopy. Fine-wire external fixation may alternatively be used in this instance, particularly for those patients with open fractures or a compromised soft-tissue envelope.[23]

Fracture-Dislocation Patterns

Fracture-dislocation patterns are relatively rare and occur when the superolateral fragment remains contiguous with the lateral wall and posterior tuberosity.[24-26] The resulting large lateral fragment dislocates laterally and is forcefully driven into the talofibular joint, often producing a fracture of the lateral malleolus. Because of the generally high-energy nature of the injury, the peroneal tendons typically dislocate anteriorly, and the lateral ligamentous complex of the ankle joint is disrupted. With recoil of the limb, there is inversion of the hindfoot through the ankle joint, which is manifest radiographically as increased lateral talar tilt. CT shows the typical fracture-dislocation pattern (**Figure 10**).

The fracture pattern is most commonly a simple two-part split fracture, such that as the dislocation is reduced, the articular fragments typically align anatomically. As with most dislocations, the sooner the reduction, the easier the reduction tends to be. If treatment is delayed, a formal open reduction usually is required. The patient is placed in the lateral decubitus position. A blunt periosteal elevator is introduced through a small stab incision at the superior edge of the lateral tuberosity fragment and advanced inferiorly along the medial surface of the fragment until positioned at the inferolateral edge of the talus within the subtalar joint.

The lateral tuberosity fragment is then gently levered plantarward; the fragment will typically reduce once it clears the inferolateral edge of the talus. Definitive fixation of the fracture is typically completed in percutaneous fashion with cortical lag screws, in combination with repair of the lateral ligamentous complex of the ankle and superior peroneal retinaculum. The limb is immobilized for 6 weeks postoperatively to allow healing of the soft-tissue repair; weight bearing is initiated at 10 to 12 weeks.

Open Calcaneus Fractures

Open fractures of the calcaneus are distinct injuries relative to closed fractures and are generally associated with a higher complication rate, including deep infection, osteomyelitis, and amputation.[27-30] The degree of soft-tissue injury is the most important variable predicting outcome, and the incidence of major complications seems to increase with the increasing severity of the soft-tissue injury.[29,30] Open fractures of the calcaneus may present with a puncture wound medially from a spike of bone or with a more significant soft-tissue injury, typically laterally or posteriorly.

Treatment includes antibiotic prophylaxis, irrigation, and débridement of the wound. All open type I fractures and type II fractures with a medial wound are

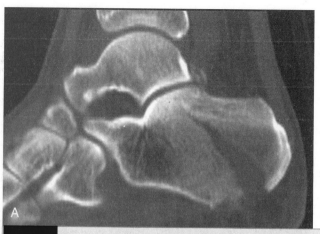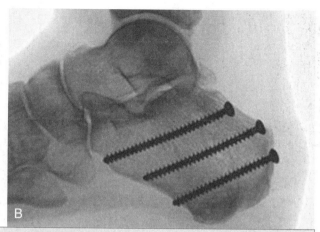

Figure 11 **A,** Sagittal CT image showing a calcaneal beak fracture. **B,** Lateral radiograph following fixation with multiple small fragment screws.

treated with delayed open reduction and internal fixation (ORIF) once the soft tissues are suitably healed for surgery. Open type II fractures with a nonmedial wound and all open type IIIA wounds are treated with percutaneous stabilization and/or external fixation; all open type IIIB wounds are best managed by late reconstruction.[29]

ORIF and Primary Arthrodesis for Sanders Type IV Fractures

ORIF with primary subtalar arthrodesis is indicated only for highly comminuted intra-articular fractures in which the articular surface is determined to be nonreconstructable.[11,31] Standard ORIF techniques are used, such that calcaneal height, length, and overall morphology are fully reestablished. The remaining articular cartilage is removed from the corresponding surfaces of the posterior facet, the subchondral surfaces are drilled with a 2.5-mm drill bit for vascular ingrowth, and supplemental cancellous allograft is placed within the subtalar joint. With the subtalar joint held in neutral alignment, definitive fixation for the arthrodesis is obtained with two large (6.5-mm to 8.0-mm) cannulated screws placed from posterior to anterior in diverging fashion perpendicular to the plane of the posterior facet. One of the 3.5-mm cortical lag screws may need to be removed and subsequently redirected to allow placement of the larger cannulated screws; ideally, the lag screw placed through the plate is preserved to maintain continuity between the posterior facet and the remainder of the calcaneus. Serial short leg casts are used for 10 to 12 weeks, after which radiographic union of both the fracture and the arthrodesis should be confirmed.

Extra-articular Fractures

Extra-articular fractures, which account for up to 30% of all calcaneal fractures, are typically the result of lower energy injuries, such as a twisting injury or avulsion of bone from strong pull of a ligament or tendon. Because of the lower energy involved, pain and swelling tend to be more localized directly over the fracture. Treatment is generally based on the size, location, and overall displacement of the involved fracture fragments.

Calcaneal Beak and Tuberosity Fractures

Fractures of the calcaneal tuberosity usually result from a violent pull of the gastrocnemius-soleus complex, such as occurs with forced dorsiflexion following a stumble and fall. The resulting fragment is of variable size and typically includes the entire Achilles tendon insertion[2,32,33] (**Figure 11,** *A*). Patients have weakness with resisted plantar flexion and a positive Thompson test because of the shortened Achilles tendon. Marked displacement of the fracture fragment may endanger the surrounding skin, which may necessitate expedient care of the fracture to avoid skin slough. This fracture is distinct from a tongue-type fracture because there are no other fracture lines within the calcaneus.

Nondisplaced fractures may be treated with non–weight-bearing cast immobilization in equinus for 6 weeks, followed by range-of-motion exercises and progressive weight bearing. Surgical treatment is indicated if the posterior skin is at risk for skin slough because of pressure from displacement of the fragment or if displacement and shortening of the fragment results in incompetence of the gastrocnemius-soleus complex. Because of the potential for soft-tissue interposition, this fracture requires an open anatomic reduction through a lateral paratendinous approach, and lag screw fixation either with large cannulated screws or small fragment screws (**Figure 11,** *B*). Fixation may be further supplemented with a tension-band construct. The limb is immobilized in equinus to neutralize the pull of the Achilles tendon. At 2 weeks postoperatively, the immobilization method is converted to a compression stocking and fracture boot with a 1.5- to 2-inch heel lift to allow range-of-motion exercises; weight bearing is initiated at 8 to 10 weeks postoperatively.

Body Fractures (Sanders Type I)

Fractures of the calcaneal body are true extra-articular fractures and generally are the result of similar injury mechanisms to those that cause intra-articular fractures, but with lower energy involved. CT usually is necessary to confirm the absence of intra-articular extension and the extent of displacement. Nonsurgical treatment is indicated for nondisplaced or minimally displaced fractures.[2] Surgical treatment is reserved for fractures with significant displacement, such as varus or valgus malalignment of more than 30° or more than 1 cm medial or lateral translation of the calcaneal tuberosity; those with sufficient expansion of the lateral calcaneal wall to cause peroneal tendon impingement; or fractures with loss of calcaneal height that affects gastrocnemius function.[2,18,19] In these instances, allowing the fracture to heal in situ would result in unacceptable calcaneal malunion, even in the absence of intra-articular extension.

Sustentaculum Fractures

Sustentaculum fractures are the result of axial load and forced inversion of the hindfoot and are rare. The fracture can be difficult to visualize on standard radiographs; CT evaluation typically is necessary to determine intra-articular extension and the extent of displacement. Surgical treatment is indicated for fractures with more than 2 mm of displacement or extension into the posterior facet[34] (Figure 12).

The sustentaculum is exposed through the floor of the flexor digitorum longus tendon sheath; the adjacent neurovascular bundle is protected and the tibiocalcaneal portion of the deltoid ligament is preserved to avoid destabilization of the medial hindfoot. The fracture is provisionally reduced and held with 1.2- to 1.6-mm K-wires; the reduction is confirmed with fluoroscopic lateral and Broden views. Definitive fixation is achieved with small or minifragment lag screws (depending on the size of the fragment) placed parallel to the posterior facet. A meticulous, layered closure is completed and range-of-motion exercises are started at 2 weeks postoperatively; weight bearing is initiated at 10 to 12 weeks postoperatively.

Anterior Process Fractures

Anterior process fractures typically result from forced inversion and plantar flexion of the foot, which produces an avulsion fracture through tension on the bifurcate ligament.[35,36] The fracture line exits in the calcaneocuboid joint and typically involves only a minimal portion of the articular surface. These fractures also may result from forced abduction of the foot, which produces a higher energy impaction injury to the calcaneocuboid articular surface.[37] With this particular mechanism, there is more involvement of the articular surface and the fragment is typically larger and may

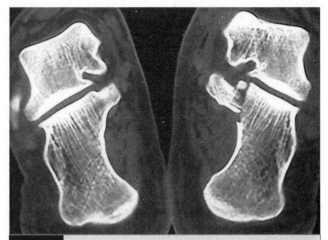

Figure 12 Coronal CT image showing a sustentaculum fracture. Note more than 2 mm of displacement and slight extension into the posterior facet.

displace superiorly. CT evaluation is often necessary to determine the extent of intra-articular involvement. Smaller fragments with minimal intra-articular involvement can be treated nonsurgically; surgical treatment is reserved for larger, displaced fragments with significant intra-articular involvement (> 25% of calcaneocuboid articulation) or those fractures that occur as part of an unstable midfoot injury.[7,34,38]

With the patient supine, the anterior process of the calcaneus is identified just distal to the sinus tarsi. The extensor digitorum brevis muscle is mobilized, exposing the calcaneocuboid joint. The fracture is reduced and provisionally stabilized with 1.2- to 1.6-mm K-wires. Definitive fixation is obtained with small or minifragment screws. Excessively comminuted fragments too small to accept fixation may be primarily excised; however, every attempt should be made to preserve as much articular surface as possible. Range-of-motion exercises are initiated at 2 weeks postoperatively; weight bearing is not permitted for 8 to 10 weeks postoperatively.

Complications

Delayed Wound Healing and Wound Dehiscence

The most common complication following surgical treatment of a calcaneal fracture is wound dehiscence, which occurs in up to 25% of patients.[11,21,28,30,39-42] Despite relatively easy approximation at the time of surgical closure, the wound may later separate, typically at the apex of the incision; dehiscence may occur at up to 4 weeks following surgery. Most wounds ultimately heal. Deep infection and osteomyelitis develops in 1% to 4% of closed fractures.[11,28,39-41,43]

If wound dehiscence occurs, all range-of-motion exercises are discontinued to prevent further wound separation. The wound is treated with serial whirlpool treat-

2: Foot and Ankle Trauma

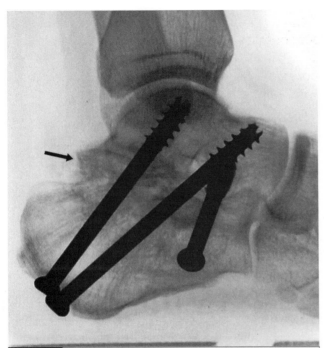

Figure 13 Lateral radiograph showing definitive stabilization of a type II calcaneal malunion. Note position of the subtalar autograft bone block (*arrow*).

pared and the resected lateral wall fragment is placed within the subtalar joint as an autograft bone block and stabilized with two large cannulated screws as previously described.[13,51,54] A third screw may be placed extending from the anterior process region into the talar neck and head (**Figure 13**). For a type III malunion, correction of angular malalignment in the calcaneal tuberosity is completed before implant placement. A Dwyer-type closing wedge osteotomy is used for varus malalignment and a medial displacement calcaneal osteotomy is used for valgus malalignment.[13,54] Weight bearing and range-of-motion exercises are begun for type I malunions after the incision has healed, whereas those with type II or type III malunions are not permitted to bear weight for 10 to 12 weeks postoperatively.

Compartment Syndrome of the Leg and Foot

The Leg

Compartment syndrome of the leg is a well known condition that is caused by increased pressure in the structurally limited compartments of the leg. The increased intracompartmental pressure that leads to clinical compartment syndrome is generally initiated by trauma, with the increased pressure occurring secondary to intracompartmental swelling or bleeding. The disease state is generally initiated by high-energy trauma, such as a displaced tibial fracture, or from cumulative repetitive stress in the leg, such as occurs in marathon runners. Compartment syndrome also has been initiated by certain types of positioning in comatose patients or those with altered or impaired mental status, or by surgical positioning in the lithotomy or prone positions.

The resultant pathophysiology of compartment syndrome is caused by increased tissue pressure within a closed compartmental space. At some point, the increased venous pressure exceeds the arterial pressure and occludes arterial inflow, leading to ischemic death of muscle tissue within the involved compartment. The classic five "Ps" (pain, pallor, paresthesia, paralysis, and a pulseless limb) should cause a heightened index of suspicion for compartment syndrome. Symptoms progress from pain in the involved extremity, followed by the nebulous finding of pallor. Irreversible muscle damage has occurred by the time paresthesia develops. Compartmental paralysis affects the muscles before the limb becomes pulseless.

Pain elicited by passively extending or stretching a muscle within the involved compartment is the classic physical finding of compartment syndrome. Pressures in the compartments of the leg or arm can be measured with a mercury manometer, commercial pressure-sensing catheter, or pressure transducer attached to a catheter placed within the suspected compartment. Treatment involves urgent surgical fasciotomy of any involved compartments to alleviate intracompartmental pressure and restore arterial inflow. The end result of

ments, damp-to-dry dressing changes, and oral antibiotics. Alternatively, cast immobilization may be instituted with window access for dressing changes. Once the wound heals, range-of-motion exercises are reinstituted. A negative pressure device (Vacuum-Assisted Closure, KCI, San Antonio, TX) may be used for recalcitrant wounds.[43]

Posttraumatic Arthritis

A principal goal of internal fixation is anatomic restoration of the posterior facet articular surface. Posttraumatic arthritis may develop even in patients in whom a truly anatomic reduction is achieved, as a result of cartilage damage at the time of injury.[10] In these instances, because calcaneal height and morphology have already been restored, implant removal and an in situ subtalar arthrodesis may be performed.[10,44-46]

Calcaneal Malunion

Nonsurgical treatment of a displaced intra-articular calcaneal fracture typically results in a calcaneal malunion with significant associated sequelae.[11,13,47-54] Standard weight-bearing radiographs show the calcaneal malunion, which is further defined by evaluation of CT scans. Treatment is based on the Stephens-Sanders classification system.[13,54]

Through an extensile lateral approach, a lateral wall exostectomy and peroneal tenolysis is completed for all three malunion types.[49] In patients with a type II or III malunion, the subtalar joint articular surface is pre-

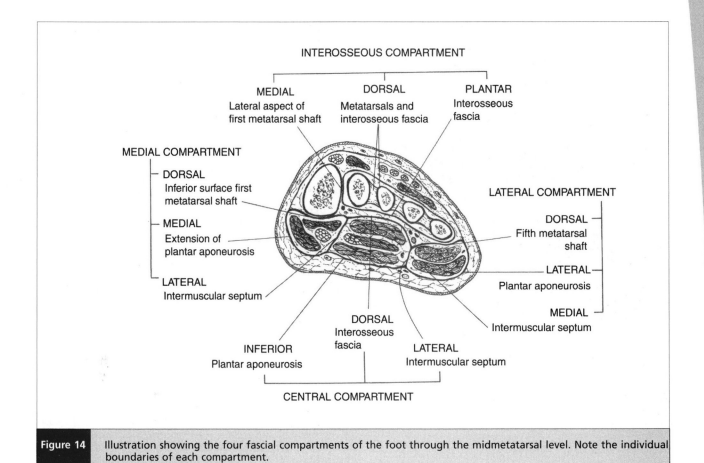

INTEROSSEOUS COMPARTMENT

MEDIAL
Lateral aspect of
first metatarsal shaft

DORSAL
Metatarsals and
interosseous fascia

PLANTAR
Interosseous
fascia

MEDIAL COMPARTMENT

DORSAL
Inferior surface first
metatarsal shaft

MEDIAL
Extension of
plantar aponeurosis

LATERAL
Intermuscular septum

LATERAL COMPARTMENT

DORSAL
Fifth metatarsal
shaft

LATERAL
Plantar aponeurosis

MEDIAL
Intermuscular septum

DORSAL
Interosseous
fascia

INFERIOR
Plantar aponeurosis

LATERAL
Intermuscular septum

CENTRAL COMPARTMENT

Figure 14 Illustration showing the four fascial compartments of the foot through the midmetatarsal level. Note the individual boundaries of each compartment.

compartment syndrome is a severe long-term negative impact on the health-related quality of life.[55]

The Foot

Four compartments of the foot have been described[56] (Figure 14). The diagnosis of compartment syndrome in the foot must be based on a high index of suspicion for the condition because passively stretching the foot is an unreliable examination technique and accepted normal compartment pressures have not been established. Surgery to relieve pressure can be performed using two dorsal incisions or one medial incision (Figures 15 and 16).

Late Reconstruction

The goal of late reconstruction following compartment syndrome of the foot is to provide a plantigrade foot without static structural deformity and to allow the patient to wear standard shoe wear. Excision of scarred muscle tenotomies and correction of structural deformities of the toes are recommended.[57]

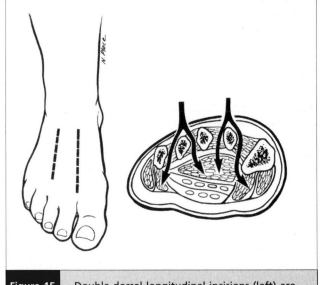

Figure 15 Double dorsal longitudinal incisions (left) are used to decompress all four compartments (right).

Summary

Calcaneal fractures are among the most challenging of the lower extremity fractures, with a variety of com-

plex, three-dimensional fracture patterns necessitating specific treatment methods and techniques. Arthroscopically controlled percutaneous fixation techniques, although technically demanding, may prove increasingly

2: Foot and Ankle Trauma

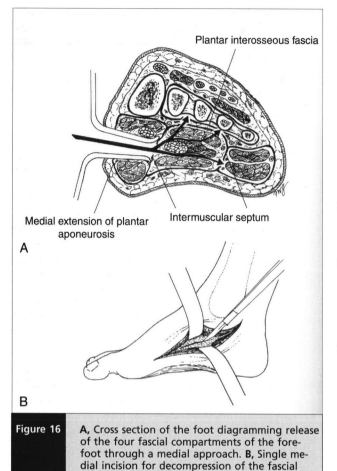

Plantar interosseous fascia

Medial extension of plantar
aponeurosis

Intermuscular septum

A

B

Figure 16 **A,** Cross section of the foot diagramming release of the four fascial compartments of the fore-foot through a medial approach. **B,** Single medial incision for decompression of the fascial compartments of the foot. Proximal extension is used for decompression of the calcaneal compartment and the tarsal tunnel.

useful, particularly in patients with certain amenable fracture patterns.

Annotated References

1. Lindsay WR, Dewar FP: Fractures of the os calcis. *Am J Surg* 1958;95:555-576.

2. Rowe CR, Sakellarides H, Freeman P, Sorbie C: Fractures of os calcis: A long term follow-up study of one hundred forty-six patients. *JAMA* 1963;184:920.

3. Burdeaux BD: Reduction of calcaneal fractures by the McReynolds medial approach technique and its experimental basis. *Clin Orthop Relat Res* 1983;177:87-103.

4. Carr JB, Hamilton JJ, Bear LS: Experimental intra-articular calcaneal fractures: Anatomic basis for a new classification. *Foot Ankle* 1989;10:81-87.

5. Essex-Lopresti P: The mechanism, reduction technique, and results in fractures of the os calcis. *Br J Surg* 1952; 39:395-419.

6. Palmer I: The mechanism and treatment of fractures of the calcaneus. *J Bone Joint Surg Am* 1948;30:2-8.

7. Isherwood I: A radiographic approach to the subtalar joint. *J Bone Joint Surg Br* 1961;43:566-574.

8. Sanders R: Displaced intra-articular fractures of the calcaneus. *J Bone Joint Surg Am* 2000;82:225-250.

9. Sanders R: Intra-articular fractures of the calcaneus: Present state of the art. *J Orthop Trauma* 1992;6:252-265.

10. Crosby LA, Fitzgibbons T: Computerized tomography scanning of acute intra-articular fractures of the calcaneus. *J Bone Joint Surg Am* 1990;72:852-859.

11. Sanders R, Fortin P, DiPasquale T, Walling A: Operative treatment in 120 displaced intraarticular calcaneal fractures: Results using a prognostic computed tomography scan classification. *Clin Orthop Relat Res* 1993; 290:87-95.

12. Herscovici D Jr , Widmaier J, Scaduto JM, Sanders RW, Walling A: Operative treatment of calcaneal fractures in elderly patients. *J Bone Joint Surg Am* 2005;87:1260-1264.

   The authors present the results of a retrospective case study of patients 65 years or older who underwent surgical treatment of a calcaneal fracture. Results and complication rates were comparable to previously published results for younger patients. Careful patient selection is recommended. Level of evidence: IV.

13. Clare MP, Lee WE III, Sanders RW: Intermediate to long-term results of a treatment protocol for calcaneal fracture malunions. *J Bone Joint Surg Am* 2005;87:963-973.

   This retrospective comparative study evaluated longer term results of a previously described CT-based classification system and treatment protocol for calcaneal malunions. The protocol was effective in improving pain and function, although restoration of calcaneal morphology proved difficult in this subset of patients. Level of evidence: III.

14. Tornetta P III: The Essex-Lopresti reduction for calcaneal fractures revisited. *J Orthop Trauma* 1998;12:469-473.

15. Broden B: Roentgen examination of the subtaloid joint in fractures of the calcaneus. *Acta Radiol* 1949;31:85-91.

16. Borrelli J Jr, Lashgari C: Vascularity of the lateral calcaneal flap: A cadaveric injection study. *J Orthop Trauma* 1999;13:73-77.

17. Gould N: Lateral approach to the os calcis. *Foot Ankle* 1984;4:218-220.

18. Sanders RW, Clare MP: Fractures of the calcaneus, in

Bucholz RW, Heckman JD, Court-Brown C (eds): *Rockwood and Green's Fractures in Adults*, ed 6. Philadelphia, PA, Lippincott Williams & Wilkins, 2006, pp 2293-2336.

A comprehensive review of calcaneal fracture pathoanatomy, evaluation, and management, including historical perspectives is presented along with current literature analysis and in-depth descriptions of surgical techniques.

19. Sanders RW, Clare MP: Fractures of the calcaneus, in Coughlin MJ, Mann RA, Saltzman CL (eds): *Surgery of the Foot and Ankle*, ed 8. Philadelphia, PA, Mosby Elsevier, 2007, pp 2017-2073.

    The authors present a comprehensive review of calcaneal fracture pathoanatomy, evaluation, and management, including in-depth descriptions of surgical techniques.

20. Eastwood DM, Langkamer VG, Atkins RM: Intra-articular fractures of the calcaneum: Part II. Open reduction and internal fixation by the extended lateral transcalcaneal approach. *J Bone Joint Surg Br* 1993;75:189-195.

21. Benirschke SK, Sangeorzan BJ: Extensive intraarticular fractures of the foot: Surgical management of calcaneal fractures. *Clin Orthop Relat Res* 1993;292:128-134.

22. Rammelt S, Amlang M, Barthel S, Zwipp H: Minimally-invasive treatment of calcaneal fractures. *Injury* 2004; 35(suppl 2):SB55-SB63.

    The authors present a review of patients with two-part intra-articular calcaneal fracture patterns treated with percutaneous reduction and screw fixation, controlled by subtalar arthroscopy. The authors report favorable results, but caution against uniform application of percutaneous techniques to all calcaneal fractures.

23. McGarvey WC, Burris MW, Clanton TO, Melissinos EG: Calcaneal fractures: Indirect reduction and external fixation. *Foot Ankle Int* 2006;27:494-499.

    The authors present the results of a series of patients treated with percutaneous reduction and fine wire external fixation. This technique is a viable alternative, particularly for patients with open fractures or a compromised soft-tissue envelope.

24. Eastwood DM, Maxwell AC, Atkins RM: Fracture of the lateral malleolus with talar tilt: Primarily a calcaneal fracture not an ankle injury. *Injury* 1993;24:109-112.

25. Ebraheim NA, Elgafy H, Sabry FF, Tao S: Calcaneus fractures with subluxation of the posterior facet: A surgical indication. *Clin Orthop Relat Res* 2000;377:210-216.

26. Turner NS, Haidukewych GJ: Locked fracture dislocation of the calcaneus treated with minimal open reduction and percutaneous fixation: A report of two cases and review of the literature. *Foot Ankle Int* 2003;24:796-800.

A case report of two fracture-dislocation patterns treated with minimal open reduction and percutaneous screw fixation is presented. Detailed surgical technique is described.

27. Aldridge JM III, Easley M, Nunley JA: Open calcaneal fractures: Results of operative treatment. *J Orthop Trauma* 2004;18:7-11.

    The authors report on a retrospective case study of patients with open calcaneal fractures managed by a standardized treatment protocol and various fixation techniques. Results included a lower complication rate than previously reported.

28. Benirschke SK, Kramer PA: Wound healing complications in closed and open calcaneal fractures. *J Orthop Trauma* 2004;18:1-6.

    The authors report on a retrospective review of wound complication rates in a large series of patients with both closed and open calcaneal fractures treated by standard fixation techniques through an extensile lateral approach. The authors concluded that patient compliance was the most important factor in preventing wound complications.

29. Heier KA, Infante AF, Walling AK, Sanders RW: Open fractures of the calcaneus: Soft-tissue injury determines outcome. *J Bone Joint Surg Am* 2003;85:2276-2282.

    In this retrospective prognostic study of patients with open calcaneal fractures treated according to a standardized protocol, definitive fixation methods were dependent on wound location and severity. The authors concluded that the extent of soft-tissue injury was prognostic of outcome. Level of evidence: II-1.

30. Folk JW, Starr AJ, Early JS: Early wound complications of operative treatment of calcaneus fractures: Analysis of 190 fractures. *J Orthop Trauma* 1999;13:369-372.

31. Clare MP, Sanders RW: Open reduction and internal fixation with primary subtalar arthrodesis for Sanders type IV calcaneus fractures. *Tech Foot Ankle Surg* 2004; 3:250-257.

    The authors of this technique-based article review surgical management of Sanders type IV calcaneal fractures.

32. Dieterle JO: A case of so-called "open-beak" fracture of the os calcis. *J Bone Joint Surg Am* 1940;22:740.

33. Rothberg AS: Avulsion fractures of the os calcis. *J Bone Joint Surg Am* 1939;21:218-220.

34. Clare MP: Occult injuries about the subtalar joint, in Nunley JA, Pfeffer GB, Sanders RW, Trepman E (eds): *Advanced Reconstruction: Foot and Ankle*. Rosemont, IL, American Academy of Orthopaedic Surgeons, 2004, pp 385-391.

    The author reviews the diagnosis and management of subtle fracture patterns about the subtalar joint.

35. Gellman M: Fractures of the anterior process of the calcaneus. *J Bone Joint Surg Am* 1951;33:382-386.

2: Foot and Ankle Trauma

36. Jahss MH, Kay B: An anatomic study of the anterior superior process of the os calcis and its clinical application. *Foot Ankle* 1983;3:268-281.

37. Hunt DD: Compression fracture of the anterior articular surface of the calcaneus. *J Bone Joint Surg Am* 1970; 52:1637-1642.

38. Rothberg AS: Avulsion fractures of the os calcis. *J Bone Joint Surg Am* 1939;21:218-220.

39. Harvey EJ, Grujic L, Early JS, Benirschke SK, Sangeorzan BJ: Morbidity associated with ORIF of intra-articular calcaneus fractures using a lateral approach. *Foot Ankle Int* 2001;22:868-873.

40. Howard JL, Buckley R, McCormack R, Pate G, Leighton R, Petrie D: Complications following management of displaced intra-articular calcaneal fractures: A prospective randomized trial comparing open reduction internal fixation with nonoperative management. *J Orthop Trauma* 2003;17:241-249.

    This large multicenter trial compared complication rates in patients with surgical versus nonsurgical treatment of displaced intra-articular calcaneal fractures. Patients treated surgically had higher outcome scores and higher complication rates; the development of posttraumatic subtalar arthritis was six times more likely in those treated nonsurgically.

41. Levin LS, Nunley JA: The management of soft-tissue problems associated with calcaneal fractures. *Clin Orthop Relat Res* 1993;290:151-160.

42. Lim EV, Leung JP: Complications of intraarticular calcaneal fractures. *Clin Orthop Relat Res* 2001;391:7-16.

43. Herscovici D Jr, Sanders RW, Scatudo JM, Infante A, DiPasquale T: Vacuum-assisted wound closure (VAC therapy) for the management of patients with high-energy soft tissue injuries. *J Orthop Trauma* 2003;17: 683-688.

    The authors report on a case study of patients with high-energy soft-tissue injuries treated with a vacuum-assisted closure device. The authors concluded that the device is a viable adjunct to treatment and may alleviate the need for free-tissue transfer in certain patients.

44. Flemister AS Jr , Infante AF, Sanders RW, Walling AK: Subtalar arthrodesis for complications of intra-articular calcaneal fractures. *Foot Ankle Int* 2000;21:392-399.

45. Sanders R, Fortin P, Walling A: Subtalar arthrodesis following calcaneal fracture. *Orthop Trans* 1991;15:656.

46. Radnay CS, Sagi HC, Clare MP, Sanders RW: Subtalar fusion after displaced intra-articular calcaneal fractures: Does initial operative treatment matter? *J Bone Joint Surg Am*, in press.

    This retrospective cohort study compares outcomes for patients initially treated by ORIF who required late subtalar arthrodesis with patients with calcaneal malunions treated according to a previously published treatment protocol. The authors report superior results in patients treated with initial surgical management.

47. Braly WG, Bishop JO, Tullos HS: Lateral decompression for malunited os calcis fractures. *Foot Ankle* 1985; 6:90-96.

48. Carr JB, Hansen ST, Benirschke SK: Subtalar distraction bone block fusion for late complications of os calcis fractures. *Foot Ankle* 1988;9:81-86.

49. Cotton FJ: Old os calcis fractures. *Ann Surg* 1921;74: 294-303.

50. Gallie WE: Subastragalar arthrodesis in fractures of the os calcis. *J Bone Joint Surg Am* 1943;25:731-736.

51. Kalamchi A, Evans J: Posterior subtalar fusion. *J Bone Joint Surg Br* 1977;59:287-289.

52. Myerson M, Quill GE: Late complications of fractures of the calcaneus. *J Bone Joint Surg Am* 1993;75:331-341.

53. Isbister JF: Calcaneo-fibular abutment following crush fracture of the calcaneus. *J Bone Joint Surg Br* 1974;56: 274-278.

54. Stephens HM, Sanders R: Calcaneal malunions: Results of a prognostic computed tomography classification system. *Foot Ankle Int* 1996;17:395-401.

55. Giannoudis PV, Nicolopoulos C, Dinopoulos H, Ng A, Adedapo S, Kind P: The impact of lower leg compartment syndrome on health related quality of life. *Injury* 2002;33:117-121.

56. Manoli A II, Weber TG: An anatomical study with special reference to release of the calcaneal compartment. *Foot Ankle* 1990;10:267-275.

57. Perry MD, Manoli A II: Reconstruction of the foot after leg or foot compartment syndrome. *Foot Ankle Clin* 2006;11:191-201.

    Compartment syndrome of the leg or foot should be treated early to avoid late complications. The goal of late reconstruction is to provide a plantigrade functional foot. Complete excision of scarred muscle appears to prevent recurrence of deformity. Early tenotomy may prevent late deformities. Deformities of the toes should be corrected to allow the use of standard shoe wear.

Chapter 8

Talus Fractures and Reconstruction: An Overview

Amy Jo Ptaszek, MD

Introduction

Talus fractures are generally the result of high-energy impact. Up to 20% of these fractures are open and 25% are associated with medial malleolus fractures.[1,2] The incidence of talus fractures, specifically talar neck fractures, is increasing secondary to the survivability of patients involved in motor vehicle collisions.

The talus is pivotally important in hindfoot mechanics and is vulnerable to injury. It relies heavily on direct blood supply, although cartilage covers 60% to 70% of its surface. These anatomic constraints pose significant risks for complications following injury. The shape of the talus controls the motion and interaction of the ankle, subtalar, and talonavicular complex joints. Vertical weight-bearing forces are transferred into the horizontal structures of the foot through articulation with the talus.

Diagnostic Evaluation

The soft-tissue envelope of the foot and ankle should be carefully evaluated for edema, fracture blistering, vascular embarrassment, and/or deformity associated with dislocation. Radiographs should include ankle mortise, AP, and lateral views, as well as a modified AP Canale view, which is obtained by pronating the foot 15° while the x-ray beam is directed 75° from the horizontal plane of the table. The Canale view provides direct AP visualization of the talar neck. Broden and Anthonsen views allow observation of the posterior and middle facets of the subtalar joint. Thin-cut CT scans in the coronal and axial planes with sagittal reconstruction help determine the surgical approach, placement of fixation, and locate impediments to reduction if fracture impaction is present. Associated injuries also should be assessed.

Anatomy

The talus relies on a direct blood supply from the posterior, anterior, and peroneal arteries. The talar head and neck are supplied with blood via an arterial sling branching from the dorsalis pedis. The talar body is supplied via an arterial sling extending from the tarsal canal to the sinus tarsi. The neck itself deviates medially and plantarly approximately 24°; this alignment should be duplicated with fracture fixation.

Talar Neck Fractures

The primary mechanism of injury in fractures of the talar neck is hyperdorsiflexion with axial loading of the foot against a fixed tibia. A cascade of injury ensues depending on the degree of dorsiflexion and the inversion force. Hawkins type II and III patterns occur as the posterior capsule and peritalar constraints rupture. Subtalar subluxation and/or dislocation (type II), ankle dislocation (type III), or both types may occur. Medial comminution increases with inversion stress and/or osteopenia or osteoporosis. This type of injury also may be associated with talar head subluxation or dislocation (type IV).

Classification

The Hawkins classification system is based on the degree of displacement and congruity of the subtalar, tibiotalar, and talonavicular joints (**Table 1**). The Hawkins system is a prognostic classification system because

Table 1

Hawkins Classification System for Talar Neck Fractures

Type I	Nondisplaced fracture (includes incomplete fractures)
Type II	Displaced fracture with subtalar subluxation or dislocation; the ankle mortise remains intact
Type III	Displaced fracture with the body subluxated or dislocated from both the subtalar and tibiotalar joints
Type IV	Same as type III with subluxation or dislocation of the talonavicular joint

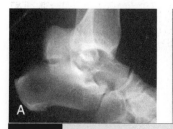
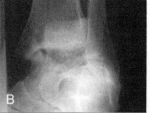

Figure 1 | Lateral (A) and AP (B) radiographs of Hawkins type III talar neck fracture-dislocations with an associated medial malleolus fracture.

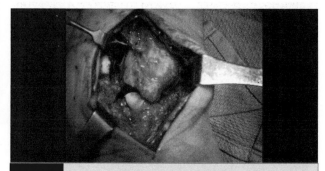

Figure 2 | Intraoperative view of the talar neck fracture-dislocation shown in Figure 1. The extensile medial approach was used.

it is capable of predicting the risks for osteonecrosis, which are approximately 50% in patients with dislocations and 13% in those without.[2-4] The risk for the development of posttraumatic arthritis also corresponds with the severity of the injury and the more severe fracture types. Anatomic alignment is necessary for optimizing patient outcomes. Incomplete or truly nondisplaced fractures can be treated closed; however, closed treatment must be carefully monitored. Any displacement warrants a conversion to surgical treatment.

Treatment

Type I fractures may be treated closed if potential displacement is radiographically monitored. A short leg cast positioned in modest equinus with transition to neutral ankle positioning is the traditional treatment protocol. A non–weight-bearing protocol is strongly advised for 6 to 8 weeks, until radiographic union is demonstrated.

Lateral subtalar dislocation (15%) is less common than medial dislocation (85%).[2-4] The posterior tibial tendon may become interposed, precluding reduction. Occasionally, the flexor digitorum longus can block reduction. Approximately 20% of lateral dislocations require open reduction and the long-term prognosis is worse than that of medial dislocations. Medial dislocations are commonly seen in basketball, occurring when one player lands on another player's foot. The talonavicular joint capsule and/or the extensor digitorum brevis may buttonhole the talar head and block reduction. CT is advised following closed reduction. Closed treatment with cast immobilization is recommended if no fractures are identified with plain radiography or CT. Stiffness ultimately will aid in outcome stability. Osteonecrosis is uncommon (**Figure 1**).

Restoration of normal alignment is critical for obtaining the most favorable patient outcomes. The gold standard of treatment is open reduction and internal fixation (ORIF) using one or two incisions. There is a limited role for closed reduction and percutaneous fixation with cannulated screws placed over fluoroscopically threaded guide wires.[5] The use of titanium screws allows follow-up MRI.[6] Comminuted fractures should not be treated with open reduction. Combined medial and lateral longitudinal incisions are the preferred surgical approach to allow longitudinal placement of

screws. Care should be taken to avoid medial compression by using fully threaded screws along with bone grafting and lateral compression (**Figure 2**).

The anteromedial and/or anterolateral approaches are commonly used. Traditionally, an incision is made medial and in line with the course of the anterior tibial tendon. Care is taken to prevent disruption of the deltoid vasculature and the talonavicular joint, unless necessary for adequate visualization and fixation. This approach allows a medial malleolar osteotomy. The anterolateral approach affords fixation in denser cortical bone. Often this approach is applicable to avoid varus alignment when medial comminution is present. The superficial branch of the peroneal nerve should be avoided and/or protected during lateral dissection.

Screws can be inserted anteroposteriorly or through a small posterolateral portal. The advantage of anteroposterior fixation is that it provides better exposure. Posteroanterior screw placement diminishes the potential for vascular disruption and improves biomechanical fixation, as evidenced in cadaver models. The strength of fixation is not as good a determinant of outcome as are adequate anatomic reduction and retention of the talar blood supply. Minifragment, contoured plate fixation has been described in the literature.[7] Plating is done on the side with predominant comminution. This technique helps buttress the bone graft and maintains the length of the medial column (**Figure 3**).

Open fractures have a deep infection rate as high as 38%.[8] Deep infection is difficult to treat in an avascular talus. Prolonged hospitalization and multiple procedures merit discussion of amputation for salvage. Smokers and patients with diabetes may be candidates for treatment with bone stimulators to assist healing in the event of nonunion.

Displaced talar neck fractures causing soft-tissue compromise require emergent reduction. Open reduction can be delayed to allow the soft-tissue zone of injury to recover. There is no definite evidence that emergent fixation affects the risk for osteonecrosis. The timing of fixation is controversial because no studies support the conclusion that early treatment affects outcome. Late osteonecrosis appears to be associated with

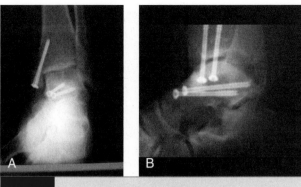

Figure 3 Immediate postoperative AP (A) and lateral (B) ankle radiographs after ORIF of the fracture-dislocation shown in Figure 1.

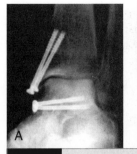
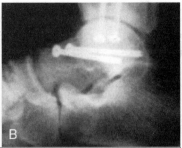

Figure 4 AP (A) and lateral (B) radiographs taken 6 months after ORIF of the fracture-dislocation shown in Figure 1 show evidence of asymptomatic osteonecrosis.

comminution, open fractures, and high-energy injuries. In a survey of orthopaedic surgeons, 60% believed that treatment after 8 hours is acceptable and 46% believed that treatment after 24 hours is acceptable.[9]

Restricted weight bearing is necessary until radiographic evidence of healing occurs. The Hawkins sign may appear after 6 to 8 weeks. A subchondral linear radiolucency on the talar dome indicates bone absorption and intact blood flow within the talus. A partial Hawkins sign also has been described and suggests partial necrosis.[10] This sign may indicate the need for further evaluation with MRI and may assist in the recommendation for restricted weight bearing (Figure 4).

Complications

Complications after treatment of talar neck fractures include skin necrosis, infection, osteonecrosis, delayed union, nonunion, malunion, and arthritis. The rate of nonunion has been reported at approximately 4%.[1,2] Skin necrosis can result from a prolonged delay until reduction with or without surgical intervention. The magnitude of the traumatic injury contributes to both fracture comminution and soft-tissue compromise. Open fractures are associated with overall increased morbidity including deep infection and delayed union or nonunion, which are secondary to the trauma and the potential disruption of the blood supply. Osteonecrosis may occur in up to 20% of talar neck fractures but is not always symptomatic. Arthritis is the most common sequelae occurring in the subtalar and/or ankle joint. Contributing factors include cartilage injury from the sustained trauma, osteonecrosis, and arthrofibrosis. Varus malunion presents the most common preventable complication. Varus malalignment of the talus leads to lateral foot overload and compensatory subtalar stress. Dorsal malunion can limit ankle dorsiflexion.

Talar Body Fractures

Fractures of the talar body are by definition intra-articular, involving the surface of both the tibiotalar and subtalar joints. Body fractures enter into the lateral process, or exit posteriorly. The mechanism of injury is dependent on foot position, but involves axial loading combined with ankle dorsiflexion. This pattern occurs in 7% to 38% of talus fractures.[11] The talar body consists of the dome, the lateral process, and posterior tubercle. The overall prognosis for talar body fractures is poor in comparison with talar neck fractures. Approximately 64% of patients with talar neck fractures report satisfactory outcomes compared with 30% of patients with talar body fractures.[4,11] Talar body fractures present a greater risk for the development of osteonecrosis and disruption of the deltoid blood supply.

Treatment

Tools for internal fixation include minifragment screws, cannulated partially and fully threaded 4.0- and 4.5-mm screws, and smaller diameter Kirschner wires or bioabsorbable pins involving the articular fragments. CT with sagittal reconstruction helps in planning the surgical approach. Although osteotomy is not always necessary, it is generally used on the side of the comminution.

Osteochondral dome injuries are classified using plain radiographs, CT scans, MRI, and arthroscopic examination. Treatment depends on the size of the lesion, displacement, and location. Primary fixation with absorbable pins is acceptable, but may require malleolar osteotomy.

Shear fractures occur in coronal, sagittal, and horizontal patterns. Truly nondisplaced fractures are treated closed if less than 2 mm of gap is identified. Serial CT and/or plain radiographs should document the continued alignment. ORIF is advised for fractures with 1 to 2 mm of dome displacement. The anteromedial approach with or without medial malleolar osteotomy is used. If necessary, the anterolateral approach is added for visualization. Retrospective studies report tibiotalar arthritis in 65% of patients, osteonecrosis in 38%, and subtalar arthritis in 35%.[2,11] Weight bearing is restricted until fracture healing is demonstrated.

Comminuted body fractures have the highest level of reported osteonecrosis and arthritis (up to 88%).[2,4,11]

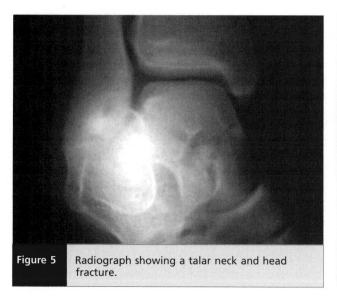

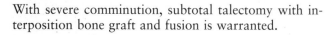

Figure 5 Radiograph showing a talar neck and head fracture.

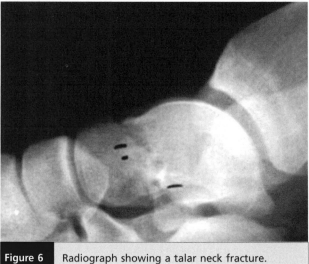

Figure 6 Radiograph showing a talar neck fracture.

With severe comminution, subtotal talectomy with interposition bone graft and fusion is warranted.

Posterior Process Fractures

The posterolateral (Stieda process, os trigonum) and the posteromedial tubercles together compose the posterior process of the talus. A Cedell fracture involves the posteromedial tubercle and a Shepherd fracture involves the posterolateral tubercle. An acute fracture of the posterior tuberosity is transverse and irregular as opposed to a smooth, rounded os trigonum. The mechanism of injury is either marked ankle inversion, ankle dorsiflexion with inversion, or marked plantar flexion with impingement of the tubercle against the plafond. The posterolateral tubercle is most commonly involved, with avulsion of the posterior talofibular ligament as the mechanism of injury.

Cedell fractures caused by a direct blow or with a pronation load can be missed; a CT scan should be obtained to evaluate the extent of the fracture. Nondisplaced or minimally displaced fractures are treated nonsurgically with a non–weight-bearing cast or boot for 4 to 6 weeks, followed by progressive rehabilitation and symptomatic weight bearing. Symptomatic lesions that present after 3 to 6 months are treated with excision through a parasagittal approach. Displaced fracture fragments should be fixed or excised because immobilization alone is ineffective.

Lateral Process Fractures

The primary mechanism of injury in fractures of the lateral process is ankle inversion with dorsiflexion. This type of fracture accounts for approximately 25% of talar body fractures. These fractures are often missed, but can be seen on plain radiographs, specifically ankle mortise and AP views. CT can be used to determine the extent and displacement of the fracture. This injury is commonly referred to as a snowboarder's fracture.

Hawkins has classified these fractures as type I, simple two part fractures; type II, comminuted fractures; and type III, avulsion fractures of the anteroinferior lateral process. Nondisplaced type I and type III fractures are managed in a non–weight-bearing short leg cast or boot for 4 to 6 weeks with progressive rehabilitation. If the fracture does not heal or symptoms persist, fragment excision is performed. Type II or displaced type I and type III fractures are treated surgically with excision or ORIF. Fragments of at least 1 cm in size are preferred for ORIF. Surgically treated patients had better outcomes in a small reported study, with rates of subtalar arthritis at 5% compared with 10% for patients who were treated nonsurgically.[12] Fragmentation and joint debris should be evacuated if noted on CT scans and/or at the time of surgery.

Talar Head Fractures

Fractures of the talar head account for approximately 10% of all talus fractures and often are accompanied by subtalar dislocation or lateral column injury. An axial load through the navicular can produce a shearing injury, whereas compressive loads through the sustentaculum tali, primarily the middle facet, occur with crush injuries. Shear fractures are predominantly medial and indicative of inversion of the foot before the load (**Figures 5** and **6**).

Isolated talar head fractures occur, but usually accompany lateral column injuries, specifically a fracture of the cuboid. Subtalar instability and/or dislocation may develop. Displacement produces medial column shortening, which may impede subtalar joint reduction.

Treatment

Surgical reduction restores subtalar complex motion. The surgical approach to the middle facet is achieved in

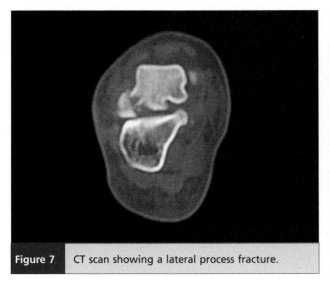

Figure 7 CT scan showing a lateral process fracture.

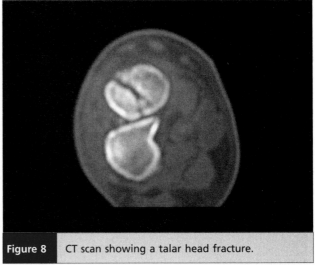

Figure 8 CT scan showing a talar head fracture.

the interval between the tibialis posterior and tibialis anterior, extending from the medial malleolus to the navicular bone. The relatively dorsal incision can be positioned over the talonavicular joint and fracture. A small or mini-external fixator may be used to distract the joint for visualization with proximal pins in either the calcaneus or talus, and distal pins in the medial cuneiform. Care should be taken to prevent dissection of the capsule off the talar neck. Fixation from the more dorsal approach is percutaneous from either the medial or lateral cortex. Elevation of the depressed fragment is maintained with bone graft and appropriate internal fixation (usually bioabsorbable fixation in this location); however, low-profile screws can be used. Fragments in the joint should be excised.

Postoperative Management

Postoperatively, the patients should not bear weight for 10 to 12 weeks. The external fixator is used for approximately 6 weeks. Talar head fractures can be treated closed if they are nondisplaced and stable during fluoroscopic imaging with motion of the talonavicular joint. Alternatively, maximal inversion and eversion AP views of the foot can show an unstable fracture pattern. Simple, nondisplaced injuries can be treated with cast immobilization for approximately 4 weeks followed by non–weight-bearing range-of-motion exercises, and then protected weight bearing. Patients with fracture patterns that are stabilized with surgery may begin early active motion after 4 to 6 weeks. No specific outcome studies have reported on the incidence of arthritis. Improved outcomes are anticipated with internal fixation and débridement. Disability and malunion are treated with arthrodesis (Figures 7 and 8).

The treatment plan should ensure restoration of medial column length either through external fixation while the head lesion heals, or bridging plate fixation with planned removal. Osteonecrosis may develop in up to 10% of patients[13,14] (Figure 9).

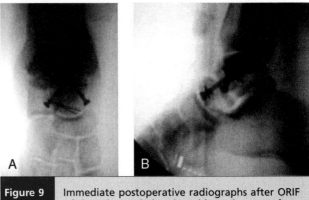

Figure 9 Immediate postoperative radiographs after ORIF of the talar neck, head, and lateral process fracture. **A,** AP view of the foot. **B,** Lateral view of the ankle.

Summary

Talus fractures can be challenging to treat. A thorough preoperative evaluation, technically appropriate fixation, and patient participation in a rehabilitation program will contribute to improved outcomes.

Annotated References

1. Higgins TF, Baumgaertner MR: Diagnosis and treatment of fractures of the talus: A comprehensive review of the literature. *Foot Ankle Int* 1999;20:595-605.

2. Ahmad J, Raikin SM: Current concepts review: Talar fractures. *Foot Ankle Int* 2006;27:475-482.

   The authors present a thorough review of talar injuries, including classification, treatment, and a review of the literature citing level of evidence.

3. Berlet GC, Lee TH, Massa EG: Talar neck fractures. *Orthop Clin North Am* 2001;32:53-64.

4. Vallier HA, Nork SE, Barei DP, Benirschke SK, Sangeorzan BJ: Talar neck fractures: Results and outcomes. *J Bone Joint Surg Am* 2004;86:1616-1624.

   The authors note no correlation between timing of surgery and development of osteonecrosis in patients with talar neck fractures. The authors report that 54% of patients had posttraumatic arthritis and that there is a 49% rate of osteonecrosis associated with fracture comminution and open injury. Level of evidence: II.

5. Juliano PJ, Dabbah M, Harris TG: Talar neck fractures. *Foot Ankle Clin* 2004;9:723-736.

   The authors review current management and surgical fixation of talar neck fractures citing relevant recent literature.

6. Thordarson DB, Triffon MJ, Terk MR: Magnetic resonance imaging to detect avascular necrosis after open reduction and internal fixation of talar neck fractures. *Foot Ankle Int* 1996;17:742-747.

7. Fleuriau Chateau PB, Brokaw DS, Jelen BA, Scheid DK, Weber TG: Plate fixation of talar neck fractures: Preliminary review of a new technique in 23 patients. *J Orthop Trauma* 2002;16:213-219.

8. Sanders R, Pappas J, Mast J, Helfet D: The salvage of open grade IIIB and talus fractures. *J Orthop Trauma* 1992;6:201-208.

9. Patel R, Van Bergeyk A, Pinney S: Are displaced talar neck fractures surgical emergencies? A survey of orthopaedic trauma experts. *Foot Ankle Int* 2005;26:378-381.

   Surgeons were surveyed regarding the timing of treatment for displaced talar neck fractures. The authors report that 60% of surgeons believed that treatment after 8 hours was acceptable; 46% believed that treatment after 24 hours was acceptable provided that no dislocation and skin compromise was present. Level of evidence: V.

10. Tehranzadeh J, Stuffman E, Ross SD: Partial Hawkins sign in fractures of the talus: A report of three cases. *AJR Am J Roentgenol* 2003;181:1559-1563.

    The authors clarify the characteristics of the Hawkins sign and a partial Hawkins sign used in the postoperative evaluation of osteonecrosis.

11. Vallier HA, Nork SE, Benirschke SK, Sangeorzan BJ: Treatment of talar body fractures. *J Bone Joint Surg Am* 2003;85:1716-1724.

    The authors explore issues surrounding fixation and osteotomy as well as surgical timing for talar body fractures. Level of evidence: II.

12. Valderrabano V, Perren T, Ryf C, Rillmann P, Hintermann B: Snowboarder's talus fracture. *Am J Sports Med* 2005;33:871-880.

    A review of the classification of injuries and outcomes of lateral process fractures is presented. Level of evidence: II.

13. Early JS: Management of fractures of the talus: Body and head regions. *Foot Ankle Clin* 2004;9:709-722.

    A review of associated pathology, diagnostic measures, and surgical recommendation and techniques for the treatment of talar head and body fractures are presented.

14. Hansen ST (ed): *Functional Reconstruction of the Foot and Ankle*. Philadelphia, PA, Lippincott Williams & Wilkins, 2000, pp 65-76.

Chapter 9

Lisfranc, Forefoot, Sesamoid Turf Toe Injuries

J. Chris Coetzee, MD, FRCSC   Patrick Ebeling, MD

Introduction

Midfoot and forefoot injuries, including tarsometatarsal and great toe injuries, are fairly common and frequently occur at all levels of sports participation. Such injuries have a profound influence on a patient's ability to retain normal function.

Lisfranc Injuries

Fractures and/or dislocations of the tarsometatarsal (TMT) joint complex are referred to as Lisfranc injuries and are named after the French war surgeon, Jacques Lisfranc de St. Martin. Lisfranc injuries are relatively uncommon; however, if undetected, untreated, or undertreated, these injuries can cause significant morbidity and disability. The situation is further complicated by the fact that a Lisfranc injury can be part of a wide and poorly defined spectrum of injuries. The injury sustained at the TMT joints during a hyperplantarflexion injury caused by walking down a flight of stairs is different than an injury sustained during a high-energy motor vehicle crash. A high index of suspicion of TMT joint injury is required when a patient reports midfoot pain following trauma.

Anatomy

Stability of the TMT joint complex is maintained by the unique wedge-shaped anatomy of the metatarsal bases and their corresponding cuneiform articulations (Figure 1). The second metatarsal is recessed between the medial and lateral cuneiform articulations; the strong plantar ligaments "lock" the metatarsals to the midfoot.

The Lisfranc ligament is a thick structure composed of three portions running from the medial cuneiform to the base of the second metatarsal. The plantar portion of the ligament is the thickest and strongest part and is the main stabilizing component of the first and second metatarsal interspace. There is little motion at the second and third TMT joints, 10° to 20° at the fourth and fifth metatarsocuboid junction, and 5° to 10° at the first TMT joint.

Mechanism of Injury

Injuries to the TMT joints can be caused by direct or indirect forces. With direct injuries, the direction of displacement depends on the point of application of the injuring force.[1] The direct force or axial load is usually centered around the dorsum of the foot, creating a tensile force on the plantar side of the TMT joints. If the joints tear, the Lisfranc complex is unstable. The intensity and angle of the force will determine whether fractures and/or ligamentous injuries occur. Indirect forces, such as bending or twisting moments applied to the midfoot, are more common. The history and mechanism of injury can help determine the severity, stability, and prognosis of the injury.

A "friendly" or benign injury occurs when the ankle and toes are plantar flexed and an axial load is applied (such as during football or soccer play, or missing a step when descending a flight of stairs). If the force is mild to moderate, only the dorsal ligaments are torn, leaving the strong plantar structures intact. In such situations, the injury is painful, but benign. There is seldom any widening of the intermetatarsal space; return to activity is determined by the level of pain and discomfort. In an "unfriendly" or serious injury, the force is continuous and the strong plantar ligaments also are torn, leaving the TMT complex very unstable and usually causing dorsal dislocation of the metatarsals.

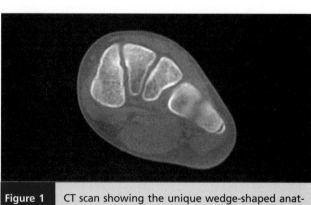

Figure 1 CT scan showing the unique wedge-shaped anatomy of the metatarsal bases and their corresponding cuneiform bones that contribute to the stability of the Lisfranc joints.

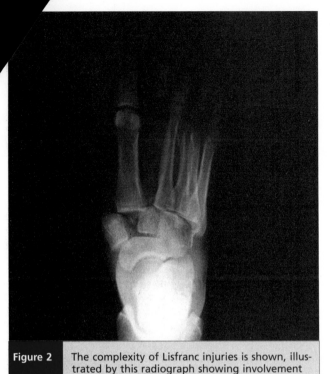

Figure 2 The complexity of Lisfranc injuries is shown, illustrated by this radiograph showing involvement of the TMT joints and disruption of the intercuneiform and naviculocuneiform articulations.

A variety of injury patterns is possible, depending on the position of the foot during maximal force. For example, the injury pattern in the foot of a horseback rider who loses control with the foot fixed in the stirrup will differ from the injury pattern caused by an axial loading force. The foot of the horseback rider probably will be subjected to a twisting force, pronation, and abduction on the midfoot, which may lead to a windswept deformity with the metatarsals abducted. The more classic injury pattern occurs in football players: the ankle is plantar flexed, the toes are dorsiflexed, and an axial load is placed on the midfoot, resulting in a disruption of the plantar ligaments, with or without bony fragments.

Patients with Lisfranc injuries typically report pain and swelling in the midfoot and difficulty bearing weight. The presence of plantar ecchymosis is indicative of severe soft-tissue disruption, even if plain radiographs do not show a fracture. Any midfoot sprain characterized by greater than expected swelling, pain, and tenderness should be considered a Lisfranc injury until proven otherwise.

Weight-bearing AP and lateral radiographs are good initial imaging studies. If radiographic results are normal, a CT scan (weight bearing if possible) or examination under anesthesia should be considered. The latter assessment may be the most reliable method to evaluate instability in the absence of fractures.

Classification

Hardcastle's classification of TMT joint injuries is often used. Type A injuries have total incongruity, type B

have partial incongruity, and type C are characterized by a divergent incongruity based on the three-column concept of the midfoot.[2] The medial column consists of the first metatarsal, medial cuneiform, and its navicular facet. The middle column consists of the second and third metatarsals, their corresponding cuneiform bones, and the central and lateral facets of the navicular. The fourth and fifth metatarsals and their articulations with the cuboid make up the lateral column. This classification system is important because injury to one portion of a column usually indicates injury to other portions of that column. Knowledge of this concept will reduce the likelihood of an undiagnosed propagation of a fracture or dislocation through the cuneiform or navicular-cuboid-calcaneal articulation (Figure 2).

Myerson and associates[1] proposed a more complete classification system that subdivided types B and C into types B1, B2, C1, and C2 based on the complexity of the injury. However, it should be emphasized that it is difficult to accurately organize Lisfranc injuries into neatly organized groups because of the many variations and levels of severity of this injury.[3]

Treatment

Weight-bearing radiographs (as can be tolerated) should be obtained when a midfoot injury is suspected. To provide a comparative study, radiographs should be taken of both feet. AP, 30° medial oblique, and lateral views of the foot are needed. On the AP view, the TMT joints should all be congruent with no overhang of the first metatarsal-cuneiform articulation. The medial aspect of the second metatarsal should be in continuity with the medial aspect of the middle cuneiform. On the oblique view, the fourth metatarsal should be in continuity with the medial aspect of the cuboid. On the lateral view, there should be no dorsal subluxation of the metatarsals in relationship to the cuneiform bones (Figure 3).

If the results of initial radiographs are normal but a high index of suspicion for injury is present, several options are available. Stress radiographs may be obtained with the patient under anesthesia with a supination and abduction force applied to the forefoot, followed by a pronation and adduction force; any abnormal widening or displacement at the TMT joints should be noted. Alternatively, the patient may be reevaluated after 10 days, with another series of weight-bearing radiographs, or with MRI and/or CT scanning. A CT scan is especially helpful in determining associated fractures. The presence of a "fleck sign" is sometimes indicative of an intact Lisfranc ligament, but may indicate instability of the Lisfranc complex caused by an interruption of the stabilizing complex (Figure 4). An MRI scan can accurately identify a disruption of the Lisfranc ligament; however, its usefulness in acute injuries is limited. Good initial radiographic studies are still necessary.

Lisfranc injuries require a range of treatment options. If a patient has a partial dorsal disruption that is painful but stable on weight-bearing radiographs, no treatment other than management of symptoms is re-

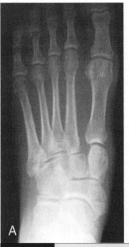
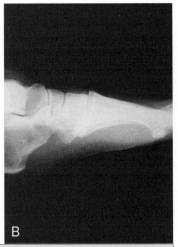

Figure 3	**A,** On an AP view, the medial border of the second metatarsal should line up with the medial border of the middle cuneiform. This radiograph shows an obvious displacement that contributes to the instability of the first TMT joint. **B,** On a lateral radiograph, the metatarsal should be in the same line as the cuneiform bones. This radiograph shows a dorsal subluxation.

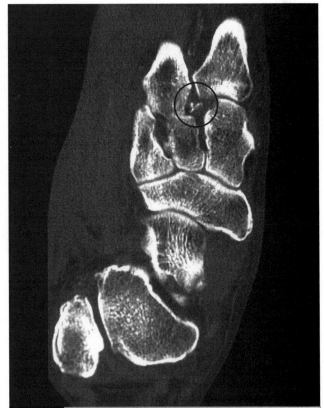

Figure 4	The fleck sign is a bony fragment seen at the plantar medial base of the second metatarsal and represents a Lisfranc ligament avulsion (circle). Note the subtle lateral subluxation of the second tarsometatarsal joint.

quired. At the opposite end of the injury spectrum is the patient with a severely comminuted fracture-dislocation with extensive joint damage. These injuries are probably better treated with formal open reduction and internal fixation (ORIF), which can be performed through one or two longitudinal dorsal incisions. If only the medial column is involved (whether TMT, intercuneiform, or cuneiform-navicular) one incision will suffice. If the fracture-dislocation involves more than the medial column, an approach using two longitudinal incisions is preferred (**Figure 5**). The first incision is made over the first intermetatarsal space. The neurovascular bundle is located immediately lateral to the incision and should be protected. This incision provides access to the first and second TMT joints. The second incision is made over the third TMT joint. This incision is always more lateral than is expected, and at least a 3-cm bridge between the incisions is needed. This approach provides access to the lateral side of the second, third, and fourth TMT joints.

The gold standard of treatment for fracture-dislocations is open reduction, débridement of the joints, anatomic reduction, and screw fixation of the medial three metatarsals. The sequence of fixation can vary, but as a rule the medial column is first reduced and stabilized with a screw from the metatarsal into the medial cuneiform. If there is intercuneiform or cuneiform–navicular instability, those joints also are débrided, reduced, and fixed with screws. With the medial column stabilized, a pointed reduction clamp is placed over the lateral aspect of the second metatarsal base and the medial aspect of the medial cuneiform. This allows the second metatarsal to be reduced in its

position between the medial and lateral cuneiform bones. The "home-run" screw secures the second metatarsal into the recess between the medial and lateral cuneiform bones and is usually inserted from the medial cuneiform into the base of the second metatarsal. Direct visualization as well as radiographic control should be used to confirm reduction (**Figure 6**). Kirschner wires (K-wires) can be used to maintain reduction but are inadequate for permanent fixation of the medial three rays. With the use of K-wires, initial stability is inadequate and the wires must be removed before adequate stability and healing of the joints is achieved.[4]

In traditional ORIF, 3.5-mm cortical screws are used in a noncompression fashion. If there is significant comminution of the metatarsals, low-profile plating across the joints is indicated to maintain alignment and length while the fractures and joints heal.[5] The lateral metatarsal-cuboid joint usually reduces with reduction of the medial three rays. If there is still appreciable instability, the lateral rays are reduced and immobilized with percutaneous K-wires. The lateral two rays should not be fused.

In some situations, primary fusion of the medial Lisfranc joints is indicated. If there is significant articular cartilage damage, severe intra-articular comminution

2: Foot and Ankle Trauma

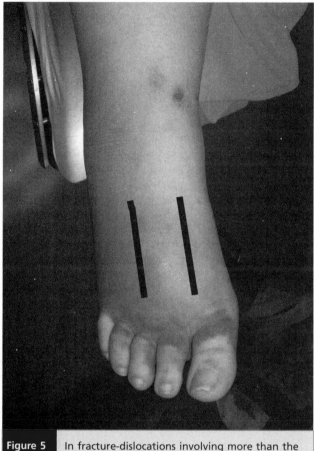

Figure 5   In fracture-dislocations involving more than the medial column of the TMT joints, two longitudinal incisions are used. The dorsomedial incision is made over the first intermetatarsal space and the dorsolateral incision is made between the third and fourth metatarsals.

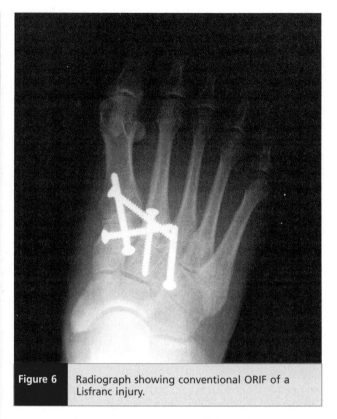

Figure 6   Radiograph showing conventional ORIF of a Lisfranc injury.

caused by high impact or high force, or a complete ligamentous dislocation, a primary fusion will lead to a more reliable and satisfactory result than conventional ORIF. If the bone structure is well maintained, the joints are prepared by removing the cartilage, reducing the joints, and placing the screws in exactly the same manner as is used in ORIF, but under compression. In patients with significant fractures, screw fixation may be impossible and plating is used across the joints.

A "nutcracker" fracture of the cuboid secondary to a severe abduction force on the foot is best appreciated with a 30° medial oblique radiographic view. The congruity of the joint should be restored and the cuboid compression elevated, which often requires bone grafting to fill the void and plating to stabilize the fracture. Occasionally the lateral border can be reduced and the length maintained with a mini-external fixator that should be removed after 6 weeks. Half pins are placed in the calcaneus and the fifth metatarsal to maintain length during healing.

Occasionally there is very severe comminution and fracture of the TMT joints and the cuneiform bones and/or the navicular. A spanning plate from the talus to the metatarsals can restore alignment and length. The plate must be removed after ligamentous and bony healing are achieved, usually at 3 to 6 months. An alternative method is the use of a spanning mini-fixator. Severe crush injuries require adequate soft-tissue management to minimize complications. In crush injuries, the potential for compartment syndrome should be recognized and fasciotomies should be performed if needed.

Rehabilitation

A bulky dressing and cast splint are applied after surgery. The extremity is elevated most of the first week to control pain and reduce swelling. Sutures are removed after 14 days and a pneumatic walking boot can be used instead of a cast. Patients should be encouraged to move their toes as much as possible to reduce swelling, limit ultimate stiffness, and reduce the risk for deep venous thrombosis. Ankle range-of-motion exercises can be started. Minimal (if any) weight bearing should be allowed in the first 6 weeks. Depending on the individual patient, protected weight bearing in a walking boot can begin at 6 weeks and generally is continued for an additional 6 weeks.

The timing and need for hardware removal is debatable. Some physicians advocate leaving the hardware in place indefinitely, even in patients treated with ORIF. The hardware is removed only if it causes adverse symptoms or if the Lisfranc complex is completely healed and screw removal may improve midfoot range of motion. For those physicians who routinely remove hardware, removal should be done before 4 months.

Outcome

The only prospective randomized outcome study on Lisfranc injuries suggests that severe ligamentous disruption with very unstable joints is better treated with primary fusion than with conventional ORIF.[6] However, the authors of this study do not suggest that primary fusion is the best treatment option for all Lisfranc injuries. More research is needed to determine which injuries do best with a specific treatment. As previously mentioned, Lisfranc injuries have a wide spectrum of severity and complexity and it may be difficult to place such injuries into neatly organized groups.

Surgical outcomes are affected by the accuracy of the reduction, with an anatomic reduction providing the best chance for good to excellent results.[7] Even with careful initial treatment, the prevalence of symptomatic degenerative changes after Lisfranc injuries can be as high as 58%. Patients with such complications are usually treated with reduction and fusing of the involved TMT joints.[8]

Forefoot Trauma

First Metatarsal Fractures

Fractures of the first metatarsal most often result from direct trauma. Nondisplaced, extra-articular fractures of the first metatarsal should be immobilized for 4 to 6 weeks in a stiff-soled shoe, walking boot, or cast, with progressive weight bearing as tolerated. Patients with displaced fractures can be treated with closed reduction and a short leg cast if adequate reduction can be achieved. Little residual displacement should be tolerated because of the important weight-bearing properties of the first metatarsal. If the fracture is unstable or the reduction is inadequate, ORIF is required. Shaft fractures are approached through a dorsal incision and stabilized with either a 2.7-mm or 3.5-mm plate, depending on the size of the bone. On occasion, a long spiral fracture can be adequately stabilized with multiple lag screws placed through either a medial or dorsal incision. External fixation can be useful in injuries with more significant soft-tissue damage, such as severe crush injuries. Fractures at either end of the first metatarsal may require a T-plate for optimal stabilization. Intra-articular fractures must be anatomically reduced. Comminuted fractures of the base of the first metatarsal can be treated with a spanning plate across the TMT joint or primary arthrodesis.[9]

Postoperatively, the foot is placed in a splint or well-padded short leg cast. Sutures are removed at 2 weeks and heel weight bearing is permitted in a walking boot. If possible, early range of motion of the metatarsophalangeal joint is initiated. Progressive weight bearing can usually be started between 4 and 6 weeks; full healing is expected at 8 to 12 weeks.

Middle Metatarsal Fractures

In the second, third, and fourth metatarsals, injuries can result from direct forces, indirect forces, or cumulative stress. Direct forces most often produce transverse or comminuted fractures, whereas indirect forces usually result in spiral fractures. Closed fractures that are minimally displaced or nondisplaced are treated in a short leg cast for 4 to 6 weeks, followed by the use of a stiff-soled shoe. Healing is usually complete in 6 to 8 weeks. Open, unstable, or displaced fractures should be reduced and stabilized. Three to 4 mm of transverse displacement can be tolerated in the middle metatarsals, but any shortening or sagittal displacement should be corrected. Failure to do so can result in painful transfer metatarsalgia. When multiple metatarsals are fractured, the tendency for instability increases and surgical fixation is often indicated. Midshaft fractures with minimal comminution are adequately treated with intramedullary K-wire fixation. If a closed reduction is possible, the K-wire can be placed retrograde through the metatarsal head. If open reduction is necessary, the K-wire is first driven antegrade through the distal fragment and then passed retrograde across the fracture under direct visualization. Comminuted or otherwise unstable fractures are treated with plate fixation using 2.7-mm or smaller plates, depending on the size of the bone. Displaced metatarsal head fractures should be reduced and stabilized with K-wires or small lag screws.[10]

Postoperatively, a splint or well-padded short leg cast is used. Heel weight bearing is permitted with crutches or a walker. After 2 weeks, a walking boot is placed and range of motion is initiated when possible. Progressive weight bearing usually can begin between 4 and 6 weeks. If K-wires are used, they are removed when early radiographic healing is evident, usually at 4 to 6 weeks after surgery. Full healing is expected by 8 to 12 weeks.

Stress fractures of the middle metatarsals result from cumulative trauma and often are precipitated by an abrupt increase in the patient's activity level; therefore, the medical history should document any new activities or changes in activity level. Patients also should be evaluated for contributing anatomic factors including malalignment, osseous variants, and soft-tissue factors. Examples of such contributing factors include cavus foot position, a long second metatarsal, and gastrocnemius contracture. A stress fracture often can be clinically diagnosed. Radiographs are usually negative in the first few weeks after such a fracture, but cortical sclerosis or thickening may be seen in patients with acute-on-chronic stress fractures. Bony healing may later be seen at the fracture site. MRI or bone scanning may occasionally be necessary to confirm the diagnosis.

The mainstay of treatment for stress fractures is rest and elimination of the inciting cause. Internal fixation is indicated for recurrent or recalcitrant fractures and for symptomatic nonunions. Contributing bony or soft-tissue factors should be treated when identified. A recent small collection of case reports showed successful treat-

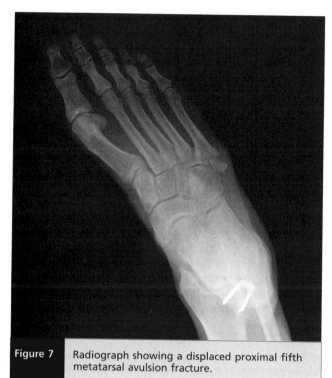

Figure 7 | Radiograph showing a displaced proximal fifth metatarsal avulsion fracture.

ment of second and third metatarsal stress fractures in college-level athletes using a fracture brace and a modified shoe while continuing athletic participation.[11]

Fifth Metatarsal Fractures

The fifth metatarsal is the most frequently fractured metatarsal bone.[12] It is unique because of its extrinsic muscle and plantar fascia attachments and border position. Four fracture types are typically described in the fifth metatarsal: proximal metatarsal avulsion fractures, fractures of the proximal metaphyseal-diaphyseal junction, stress fractures, and acute fractures of the shaft. Although uncommon, fractures of the metatarsal head can occur with direct trauma.

Proximal metatarsal avulsion fractures compose up to 90% of all fifth metatarsal fractures and result from an inversion injury (**Figure 7**). There is debate, however, concerning whether the bony fragment is avulsed by the peroneus brevis or the lateral plantar aponeurosis. Patients with small, nondisplaced, extra-articular fractures are treated with a walking boot for 4 weeks; weight bearing is allowed as tolerated.[13] Because radiographic healing can be prolonged, return to activity is based on clinical recovery. In a recent cohort study, 85% of patients reported being at their preinjury functional level 6 months after injury.[14] Rare symptomatic nonunion can be treated by excision of the fragment or delayed internal fixation. Large, displaced, or intra-articular fractures may be more appropriately treated by primary internal fixation with tension band wiring or bicortical screws.[15]

Acute fractures of the proximal metaphyseal-diaphyseal junction (Jones fractures) should be care-fully distinguished from proximal avulsion fractures. The Jones fracture exits the bone in the intermetatarsal area whereas the avulsion fracture enters the fifth metatarsal-cuboid articulation. Jones fractures are acute injuries and also must be distinguished from stress fractures in the same area. Nondisplaced Jones fractures are treated in a non–weight-bearing short leg cast for 6 weeks, followed by the use of a stiff-soled shoe until there is clinical and radiographic evidence of healing. Traditionally, internal fixation has been reserved for symptomatic nonunions and high-level athletes; however, several recent studies suggest that primary internal fixation should be considered an option for most patients. In a 2005 study, nonsurgical treatment had a failure rate of 44% and a median healing time of 15 weeks. In contrast, early screw fixation had a 5% failure rate with fracture union at a mean follow-up of 8 weeks.[16]

Although tension band wiring and external fixation may be used in some circumstances, internal fixation of Jones fractures is most often achieved with an intramedullary screw.[17] Cannulated, solid, and variable pitch screws all have been used with good results. The screw should be placed through a "high and inside" starting point and, except for variable pitch screws, need only be long enough to advance all the threads beyond the fracture site. If a fully threaded screw is used with a traditional long technique, the screw should be as long as possible, while still avoiding straightening the bone, which results in lateral gaping at the fracture side. Postoperatively, patients use touch-down weight bearing with the foot in a cast, walking boot, or stiff-soled shoe for 6 weeks. Return to full activity is allowed with radiographic evidence of healing (**Figure 8**).

Stress fractures of the proximal fifth metatarsal often occur in the same region as the Jones fracture, but do not result from a single acute injury. The patient's history usually reveals prodromal symptoms, and radiographs often show a sclerotic fracture line and cortical thickening. These fractures have a high rate of delayed union or nonunion. Nonsurgical treatment often involves a lengthy period of limited weight bearing; therefore, surgical treatment with intramedullary screw placement and bone grafting often is warranted. The technique for screw placement is the same as previously described for acute fractures. Bone grafting through a limited incision is recommended for surgical nonunions and any nonunion with sclerotic margins. Autograft should be used in most instances.

Fractures of the shaft of the fifth metatarsal are generally treated nonsurgically. Most fractures can be managed successfully, allowing weight bearing as tolerated with the foot in a walking boot or stiff-soled shoe for 6 weeks. Internal fixation is necessary only for significant displacement and symptomatic nonunion. Sagittal displacement and shortening are more poorly tolerated, but also are less common. If internal fixation is warranted, it is accomplished with plate fixation. Multiple lag screws are used in long, oblique fractures.

Treatment of proximal fifth metatarsal fractures may result in multiple complications. The sural nerve can be injured during surgical exposure, especially when treating proximal fractures. Delayed union or nonunion is common in Jones fractures and proximal stress fractures because of the tenuous blood supply to this portion of the bone. Technical errors can contribute to nonunion. Failure to completely cross the fracture site with all of the screw threads will result in a lack of compression and can lead to nonunion. Because the bone is curved, placement of a screw that is too long will cause distraction at the lateral cortex, which also can increase the risk of nonunion. Refracture is most common after nonsurgical treatment but also can occur after removal of an intramedullary screw. Some authors recommend leaving the screw in place for the remainder of an athlete's career. Subtle foot deformity also may contribute to refracture. In a recent study of 21 consecutive patients with Jones fractures, 18 had a varus hindfoot position.[18] These patients were treated with a lateral heel wedge; no refractures had occurred at a mean follow-up of 4 years. Prominence of the instrumentation also can cause complications, especially when the patient is thin or if a 6.5-mm screw is used. Initially, the area can be padded or the patient's shoes can be modified. If symptoms persist, the screw can be removed after full healing.

Metatarsophalangeal and Interphalangeal Dislocations

Metatarsophalangeal dislocations most commonly occur at the great toe. These injuries are almost uniformly dorsal in direction. Jahss classified these injuries into two types.[19] The radiographic appearance of the sesamoids is the key to differentiating the two types. In type I injuries the sesamoid complex is intact and blocks closed reduction. Open reduction is performed through a dorsal approach. Release of the adductor hallucis and/or intersesamoid ligament may be necessary to achieve reduction. Type II injuries are amenable to closed reduction with gentle traction and hyperextension. Type IIB injuries require open débridement of the joint if postreduction imaging shows an intra-articular fragment from the sesamoid fracture. After either open or closed reduction, metatarsophalangeal dislocations are usually stable and weight bearing (as tolerated) is allowed with the foot in a cast or stiff-soled shoe for 3 to 4 weeks.

Dislocations of the lesser metatarsophalangeal joints are uncommon; if they occur, closed reduction usually can be achieved with axial traction. If open reduction is necessary, it is done through a dorsal approach. After reduction, the adjacent toe is buddy taped for 2 to 3 weeks. Interphalangeal joint dislocation at the great toe most often results from an axial force. The distal phalanx displaces dorsally and closed reduction usually is easily accomplished. For 2 to 3 weeks after surgery, weight bearing (as tolerated) is allowed with the foot in a stiff-soled shoe.

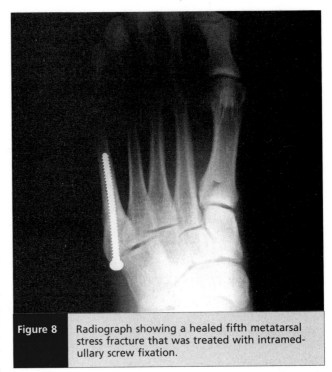

Figure 8 Radiograph showing a healed fifth metatarsal stress fracture that was treated with intramedullary screw fixation.

Phalangeal Fractures

Phalangeal fractures of the lesser toes usually are the result of axial trauma, the "nightwalker's" fracture, or a crush injury. These fractures almost universally are treated nonsurgically. Closed reduction under a digital block is indicated if there is significant displacement, but mild angulation is well tolerated. For the middle and distal phalanx especially, acceptable position should be based more on the clinical appearance of the toe than on the radiographic reduction. When acceptable position is achieved, the toe is buddy taped for 3 to 4 weeks and weight bearing is allowed as tolerated. A stiff-soled shoe may be helpful initially because these injuries can be quite swollen and painful.

Fractures of the proximal phalanx of the great toe most often result from axial injury (**Figure 9**). Imaging studies must be carefully evaluated for fracture extension into the surrounding joints, especially proximally. Surgical treatment is indicated for any significant articular displacement. The fracture is approached through a dorsal longitudinal or L-shaped incision and fixation is achieved with either K-wires or minifragment screws. Patients with nondisplaced fractures should use a walking boot or stiff-soled shoe for 3 to 4 weeks.

Distal phalanx fractures of the great toe are most often treated nonsurgically and weight bearing (as tolerated) is allowed with the foot in a stiff-soled shoe for 3 to 4 weeks. Significant displacement at the interphalangeal joint usually can be treated with closed reduction. These fractures are, however, more likely to result from crush injuries and may be complicated by significant soft-tissue trauma. The associated soft-tissue injuries, including open fractures, nail bed injury, or tissue loss, may independently require surgical treatment.

2: Foot and Ankle Trauma

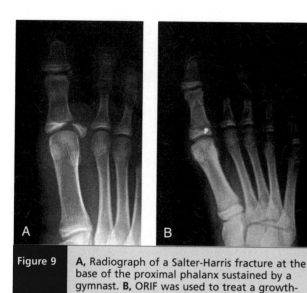

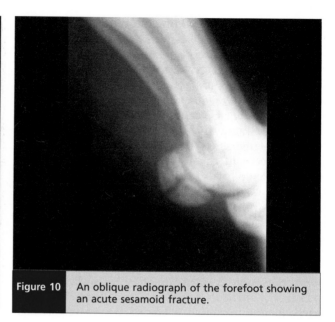

Figure 9   **A**, Radiograph of a Salter-Harris fracture at the base of the proximal phalanx sustained by a gymnast. **B**, ORIF was used to treat a growth-plate fracture.

Figure 10   An oblique radiograph of the forefoot showing an acute sesamoid fracture.

Sesamoid Injuries

The sesamoids function as a fulcrum to increase the mechanical force of the flexor hallucis brevis, protect the flexor hallucis longus, and absorb and distribute weight-bearing pressure. Because more than 50% of body weight is transmitted through the first metatarsophalangeal joint, the sesamoids are vulnerable to injury. Some changes in athletic playing surface, especially artificial turf in football, have resulted in an increase in toe and sesamoid injuries. The general surge in athletic activity in all age groups also has contributed to an increase in stress-related sesamoid disorders.

Anatomy

The sesamoids form an integral part of the first metatarsophalangeal joint complex and are located within the tendons of the flexor hallucis brevis. The medial sesamoid also is the attachment site for the abductor hallucis, whereas the lateral sesamoid is the attachment site for the oblique head of the adductor hallucis and the deep transverse metatarsal ligament. The medial sesamoid is usually larger than the lateral sesamoid and is more prone to injury. The medial sesamoid is bipartite in approximately 10% of the population, whereas the lateral sesamoid is rarely bipartite. In 25% of patients with a bipartite sesamoid, the condition is bilateral.

Clinical Presentation of Acute Injuries

Acute sesamoid injuries are less common than typical overuse, stress-related, chronic sesamoiditis. There is usually a history of a specific injury, immediate pain, discoloration, swelling, and difficulty in continuing an intended activity. These injuries usually result from hyperdorsiflexion during high-impact activities such as high jumping, long jumping, and sprinting.

Radiographic Examination

The usual AP, lateral, medial, lateral oblique, and axial sesamoid views should be obtained (**Figure 10**). If there is a question about a possible fracture versus a bipartite sesamoid, an AP and lateral radiograph of the unaffected side should be obtained. An acute fracture usually has ragged edges versus the sclerotic rounded edges of a bipartite sesamoid. If results are inconclusive, a bone scan and/or fine cut CT scan can help in determining the character and acuteness of the injury.

Treatment

The conventional treatment for sesamoid injuries includes non–weight-bearing activities for at least 6 weeks with the foot in a stiff-soled shoe or a cast. Fracture healing can be slow and it may take 6 months for complete recovery. Some sesamoids do not heal, but may have a pain-free nonunion. Excision of the medial sesamoid is recommended if there is ongoing debilitating pain after 6 months.

ORIF is the alternative treatment for a transverse sesamoid fracture, especially in high-profile athletes, which is similar to the principle used to treat patellar fractures. Surgery for the medial sesamoid can be safely performed through a plantar medial approach and may lead to more reliable healing of the fracture and quicker return to activity.[20] Some authors recommend bone grafting of sesamoid nonunions, even 6 months after injury[21] (**Figure 11**).

The fibular sesamoid is approached through a plantar incision just lateral to the weight-bearing area of the first metatarsophalangeal joint. The neurovascular bundle is carefully identified and retracted laterally. This provides access to the sesamoid for bone grafting or fracture treatment. To complete a sesamoidectomy, the intersesamoid ligament is released and the bone is carefully removed, preserving the flexor hallucis brevis tendon attachment to the extent possible. The resulting defect in the flexor hallucis brevis also should be repaired to the extent possible.

Clinical Presentation: Chronic Injuries

Patients with chronic sesamoid injuries present with generalized pain around the hallux with an insidious onset over many weeks. There is a gradual progression of pain with motion, especially hyperdorsiflexion. Patients often report difficulty walking or running and shift their weight to the outside border of the foot. There may be an objective or subjective feeling of swelling, which could result in neuritic symptoms if the digital nerve is compressed.

Because the sesamoids are close together it can be difficult to localize the painful sesamoid with palpation. Palpation with hyperdorsiflexion of the hallux may help determine which sesamoid is involved. In patients with flexor hallucis longus tenosynovitis, there is increasing pain with resisted plantar flexion of the interphalangeal joint of the hallux. Patients with cavovarus deformities often have a plantar-flexed first ray, which in turn places more axial load on the sesamoids, making them more prone to injury.

Radiographic Examination

Radiographs should include weight-bearing AP and lateral views, medial and lateral oblique views, and axial sesamoid views. The AP and lateral views are useful for the detection of fractures, bipartite sesamoids, and proximal retraction of the sesamoids that occur with turf toe injuries. The lateral oblique view is best for viewing the lateral sesamoid, whereas the medial sesamoid is best seen on the medial oblique view. The axial sesamoid view is useful in showing osteochondritis of the sesamoid and degenerative changes between the sesamoids and metatarsal head.

If there is ongoing pain and negative radiographic findings, a bone or MRI scan may be helpful. A bone scan always should compare the symptomatic side to the contralateral side before the painful side is determined to be abnormal. Increased bone scan activity in the sesamoids has been reported in up to 29% of asymptomatic athletes; therefore, a significant difference in uptake between the feet should be present before injury is diagnosed. An MRI may be helpful for determining the presence of soft-tissue injury, flexor hallucis longus tendinitis, and osteochondritis.

Treatment

Nonsurgical treatment is indicated for most chronic sesamoid disorders. The initial treatment goal is to limit stress on the sesamoid with activity and footwear modifications. Activities involving repetitive pounding and hyperdorsiflexion should be avoided. The hallux can be taped or splinted to avoid dorsiflexion. Comfortable shoe wear with a low heel and wide toe box is recommended. Orthotics with a recessed area under the first metatarsophalangeal joint may help to unload the sesamoids.[22]

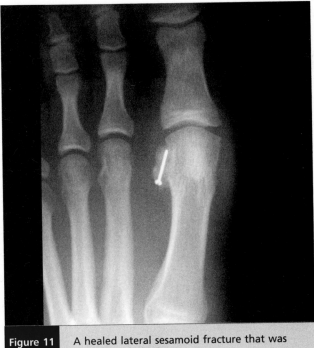

| Figure 11 | A healed lateral sesamoid fracture that was treated with ORIF. |

If there is a confirmed structural reason for chronic sesamoiditis, surgical treatment is indicated if conservative management fails. For chronic sesamoiditis secondary to a plantar-flexed first ray in a cavovarus foot, dorsiflexion osteotomy at the base of the first metatarsal is indicated. In patients with a hypertrophied medial sesamoid, sesamoid height can be reduced by shaving the plantar half through a medial approach.

If all conservative efforts fail, a sesamoidectomy should be performed.[23] The medial sesamoid is removed through a medial approach, incising the capsule in-line with the metatarsal-sesamoid joint to access the bone. The lateral sesamoid is removed through a plantar approach as was previously described. In both situations, any resulting defect in the flexor hallucis brevis tendon or plantar plate should be repaired to the extent possible. The digital nerves are in close proximity to the sesamoids and should be protected to avoid sensory loss or painful neuromas.

As a general rule, only one sesamoid should be excised to avoid a claw toe deformity. Sesamoid excision provides complete pain relief in 50% to 80% of patients; however, potential complications include plantar flexion weakness, loss of motion, pain over the remaining sesamoid, and neuroma formation.

Turf Toe Injuries

Turf toe is a term used to describe injuries to the first metatarsophalangeal joint that vary in both severity and structures involved. These injuries include minor sprains, traumatic osteochondral injuries, disruption of the plantar plate, traumatic hallux valgus deformities, and any other injury related to the hallux metatarsophalangeal complex.[19,24] Etiologic factors commonly include the type of athletic playing surface and the flexibility of the athlete's shoe. Most turf toe injuries occur on artificial turf and may be caused by the hard surface or the fact that shoes used on these surfaces are usually lighter and less protective than those used on grass surfaces. Traditional shoe wear used on grass playing surfaces has a steel plate in the sole for the attachment of cleats; this plate limits forefoot motion and protects the metatarsophalangeal joint.

Mechanism of Injury

The injury mechanism can be an excessive force in any direction, with hyperdorsiflexion most commonly reported. Depending on the direction and magnitude of the force, a spectrum of injuries can result, including partial or complete tearing of the plantar plate or complete dislocation. With disruption of the plantar plate, push-off strength is not only severely limited but also is extremely painful. An untreated plantar plate disruption will lead to early degenerative changes of the metatarsophalangeal joint caused by excessive shear forces, primarily over the dorsal aspect of the joint.

Hyperplantarflexion injuries are the second most common injury mechanism and are termed sand toe injuries because of their frequent occurrence in beach volleyball players, although they occur in participants in other sports activities as well. The hyperplantarflexion causes a tear in the dorsal capsule of the joint and can lead to shear forces on the plantar aspect of the metatarsophalangeal joint complex.

A valgus force applied to the metatarsophalangeal joint when the forefoot is firmly planted and then internally rotated during push-off to suddenly decelerate or change direction is the third most common injury mechanism. This injury can lead to a completely unstable, painful, traumatic hallux valgus deformity.

Physical Examination

A complete evaluation should be performed immediately after the injury while swelling and pain are at a minimum. The patient's ability to ambulate on the injured toe either comfortably or with difficulty is helpful in determining the severity of the injury. An intrinsic minus or clawed hallux is always indicative of a severe injury. The plantar plate can be avulsed from the base of the proximal phalanx, or one or both flexor hallucis brevis tendon insertions into the sesamoids can be avulsed.

The radiographic evaluation is the same as that performed for potential sesamoid injuries. Plantar evaluation should check for proximal migration of the sesamoids. The distance from the distal aspect of the sesamoids to the metatarsophalangeal joint on the injured side should be measured and compared with the contralateral side. The difference between the right and left foot should be less than 3 mm for the medial sesa-

moid and 2.7 mm for the lateral sesamoid. Evaluation of joint motion under fluoroscopic control can be helpful in determining plantar plate avulsions and other instabilities of the metatarsophalangeal joint. MRI is useful for determining the extent of soft-tissue and chondral injuries.[25]

Nonsurgical Treatment

Treatment of metatarsophalangeal joint injuries depends on the nature and severity of the injury. Grade 1 injuries (incomplete tear/sprain of the capsule) can be treated with rest, ice, compression, and elevation (RICE protocol), anti-inflammatory medication, early protected joint motion after 3 to 5 days, and taping of the toe to prevent the direction of movement that caused the injury. Athletes with grade 1 injuries usually can return to sports activities with little or no loss of playing time. The use of a spring, carbon-fiber steel plate in the shoe may be beneficial.

Athletes with grade 2 injuries (partial tear of the capsule) should not return to sports participation for approximately 3 to 14 days. Treatment is the same as that used for grade 1 injuries. Grade 3 injuries (complete tear of the capsuloligamentous complex) may result in 4 to 6 weeks of lost playing time. Patients with grade 3 injuries are immobilized in a walking boot or short leg cast with a toe extension. The toe is immobilized until the joint is stable. Return to activity is based on comfort level and type of activity. Generally, 50° to 60° of pain-free dorsiflexion is required before the athlete returns to competitive play.

Surgical Treatment

Surgical treatment is seldom necessary for patients with acute grade 1 and 2 injuries, but is performed in the presence of loose bodies, large cartilage flaps, or for certain sesamoid fractures. Late reconstruction of grade 3 injuries, especially complete plantar plate avulsions, is difficult; therefore, these injuries can be repaired through a J or L plantar incision. The sesamoids are advanced and the soft tissues repaired to the base of the proximal phalanx. The abductor hallucis can be transferred into the proximal phalanx to increase plantar flexion strength. The recovery period is long.

Chronic situations that may require surgical treatment include diastases of a bipartite sesamoid, osteochondritis of a sesamoid, and traumatic hallux valgus and hallux rigidus. A diastasis of a bipartite sesamoid often can be treated by excising the smaller (usually distal) pole and reattaching the soft tissue to the proximal pole. If a sesamoid is significantly fragmented or obvious degenerative changes have occurred, excision may be the best option. A traumatic hallux valgus can be difficult to treat surgically. The medial eminence is removed to provide a fresh surface for adherence of the capsular repair and an abductor hallucis transfer is used to augment the repair. More information on turf toe and sesamoid injuries is available in chapter 12.

Summary

Lisfranc injuries can be debilitating, especially if undiagnosed or undertreated; therefore, a high index of suspicion is necessary when evaluating patients with midfoot trauma. The severity of injury determines the necessary treatment, but a stable anatomic reduction offers the best opportunity for a good outcome. Unless minimally displaced, first metatarsal fractures should be reduced and stabilized. Open treatment is necessary for unstable fractures. The middle metatarsals can often be treated nonsurgically, but any shortening or sagittal displacement should be corrected. Proximal fifth metatarsal avulsion fractures are common and rarely require surgical treatment. Metaphyseal-diaphyseal junction fractures, however, are more prone to delayed union or nonunion; therefore, early fixation of these fractures should be considered. Dislocations of the metatarsophalangeal and interphalangeal joints are usually stable after reduction and early weight bearing is possible. In the lesser toes, phalangeal fractures can be treated nonsurgically.

Significant displacement at the joint surfaces should be reduced, especially in the hallux. Acute sesamoid fractures are often amenable to nonsurgical treatment, although healing can be prolonged. Transverse fractures may benefit from surgical fixation. Chronic injuries to the sesamoids are usually treated nonsurgically, but prolonged symptoms may require excision. Turf toe injuries vary in severity and can require a prolonged period of nonsurgical care. Relatively few acute injuries require surgery. Reconstruction of chronic injuries can be challenging.

Annotated References

1. Myerson MS, Fisher RT, Burgess AR, Kenzora JE: Fracture dislocations of the tarsometatarsal joints: End results correlated with pathology and treatment. *Foot Ankle* 1986;6:225-242.

2. Hardcastle PH, Reschauer R, Kutscha-Lissberg E, Schoffmann W: Injuries to the tarsometatarsal joint: Incidence, classification and treatment. *J Bone Joint Surg Br* 1982;64:349-356.

3. Talarico RH: Hamilton GA, Ford LA, Rush SM: Fracture dislocations of the tarsometatarsal joints: Analysis of interrater reliability in using the modified Hardcastle classification system. *J Foot Ankle Surg* 2006;45:300-303.

   The authors of this study reported moderate interrater agreement among clinicians interpreting the modified Hardcastle classification system for Lisfranc fracture-dislocations.

4. Lee CA, Birkedal JP, Dickerson EA, Vieta PA Jr, Webb LX, Teasdall RD: Stabilization of Lisfranc joint injuries: A biomechanical study. *Foot Ankle Int* 2004;25:365-370.

   Cortical screw fixation provides a more rigid and stable method of fixation for Lisfranc injuries compared with K-wire fixation. Cortical screw fixation allows maintenance of anatomic reduction and possibly earlier mobilization with a decreased risk of posttraumatic arthrosis.

5. Alberta FG, Aronow MS, Barrero M, Diaz-Doran V, Sullivan RJ, Adams DJ: Ligamentous Lisfranc joint injuries: A biomechanical comparison of dorsal plate and transarticular screw fixation. *Foot Ankle Int* 2005;26: 462-473.

   Dorsal plating is an alternative to transarticular screws in the treatment of displaced Lisfranc injuries and is advantageous because correct length and alignment can be maintained in comminuted fractures.

6. Ly TV, Coetzee JC: Treatment of primarily ligamentous Lisfranc joint injuries: Primary arthrodesis compared with open reduction and internal fixation. A prospective, randomized study. *J Bone Joint Surg Am* 2006;88: 514-520.

   The authors of this study concluded that primary stable arthrodesis of the medial two or three rays appears to have better short- and medium-term outcomes than ORIF of ligamentous Lisfranc joint injuries. Level of evidence: I.

7. Kuo RS, Tejwani NC, Digiovanni CW, et al: Outcome after open reduction and internal fixation of Lisfranc joint injuries. *J Bone Joint Surg Am* 2000;82:1609-1618.

8. Desmond EA, Chou LB: Current concepts review: Lisfranc injuries. *Foot Ankle Int* 2006;27:653-660.

   This article presents of review of the literature regarding the current treatment of Lisfranc injuries.

9. Schenck RC Jr, Heckman JD: Fractures and dislocations of the forefoot: Operative and nonoperative treatment. *J Am Acad Orthop Surg* 1995;3:70-78.

10. DiGiovanni CW, Benischke SK, Hansen ST Jr: Foot injuries, in Browner BD, Trafton PG, Green NE, Swiontkowski MF, Jupiter JB, Levine AM (eds): *Skeletal Trauma* Philadelphia, PA, Elsevier Science, 2003, pp 2455-2473.

    Injuries to the metatarsals, phalanges, and metatarsophalangeal and interphalangeal joints are discussed.

11. Queen RM, Crowder TT, Johnson H, Ozumba D, Toth AP: Treatment of metatarsal stress fractures: Case reports. *Foot Ankle Int* 2007;28:506-510.

    Stress fractures of the lower extremity are common in athletes and can result in lost practice and playing time. The authors review case reports showing successful treatment of second and third metatarsal stress fractures in college-level athletes using a fracture brace and a modified shoe. Athletic participation continued during treatment.

12. Petrisor BA, Ekrol I, Court-Brown C: The epidemiology of metatarsal fractures. *Foot Ankle Int* 2006;27:172-174.

    The authors of this study reported a higher proportion

of metatarsal fractures in older women, that fifth metatarsal fracture was the most common type, multiple metatarsal fractures occurred in contiguous metatarsals, and 63% of third metatarsal fractures were associated with a fracture of either the second or fourth metatarsal.

13. Konkel KF, Menger AG, Retzlaff SA: Nonoperative treatment of fifth metatarsal fractures in an orthopaedic suburban private multispecialty practice. *Foot Ankle Int* 2005;26:704-709.

   By using closed treatment techniques for fifth metatarsal fractures, bony union was predictable with minimal cost and a high rate of satisfaction. The authors recommend nonsurgical treatment of fifth metatarsal fractures when time for return to full activity level is not critical. The authors reported a union rate of 98.5% and a satisfaction rate of 100%.

14. Egol K, Walsh M, Rosenblatt K, Capla E, Koval K: Avulsion fractures of the fifth metatarsal base: A prospective outcome study. *Foot Ankle Int* 2007;28:581-583.

   This prospective study was done to evaluate functional outcomes after acute avulsion fractures of the fifth metatarsal base. Although patients can be expected to return to their preinjury level of function, recovery may take 6 months or longer. Level of evidence: III.

15. Sarimo J, Rantanen J, Orava S, Alanen J: Tension-band wiring for fractures of the fifth metatarsal located in the junction of the proximal metaphysis and diaphysis. *Am J Sports Med* 2006;34:476-480.

   The tension-band wire technique seems to provide good results in the treatment of proximal metaphyseal/diaphyseal fractures of the fifth metatarsal in cases of primary unsuccessful nonsurgical treatment or primary unsuccessful intramedullary screw fixation. Level of evidence: IV.

16. Mologne TS, Lundeen JM, Clapper MF, O'Brien TJ: Early screw fixation versus casting in the treatment of acute Jones fractures. *Am J Sports Med* 2005;33:970-975.

   A high incidence of failure (44%) occurs after cast treatment of acute Jones fractures. Early screw fixation results in faster time to union and return to sports activities compared with cast treatment. Level of evidence: I.

17. Porter DA, Duncan M, Meyer SJ: Fifth metatarsal Jones fracture fixation with a 4.5-mm cannulated stainless steel screw in the competitive and recreational athlete: A clinical and radiographic evaluation. *Am J Sports Med* 2005;33:726-733.

   The authors report that 4.5-mm cannulated screws can yield reliable and effective healing as evidenced by clinical assessment and radiographs of fifth metatarsal Jones fractures in athletes.

18. Raikin SM, Slenker N, Ratigan B: The association of a varus hindfoot and fracture of the fifth metatarsal metaphyseal-diaphyseal junction: The Jones fracture *Am J Sports Med* 2008;36:1367-1372.

   In this study, 18 of 21 patients with a Jones fracture had varus hindfoot position, a possible predisposing factor for developing the fracture. Varus unloading may be helpful in preventing injury or refracture in these patients.

19. Jahss MH: Classic article: Foot & ankle 1:15, 1980 traumatic dislocations of the first metatarsophalangeal joint. *Foot Ankle Int* 2006;27:401-406.

   In this reprint of his classic article, Jahss describes the pathophysiology and classification system for traumatic dislocations of the first metatarsophalangeal joint.

20. Blundell CM, Nicholson P, Blackney MW: Percutaneous screw fixation for fractures of the sesamoid bones of the hallux. *J Bone Joint Surg Br* 2002;84:1138-1141.

21. Anderson RB, McBryde AM Jr : Autogenous bone grafting of hallux sesamoid nonunions. *Foot Ankle Int* 1997;18:293-296.

22. Dedmond BT, Cory JW, McBryde A Jr : The hallucal sesamoid complex. *J Am Acad Orthop Surg* 2006;14:745-753.

   A review of the evaluation and treatment options for various disorders of the sesamoid is presented.

23. Lee S, James WC, Cohen BE, Davis WH, Anderson RB: Evaluation of hallux alignment and functional outcome after isolated tibial sesamoidectomy. *Foot Ankle Int* 2005;26:803-809.

   Isolated tibial sesamoidectomy is a safe and effective treatment for recalcitrant tibial sesamoiditis. Hallux malalignment and deformity resulting in functional loss and change in hallux alignment can be avoided by meticulous surgical technique with repair of the soft tissues.

24. Watson TS, Anderson RB, Davis WH: Periarticular injuries to the hallux metatarsophalangeal joint in athletes. *Foot Ankle Clin* 2000;5:687-713.

25. Tewes DP, Fischer DA, Fritts HM, Guanche CA: MRI findings of acute turf toe: A case report and review of anatomy. *Clin Orthop Relat Res* 1994;304:200-203.

Chapter 10

Fractures and Dislocations of the Midfoot

James R. Ficke, MD

2: Foot and Ankle Trauma

Introduction

Injuries of the first and second tarsometatarsal joint, commonly known as the Lisfranc complex, are well described in the literature. This chapter will focus on current concepts in the treatment of fractures and dislocations to the midfoot area, including the navicular, cuneiform, and cuboid bones. Trauma to the midfoot area from crush injuries often results in severe open injuries to the midfoot, which can be life threatening. Treatment strategies for such traumatic injuries also will be discussed.

Navicular Injuries

Anatomy

The navicular bone has a complex shape: concave posteriorly to match the head of the talus; convex anteriorly, with three facets to match each cuneiform; wider laterally, where it receives the bifurcate ligament; and tapering medially to its tuberosity, where the posterior tibial tendon (the only tendon attached to the navicular) contributes one of its insertions. Much of the bone is covered with articular cartilage; therefore, vascularity is primarily supplied dorsally and is supplied to a lesser extent through the plantar ligamentous complex. Insufficiency fractures in an area of relative hypovascularity in the central body can lead to fracture nonunion. Because peripheral vascularity diminishes with age, there is an increasing incidence of nonunion in older patients.

The navicular bone forms the keystone of the midfoot and provides a transition zone between the mobile talonavicular joint and the relatively immobile naviculocuneiform joints. In conjunction with the anterior and middle calcaneal facets, the navicular comprises the acetabulum pedis and accounts for essentially all of the transverse tarsal rotatory motion. Navicular injuries include dorsal lip, tuberosity, body, and stress fractures.

Avulsion Fractures

Injuries to the navicular include avulsion injuries and fractures of the body and tuberosity. Dorsal avulsion is

the most common pattern, occurring in nearly 50% of navicular fractures, and is produced by an acute plantar flexion force combined with inversion. When significant articular surface is avulsed (≥ 25%), open reduction and screw fixation will accelerate the patient's return to sports activities. These uncommon injuries usually result from a high-energy force and often are associated with cuboid fractures or other midfoot injuries. Imaging studies for these injuries should include AP, lateral, and oblique plain radiographs and CT to assess often subtle secondary injuries. Coronal and transverse plane images are used in preoperative planning and are valuable for determining reconstruction options.

Body Fractures

Navicular body fractures have been categorized by Sangeorzan and associates[1] into types I, II, and III (Figures 1 through 3). Type I navicular fractures are oriented in a coronal plane and most often have no medial displacement. Type II fractures have an oblique pattern with midfoot instability and usually require open reduction and internal fixation. Type III fractures are comminuted with forefoot displacement and gross instability. This type of fracture has a poor prognosis regarding successful fixation. Recent investigations have demonstrated improved outcomes for large or displaced intra-articular fractures with anatomic reduction

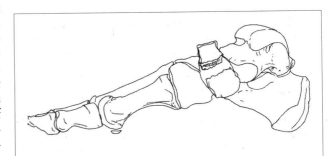

| Figure 1 | Type I navicular fractures are characterized by no midfoot instability and variable dorsal displacement. This fracture is best seen on a lateral view. The fracture line is in the coronal plane. |

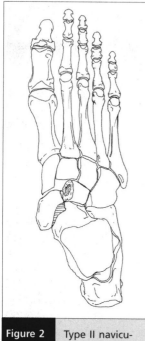

Figure 2 Type II navicular fractures are best seen on AP or oblique views. The fracture line is in the dorsolateral to plantar medial plane with medial displacement from the posterior tibial tendon.

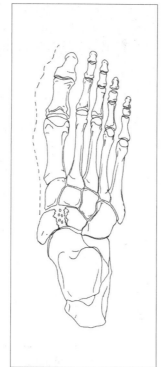

Figure 3 Type III navicular fractures are best seen on AP views and are characterized by midbody comminution and varus foot angulation.

and internal fixation.[2] Fractures should be approached in the plane of the fracture to allow maximal visualization of the reduction. The insertions of the tibialis anterior and posterior should be protected, with minimal soft-tissue stripping. Timing of the surgical procedure must respect restoration of a stable soft-tissue envelope. If the foot is globally unstable, external fixation or splints can be used until the patient is medically stable or the condition of the soft-tissue envelope will permit a safe surgical approach and definitive closure. CT is assistive in confirming reduction of the intertarsal (Chopart) and tarsometatarsal (Lisfranc) joints. Dislocation or subluxation of these joints further compromises the tenuous soft tissue and the vascularity of the forefoot. These injuries require early reduction and stabilization, often with temporary external fixation. The technique of medial column bridge plating has shown reliable results in retaining both length and alignment.[3]

The posttraumatic sequelae of pain, deformity, and loss of function are increasingly common with progressive severity of comminution and loss of talonavicular articular congruity. The same factors that make primary treatment challenging will often increase the dif-

ficulty in managing chronic deformity and pain. Few studies in the literature support specific treatments; therefore, treatment choices must be individualized to the patient. Evaluation should assess hindfoot alignment, medial arch configuration, and dynamic midfoot function. Osteonecrosis has been reported in up to 25% of navicular body fractures. Functional assessment of the patient's skin condition, grafting or flap scars, claw toes, and the presence of soft-tissue contractures (such as Achilles tendon contractures) is needed. Nerve injury, allodynia, and vascular conditions are important to evaluate before surgery. Symptomatic treatment with foot orthoses and activity modification often can delay arthrodesis of the critical talonavicular complex.[4] When medial column collapse is present, restoration through naviculocuneiform arthrodesis with bone grafting can restore hindfoot mechanics and forefoot alignment, either acutely or in delayed fashion after soft-tissue coverage is ensured (**Figure 4**).

Stress Fractures

Stress reactions and complete fractures through the navicular body are relatively common; treatment guidelines have been described in the literature. These sports injuries are somewhat difficult to diagnose with plain radiographs. These fractures should be suspected in athletes with clinical examination results showing point tenderness in a dorsal medial location over the navicular body (the N spot). CT, bone scanning, or MRI is often needed to confirm the diagnosis. The standard treatment for a patient with a navicular stress fracture has been the use of a short leg cast for 6 weeks without weight bearing. Recent studies have questioned the outcomes of this traditional treatment compared with surgery.[5,6] Because most physicians do not use traditional cast-immobilization practices, outcomes that measure return-to-sport activities are not comparable. Surgical treatment does not appear to provide better results than traditional immobilization in a cast. Current recommendations for early stress fracture diagnosis and strict adherence to non–weight-bearing restrictions in a plaster or fiberglass cast continue to be the best treatment to allow athletes to return to sports activities.

Cuboid Injuries

The cuboid bone forms the base of the mobile lateral column of the foot. With the relatively stable and immobile medial column, the calcaneocuboid joint is a biconcave saddle joint, permitting motion in coronal and sagittal planes. The articulations between the cuboid and the fourth and fifth metatarsals are similarly quite mobile, and thereby permit the lateral foot to accommodate irregular surfaces and to correct hindfoot position in varus or valgus to create a level forefoot. Cuboid injuries most commonly involve capsular avulsions or ligamentous sprains and are treated nonsurgically with plaster cast immobilization. Fractures of the body of the cuboid are

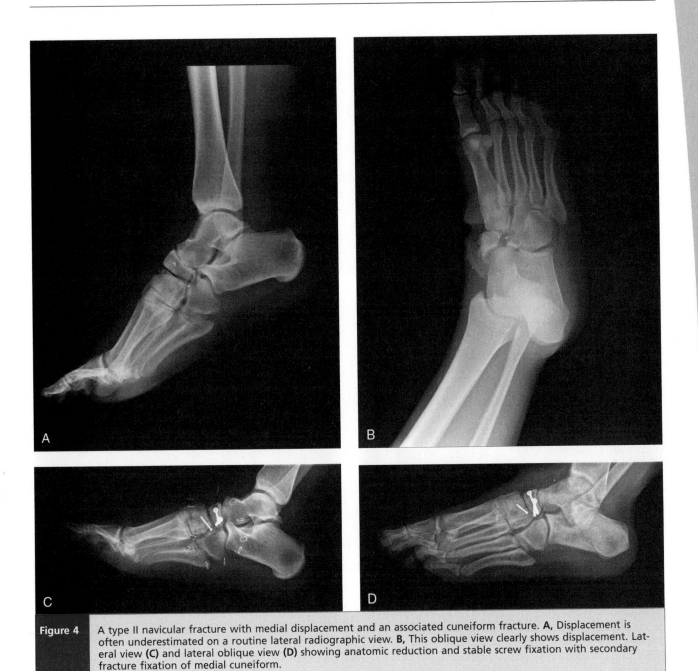

Figure 4 A type II navicular fracture with medial displacement and an associated cuneiform fracture. **A,** Displacement is often underestimated on a routine lateral radiographic view. **B,** This oblique view clearly shows displacement. Lateral view **(C)** and lateral oblique view **(D)** showing anatomic reduction and stable screw fixation with secondary fracture fixation of medial cuneiform.

most often associated with other midfoot injuries; the term "nutcracker" has been used to describe the effect of axial compression to the cuboid. In this injury, the lateral column is acutely shortened by a sharp abduction or plantar flexion mechanism. These injuries have recently been described in children.[7,8]

Because of the frequent occurrence of associated injuries, the entire foot should be imaged with plain radiography, CT, or MRI to assess for other injuries (Figure 5). A high index of suspicion for injury is needed in patients with a massively swollen midfoot and lateral tenderness. The primary goals of treatment are restoration of articular congruity and lateral column length. Stable or simple avulsion fractures can be treated with immobilization and protected weight bearing. Lateral

column injuries carry a high risk of collapse, deformity, and painful malunion; therefore, open reduction, bone grafting, and internal buttress plating often are necessary to stabilize these fractures.[9] The bridge plating technique for severely comminuted medial column injuries has been described and is also useful for open or comminuted lateral column injuries. Alternatively, external fixation can be applied using monolateral or hybrid circular frames.

Cuneiform Injuries

Taken as a complex, the cuneiform bones articulate with the navicular over a common synovial joint and

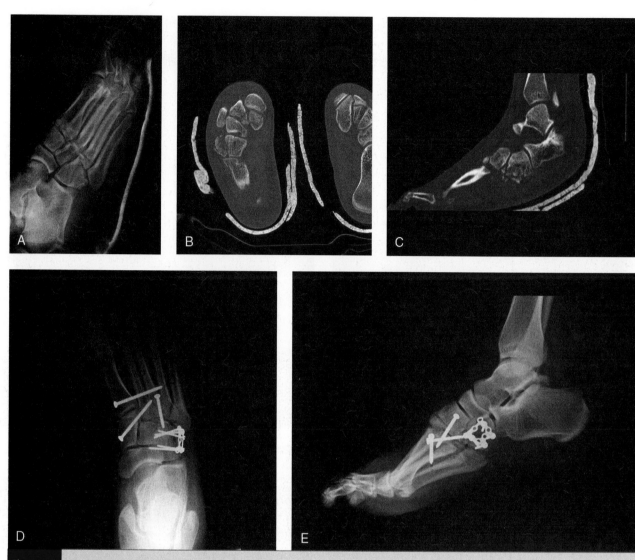

Figure 5 A patient sustained indirect trauma to multiple systems. A tertiary survey performed in the surgical intensive care unit with the patient intubated showed massive foot swelling. **A,** This oblique view shows very little displacement or shortening of the longitudinal foot architecture, but is often the ideal plain radiographic view for imaging the lateral wall of the cuboid when there is suspicion of a lateral column fracture. **B** and **C,** Biplanar CT scans often show loss of articular congruity, subluxation of the surrounding joints, and midfoot alignment, and are essential for preoperative planning in cuboid injuries. **D,** Postoperative oblique radiographic view shows restoration of lateral column height and midfoot alignment with stabilized secondary midfoot injuries. **E,** Postoperative lateral view confirms restoration of sagittal alignment.

share the distal facet of that bone. With little motion at this articulation, intra-articular injuries can tolerate transarticular screw fixation and primary arthrodesis better than the talonavicular joint. Isolated cuneiform fractures are quite rare, but often are a result of direct impact. Cuneiform injuries are diagnosed by AP, lateral, and oblique radiographs, biplanar CT, and exclusion of associated collateral injury. Current treatment recommendations involve restoration of articular congruity when possible, absolute restoration of medial column stability and alignment, and prevention of secondary complications such as skin loss, planovalgus deformity, and infection. When reduction is possible, stabilization with transarticular screws is the method of

choice. Primary arthrodesis is often an acceptable alternative in purely ligamentous injuries or severely comminuted midfoot crush-type injuries. Dislocations have been reported but appear to be quite rare. In a patient with a dislocation, open reduction is indicated.

Crush Injuries and Severe Trauma

Recently, significant attention has been directed to strategies designed to improve outcomes following severe open foot injuries (**Figure 6**). With limited soft tissue covering the midfoot, open fractures, extensive comminution, and contamination often occur. After the

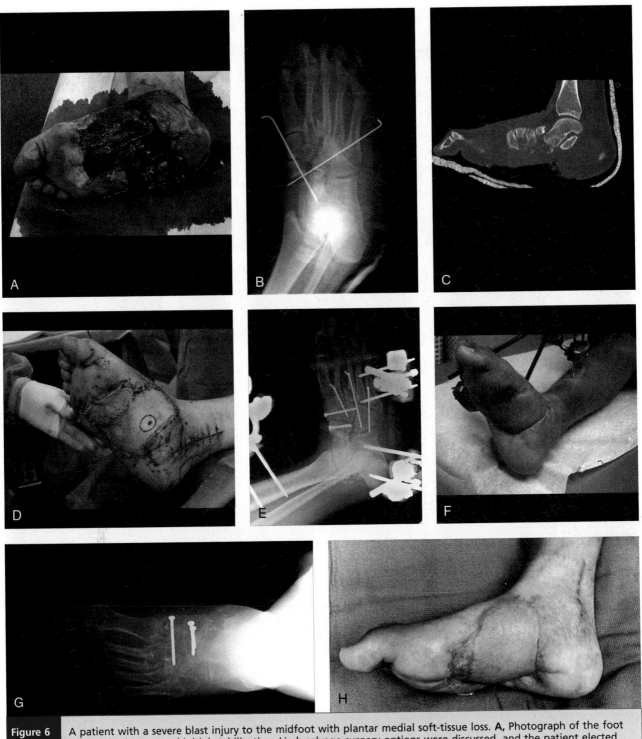

Figure 6   A patient with a severe blast injury to the midfoot with plantar medial soft-tissue loss. **A,** Photograph of the foot after débridement and initial stabilization. Limb-salvage surgery options were discussed, and the patient elected stabilization and flap coverage. **B,** Presentation radiograph after initial damage-control débridement and temporizing stabilization for transportation from a combat zone. **C,** Preoperative CT scan showing significant talonavicular subluxation and extensive comminution. **D,** Immediate postoperative photograph after bony stabilization, free innervated radial forearm flap coverage, and anastomosis of the tibial artery and medial plantar nerve. **E,** Immediate postoperative radiograph. External fixation prevents equinus contracture, supports the free tissue transfer, and permits access to the wound. **F,** Photograph at short-term follow-up shows flap survival and foot position. **G,** Radiograph at long-term follow-up shows the healed fractures and satisfactory foot alignment. **H,** Clinical photograph at long-term follow-up shows a plantigrade foot. The patient had improved sensation and a painless stable skeleton.

2: Foot and Ankle Trauma

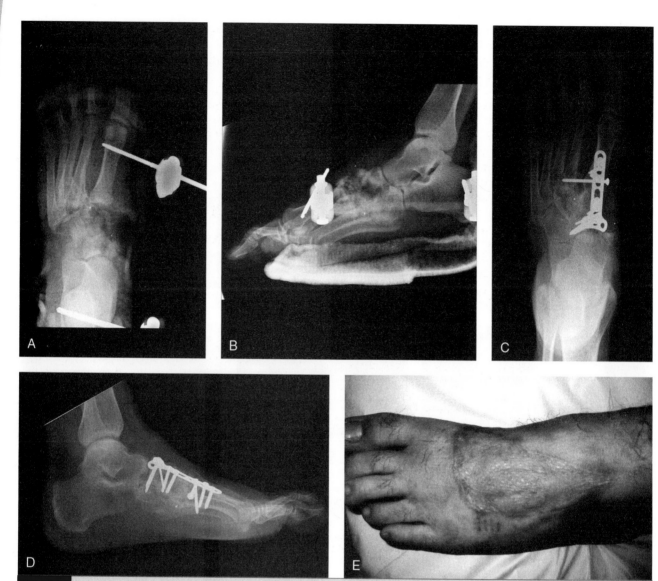

Figure 7 AP **(A)** and lateral **(B)** radiographs of a 23-year-old man with a gunshot wound to the midfoot following serial débridements and initial stabilization with external fixation. The patient had no clinical infection and had viable soft tissue, including the short anterior tibialis and posterior tibial tendon with a small residual bone fragment. Most of the navicular body and all of the medial and middle cuneiforms were missing, along with severe articular loss of the proximal first and second metatarsals. AP **(C)** and lateral **(D)** views of the foot after initial débridement before definitive treatment. Primary arthrodesis of the navicular to the first, second, and third metatarsals was performed using a T plate, iliac crest structural graft, and rotation pedicle flap coverage. The anterior tibialis and posterior tibialis were reattached into the fusion mass. These views demonstrate solid midfoot fusion at 6 months. **E,** Photograph of the foot at 8-month follow-up. After solid fusion was achieved, the patient returned to limited duty as a soldier. The patient used a padded semirigid foot orthosis for full weight bearing and ambulation.

initial trauma survey and treatment of life-threatening injuries, early aggressive wound débridement and determination of foot viability are top priorities. The ultimate treatment goal is to provide a stable, painless foot with flexibility and sensation. In the severely injured foot, extensive bony and/or soft-tissue injury may result in early amputation. Radiographic and photographic documentation and a discussion with the patient (when possible) are advisable. When amputation is necessary, the surgeon should attempt to preserve maximal function. Amputations at levels proximal to the Lisfranc joint are controversial. The Syme amputation, classi-

cally described as an ankle disarticulation, requires an intact heel pad and provides an end-bearing surface that can be fitted with a low-profile prosthetic socket and modern dynamic response foot. Recent use of the Syme amputation in patients with severe trauma and blast injuries has achieved mixed results. Current prosthetic technology often supports higher function with transtibial level amputation. In young athletes, a transtibial amputation can provide better socket fit and improved return to sports activities that require running. Partial foot amputation should be considered and can provide good function in young patients with traumatic

2: Foot and Ankle Trauma

limb loss. Soft-tissue balance is one of the most important factors in good outcomes. Ideally, after initial débridement, the patient should be informed of treatment options and included in the decision-making process.

When salvage is determined to be a possible option after adequate débridement, reconstruction requires a team approach, often including a microvascular surgeon skilled in free tissue transfer and a foot or trauma surgeon skilled in complex reconstruction. The surgeons must be prepared to use a spectrum of instrumentation to achieve articular congruity in the essential joints (ankle, talonavicular, and metatarsophalangeal); hindfoot, midfoot, and forefoot alignment and stability; and early wound coverage.[10] Often, the bones readily unite, but motion and stability are critical to successful return to function. There are no clear prognostic factors to predict outcome in the multiply injured trauma patient with associated foot injuries; treatment guidelines are lacking.[11,12] However, early restoration of functional weight bearing with a plantigrade foot and adaptive motion appear to be most predictive of successful outcomes. Avoiding late equinus deformity is a crucial factor in allowing patients to recover function. Treatment options include definitive external fixation, open reduction and internal fixation, and early arthrodesis. External fixation can be circular or hybrid, or a monolateral frame for limited stability. Indications for external fixation include extensively traumatized soft tissue, severe comminution, and unreconstructible articular surfaces in which alignment can be maintained and stability is the primary consideration. Open reduction and internal fixation continues to be an option when the condition of the soft tissue permits such surgery and articular surfaces are amenable to reduction. As earlier described, several techniques preserve vital capsular or periosteal attachments, including bridge plating or indirect reduction and percutaneous fixation. Primary arthrodesis provides a potentially stable foot and may be preferable when severe articular damage or bone loss is present and the zone of injury can be adequately covered (**Figure 7**). Probably, the single most important factor in successful outcomes for patients with these severe injuries is the ability to achieve early soft-tissue coverage.

Summary

Midfoot injuries can be mild and easily treated but are often subtle and difficult to diagnose. The key characteristic in successful management is a high index of suspicion for injury and attention to the mechanism of injury and physical examination findings. Treatment of increasingly severe injuries requires restoration of articular surfaces when possible, achieving bony and soft-tissue stability, and prevention of soft-tissue complications. Because severe midfoot injuries are relatively uncommon, understanding the patterns of these injuries, the varying prognoses, and choosing optimal treat-

ment is difficult. Progress is being made to categorize the outcomes of these injuries, especially in the patient with multiple traumatic injuries.

The views expressed in this article are those of the author and do not reflect the official policy or position of the United States Army, Department of Defense, or the US government.

Annotated References

1. Sangeorzan BJ, Benirschke SK, Mosca V, Mayo KA, Hansen ST: Displaced intra-articular fractures of the tarsal navicular. *J Bone Joint Surg Am* 1989;71:1504-1510.

2. DiGiovanni CW: Fractures of the navicular. *Foot Ankle Clin* 2004;9:25-63.

   The authors review the current literature concerning classification, diagnosis, treatment, and outcomes of tarsonavicular fractures. Key points in management include proper medial column length, maintaining posterior tibial tendon function and articular congruity of the talonavicular joint, and preserving stability of naviculocuneiform joints.

3. Schildhauer TA, Nork SE, Sangeorzan BE: Temporary bridge plating of the medial column in severe midfoot injuries. *J Orthop Trauma* 2003;17:513-520.

   The authors evaluate seven patients with severe midfoot trauma and review treatment techniques. All patients were treated with open bridge plating across the talonavicular joint or distally to stabilize the medial column. All patients retained length and alignment without secondary wound complications or infections.

4. Penner MJ: Late reconstruction after navicular fracture. *Foot Ankle Clin* 2006;11:105-119.

   Navicular fractures are uncommon injuries, and there is extremely limited literature on management of significant posttraumatic sequelae from navicular injuries. The author describes complications and presents management recommendations for nonunion, osteonecrosis, posttraumatic arthritis, and medial column deformity.

5. Burne SG, Mahoney CM, Forster BB, Koehle MS, Taunton JE, Khan KM: Tarsal navicular stress injury: Long term outcome and clinicoradiological correlation using both computed tomography and magnetic resonance imaging. *Am J Sports Med* 2005;33:1875-1881.

   Patients with navicular stress fracture were treated with traditional cast management, surgery, or weight-bearing limitations without casting. Results showed that 18% received treatment protocols recommended in the literature and 55% returned to previous activity levels. Imaging parameters did not correlate with function or clinical assessment at long-term follow-up. Level of evidence: IV.

6. Potter NJ, Brukner PD, Makdissi M, Crossley K, Kiss ZS, Bradshaw C: Navicular stress fractures: Outcomes of surgical and conservative management. *Br J Sports Med* 2006;40:692-695.

Navicular stress fractures are relatively common sports injuries and are generally effectively treated by cast immobilization and weight-bearing restrictions. Tenderness over the N spot is a reliable factor indicating the need for additional imaging studies (usually CT). Surgical fixation is an equally effective treatment as casting over the long term. Level of evidence: IV.

7. Senaran H, Mason D, De Pellegrin M: Cuboid fractures in preschool children. *J Pediatr Orthop* 2006;26:741-744.

Retrospective analysis of 28 consecutive children with cuboid fractures at an average follow-up of 39 months is presented. After treatment with plaster cast immobilization, all fractures healed. Eight patients had an underlying medical or genetic disorder.

8. Ceroni D, De Rosa V, De Coulon G, Kaelin A: Cuboid nutcracker fracture due to horseback riding in children. *J Pediatr Orthop* 2007;27:557-561.

The authors present a review of four patients with compression fractures of the cuboid as a result of forced abduction of the forefoot. The surgical technique using allograft to restore lateral column length is described.

9. Weber M, Locher S: Reconstruction of the cuboid in compression fractures: Short to midterm results in 12 patients. *Foot Ankle Int* 2002;23:1008-1013.

10. Wülker N, Stukenborg C, Savory KM, Alfke D: Hindfoot motion after isolated and combined arthrodeses: Measurements in anatomic specimens. *Foot Ankle Int* 2000;21:921-927.

11. Turchin DC, Schemitsch EH, McKee MD, Waddell JP: Do foot injuries significantly affect the functional outcome of multiply injured patients? *J Orthop Trauma* 1999;13:1-4.

12. Richter M, Wippermann B, Krettek C, et al: Fractures and fracture dislocations of the midfoot: Occurrence, causes and long-term results. *Foot Ankle Int* 2001;22:392-398.

Chapter 11

Disorders of the Anterior Tibial, Peroneal, and Achilles Tendons

Jeff Feinblatt, MD   Stanley C. Graves, MD

The Anterior Tibial Tendon

Arising from the anterolateral tibia, the anterior tibial tendon passes beneath the superior extensor retinaculum and both limbs of the inferior extensor retinaculum before inserting into the medial cuneiform and first metatarsal. The muscle functions concentrically during the swing phase of gait to dorsiflex the ankle, allowing clearance of the foot. With heel strike, the muscle functions eccentrically, slowing progression to a foot flat position. Isolated loss of the anterior tibial tendon can result in a steppage gait and foot slap. These findings are not as dramatic as those associated with common peroneal nerve dysfunction because a patient with isolated anterior tibial tendon loss will partially compensate with the remaining extensors.

Diagnosing Injuries

Brüning first reported anterior tibial tendon rupture in 1905.[1] The English literature reflects the relative rarity of this diagnosis. Most clinical studies involve small cohorts or case reports.

Acute injuries can be divided by etiology. Laceration can result from penetrating injuries or fracture of the tibia, blunt trauma causing contusion, or forceful contraction of the tibialis anterior muscle causing spontaneous rupture of the tendon in a younger patient. Tendon rupture resulting from underlying tendinosis after minimal trauma in patients 60 to 80 years of age is the most common presentation. Delayed presentation in these instances is usually the norm. A review of 12 anterior tibial tendon injuries showed that only two patients sought immediate medical attention.[2] Six patients did not present for medical evaluation until 3 to 8 months after tendon rupture. Symptoms include an initial bout of pain and weakness, which is often tolerated because of partial compensation provided by the extensor hallucis longus and extensor digitorum longus.

An avascular region exists in the anterior half of the tendon as it passes under the superior and inferior extensor retinacula. Chondroid cells are present as an adaptation to compressive and shearing forces. This region corresponds to the location of most spontaneous ruptures. Although gout, rheumatoid arthritis, diabetes, vascular disorders, and steroid injections have been associated with spontaneous rupture, most patients have no identifiable, underlying, predisposing factors. Thickening of the superomedial limb of the inferior extensor retinaculum and enhancement with contrast on MRI are associated with anterior tibial tendon rupture[3] (Figure 1).

Increased internal rotation, plantar flexion, and inversion of the talus and calcaneus have been reported in a cadaveric model of anterior tibial tendon deficiency. Reduction of heel pressure occurring during the first half of stance phase caused by loss of the eccentric deceleration of the foot also was reported.[4] Because these subtle changes can be difficult to detect in a patient who is wearing shoes, barefoot examination is recommended to reveal compensatory hyperextension of the toes during the first half of the stance phase. Inability to heel walk on the affected side is common. L5 radiculopathy or a peroneal nerve lesion should be considered in the differential diagnosis.[5] Gait abnormalities combined with a palpable defect or balled-up proximal stump appearing as a mass at the anteromedial ankle clarifies the diagnosis (Figure 2).

Treatment

Nonsurgical treatment may be appropriate for older sedentary patients or patients with significant medical comorbidities. An ankle-foot orthosis to prevent tripping over plantar-flexed toes during the swing phase of gait is often tolerated. Indications for surgical repair include lacerations involving most of the tendon width, traumatic ruptures in young patients, and spontaneous ruptures resulting in weakness in a patient who does not want to use an orthosis.

End-to-end anastomosis using a grasping type stitch (such as the Krackow, Kessler, or Bunnell stitches) is appropriate if allowed by the tendon excursion. In patients who present for delayed treatment, the tendon may not be sufficiently mobile; therefore, lengthening (V-Y or hemisection slide), interposition with autograft or allograft, or local tendon transfer (extensor hallucis longus) may be necessary (Figure 3).

Successful use of a free hemisection of the proximal anterior tibial tendon stump up to 7 cm in length has been reported.[5] Functional recovery following surgical

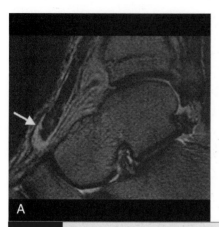
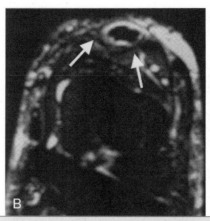
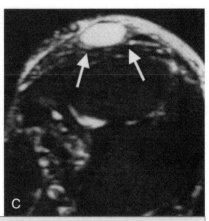

Figure 1 Rupture of the anterior tibial tendon. **A,** Sagittal proton density-weighted MRI shows rupture at the level of the oblique superomedial limb of the inferior extensor retinaculum (*arrow*). Coronal T2- weighted MRI scan (**B**) and coronal T2-weighted MRI scan distal to rupture (**C**) show the fluid-filled tendon sheath (*arrows*). (*Reproduced with permission from Lee MH, Chung CB, Cho JH, et al: Tibialis anterior tendon and extensor retinaculum: Imaging in cadavers and patients with tendon tear. AJR Am J Roentgenol 2006;187:W161-168.*)

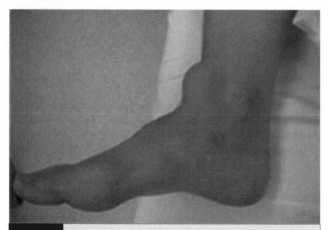

Figure 2 Clinical photograph of an anterior tibial tendon rupture. (*Reproduced with permission from Coughlin MJ, Schon LC: Disorders of tendons, in Coughlin MJ, Mann RA, Saltzman CL: Surgery of the Foot and Ankle, ed 8. St Louis, MO, Mosby, 2007, p 1159.*)

repair 3 months or more after injury is possible, although earlier treatment yields more consistent results.[6,7]

Closure of the extensor retinaculum is performed to prevent bowstringing. This procedure should be considered before incising the retinaculum. If added bulk of the repair will prevent primary closure of the retinaculum, an incision to allow V-Y or a step-cut lengthening can be performed.

The Peroneal Tendons

Anatomy

The peroneal tendons are the main evertors of the hindfoot. Because injury to these tendons is strongly associated with concomitant ankle and hindfoot pathology, contributing factors should be determined and treated to prevent recurrent injury. The peroneal tendons originate from the lateral fibula, with the peroneus brevis (PB) muscle belly continuing further distally than the peroneus longus (PL). The PB tendon lies deep to the PL tendon at the retromalleolar sulcus. Because this sulcus is variable in terms of its shape and depth, patients may be predisposed to subluxation of the tendons. The sulcus is further deepened by a fibrocartilaginous ridge, which may be avulsed along with the superior peroneal retinaculum during a dislocation event. Both structures act as restraints to lateral displacement of the tendons. The tendons continue their course along the hindfoot, separated by the peroneal tubercle on the lateral wall of the calcaneus. The PB tendon inserts into the base of the fifth metatarsal. The PL tendon abruptly turns under the foot at the cuboid tunnel and inserts plantarly on the medial cuneiform-first metatarsal base and variably to surrounding structures. Recent studies have focused on examining the factors contributing to degeneration and rupture of the peroneal tendons and to the surgical management of these lesions.

Diagnosing Injuries

Diagnosing longitudinal tears of the peroneal tendons can be difficult. Often tenderness and swelling occur; however, concomitant injury to the lateral ankle can make diagnosis more difficult. MRI can assist with the diagnosis and is often performed preoperatively. The surgeon should be aware of the "magic angle phenomenon," which is an increase in signal present in certain tissue such as tendons at an approximate 55° angle to the MRI coil (**Figure 4**). Because of their curving nature around the fibula, the peroneal tendons are especially susceptible to this phenomenon, potentially leading to an erroneous interpretation of tendon pathology. In a

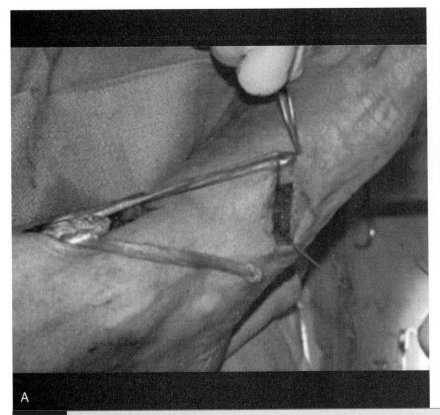
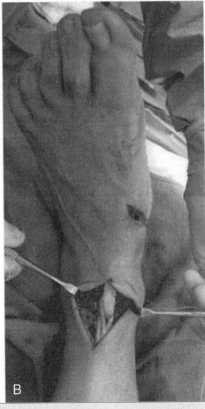

Figure 3 Free graft is used to bridge the gap during a delayed reconstruction. **A,** Medial view of free graft looped through the anterior tibial tendon stump. **B,** Anterior view after tensioning and anchoring the graft distally. (*Reproduced with permission from Coughlin MJ, Schon LC: Disorders of tendons, in Coughlin MJ, Mann RA, Saltzman CL: Surgery of the Foot and Ankle, ed 8. St Louis, MO, Mosby, 2007, pp 1165-1166.*)

recent study, 30 asymptomatic volunteers and 5 cadaveric specimens were imaged in a supine ankle neutral position and in a prone plantar-flexed position.[8] The supine position produced a high prevalence (77% to 100%) of the magic angle phenomenon in tendons coursing past the ankle, with the exception of the anterior tibial tendon (20%). The magic angle phenomenon was almost absent from tendons imaged in the prone, plantar-flexed position.

Peroneus Brevis Tears
Risk factors for PB tears include a local decrease in vascularity, ankle inversion injuries, recurrent dislocation or subluxation of the tendon out of the retromalleolar sulcus, and any mass or anatomic factor that decreases available space in the retromalleolar region (such as a low-lying PB muscle belly, peroneus quartus, tendinosis, or anatomic contour of the retromalleolar sulcus). Two types of painful intrasheath pseudosubluxation in which the tendons remain in the retromalleolar sulcus have been reported. In the first type, the PL subluxates through a longitudinal tear in the PB. In the second type, the PL subluxates around the PB, coming to rest deep to the PB intimate with the fibula.[9] The association of posterior antiglide plates used for lateral malleolar fracture and peroneal tendon pathology recently

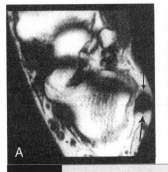
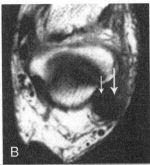

Figure 4 **A,** MRI scan shows the magic angle phenomenon. Increased signal in the PB mimics the disease state (*short arrow*). The long arrow points to the PL. **B,** MRI scan showing increased signal intensity in concomitant tears of the PB (*short arrow*) and PL (*long arrow*) tendons. (*Reproduced with permission from Wang XT, Rosenberg ZS, Mechlin MB, Schweitzer ME: Normal variants and diseases of the peroneal tendons and superior peroneal retinaculum: MR imaging features. Radiographics 2005;25:587-602.*)

has been examined. Low plate positioning with a prominent screw head in the distal hole of the plate was a risk factor for tendon lesions. Distal plate position alone was not correlated with tendon lesions.[10]

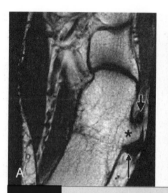
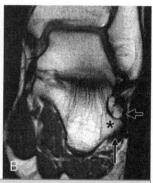

Figure 5 Hypertrophic peroneal tubercle. Axial **(A)** and coronal **(B)** T1-weighted MRI scans showing bone protuberance (*) between the PB (*short arrow*) and PL (*long arrow*) tendons. (*Reproduced with permission from Wang XT, Rosenberg ZS, Mechlin MB, Schweitzer ME: Normal variants and diseases of the peroneal tendons and superior peroneal retinaculum: MR imaging features. Radiographics 2005;25:587-602.*)

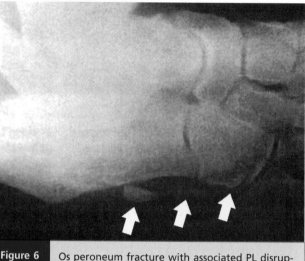

Figure 6 Os peroneum fracture with associated PL disruption (note diastasis). Os peroneum fracture fragments (*arrows*). (*Reproduced with permission from Brigido MK, Fessell DP, Jacobson JA, et al: Radiography and US of os peroneum fractures and associated peroneal tendon injuries: Initial experience. Radiology 2005;237:235-241.*)

Several recent studies have examined the relationship between a low-lying PB muscle belly and the incidence of PB tendon tears.[11-13] Preoperative MRIs in a group of patients with a surgically confirmed tear were compared with MRIs in a group of patients without tears at the time of surgery.[11] The distance between the distal extent of the PB muscle belly and the tip of the lateral malleolus was statistically smaller in patients with tears. A cadaveric examination of 30 specimens also found a significantly more distal musculotendinous junction and thicker tendon in specimens with PB tears.[12] However, an MRI study of patients with asymptomatic ankles reported that the musculotendinous junction of the PB extended to the tip of the lateral malleolus in 38% of the asymptomatic ankles.[13]

Longitudinal splitting of the PB can occur with recurrent dislocations or subluxations. The goal of surgical reconstruction is to prevent pain and further subluxation and degeneration of the tendon. Peroneal groove-deepening has been shown to decrease pressure within the middle and distal peroneal groove.[14] Groove deepening and retinacular reconstruction in 14 ankles of athletes resulted in no recurrent subluxation or dislocations at 3-year follow-up. All patients were able to return to sports activities 3 months postoperatively.[15]

Peroneus Longus Tears

The PL is at risk for degenerative changes in the retromalleolar sulcus, in a similar manner to the PB. The PL is relatively avascular in this area, with the avascular area extending to the cuboid tunnel.

An enlarged peroneal tubercle of the calcaneus is associated with PL tears (**Figure 5**). Peroneal tubercle morphology was examined in a study of 114 calcanei from an osteologic collection.[16] Presence of the tubercle was reported in 90% of specimens. Morphology was classified as flat in 42.7%, prominent in 29.1%, con-

cave in 27.2%, and as a tunnel in 1.0%. MRI scans of asymptomatic ankles showed a peroneal tubercle in 55% of patients, with 90% having a height of 4.6 mm or less.[13]

Rupture of the PL occurs most commonly just distal to the os peroneum and also can occur via fracture of an os peroneum (**Figure 6**). Discontinuity of the PL is associated with displacement of the proximal fracture fragment 10 mm from the calcaneocuboid joint on lateral radiographs, 20 mm on oblique radiographs, and with diastasis between os peroneum fragments greater than 6 mm.[17] Although both attritional and traumatic rupture of the PL occurs most commonly in this area, rupture can occur at the musculotendinous junction. Lateral compartment syndrome was reported in a 16-year-old football player after rupture of the PL at the musculotendinous junction.[18]

Combined PB and PL Tears

An algorithm has been defined for the rare clinical situation of concomitant tears of both peroneal tendons. If both tendons are grossly intact, the lesions are excised and the tendons are each tubularized. If one tendon is unusable, tenodesis is performed. If both tendons are unusable with proximal degeneration such that the tendon has no excursion, tendon transfer is performed. If both tendons are unusable but excursion of the proximal tendon is preserved, an interposition allograft or tendon transfer can be performed. In situations with significant scarring about the tendon bed, placement of a Hunter rod with delayed allograft reconstruction is suggested. Anatomic factors that predispose the patient to peroneal tears or recurrent injury, such as ankle instability or hindfoot varus, should be treated.[19]

The results of a 2003 study suggested that there was no significant difference in return to activity or American Orthopaedic Foot and Ankle Society (AOFAS) ankle-hindfoot scores in patients with an isolated PB tear, an isolated PL tear, or combined tears.[20] Return to activities averaged 3.5 months, with 14 of 16 athletes able to return to preinjury activity levels. Good results also have been reported in long-term follow-up (mean, 8.5 years) for chronic rupture of both peroneal tendons treated with staged reconstruction with flexor hallucis longus (FHL) transfer after placement of a Hunter rod.[21]

Postoperative surgical adhesion formation remains a complication after any tendon repair. Lubricin is a principal lubricant of synovial fluid and is responsible for boundary lubrication of articular cartilage. In a recent in vitro extrasynovial canine tendon model, significant reduction in gliding resistance was reported after application of lubricin and carbodiimide derivatized gelatin (hypothesized to allow increased covalent bonding of lubricin to the tendon surface through exposure of carboxyl groups) compared with controls.[22] Continued research could provide pharmacologic methods for preventing postoperative adhesion formation.

The Achilles Tendon

Anatomy

The Achilles tendon, the confluence of the triceps surae, is the largest tendon in the body. Although a synovial sheath is not present, the tendon is encased in a paratenon, which decreases friction during excursion. The blood supply to the tendon arises distally from interosseous arterioles in the calcaneus, proximally through intramuscular arterioles, and through the paratenon. There is a relative avascular area 2 to 6 cm above the calcaneal insertion, predisposing this area to degenerative changes. Two bursae are intimate with the insertion: the retrocalcaneal bursa between the calcaneal tuberosity and the Achilles tendon, and the Achilles tendon bursa, which is variably found between the tendon and the skin. A 90° rotation of the Achilles fibers occurs such that medial gastrocnemius fibers insert posteriorly on the calcaneus. The Achilles tendon is the primary plantar flexor of the ankle and it also can act as an invertor of the heel because of its relatively medial insertion. During normal activities, the Achilles tendon can be subjected to 2,000 to 7,000 N of force or 6 to 10 times body weight during the single-stance phase of running. The collagen orientation and spiral of the Achilles tendon before insertion enables it to elongate 7% to 15%. Ultimate strength has been estimated at 70% of bone; therefore, Achilles tendon rupture occurs more frequently than an avulsion fracture.

Imaging

Although the diagnosis of Achilles tendon injury is often made based on the patient history and examination,

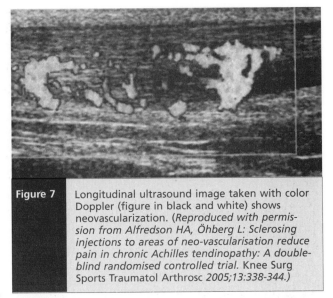

Figure 7 Longitudinal ultrasound image taken with color Doppler (figure in black and white) shows neovascularization. (*Reproduced with permission from Alfredson HA, Öhberg L: Sclerosing injections to areas of neo-vascularisation reduce pain in chronic Achilles tendinopathy: A double-blind randomised controlled trial.* Knee Surg Sports Traumatol Arthrosc *2005;13:338-344.*)

additional information is often required. Plain radiographs can show calcification of the tendon near the insertion (indicating chronicity), a Haglund deformity associated with retrocalcaneal bursitis, and signs of systemic inflammatory arthropathies (indicated by cortical erosion or indistinct borders).

Ultrasonography also is used for diagnosing Achilles tendon disorders. It is cost effective, can be performed in the physician's office, allows dynamic evaluation, and can be used to confirm localization for invasive procedures such as injections. Because most US surgeons are unfamiliar with ultrasonography techniques, this imaging modality is used more often in Europe. Recently, color Doppler and power Doppler have been used to examine neovascularization associated with tendinosis (**Figure 7**). More information on ultrasonography is available in chapter 3.

MRI allows evaluation of both bony and soft-tissue detail, and localized reactive and degenerative changes are easily assessed. A large field of view aids in evaluating surrounding structures and eliminating other potential sources of pathology. More information on MRI is available in chapter 3.

Pathologic Conditions

Acute Achilles tendon disruption, chronic disruption, bursitis, Haglund deformity, paratenonitis, paratenonitis with tendinosis, and tendinosis are commonly occurring disorders. The literature on these disorders is often vague, referring only to the clinical presentation of tendinopathy rather than the underlying diagnosis. Changes in the understanding of underlying pathologic and histologic characteristics of each disease have translated into changes in terminology. Continued research and increasingly specific tests will continue to redefine these disease entities and their progression from normal to pathologic.

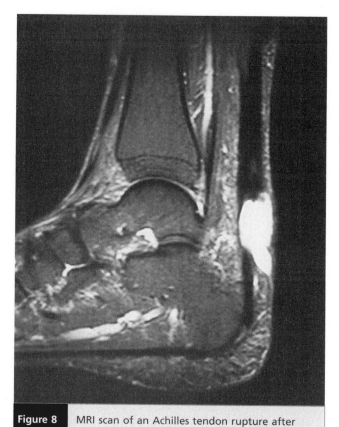

Figure 8 MRI scan of an Achilles tendon rupture after corticosteroid injection. (*Reproduced with permission from Solan M, Davies M: Management of insertional tendinopathy of the Achilles tendon. Foot Ankle Clin 2007;12:597-615.*)

Acute Ruptures

Clinical Presentation

The peak incidence of acute Achilles tendon rupture occurs during the third to fifth decades of life, with sporadically active individuals most often affected. It is believed that some underlying intratendinous degeneration is present at the time of overt failure. Although rupture can occur anywhere along its course, Achilles tendon rupture most commonly occurs from 2 to 6 cm proximal to the calcaneal insertion. Direct injury, such as a laceration or blow to the posterior leg, can cause acute disruption, although most injuries occur indirectly as a result of longitudinal overloading of the tendon during attempted plantar flexion against an immobile object or violent dorsiflexion of the ankle (during jumping and landing). Fluoroquinolone and local corticosteroid administration, underlying systemic inflammatory conditions, endocrine dysfunction, and infection can predispose patients to acute rupture (**Figure 8**). Patients often report hearing and feeling the sensation of "getting shot" or of being kicked. Pain and difficulty walking occur immediately. Swelling and ecchymosis occur rapidly and can obscure the initially palpable defect. Lack of plantar flexion with squeezing of the calf (Thompson test) is positive in complete ruptures. With the patient in a prone position and the knee flexed to 90°, increased ankle dorsiflexion will occur from loss of resting tension of the triceps surae. Active plantar flexion strength is decreased, but is still present because of recruitment of secondary flexor muscles. Because of delayed presentation for treatment, up to 25% of Achilles tendon ruptures may be undetected in the emergency department because the tendon outline is obscured by edema and active plantar flexion is retained.

Treatment

There is no uniformly accepted algorithm for the treatment of acute Achilles tendon disruption. Investigators have reported lower rerupture rates and better functional outcomes with surgical treatment compared with nonsurgical management.[23] Historically, apposition of the tendon ends during nonsurgical treatment has not been examined. Prolonged periods of immobilization and non–weight-bearing protocols also were prescribed for nonsurgically treated patients. Basic science and clinical studies in the literature concerning the hand have shown significant improvements in tendon strength and gliding movement with early motion and controlled loading. The available literature shows that the benefits of early motion and weight bearing are beginning to be recognized for patients treated with Achilles tendon surgery.

Nonsurgical Treatment and Outcomes

Nonsurgical management consists of serial casting beginning in a plantar-flexed position to allow closer apposition of the tendon ends, with progression over time to a plantigrade position. A boot walker with heel inserts also can be used to obtain the same progression (over time) from plantar flexion to plantigrade, while allowing the patient controlled motion. Many recent reports focus on early functional rehabilitation for patients treated surgically or nonsurgically; however, no working definitions of "early" and "functional" currently exist.[24,25] Many physicians use a shortened period of absolute immobilization, with subsequent progression into a walking boot or dorsiflexion-limiting orthosis. Variables that should be considered include time of absolute immobilization, the range of motion limited by an orthosis, and time progression until unlimited range of motion is allowed. Weight-bearing status and duration until full weight bearing also varies among physicians.

A 2006 study compared immediate weight bearing with non–weight-bearing cast immobilization in a group of nonsurgically treated patients.[24] Three 1.5-cm heel lifts were used initially and decreased by one heel lift every 2 weeks in the weight-bearing group. The weight-bearing group was not predisposed to a higher complication rate. No tendon lengthening or higher rerupture rate was reported. Strength, as determined by dynamometry, did not differ between the two groups.

In a 2007 randomized control trial, outcomes of 50 patients treated nonsurgically or with open repair using nonabsorbable suture were evaluated.[25] Both patient groups were immobilized in an equinus cast for 10 days followed by an orthosis (initially at 20° plantar flexion). At 4 weeks, the orthosis was brought to neutral, and at 6 weeks weight bearing commenced. Patients were weaned from crutches at 8 weeks. Patients were instructed to remove the orthosis and perform active dorsiflexion and passive plantar flexion every hour during orthosis use. No significant difference in motion, calf circumference, strength, rerupture rate, or complications were reported at 1-year follow-up.

Surgical Treatment Outcomes

Surgical treatment of Achilles tendon rupture has a higher rate of all types of complications (with the exception of rerupture) compared with nonsurgical treatment. Less invasive methods have been devised to avoid these complications, with a focus on early functional rehabilitation and weight bearing (**Figure 9**).

In a 2007 study, 50 patients were randomized to receive early movement of the ankle (between neutral and plantar flexion) in a brace, or immobilization in a cast with the foot in neutral position for 6 weeks.[26] Weight bearing was allowed by the third postoperative week in both groups. Results showed tendon elongation during the first 6 weeks followed by some tendon shortening; however, less tendon elongation (2 mm) occurred in the early movement group compared with the group treated with immobilization (5 mm of tendon elongation). Measurements were based on intraoperatively placed markers. Patients with less elongation had better clinical outcomes, although peak isokinetic torque was not greater.

In a 2003 study, a group of patients treated for acute midsubstance tears of the Achilles tendon were allowed immediate weight bearing to tolerance after immobilization in equinus for 2 weeks, followed by immobilization with an ankle neutral dorsiflexion stop.[27] Another group of patients did not bear weight for 4 weeks. Comparison of the groups showed higher patient satisfaction but no increase in isometric strength in the early weight-bearing group. No incidents of rerupture were reported in either group.

Another study showed a reduction in time to normal walking and stair climbing in patients treated with immediate weight bearing.[24] No difference in return to sports activities or work was reported. Two patients in the immediate weight-bearing group sustained rerupture during activities in violation of the study's protocol. The authors commented that patients mobilized immediately after repair may be more vulnerable to injury because some patients return to strenuous activities too quickly.

Augmentation of end-to-end anastomosis with various grafts for Achilles tendon rupture has been described in the literature. A 2007 study reported no clinical difference at 17-month follow-up in patients treated with end-to-end repair compared with those treated with end-to-end repair and augmentation using

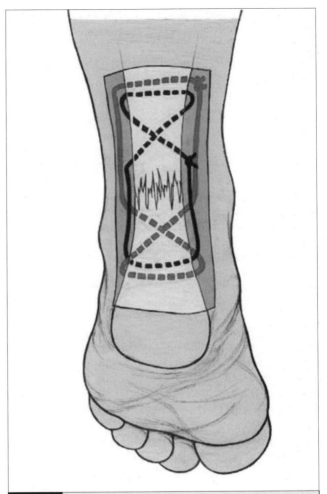

Figure 9 Illustration showing the modified Ma and Griffith percutaneous repair method for Achilles tendon rupture. (*Reproduced with permission from Halasi T, Tállay A, Berkes I: Percutaneous Achilles tendon repair with and without endoscopic control. Knee Surg Sports Traumatol Arthrosc 2003;11:409-414.*)

plantaris tendon.[28] The additional time and potential morbidity of tendon augmentation is usually unnecessary when repairing acute tendon ruptures.

The role of percutaneous repair for acute Achilles tendon ruptures has been examined in several studies.[29-31] Compared with open surgical repair, percutaneous or minimally invasive repair is reportedly simpler to perform and yields more favorable cosmetic results; however, some clinical studies have reported a higher rerupture rate and sural nerve complications. A recent study compared 132 patients treated with percutaneous repair with 105 patients treated with open repair.[29] Fewer major complications were noted in the percutaneous group (4.5% versus 12.4%); however, a higher rerupture rate (3.7% versus 2.8%) and sural nerve dysfunction rate (4.5% versus 2.8%) were reported in the group treated with percutaneous repair.

Another study examined the outcome differences in

patients treated with a commercially available percutaneous technique (Achillon, Newdeal, Lyon, France) and a minimally invasive technique (modified Ma and Griffith).[30] Twelve patients in each group were followed for a minimum of 2 years. Both groups had no reruptures and similar AOFAS scores, return to work and sports times, and isokinetic strength.

Although the historic rerupture rate after percutaneous repair has been higher than after standard open repair, a low rerupture rate (2.5%) was reported in 163 patients after minimally invasive repair using absorbable sutures and a postoperative functional rehabilitation protocol (5 days in a non–weight-bearing cast, followed by full weight bearing, and semirigid taping or a soft cast for a total of 6 weeks).[31]

With percutaneous techniques, coaptation of the tendon ends is not ensured. The higher reported Achilles tendon rerupture rates can result from the remaining gap. A recent study of MRI findings showed that it took a significantly longer time for the tendon gap to disappear in patients treated with percutaneous repair (11.6 weeks) compared with those treated with open repair (8.6 weeks).[32] The potential gap between tendon ends can be evaluated with endoscopy and treated at the time of percutaneous repair. In a 2003 study, the rerupture rate was lower when endoscopy was used to ensure tendon coaptation compared with percutaneous repair alone.[33]

A Cochrane database meta-analysis of 14 recent studies examined Achilles tendon rupture management.[34] Pooled results showed that the rerupture rate was 3.5% in the surgically treated group compared with 12.6% in the nonsurgically treated group. Complication rates (other than rerupture) were reported as 34% in the surgical group and 2.7% in the nonsurgical group. The most common complications were adhesions, altered sensation, and infection. The overall wound infection rate was 4.0% in the surgical group. Comparison of casting versus the use of a functional splint after surgery revealed no significant difference in rerupture rates. Complications excluding rerupture were higher in the cast group (35.7%) compared with the group treated with a functional splint (19.5%). Comparison of open versus percutaneous repair showed no difference in the rerupture rate; however, only two studies qualified for review. A higher infection rate was reported in the group treated with open repair, although the infection rate was exceedingly high (19.6%) compared with historic infection rates. It was concluded that open treatment significantly reduces the risk of rerupture compared with nonsurgical treatment but results in a higher rate of other complications. Complications may be decreased by performing percutaneous repair; however, this assumption is based on data from a small number of patients. Use of a functional brace postoperatively rather than a cast appears to reduce the overall complication rate.

In a meta-analysis of six studies comparing early functional protocols with postoperative immobilization after Achilles tendon reconstruction, no difference in rerupture rates (2.5% functional rehabilitation versus 3.9% immobilization) were found.[35] No differences in superficial or deep infection rates were noted, but decreased scar adhesion and sural deficits were reported in the functional rehabilitation group. Improved subjective results were reported for the early functional rehabilitation group.

The need for prophylaxis to prevent deep venous thrombosis (DVT) in patients undergoing surgery to the lower extremity was examined in a recent study. Distal DVT was diagnosed in 34% of patients after end-to-end repair and casting within 72 hours of Achilles tendon rupture despite treatment with dalteparin. A placebo group had a similar rate of distal DVT. The rate of proximal DVT was 2% in the treated group and 6% in the placebo group. No pulmonary embolisms or bleeding complications occurred.[36] The timing of DVT prophylaxis and appropriate patient selection for this preventive treatment remain controversial.

Chronic Ruptures

No uniform definition or point in time exists to differentiate acute and chronic ruptures. Some authors confine acute injuries to patients treated in the initial 48 hours after tendon rupture. Other authors use a definition based on the required surgical treatment, although primary repair techniques may be successful at obtaining end-to-end anastomosis as late as 3 months after injury. Contracture of the triceps surae occurs within 3 to 4 days of injury. After 6 weeks, collagen reorientation occurs with more haphazard scar formation. Reestablishment of tendon continuity occurs as the void is filled with maturing scar tissue. A once palpable defect may disappear and the Thompson test may be negative. As the scar matures, a patient can regain the strength to perform a single leg heel raise, although endurance is rarely regained. Clinical outcome can be predicated based on the functional muscle-tendon unit length. In Achilles tendons that heal in an elongated position, patients will have weakened plantar flexion and an altered gait.

Nonsurgical Treatment

In patients electing nonsurgical treatment, such as those with minimal pain and good function or those who are poor surgical candidates because of medical comorbidities, an ankle-foot orthosis can be used. Some patients have been successfully treated with immobilization in plantar flexion despite a prolonged elapsed period from the time of injury. Physical therapy is needed to maximize strength of the triceps surae and the secondary plantar flexors.

Surgical Treatment

The decision to proceed with surgical treatment is based on a patient's pain and functional disability. Patients should be counseled that calf circumference and strength will not be equal to that of the uninjured leg.

Because of the extensive exposure often needed, the complication rate after reconstruction for a chronic rupture is theoretically higher than for an acute repair. Methods to eliminate the tendon gap, such as gastrocnemius-soleus recession, V-Y advancement, a Bosworth turndown flap, or augmentation with FHL transfer, free autograft, or allograft may be needed. MRI is useful for evaluating the length of degenerative changes and fibrous scarring, allowing appropriate surgical planning. Gaps measuring 1 to 2 cm after débridement can often be repaired by end-to-end anastomosis after mobilization of the tendon. Gaps of 2 to 5 cm can be reconstructed with a V-Y advancement, a Bosworth turndown, tendon transfer, or a combination of these techniques. The limbs of the V in the V-Y advancement should be 1.5 times the length of the tendon defect. Advancement beyond 3 to 5 cm is not possible because the muscle insertion onto the tendon becomes disrupted. In a Bosworth turndown, the central 1.5 cm of Achilles tendon is harvested proximally, turned on itself distally after suture placement to prevent disruption of the remaining tendon, and inserted into the distal tendon stump. If tendon transfer is performed, the FHL is most commonly used, although the flexor digitorum longus and PB have been studied (**Figure 10**). The FHL is in phase with the Achilles tendon, has approximately 30% of the plantar flexion power of the Achilles tendon, and improves blood supply to the Achilles tendon because of its distal muscle belly. No significant clinical or pedobarographic changes that suggest morbidity of FHL tendon harvest have been reported in patients after FHL transfer for chronic Achilles tendon rupture or tendinosis.[37] FHL harvest can be performed distally, providing additional tendon length through a medial approach to the midfoot, or proximally through a posteromedial incision at the hindfoot. To bridge gaps of 5 cm or more, turndown, tendon transfer, free autograft or allograft, or a combination of these techniques can be used. The use of a free gracilis tendon to bridge the defect was reported in 21 patients with neglected Achilles tendon ruptures.[38] No reruptures were reported. Patients had significantly less strength in the operated limb but walked without a limp.

Achilles Tendinopathy

Tendinopathy of the Achilles tendon can occur at the insertion of the tendon into the calcaneus and within the substance of the tendon. The distinction between insertional and noninsertional tendinopathy is important because nonsurgical management is typically successful in patients with noninsertional tendinopathy whereas insertional tendinopathy is more likely to require surgical treatment.

Noninsertional Achilles Tendinopathy

Patients with noninsertional tendinopathy present with activity-related pain over the Achilles tendon. Squeezing the tendon between two fingers allows localization of the pain. Thickening or nodularity may be present.

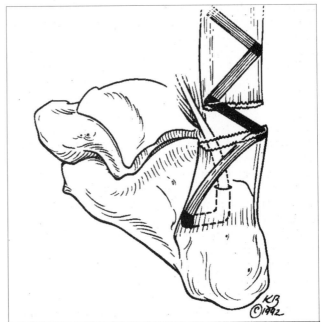

Figure 10 Illustration showing FHL transfer. A drill hole is placed just deep to the Achilles insertion directed plantarward. A second drill hole is made from medial to lateral to intersect the first drill hole midway through the posterior body of the calcaneus. These are then interconnected using a towel clip. The FHL tendon is transferred from proximal to distal and weaved through the remaining Achilles tendon. (*Reproduced with permission from Wapner KL, Pavlock GS, Hecht PJ, Naselli F, Walther R: Repair of chronic Achilles tendon rupture with flexor hallucis longus tendon transfer.* Foot Ankle *1993;14:443-449.*)

A nodule that moves with ankle motion is within the tendon (tendinosis), whereas thickening that remains stationary is located in the paratenon (paratenonitis). Multiple treatment methods have been evaluated for noninsertional tendinopathy, including extracorporal shock wave therapy (ESWT), eccentric exercises, splinting, bracing, and topical nitric oxide.

The use of ESWT for tendinopathy is controversial with many questions concerning the ideal level of energy needed and the number and frequency of treatments. In a study with up to 1 year of follow-up, significant improvements in the visual analog scale were reported in a group of patients who were treated with a single dose of high-energy ESWT (3,000 pulses of 0.21 mJ/mm²; total energy flux density, 604 mJ/mm²) compared with a control group.[39] No significant improvements were reported in a double-blinded, placebo-controlled study of patients with chronic tendinopathy (most with noninsertional tendinopathy) using low-energy ESWT (1,500 pulses of maximum 0.2 mJ/mm² repeated monthly for 3 months).[40] In another study, patients were treated with low-energy ESWT (2,000 pulses of 0.1 mJ/mm² repeated weekly for 3 weeks) or eccentric exercises. Both treatment groups had similar improvement and

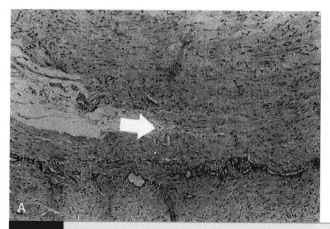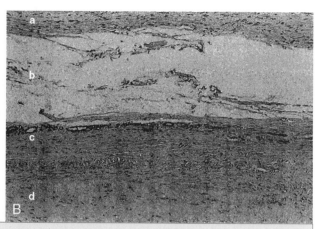

Figure 11 Histopathologic images of paratenonitis. **A,** The parietal and visceral paratenon appear fused (*arrow*). **B,** Image shows (a) thickening of the parietal paratenon; (b) space between parietal and visceral paratenon is preserved; (c) capillary proliferation within the visceral paratenon with fibrosis near small vessels; and (d) normal tendon tissue. (*Reproduced with permission from Puddu G, Ippolito E, Postacchini F: A classification of Achilles tendon disease. Am J Sports Med 1976;4:145-150.*)

had better outcomes than patients treated with an observational approach.[41] Another study examined the role of eccentric training for noninsertional tendinopathy in sedentary patients and found that training was effective in 56% of patients.[42] However, the 44% failure rate is significantly higher than previous reports that studied an athletic population. It was concluded that eccentric programs probably are not as beneficial in a sedentary population as in an athletic population.

Many studies have been performed over the past 5 years on the role of eccentric exercises in the treatment of patients with Achilles tendinopathy. Altered vascularization of the tendon and paratenon occur in Achilles tendinopathy. Paratenon microcirculation was examined before and following a 12-week course of eccentric training in 20 patients with either insertional or noninsertional tendinopathy.[43] Pain was significantly reduced after the eccentric training program. Several areas of decreased blood flow and postcapillary venous filling pressures were found, but no changes in oxygenation were reported. The reduction in pain was correlated with the reduction in blood flow.

A 2007 study examined the difference between an eccentric training program and a simple stretching program for patients with either insertional or noninsertional Achilles tendinopathy followed for 1 year.[44] Significant improvements occurred in both groups as early as 3 weeks after initiation of treatment but no differences were reported between the stretching or eccentric training groups.

The addition of a night splint did not improve symptoms when compared with eccentric training alone.[45] In another study, an AirHeel brace (Aircast, Vista, CA) was as effective as eccentric exercises when used alone, but provided no additional benefit when combined with eccentric training for moderately active patients (recreational athletes).[46] Another study showed an improved rate of return to sports activities after eccentric

training compared with eccentric training and night splinting or night splinting alone.[47] Pain at 1-year follow-up was similarly improved in the three groups.

Topical glyceryl trinitrate combined with therapy showed efficacy in a 3-year follow-up study, with 88% of patients reporting they were asymptomatic compared with 67% of patients treated with rehabilitation and a placebo.[48] Those treated with glyceryl trinitrate also had better scores on a functional assessment questionnaire; however, scores on a commonly used questionnaire had poor correlation with a battery of muscle-tendon function tests in another study.[49] Further studies are needed to confirm the role of glyceryl trinitrate. Theories behind the mechanism of action of glyceryl trinitrate include stimulation of collagen production by fibroblasts or modulation of programmed cell death.

In the competitive athletic population, it is necessary to determine if and when an athlete with Achilles tendinopathy can return to play. One study found no negative effects of continued running and jumping activities during treatment of tendinopathy.[50] Patients were allowed to perform activities that resulted in pain scores of up to 5 (of 10) on a visual analog scale if pain had subsided by the following morning. Details of the patient's diagnosis (such as insertional versus noninsertional tendinopathy) were not included in the study. Patients with isolated paratenonitis are believed to have a low risk for tendon rupture. This risk increases with tendon involvement and degeneration.

Paratenonitis
The term Achilles tendinitis is inappropriate. It is not the relatively avascular tendon that becomes inflamed but rather the paratenon (**Figure 11**). Overuse, altered training regimens, or altered mechanics caused by shoe wear or running surfaces initiates the inflammatory response most commonly seen in athletes. A study of in-

fantry recruits showed a significant seasonal effect in the incidence of paratenonitis, with a 3.6% incidence in the summer and 9.4% in the winter.[51] It was hypothesized that a temperature-associated change in viscosity of the mucopolysaccharides, which function as a lubricant in the paratenon, lead to a higher propensity for the condition during cold-weather training. Symptoms involve pain with activities and warmth and swelling with localized tenderness. Pain can be elicited by reproducing friction between the paratenon and the examiner's fingers. Treatment includes reducing the inciting factors along with rest, icing, stretching, and the administration of nonsteroidal anti-inflammatory drugs. Most patients improve rapidly. In those with refractory paratenonitis, formalized physical therapy, cross training, or discontinuation of sports activities may be appropriate.

If symptoms persist or recur, the paratenon can thicken and adhesions can form between the paratenon and the tendon. Brisement, the rapid instillation of saline or anesthetic between the paratenon and tendon, may break up these adhesions. Clinical improvement has occurred in approximately 30% to 50% of patients treated with brisement.[52,53] Surgery is typically reserved for patients with chronic refractory paratenonitis. The thickened, scarred paratenon is excised, with rapid reinstitution of motion to minimize postoperative scarring. Surgical success has been reported in 70% to 100% of patients and has resulted in better symptom resolution than surgery for tendinosis.[52,53]

Achilles Tendinosis
Degenerative lesions of the tendon alone are not painful, which may explain the spontaneous rupture of the Achilles tendon without a significant traumatic event. Often, however, degeneration of the tendon is associated with changes in the paratenon, which may be painful (paratenonitis with tendinosis) (**Figure 12**).

Clinically, patients with tendinosis are typically older than patients with isolated paratenonitis. Localized thickening and nodularity of the tendon may be present, usually 2 to 6 cm above the calcaneal insertion (**Figure 13**). This nodularity moves with excursion of the tendon. Patients may report loss of motion caused by fibrosis or gradual onset of weak plantar flexion as cyclical tearing and a blunted healing response lead to elongation of the muscle-tendon unit. A clinical finding of increased dorsiflexion is often reported. Acute onset of weakness may signal complete or partial rupture of the Achilles tendon. Surgical visualization of tendinosis often shows at the tendon with loss of normal luster and striations. The tendon becomes yellowed and soft-

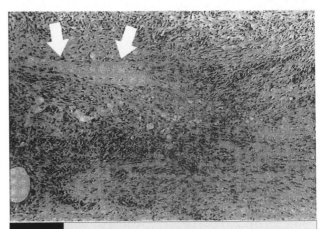

Figure 12 Histopathologic image of paratenonitis with tendinosis. Areas of fatty degeneration (appear as spaces) and hyaline degeneration (*arrows*) associated with marked vascular proliferation. Histiomonocytes are present near the small vessels. (*Reproduced with permission from Puddu G, Ippolito E, Postacchini F: A classification of Achilles tendon disease. Am J Sports Med 1976;4:145-150.*)

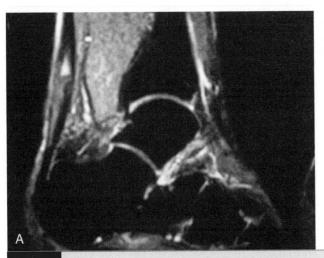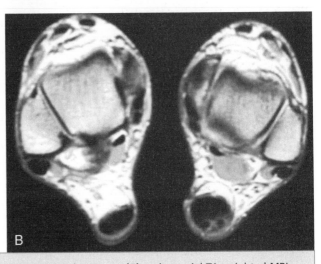

Figure 13 Noninsertional Achilles tendinosis shown on a sagittal T2-weighted MRI scan (**A**) and an axial T1-weighted MRI scan (**B**). (*Reproduced with permission from Holmes GB, Lin J: Etiologic factors associated with symptomatic Achilles tendinopathy. Foot Ankle Int 2007;28:660.*)

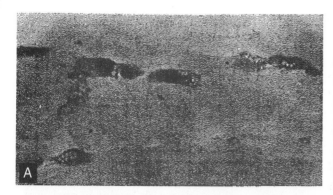

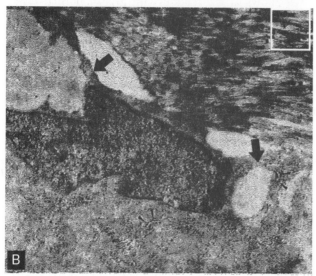

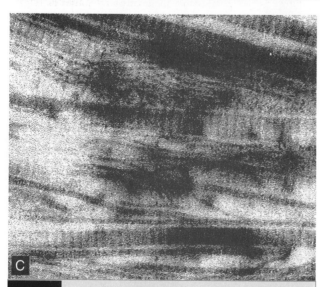

Figure 14 Tendinosis. **A,** Light microscopy reveals fatty degeneration of the tenocytes (×1,000). **B,** Electron microscopy shows residuals of the rough endoplasmic reticulum (×10,000). **C,** Field (indicated by square in part B): the parallel collagen fibrils show the normal axial periodicity; nearby, others appear completely disorganized and frayed (×40,000). (*Reproduced with permission from Puddu G, Ippolito E, Postacchini F: A classification of Achilles tendon disease. Am J Sports Med 1976;4:145-150.*)

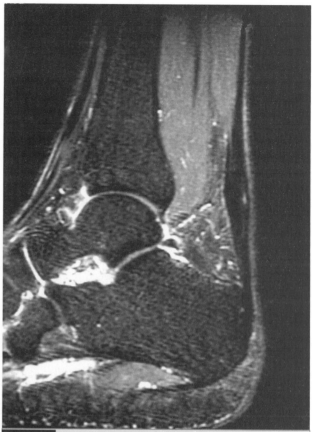

Figure 15 T2-weighted MRI scan of Achilles tendinosis with thickening and high signal within the tendon. (*Reproduced with permission from Hennessy MS, Molloy AP, Sturdee SW: Noninsertional Achilles tendinopathy. Foot Ankle Clin 2007;12:617-641.*)

ened. Microscopically, fatty or mucoid degeneration and chondroid metaplasia with decreased cellularity is seen (Figure 14). In comparison with the population norms, there is a significant association with Achilles tendinopathy and obesity in men and women, hypertension in women, hormone replacement therapy and oral contraceptives use in women, and diabetes mellitus in men younger than 44 years.[54] Imaging with sonography or MRI reveals areas of degeneration and can assist in surgical planning (Figure 15).

Initial treatment of Achilles tendinosis is nonsurgical and includes immobilization, use of a rocker-bottom shoe or heel lift, and physical therapy with a focus on modalities such as iontophoresis and electrical stimulation. Eccentric exercises can improve symptoms in most patients. These exercises require significant compliance because the exercises are performed to recreate pain with increasing loads placed on the leg as tolerance allows. The mechanism by which eccentric exercises relieve symptoms is unclear, but theories include an alteration in the tension of the Achilles tendon and promotion of vascular ingrowth that improves the healing response and disrupts neovascularization with the associated nerve endings. ESWT, nitric oxide (glyceryl trinitrate patches), and sclerosing agents have been studied and are promising nonsurgical modalities. In a recent double-blind study that used sonography to target areas of neovascularization within the tendon, local injection of polidocanol, a sclerosing agent that also has an anesthetic effect, was compared with injection of lidocaine.[55] At 3-month follow-up, the polidocanol group reported more outcome satisfaction and had a significant reduction in tendon pain compared with the group treated with lidocaine. Neovascularization was absent in the pain-free tendons, but not in the painful tendons. Sclerosant therapy appears to have good potential for symptom resolution. Nitric oxide plays an important role in collagen synthesis and tendon healing. The use of a transdermal nitric oxide patch was reported to be effective for treating tennis elbow, supraspinatus tendinosis, and Achilles tendinosis in four separate, randomized, double-blind, clinical trials.[56-59]

Surgery may be considered in patients with refractory Achilles tendinosis despite appropriate nonsurgical management for 3 to 6 months. Minimally invasive surgery is performed with multiple longitudinal percutaneous incisions in the tendon to promote vascular ingrowth. Traditional surgical treatment involves excising the most diseased portion of the tendon (the tendon in its entirety is usually abnormal microscopically). The most degenerative portion of tendon is typically centrally located, with a relatively normal-appearing peripheral tissue. Addition of a tendon transfer, most commonly a FHL transfer, improves local vascularity and increases the amount of collagen present. Tendon transfer is recommended if 50% of the Achilles tendon is resected. Time to maximal improvement after Achilles tendon débridement and FHL transfer is prolonged, with reports of continued improvement at 8 months and up to 2 years. Previous studies had reported better results in younger patients, but a recent study using a single incision with proximal harvest of the FHL tendon reported a greater increase in AOFAS scores in patients older than 50 years compared with patients younger than 50 years.[60] Complete excision of the Achilles tendon with transfer of the FHL resulted in decreased pain and an 86% patient satisfied rate; however, plantar strength was reduced by 30%.[61]

Insertional Achilles Tendinopathy

Insertional tendinopathy commonly refers to multiple diagnoses including retrocalcaneal bursitis, Haglund deformity, insertional paratenonitis, insertional tendinosis, and systemic enthesopathies. From a clinical perspective, differentiating these diagnoses helps in determining the cause of the patient's disability. It is important to understand that clinical overlap and progression from inflammatory to degenerative changes can occur.

Haglund deformity alone is not a pathologic condition but can predispose the patient to retrocalcaneal bursitis, which typically can be treated conservatively with shoe wear and activity modifications until symptoms resolve. Haglund deformity also predisposes the patient to localized mechanical irritation leading to paratenonitis, and in long-standing disorders, to insertional tendinosis. A lateral radiograph that shows calcification of the tendon indicates chronicity of the disease and, to date, has resulted in inferior results with nonsurgical management.

Isolated insertional paratenonitis can occur in athletically active patients as a result of overuse, hill running, training on hard surfaces, or using shoe wear with a firm heel counter. Systemic causes for enthesopathy, such as psoriasis, spondyloarthropathies, gout, and Reiter syndrome, should be evaluated (especially in patients with bilateral involvement).

Isolated Achilles tendinosis represents an end-stage disease and can be difficult to manage. After significant degeneration is seen on imaging studies, especially in the presence of calcification of the tendon, patients should be counseled that recovery may be prolonged and that nonsurgical treatment may be unsuccessful.

Nonsurgical Treatment

Initial management of insertional tendinopathy can include nonsteroidal anti-inflammatory drugs, shoe wear modifications (soft or absent heel counter), activity modifications, and stretching and eccentric exercises. Corticosteroid administration should be avoided because of the risk of further weakening the tendon. Unlike noninsertional tendinopathy that responds well to a stretching program, only one third of patients with insertional tendinopathy will improve with stretching. In one study, low-energy ESWT was superior to an eccentric training program for treating patients with chronic insertional Achilles tendinopathy; improvement was maintained at 1-year follow-up.[62] There are only a few reports in the literature on ESWT and sclerosing injections for treating insertional Achilles tendinopathy; however, these reports are promising.[39-41,55] The success rate with nonsurgical treatment decreases significantly once intrasubstance changes consistent with tendinosis are present on MRI scans.[63]

Surgical Treatment

The choice of surgical treatment for patients with refractory disease (typically after more than 6 to 12 months of nonsurgical management) depends on the underlying diagnosis. Options include open or endoscopic resection of the Haglund deformity to remove the mechanical source of irritation, excision of the inflamed retrocalcaneal bursa if present, and débridement of the Achilles paratenon and tendon as needed. In general, patients with disease arising from the Haglund deformity and retrocalcaneal bursa recover more quickly and have better functional outcomes than patients in whom the tendon itself is involved. In patients with extensive degenerative changes requiring substantial tendon excision, reconstruction with tendon transfer (usually FHL transfer) should be consid-

2: Foot and Ankle Trauma

ered. These patients typically require at least 6 months for full recovery.

Summary

Recent advances in the treatment of tendon disorders have focused on decreasing morbidity associated with surgical treatment and rapid mobilization of the patient. Although current surgical management of tendinosis involves excising and replacing the most degenerative area of tendon, a better understanding of the disease process on a cellular and genomic level may enable physicians to prevent, modify, or even reverse the changes that lead to pain and loss of function.

Annotated References

1. Brüning F: Zwei seltene Fälle von subcutaner Sehnenzerreißung. *Münchner Med Wochenschr.* 1905;52:1928-1930.

2. Ouzounian TJ, Anderson R: Anterior tibial tendon rupture. *Foot Ankle Int* 1995;16:406-410.

3. Lee MH, Chung CB, Cho JH, et al: Tibialis anterior tendon and extensor retinaculum: Imaging in cadavers and patients with tendon tear. *AJR Am J Roentgenol* 2006; 187:W161-W168.

   MRI examinations of cadaveric specimens were compared with scans of tendon tears in seven patients with clinical rupture of the anterior tibial tendon. Both partial tears and complete tears were noted at the level of the oblique superomedial limb of the inferior extensor retinaculum. Thickening or enhancement of this structure was associated with clinical tears. Level of evidence: IV.

4. Negrine JP: Tibialis anterior rupture: Acute and chronic. *Foot Ankle Clin* 2007;12:569-572.

   The author presents a brief review of the anatomy, clinical presentation, and treatment of patients with anterior tibial tendon rupture.

5. van Acker G, Pingen F, Luitse J, Goslings C: Rupture of the tibialis anterior tendon. *Acta Orthop Belg* 2006;72: 105-107.

   The authors present a case report of an active 68-year-old patient treated with end-to-end anterior tibial tendon reconstruction 6 weeks after rupture. A good functional recovery was reported.

6. Wong MW: Traumatic tibialis anterior tendon rupture-delayed repair with free sliding tibialis anterior tendon graft. *Injury* 2004;35:940-944.

   The authors present a case report of a 45-year-old patient who underwent anterior tibial tendon reconstruction 1 year after injury. At the time of surgery, a 7-cm defect was bridged using a 7-cm hemisection slide of the anterior tibial tendon. At 1-year follow-up, no compen-

satory hyperextension of the toes was reported during ankle dorsiflexion.

7. Wülker N, Hurschler C, Emmerich J: In vitro simulation of stance phase gait part II: Simulated anterior tibial tendon dysfunction and potential compensation. *Foot Ankle Int* 2003;24:623-629.

   Cadaver specimens were used to examine the effect of anterior tibial tendon deficiency on tarsal motion and plantar pressure. Increased internal rotation, plantar flexion, and inversion of the talus and calcaneus were reported. Decreased plantar heel pressures were noted during the first half of the stance phase.

8. Mengiardi B, Pfirrmann CW, Schöttle PB, et al: Magic angle effect in MR imaging of ankle tendons: Influence of foot positioning on prevalence and site in asymptomatic subjects and cadaveric tendons. *Eur Radiol* 2006; 16:2197-2206.

   MRI was used to examine 30 asymptomatic volunteers and 5 cadaveric specimens in supine ankle neutral and prone, plantar-flexed positions. A high prevalence of examinations showed the magic angle phenomenon (effect) in the supine position, whereas this effect was almost nonexistent in the prone plantar-flexed position. Level of evidence: IV.

9. Raikin SM, Elias I, Nazarian LN: Intrasheath subluxation of the peroneal tendons. *J Bone Joint Surg Am* 2008;90:992-999.

   Subluxation of the PL through a longitudinal tear in the PB or around the PB but remaining in the retromalleolar sulcus was reported. Surgical repair provided good pain relief.

10. Weber M, Krause F: Peroneal tendon lesions caused by antiglide plates used for fixation of lateral malleolar fractures: The effect of plate and screw position. *Foot Ankle Int* 2005;26:281-285.

    The authors present a review of 70 patients who underwent removal of a posterior antiglide plate used for fixation of a lateral malleolar fracture. Peroneal lesions were reported in nine patients. The location of the plate was not correlated with the lesion; however, a prominent screw head in the distal hole of a low-lying plate was correlated with a peroneal tendon lesion. Level of evidence: IV.

11. Freccero DM, Berkowitz MJ: The relationship between tears of the peroneus brevis tendon and the distal extent of its muscle belly: An MRI study. *Foot Ankle Int* 2006; 27:236-239.

    A retrospective review of 59 patients who underwent surgical exploration of the peroneal tendons is presented. Preoperative sagittal MRI scans were examined to determine the distance of the musculotendinous junction to the tip of fibula. The distance was significantly less in the group with confirmed tears (33.1 mm) compared with a control group of patients without lateral ankle disorders. Level of evidence: IV.

12. Geller J, Lin S, Cordas D, Vieira P: Relationship of a low-lying muscle belly to tears of the peroneus brevis

tendon. *Am J Orthop* 2003;32:541-544.

In this cadaveric study of 30 specimens, the distance from the musculotendinous junction to the fibula tip was measured in a group of specimens with longitudinal tears and compared with a group without tears. The musculotendinous junction was more distal and the tendon thicker in specimens with tears.

13. Saupe N, Mengiardi B, Pfirrmann CW, Vienne P, Seifert B, Zanetti M: Anatomic variants associated with peroneal tendon disorders: MR imaging findings in volunteers with asymptomatic ankles. *Radiology* 2007;242: 509-517.

    MRI was used to study 65 asymptomatic patients (median age, 45 years) to examine the prevalence of anatomic risk factors commonly associated with peroneal disease. The authors concluded that variants believed to predispose patients to peroneal tendon disorders are found in asymptomatic patients.

14. Title CI, Jung HG, Parks BG, Schon LC: The peroneal groove deepening procedure: A biomechanical study of pressure reduction. *Foot Ankle Int* 2005;26:442-448.

    The authors of this cadaveric study reported that after groove deepening by posterior wall osteotomy, the mean pressure over the calcaneofibular ligament increased; however, the increase was not significant. Pressure within the proximal groove increased in all but one ankle position. A decrease in pressure occurred at the middle and distal groove. This redistribution of stress may be responsible for the success of groove deepening procedures.

15. Porter D, McCarroll J, Knapp E, Torma J: Peroneal tendon subluxation in athletes: Fibular groove deepening and retinacular reconstruction. *Foot Ankle Int* 2005;26: 436-441.

    In this case study, 14 ankles underwent fibular groove deepening by posterior fibular osteotomy and superior peroneal retinaculum reconstruction. At final follow-up (average follow-up, 35 months) no recurrence of subluxation or dislocation had occurred. Eight patients returned to their previous level of sports activities. Level of evidence: IV.

16. Hyer CF, Dawson JM, Philbin TM, Berlet GC, Lee TH: The peroneal tubercle: Description, classification, and relevance to peroneus longus tendon pathology. *Foot Ankle Int* 2005;26:947-950.

    The authors of this study examined 114 calcanei from an osteologiccollection to determine the presence and morphology of the peroneal tubercle. The tubercle was noted in 90% of specimens, with an average length, height, and depth of 13.04 mm, 9.44 mm, and 3.13 mm, respectively. Morphology was considered flat in 43%, prominent in 29%, concave in 27%, and tunnel in 1%.

17. Brigido MK, Fessell DP, Jacobson JA, et al: Radiography and US of os peroneum fractures and associated peroneal tendon injuries: Initial experience. *Radiology* 2005;237:235-241.

    A review of the radiographs of nine patients with os peroneum fractures showed that complete disruption of the PL (as seen with ultrasonography, MRI scans, or confirmed at surgery) was associated with os peroneum fragment separation of 6 mm or more, displacement of the proximal fragment of 10 mm or more on lateral radiographs, and 20 mm or more on oblique radiographs. Level of evidence: IV.

18. Mendelson S, Mendelson A, Holmes J: Compartment syndrome after acute rupture of the peroneus longus in a high school football player: A case report. *Am J Orthop* 2003;32:510-512.

    The authors present a case report of a 16-year-old athlete with a PL rupture at the musculotendinous junction, which occurred during a football scrimmage. Lateral compartment syndrome developed, making fasciotomy necessary.

19. Redfern D, Myerson M: The management of concomitant tears of the peroneus longus and brevis tendons. *Foot Ankle Int* 2004;25:695-707.

    The authors of this cohort study evaluated 29 feet with concomitant tears of the PL and PB tendons (mean follow-up, 4.6 years). The average age of the patients was 36 years at time of surgery for tears of both peroneal tendons. An algorithm for treatment based on tear severity is presented. Level of evidence: IV.

20. Saxena A, Cassidy A: Peroneal tendon injuries: An evaluation of 49 tears in 41 patients. *J Foot Ankle Surg* 2003;42:215-220.

    Forty-nine tears of the peroneal tendons were evaluated at a minimum follow-up of 1 year postoperatively. No significant difference in return to activity or postoperative AOFAS scores were reported when comparing patients with an isolated PB tear, an isolated PL tear, or combined tears. Level of evidence: IV.

21. Wapner KL, Taras JS, Lin SS, Chao W: Staged reconstruction for chronic rupture of both peroneal tendons using Hunter rod and flexor hallucis longus tendon transfer: A long-term followup study. *Foot Ankle Int* 2006;27:591-597.

    The authors present the outcomes of seven patients treated with staged reconstruction of combined peroneal tendon rupture. At more than 5-years follow-up, one fair, one good, and five excellent results were reported. One patient required a Broström procedure 2 years after the peroneal reconstruction. Level of evidence: IV.

22. Taguchi M, Sun YL, Zhao C, et al: Lubricin surface modification improves extrasynovial tendon gliding in a canine model in vitro. *J Bone Joint Surg Am* 2008;90: 129-135.

    Exogenously applied lubricin combined with carbodiimide derivatized gelatin significantly decreased gliding resistance compared with saline, lubricin alone, or carbodiimide derivatized gelatin alone. The authors concluded that lubricin preferentially adheres to the tendon surface pretreated with carbodiimide derivatized gelatin and may improve clinical results of extrasynovial tendon grafting.

2: Foot and Ankle Trauma

23. Möller M, Movin T, Granhed H, Lind K, Faxen E, Karlsson J: Acute rupture of tendon Achilles: A prospective randomised study of comparison between surgical and non-surgical treatment. *J Bone Joint Surg Br* 2001; 83:843-848.

24. Costa ML, MacMillan K, Halliday D, et al: Randomised controlled trials of immediate weight-bearing mobilisation for rupture of the tendo Achillis. *J Bone Joint Surg Br* 2006;88:69-77.

    Two randomized control trials of patients with Achilles tendon ruptures were used to compare immediate functional weight bearing with cast immobilization after open repair, and immediate functional weight bearing with cast immobilization with nonsurgical management. No evidence of increased tendon lengthening or rerupture rates in either of the immediate weight-bearing groups was reported. Level of evidence: I.

25. Twaddle BC, Poon P: Early motion for Achilles tendon ruptures: Is surgery important? A randomized, prospective study. *Am J Sports Med* 2007;35:2033-2038.

    Fifty patients were treated with open repair or nonsurgical management of Achilles tendon ruptures. Both groups were placed in an equinus cast for 10 days followed by an orthosis. At 6 weeks protected weight bearing commenced and at 8 weeks patients no longer used crutches. Patients performed active dorsiflexion and passive plantar flexion every hour during the orthosis period. No significant differences in motion, calf circumference, Musculoskeletal Functional Assessment Instrument scores, rerupture rates, or complications were reported at 1-year follow-up. Level of evidence: I.

26. Kangas J, Pajala A, Ohtonen P, Leppilahti J: Achilles tendon elongation after rupture repair: A randomized comparison of 2 postoperative regimens. *Am J Sports Med* 2007;35:59-64.

    Fifty patients treated with open repair with absorbable suture were divided into a group allowed early motion and a group treated with cast immobilization at neutral. Tendon elongation was greater in the immobilization group as measured by markers placed intraoperatively. Patients with less elongation had better clinical outcomes. Level of evidence: II.

27. Maffulli N, Tallon C, Wong J, Peng Lim K, Bleakney R: Early weightbearing and ankle mobilization after open repair of acute midsubstance tears of the Achilles tendon. *J Sports Med Phys Fitness* 2003;43:367-379.

    The authors present the results of 53 patients with acute midsubstance tears of the Achilles tendon who were treated with open repair with absorbable sutures. Patients were divided into two groups. One group was allowed immediate weight bearing in an equinus cast for 2 weeks, followed by an ankle neutral dorsiflexion stop orthosis. The other group was managed with a non–weight-bearing protocol with serial casting every 2 weeks for 6 weeks, progressing from equinus to ankle neutral. Level of evidence: II.

28. Aktas S, Kocaoglu B, Nalbantoglu U, Seyhan M, Guven O: End-to-end versus augmented repair in the treatment of acute Achilles tendon ruptures. *J Foot Ankle Surg* 2007;46:336-340.

    No significant differences were found at 17 months postoperatively in 30 patients treated with either an end-to-end repair or an end-to-end repair with plantaris augmentation for acute Achilles tendon ruptures. Level of evidence: II.

29. Cretnik A, Kosanovic M, Smrkolj V: Percutaneous versus open repair of the ruptured Achilles tendon: A comparative study. *Am J Sports Med* 2005;33:1369-1379.

    In this cohort study, 132 consecutive patients treated with percutaneous repair were compared with 105 patients treated with open repair for a ruptured Achilles tendon. Percutaneous repair was associated with a lower rate of major complications, with equivalent AOFAS and Holz scores, but with a higher risk of rerupture and sural nerve disturbance. Level of evidence: II.

30. Ceccarelli F, Berti L, Giuriati L, Romagnoli M, Giannini S: Percutaneous and minimally invasive techniques of Achilles tendon repair. *Clin Orthop Relat Res* 2007; 458:188-193.

    The authors compared percutaneous and minimally invasive techniques of Achilles tendon repair. No reruptures were reported in either group and similar results were found for isokinetic strength, AOFAS scores, and the amount of time needed before return to work and sports activities. Level of evidence: III.

31. Lansdaal JR, Goslings JC, Reichart M, et al: The results of 163 Achilles tendon ruptures treated by a minimally invasive surgical technique and functional aftertreatment. *Injury* 2007;38:839-844.

    One hundred sixty-three Achilles tendon ruptures were treated with minimally invasive surgery and functional rehabilitation. The authors reported a 92% patient satisfaction rate. Major complications occurred in 5.5% of patients, sural nerve dysfunction in 9.2%, rerupture in 2.5%, deep infection in 1.8%, tendon necrosis in 0.6%, and DVT in 0.6%. Level of evidence: IV.

32. Fujikawa A, Kyoto Y, Kawaguchi M, Naoi Y, Ukegawa Y: Achilles tendon after percutaneous surgical repair: Serial MRI observation of uncomplicated healing. *AJR Am J Roentgenol* 2007;189:1169-1174.

    Thirty percutaneous and 10 open repairs of Achilles tendons were evaluated at 4, 8, and 12 weeks postoperatively. Radiologists were blinded to the procedure performed. A longer interval until the disappearance of tendon gap was noted in patients treated with percutaneous repairs. The tendon gap was reported to persist longer for both groups on T1-weighted images compared with T2-weighted images. Level of evidence: III.

33. Halasi T, Tállay A, Berkes I: Percutaneous Achilles tendon repair with and without endoscopic control. *Knee Surg Sports Traumatol Arthrosc* 2003;11:409-414.

    In this study, 89 patients treated with a minimally invasive modified Ma and Griffith technique were compared with 67 patients treated with a similar technique performed with the addition of endoscopy to confirm tendon apposition. The rerupture rate was lower with endoscopy. Return to sports, plantar-flexion strength, and subjective results were similar between the groups. Level of evidence: III.

34. Khan RJ, Fick D, Brammar TJ, Crawford J, Parker MJ: Interventions for treating acute Achilles tendon ruptures. *Cochrane Database Syst Rev* 2004;3:CD003674.

The author performed a meta-analysis on 14 trials (891 patients) and reported that open treatment of acute Achilles tendon ruptures is associated with a lower risk of rerupture (relative risk = 0.27) but higher risks of other complications (relative risk = 10.60) compared with nonsurgical management. Percutaneous repair was associated with shorter surgical time and a lower risk of infection (relative risk = 10.52) versus open repair. Postoperative management with functional bracing resulted in a shorter inpatient stay, less time off work, a quicker return to sports activities, and a lower complication rate than casting. Level of evidence: II.

35. Suchak AA, Spooner C, Reid DC, Jomha NM: Postoperative rehabilitation protocols for Achilles tendon ruptures: A meta-analysis. *Clin Orthop Relat Res* 2006; 445:216-221.

In this systematic review of level II studies, the authors evaluate six studies with 315 patients. In comparing early functional treatment protocols with postoperative immobilization, the authors reported that early functional rehabilitation led to higher patient satisfaction rates but no difference in the rate of rerupture. Level of evidence: II.

36. Lapidus LJ, Rosfors S, Ponzer S, et al: Prolonged thromboprophylaxis with dalteparin after surgical treatment of Achilles tendon rupture: A randomized, placebo-controlled study. *J Orthop Trauma* 2007;21:52-57.

In this randomized, placebo-controlled, double-blind study, 105 patients received dalteparin or a placebo after end-to-end repair and casting for acute Achilles tendon rupture. The DVT rate was 34% in the treatment group (proximal DVT, 2%) and 36% in the control group (proximal DVT, 6%). No pulmonary emboli or major bleeding occurred in either group. The authors concluded that thromboprophylaxis with dalteparin is not indicated after repair of acute Achilles tendon rupture. Level of evidence: I.

37. Coull R, Flavin R, Stephens MM: Flexor hallucis longus tendon transfer: Evaluation of postoperative morbidity. *Foot Ankle Int* 2003;24:931-934.

Clinical scoring systems and pedobarographs were used to evaluate 16 patients treated with FHL tendon transfer. No increased load at the first or second metatarsophalangeal joints and no significant decrease in peak pressure on the distal phalanx were reported. Level of evidence: IV.

38. Maffulli N, Leadbetter WB: Free gracilis tendon graft in neglected tears of the Achilles tendon. *Clin J Sport Med* 2005;15:56-61.

At an average follow-up of 28 months, 21 patients had no reported reruptures after free gracilis tendon graft was used to repair neglected tears of the Achilles tendon. Plantar strength remained less than the contralateral side, but patients walked without a limp and were able to toe walk. Level of evidence: IV.

39. Furia JP: High-energy extracorporeal shock wave therapy as a treatment for chronic noninsertional Achilles tendinopathy. *Am J Sports Med* 2008;36:502-508.

In this study, 34 patients treated with single-dose ESWT (3,000 pulses of 0.21 mJ/mm^2) were compared with 34 patients treated with other nonsurgical methods. Visual analog scores and subjective results were better at 1, 3, and 12 months in the ESWT group. Level of evidence: III.

40. Costa ML, Shepstone L, Donell ST, Thomas TL: Shock wave therapy for chronic Achilles tendon pain: A randomized placebo-controlled trial. *Clin Orthop Relat Res* 2005;440:199-204.

Forty-nine patients with chronic tendinopathy (46 with noninsertional tendinopathy) were evaluated to compare shock wave therapy and placebo for chronic Achilles tendon pain. At 1-year follow-up, no difference between the groups was reported. Tendon rupture occurred in two patients in the treatment group. The authors concluded that there was no evidence to support the efficacy of shock wave therapy, but acknowledge that the study was underpowered. Level of evidence: I.

41. Rompe JD, Nafe B, Furia JP, Maffulli N: Eccentric loading, shock-wave treatment, or a wait-and-see policy for tendinopathy of the main body of tendo Achillis: A randomized controlled trial. *Am J Sports Med* 2007;35: 374-383.

In this study, 75 patients with recalcitrant, noninsertional Achilles tendinopathy were randomized into groups treated with eccentric exercises, low-energy ESWT, or observation. At 4 months, the groups receiving treatment showed no differences; however, the observed group had poorer outcomes. Level of evidence: I.

42. Sayana MK, Maffulli N: Eccentric calf muscle training in non-athletic patients with Achilles tendinopathy. *J Sci Med Sport* 2007;10:52-58.

Thiry-four sedentary patients with chronic noninsertional Achilles tendinopathy were treated with an eccentric training program. After the training period, 44% did not improve. Of those showing improvement, the rate of improvement was less than reported for an athletic population. Level of evidence: IV.

43. Knobloch K, Kraemer R, Jagodzinski M, Zeichen J, Meller R, Vogt PM: Eccentric training decreases paratendon capillary blood flow and preserves paratendon oxygen saturation in chronic Achilles tendinopathy. *J Orthop Sports Phys Ther* 2007;37:269-276.

Twenty patients including those with both insertional and noninsertional Achilles tendinopathy participated in an eccentric training program. Laser Doppler flowmetry and spectrophotometry were used to assess paratendon microcirculation, oxygenation, and postcapillary venous filling pressures. Several areas of decreased blood flow and filling pressures were reported. No significant change of superficial or deep paratendon oxygenation was found. Level of evidence: II.

44. Nørregaard J, Larsen CC, Bieler T, Langberg H: Eccentric exercise in treatment of Achilles tendinopathy. *Scand J Med Sci Sports* 2007;17:133-138.

Forty-five patients with chronic insertional or noninser-

2: Foot and Ankle Trauma

tional Achilles tendinopathy were randomly assigned to eccentric training or stretching groups. Significant improvement over baseline measurements was reported at 3 weeks and continued improvement occurred for more than 1 year. No difference in results was reported in the two groups. Level of evidence: II.

45. de Vos RJ, Weir A, Visser RJ, de Winter T, Tol JL: The additional value of a night splint to eccentric exercises in chronic midportion Achilles tendinopathy: A randomised controlled trial. *Br J Sports Med* 2007;41:e5.

The authors report on 70 tendons affected with noninsertional tendinopathy for more than 2 months. Patients were assigned to eccentric training alone or eccentric training with a night splint. After 12 weeks of treatment, no difference was found in Victorian Institute of Sport Assessment-Achilles scores or patient satisfaction. Level of evidence: I.

46. Petersen W, Welp R, Rosenbaum D: Chronic Achilles tendinopathy: A prospective randomized study comparing the therapeutic effect of eccentric training, the AirHeel brace, and a combination of both. *Am J Sports Med* 2007;35:1659-1667.

In this randomized, controlled, clinical trial, 100 recreational athletes with noninsertional tendinopathy were divided into groups using eccentric training alone, an AirHeel brace alone, or combined treatment. Similar significant improvements were reported in the three groups at 6- to 52-week follow-up. Level of evidence: I.

47. Roos EM, Engström M, Lagerquist A, Söderberg B: Clinical improvement after 6 weeks of eccentric exercise in patients with mid-portion Achilles tendinopathy: A randomized trial with 1-year follow-up. *Scand J Med Sci Sports* 2004;14:286-295.

The authors report on 45 patients with Achilles tendinopathy who were divided into groups using eccentric training alone, a night splint alone, or combined treatment. All groups were similarly improved at up to 1-year follow-up. More patients in the eccentric training group returned to participation in sports activities than the other two groups. Level of evidence: I.

48. Paoloni JA, Murrell GA: Three-year followup study of topical glyceryl trinitrate treatment of chronic noninsertional Achilles tendinopathy. *Foot Ankle Int* 2007;28: 1064-1068.

Fifty-two patients in this randomized, double-blinded, placebo-controlled, clinical trial were treated with topical glyceryl trinitrate for chronic Achilles tendinopathy. At 3 years after cessation of treatment, significantly more of the treated patients were asymptomatic compared with a placebo control group. The authors concluded that glyceryl trinitrate has an action mechanism that provides more than an analgesic effect. Level of evidence: I.

49. Silbernagel KG, Thomeé R, Eriksson BI, Karlsson J: Full symptomatic recovery does not ensure full recovery of muscle-tendon function in patients with Achilles tendinopathy. *Br J Sports Med* 2007;41:276-280.

Thirty-seven patients with noninsertional tendinopathy were evaluated with the Victorian Institute of Sport Assessment-Achilles questionnaire and underwent functional testing at 1-year after the study began. High performance on the functional battery was reported in only 25% of patients despite symptomatic recovery as reported on the assessment questionnaire. Level of evidence: IV.

50. Silbernagel KG, Thomeé R, Eriksson BI, Karlsson J: Continued sports activity, using a pain-monitoring model, during rehabilitation in patients with Achilles tendinopathy: A randomized controlled study. *Am J Sports Med* 2007;35:897-906.

Thirty-eight active patients with Achilles tendinopathy were divided into a group who received rehabilitation exercises but had to stop all running and jumping activities and a group who participated in therapy and was allowed to continue activities with the use of a pain monitoring system. No negative effects of continued activities were reported in the group monitored for pain. Level of evidence: I.

51. Milgrom C, Finestone A, Zin D, Mandel D, Novack V: Cold weather training: A risk factor for Achilles paratendinitis among recruits. *Foot Ankle Int* 2003;24:398-401.

In this clinical study of 1,405 infantry recruits, paratenonitis developed in 3.6% during summer training and 9.4% during winter training. The authors believe that a drop in external temperature increases viscosity of mucopolysaccharides in the paratenon and may be a causative factor for Achilles paratenonitis.

52. Coughlin MJ, Schon LC: Disorders of the tendons, in Coughlin MJ, Mann RA, Saltzman CL (eds): *Surgery of the Foot and Ankle*, ed 8. Philadelphia, PA, Mosby, 2007, pp 1149-1277.

The authors provide updated information regarding tendon disorders.

53. McGarvey WC: Achilles tendon injuries: Acute and chronic, in Richardson EG (ed): *Orthopaedic Knowledge Update: Foot and Ankle*, ed 3. Rosemont, IL, American Academy of Orthopaedic Surgeons, 2004, pp 91-102.

The author presents a review of acute and chronic Achilles tendon injuries including anatomy, biomechanics, classification, diagnostic imaging, and surgical treatment.

54. Holmes GB, Lin J: Etiologic factors associated with symptomatic Achilles tendinopathy. *Foot Ankle Int* 2006;27:952-959.

Eighty-two patients with Achilles tendinosis were reviewed for medical contributing factors and compared with published population norms for these diagnoses. Obesity in men and women, hormone replacement therapy or oral contraception use in women, hypertension in women, and diabetes mellitus in men younger than 44 years were associated with Achilles tendinopathy at a higher, statistically significant rate than would be expected based on population norms.

55. Alfredson H, Ohberg L: Sclerosing injections to areas of neo-vascularisation reduce pain in chronic Achilles tendinopathy: A double-blind randomised controlled trial.

Knee Surg Sports Traumatol Arthrosc 2005;13:338-344.

The authors report on 20 patients with noninsertional Achilles tendinopathy treated with either polidocanol or lidocaine using color Doppler guidance into areas of neovascularization. At 3-month follow-up, the sclerosing agent produced significant reduction in tendon pain and an increased rate of patient outcome satisfaction. Neovascularization was absent in the pain-free tendons and present in tendons that remained painful. Level of evidence: I.

56. Paoloni JA, Appleyard RC, Nelson J, Murrell GA: Topical nitric oxide application in the treatment of chronic extensor tendinosis at the elbow: A randomized, double-blind, placebo controlled clinical trial. *Am J Sports Med* 2003;31:915-920.

The authors report on 86 patients with extensor tendinosis who were randomly assigned to two groups. Both groups participated in a standard tendon rehabilitation program. One group was treated with an active glyceryl trinitrate transdermal patch and the other group received a placebo patch. At 6-month follow-up, 81% of the patients in the transdermal patch group were asymptomatic during activities of daily living compared with 60% of patients treated with the placebo patch.

57. Berrazueta JR, Losada A, Poveda J, et al: Successful treatment of shoulder pain syndrome due to supraspinatus tendinitis with transdermal nitroglycerin: A double blind study. *Pain* 1996;66:63-67.

58. Paoloni JA, Appleyard RC, Nelson J, Murrell GA: Topical glyceryl trinitrate application in the treatment of chronic supraspinatus tendinopathy: A randomized, double-blind, placebo controlled clinical trial. *Am J Sports Med* 2005;33:806-813.

The authors of this study report that topical glyceryl trinitrate treatment significantly improved pain scores, range of motion, internal rotation impingement, muscular force, and outcomes in patients with supraspinatus tendinopathy compared with those treated with rehabilitation alone.

59. Paoloni JA, Murrell GA: Three-year follow-up study of topical glyceryl trinitrate treatment of chronic noninsertional Achilles tendinopathy. *Foot Ankle Int* 2007;28:1064-1068.

A follow-up study of 52 patients (68 tendons) treated with glyceryl trinitrate therapy or placebo for 6 months was performed 3 years after cessation of therapy. The patients treated with topical glyceryl trinitrate had significantly less Achilles tendon tenderness and improved scores on the Victorian Institute of Sport Achilles tendon scale compared with those treated with a placebo. At 3-year follow-up, 88% of patients treated with glyceryl trinitrate therapy were asymptomatic compared with 67% of patients treated with rehabilitation alone

60. Den Hartog BD: Flexor hallucis longus transfer for chronic Achilles tendinosis. *Foot Ankle Int* 2003;24:233-237.

Proximal harvest of the FHL was used in treating 29 tendons (27 insertional, 2 noninsertional). Time to maximal improvement was 8.2 months. All but three patients reported good to excellent results at an average follow-up of 35 months. No functional deficit was reported in the hallux. Level of evidence: IV.

61. Martin RL, Manning CM, Carcia CR, Conti SF: An outcome study of chronic Achilles tendinosis after excision of the Achilles tendon and flexor hallucis longus tendon transfer. *Foot Ankle Int* 2005;26:691-697.

In this cohort study, 56 patients underwent excision of the entire Achilles tendon and FHL transfer. At an average 3.4-years postoperatively, 86% were satisfied with the procedure and 96% were pain free; 19 patients returned for clinical examination. Plantar flexion motion and strength deficits were noted. Level of evidence: IV.

62. Rompe JD, Furia J, Maffulli N: Eccentric loading compared with shock wave treatment for chronic insertional Achilles tendinopathy: A randomized, controlled trial. *J Bone Joint Surg Am* 2008;90:52-61.

Fifty patients with chronic insertional Achilles tendinopathy were randomly assigned to groups treated with eccentric loading or low-energy shock wave therapy. At 4-month and 1-year follow-up, the shock wave group had more favorable results for all measured outcomes. Level of evidence: I.

63. Nicholson CW, Berlet GC, Lee TH: Prediction of the success of nonoperative treatment of insertional Achilles tendinosis based on MRI. *Foot Ankle Int* 2007;28:472-476.

The authors report on 157 patients with insertional heel pain stratified by intratendon changes as seen on MRI scans. A higher ratio of patients with severe involvement of the tendon required surgery compared with patients with minimal thickening and small foci of degeneration.

2: Foot and Ankle Trauma

Chapter 12

Sports-Related Foot and Ankle Injuries

John A. Nassar, MD   Timothy M. Badwey, MD

Introduction

Both traumatic and overuse injuries to the foot and ankle are common in individuals who participate in sporting activities at both the recreational and professional level. Understanding the mechanisms of injury, performing a thorough physical examination, and obtaining appropriate imaging studies will provide the information needed to make optimal treatment choices and facilitate a return to play for most athletes.

Turf Toe and Sesamoid Injuries

First metatarsophalangeal (MTP) joint injuries, such as turf toe and sesamoid injuries, have become more common with the advent of artificial playing surfaces and lighter, more flexible athletic shoes.[1] In 1994, it was reported that foot injuries were the third most common cause (behind ankle and knee injuries) of lost playing time in university athletes.[2] These injuries can result in significant short- and long-term functional disability including impairments in push-off and running.

In 1976, the term turf toe was coined as a result of a noted increase in the incidence of first MTP joint sprains in football players associated with artificial playing surfaces and more flexible shoe wear.[1] Turf toe classically describes a hyperextension injury to the first MTP joint; however, numerous variations of the injury have been described. A valgus component to the hyperextension injury results in damage to the plantar medial ligamentous structures. This damage can cause a capsular avulsion or tibial sesamoid injury and may eventually lead to traumatic hallux valgus.[3-6] Less commonly, varus and hyperflexion mechanisms have been described.[4,7,8] Late sequelae of turf toe injuries include hallux rigidus, hallux valgus, hallux varus, hallux cockup, and flexor hallucis longus (FHL) tendon tears.

Etiology and Mechanism of Injury

Although football is the sport originally associated with turf toe, this injury also occurs in other athletic activities (such as soccer, volleyball, dance, basketball, tennis, softball, gymnastics, and wrestling) involving cutting, jumping, accelerating, and decelerating. The classic mechanism of injury occurs in a football player whose forefoot is fixed on the ground with the heel elevated. Another player lands on the back of the foot, creating a hyperextension injury that causes varying degrees of tears of the plantar plate and possibly a compression osteochondral injury across the metatarsal head[9] (**Figure 1**). Several patient factors have been studied to establish a link with turf toe injuries, but clear implications have not been established in the literature.

Sesamoid fractures have heterogenous etiologies and a relatively low incidence. Fractures may be acute injuries from direct trauma or chronic stress injuries from repetitive trauma.

Anatomy

The articulation of the shallow socket of the base of the proximal phalanx on the biconvex metatarsal head is inherently unstable. The capsuloligamentous structure provides the most significant stability to the first MTP joint. The plantar plate is the thick fibrous structure that reinforces the plantar joint capsule. It is firmly attached to the base of the proximal phalanx and more loosely attached to the plantar neck of the first metatarsal.[10] The plantar plate also contains the medial (tibial) and lateral (fibular) sesamoid bones. The sesamoids develop from multiple ossification centers, and a failure to fuse results in varying degrees of partition. Ossification becomes evident at approximately 9 years of age in girls and 11 years of age in boys. Although the medial sesamoid is more commonly bipartite, the literature is not consistent in describing the incidence and bilaterality of bipartite sesamoids. The sesamoids are buried within the flexor hallucis brevis tendons and have hyaline cartilage that articulates with the metatarsal head. The sesamoids provide increased mechanical advantage to the tendons of the flexor hallucis brevis and provide a weight-bearing surface to protect the metatarsal head and FHL tendon. The abductor hallucis tendon attaches to the medial sesamoid, and the adductor hallucis tendon attaches to the lateral sesamoid. These tendons continue to the base of the proximal phalanx via the plantar plate. The fan-shaped collateral ligaments of the first MTP joint (including

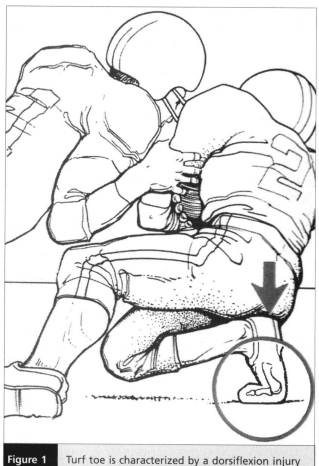

| Figure 1 | Turf toe is characterized by a dorsiflexion injury of the first MTP joint that damages the plantar structures. (*Reproduced from Sullivan JA, Anderson SJ (eds): Care of the Young Athlete. Rosemont, IL, American Academy of Orthopaedic Surgeons, 2000, p 436*). |

the MTP and metatarsosesamoid ligaments) provide significant varus and valgus stability to the joint.[11]

The first MTP joint transmits significant biomechanical forces. The first metatarsal carries twice the weight of the lesser metatarsals, with a maximum force of 40% to 60% of a person's body weight during ambulation.[9,12] This force increases twofold to threefold during running and up to eight times during jumping.[2,4,13]

Classification

In 1994, capsuloligamentous injuries of the first MTP joint were classified into three categories based on clinical presentation.[2] A grade 1 sprain involves a stretch or minor tearing injury and is characterized by mild limitation in range of motion, minimal pain with weight bearing, and mild pain with athletic activities. A grade 2 injury involves a partial tear with mild to moderate limitation in range of motion, moderate pain, a mild limp with weight bearing, and an inability to participate in athletic activities at a normal level. A grade 3 injury involves a complete tear and possibly associated injuries (osteochondral injury, sesamoid fracture, bipartite sesa-

moid diastasis, and sesamoid proximal migration). There is severe limitation in range of motion, severe pain, and an inability to bear weight on the medial forefoot.

Diagnostic Studies

Diagnostic studies include multiple radiographic views—AP, lateral, medial oblique, lateral oblique, and sesamoid views—for evaluating capsular avulsions, sesamoid fractures, osteochondral injuries, diastasis of a bipartite sesamoid, or proximal migration of the sesamoids. The appearance and position of the sesamoids should be compared with the contralateral foot. Simultaneous radiography of both feet on the same cassette has been recommended for accurate comparisons.[14] Lateral dorsiflexion stress radiographs also can help in identifying joint subluxation, sesamoid migration, or sesamoid diastasis.[4] MRI is the best modality for showing the extent of bone, cartilage, and capsuloligamentous involvement. This information is helpful in grading the injury, tailoring an appropriate treatment regimen, and anticipating the time frame for return to athletic activities.[15]

Treatment

Nonsurgical

The initial treatment of all turf toe injuries involves rest, ice, compression, and elevation (the RICE protocol). Rest is a key factor, but compliance is often an issue.[2] Nonsteroidal anti-inflammatory drugs (NSAIDs) also may be used.[9] Immobilization with a walker boot or short leg cast with toe spica extension in slight plantar flexion may be indicated for higher grade sprains during the first week after injury.[9] To avoid long-term loss of motion, early joint mobilization usually should begin as soon as symptoms permit. Shoe modifications with a carbon fiber plate or steel spring plate also will assist in returning the athlete to competition. The physician may consider an orthotic with Morton extension or toe taping and strapping. In general, athletes with grade 1 injuries can return to sports with the toe taped and a stiffened sole. Athletes with grade 2 injuries should not play for 3 to 14 days, and athletes with grade 3 injuries should not return to athletic competition for 2 to 6 weeks.[2]

Nondisplaced sesamoid fractures should be treated in a hard-sole shoe, a boot, or a cast for 4 to 6 weeks. Patients may bear weight on the heel and should avoid forced first MTP joint dorsiflexion.

Surgical

Surgical treatment is rarely indicated for turf toe injuries, and few studies are available in the literature. Because turf toe describes a wide spectrum of injuries, heterogeneous reports in the literature make comparison difficult. Surgery may be considered for patients with a large capsular avulsion with an unstable joint, diastasis of a bipartite sesamoid, a displaced sesamoid fracture, retraction of sesamoids (single or both), traumatic or progressive hallux valgus, a positive vertical

Lachman test, and the presence of a loose body or chondral injury.[15] No studies are available comparing acute versus chronic treatment of these injuries or comparing partial excision versus total excision of sesamoid fractures or diastasis. In general, it is important to repair the capsule, flexor hallucis brevis, and plantar plate defect after excision. If a primary repair is not possible, a local abductor hallucis tendon transfer to close the defect is recommended.[9,15]

It is difficult to distinguish the various entities of symptomatic bipartite/multipartite sesamoids, sesamoid fracture, and fracture through a bipartite sesamoid. Various surgical treatments, including screw fixation, sesamoidectomy, partial sesamoidectomy, and bone grafting, have been described for chronically symptomatic stress fractures for which conservative treatments have failed.[16-23] The ideal treatment method has not been established in the literature.

The authors of one study reported on the surgical treatment of diastasis of bipartite sesamoids.[4] The distal segment was excised and the capsule was repaired. All patients returned to their preinjury level of competition. One procedure was performed acutely and three were performed as late reconstruction after failed nonsurgical management.

In another study, 12 athletes were surgically treated for proximal migration or diastasis of the sesamoids.[9] Five procedures were performed acutely, and seven were performed for chronic deformities (including two valgus deformities and one varus deformity). For proximal migration, advancement and primary repair of the defect in the plantar plate found distal to the sesamoids is recommended. If a primary repair is not possible, secondary repair to the base of the proximal phalanx through drill holes or suture anchors is recommended. For progressive diastasis of a bipartite sesamoid, preservation of one pole of the sesamoid is recommended. In this study, the distal pole was usually excised, and the soft tissues were then repaired through drill holes in the remaining proximal pole. If complete sesamoidectomy was required, the authors recommended repairing the larger plantar plate defect with an abductor hallucis tendon transfer.[9]

In another study, nine surgeries on nine collegiate or professional athletes were performed, including four sesamoidectomy procedures (three tibial and one fibular).[15] All but two professional football players returned to full athletic activity. More information on turf toe and sesamoid injuries is available in chapter 9.

Other First MTP Joint and Sesamoid Injuries

Dislocations of the first MTP joint are a rare disorder that also causes fractures. First MTP joint dislocations have been classified based on sesamoid bone position and the presence of sesamoid fracture.[24] In type I dislocations, the metatarsal head buttonholes through the capsule proximal to the sesamoids and the intersesamoid ligament remains intact. Closed reduction is usually unsuccessful. In type IIA dislocations, the intersesamoid

ligament ruptures and the sesamoids migrate around both sides of the joint. In type IIB dislocations, there is a transverse fracture of the medial sesamoid. The distal fragment migrates distally and the proximal fragment remains in normal relationship with the lateral sesamoid through the intact portion of the intersesamoid ligament. Closed reduction is usually successful for treating type IIA and IIB dislocations. If there is a fracture through the sesamoids, displacement of fragments within the joint is possible.

Other sesamoid injuries, such as sesamoiditis and osteochondritis, often result from overuse. A cavus foot with a rigidly plantar flexed first ray predisposes an individual to sesamoid overload injuries. The tibial sesamoid is most often involved. Sesamoiditis is a clinical term that describes pain and swelling of the sesamoid bones/complex and includes a multitude of conditions reported in the literature, including FHL tendinitis, sesamoid bursitis, symptomatic bipartite sesamoid, MTP joint synovitis, MTP joint capsulitis, chondromalacia, and osteochondritis.[14,25,26] Osteochondritis and various related terms (osteonecrosis, osteochondrosis, aseptic necrosis) describe a histologic diagnosis.[27] Radiographically, the sesamoids appear fragmented and irregular. Clinically, the patients present with chronic repetitive injury. In general, surgery is reserved for recalcitrant disorders that have not responded to nonsurgical treatments.

Acute and Chronic Ankle Injuries

Acute Ligament Injuries

Acute ligamentous injuries of the ankle (sprains) are one of the most common sports-related injuries of the lower extremity. Lateral ankle sprains occur more often than medial ankle sprains by a ratio of at least 10:1.[28] An individual with a lateral ankle sprain will typically describe a plantar flexion/inversion mechanism of injury. Two common scenarios that result in a lateral ankle sprain are jumping for a rebound during a basketball game or struggling to control the ball during a soccer game. In both of these scenarios there are many individuals in close proximity to each other, with the focus of attention away from the playing surface. Injury typically occurs when one athlete lands on the foot of another athlete, causing the requisite hindfoot inversion with varying degrees of plantar flexion. Often, the athlete will have difficulty recalling the exact foot position or mechanism that resulted in the injury.

The anterior talofibular ligament is initially affected, which may be the extent of the injury. Greater degrees of inversion and plantar flexion result in calcaneofibular ligament involvement.

Classification

A number of classification systems are used to describe the severity of ankle sprains. Ankle sprains are commonly graded based on the severity of injury to the involved ligament. A grade I injury is indicated by a partial tear of the involved ligament, with no loss of structural integrity. A grade II injury indicates a partial tear of the affected ligament, with some degree of clinical structural instability. Grade III sprains represent a complete disruption of the ligament, with loss of structural integrity.[29] This classification system, however, is limited by the arbitrary nature of clinical examinations and interobserver variabilities among clinicians.

Patient History and Physical Examination

Although the patient's history is important, the physical examination can be critical for confirming the diagnosis of a sprain and ruling out injury to adjacent bones or tendons. By the time the patient is evaluated by the physician who will provide definitive treatment, several hours or even days may have elapsed since the traumatic event. The affected ankle may be markedly swollen and ecchymotic, and normal bony prominences and landmarks may be obscured. A thorough and accurate examination of the involved ankle is imperative.

The physician should begin by examining the uninjured ankle. By assessing pulses, range of motion (ROM), and stability of the uninjured ankle, valuable reference information can be obtained for comparison with the injured ankle. For example, if the patient has no history of an injury on the contralateral side but demonstrates significant laxity when an anterior drawer test is performed, the examiner will have a baseline for comparison with the injured ankle. Some systemic disease states, such as peripheral vascular disease, can be provisionally determined by examining the unaffected ankle. Such information may have implications in treating the injured ankle.

After evaluating the uninjured ankle, the injured ankle is examined. The basic physical diagnostic principles of inspection and careful palpation are of paramount importance in assessing the injured ankle to confirm the presence of a ligamentous sprain while simultaneously ruling out other injuries. Palpation of the ankle ligaments and bony structures will aid the examiner in detecting fractures of the medial or lateral malleoli, the fifth metatarsal base or shaft, and the anterior process of the calcaneus. This information will help to determine the need for radiographic evaluation and the location of the area to be imaged. Careful palpation over the medial and lateral ligaments of the ankle will help determine if the injury is confined to one or more ligaments, or ligaments on both the medial and lateral aspects of the ankle.

Careful examination of the muscle-tendon units about the ankle is also important. Many tendon tears, whether partial or complete, are often misdiagnosed as sprains. Assessing ankle and toe dorsiflexors (especially the tibialis anterior tendon), foot invertors and evertors (especially the posterior tibialis and peroneal tendons), and plantar flexors (the Achilles tendon) is easily accomplished. The outcome for a patient with an acute tendon injury that appears to be an ankle sprain will be much better if the diagnosis is not delayed by weeks or months.

Stress testing of the ligaments in an acute setting, unless it can be accomplished shortly after the original injury, is generally not helpful in guiding treatment. If there is a significant time lapse between the injury and the examination, the patient's ankle generally will be swollen, inflamed, and painful, which can lead to involuntary patient guarding and an unreliable stress evaluation.

Radiographic Evaluation

Radiographic examination after acute ligament injuries of the ankle is routinely performed, particularly in the emergency department. The Ottawa Rules have been developed as a tool to determine which patients require radiographic evaluation of the ankle and/or foot to rule out the presence of a fracture following an ankle sprain.[30] Ankle radiographs are required if (1) there is bone tenderness along the distal 6 cm of the posterior edge of the fibula or the tip of the lateral malleolus, (2) there is bone tenderness along the distal 6 cm of the posterior edge of the tibia or the tip of the medial malleolus, or (3) the patient is unable to bear weight both immediately after the injury and in the emergency department for at least four steps. Radiographs of the foot are required if there is bone tenderness at the base of the fifth metatarsal or the navicular, or if the patient is unable to bear weight both immediately after the injury or in the emergency department for at least four steps. The application of these rules reduces the use of ankle radiography and the cost and time spent in the emergency department.[31,32]

If needed, the radiographs are often available to the physician who will provide definitive treatment. A thorough and complete radiographic examination of the ankle should include AP, lateral, and oblique (mortise) views of the ankle and the foot. If possible, the AP and lateral images of the foot and ankle should be weight-bearing views if tolerable by the patient. Although it is important to assess all bony structures on the radiographs, attention should be directed to those areas of suspected injury based on the physical examination.

Imaging of the acutely injured ankle beyond plain radiography should be reserved for patients who, based on their history and physical and radiographic examinations, have potential injuries, such as acute osteochondral fractures, occult fractures, and partial or complete tendon ruptures that have not been adequately delineated. Routine MRI evaluation of patients with acute ligament injuries about the ankle is not necessary.

Treatment

Treatment for acute ligament injuries of the ankle is determined mainly by the severity of the injury. Grade I ligament injuries can usually be treated symptomatically with the RICE protocol. After the initial episode of pain and swelling subsides, return to activity can be initiated in conjunction with either functional bracing or by taping the ankle. The time from injury occurrence to return to activity after a grade I sprain is variable but can be immediate (with proper stabilization via taping). Typically, return to activity without symptoms can be accomplished within a few days.

Grade II ligament sprains may require, in addition to the RICE protocol, a period of protected ambulation using crutches, a walking boot, or a cast to limit weight bearing. A walking boot is preferred over a cast because it is removable for hygiene and early ROM exercises. Following a grade II sprain, a period of protected ambulation for 2 to 4 weeks may be required before return to sports activities. Return to full activity may be delayed by residual joint stiffness and weakness depending on whether the ankle has been immobilized continuously, such as with casting. A course of physical therapy focusing on ROM, strengthening exercises, and proprioceptive retraining may be necessary to enable an athlete to return to sports activites without a functional deficit. Functional bracing or taping may be beneficial.

The treatment of a grade III ligament sprain is not as straightforward as the treatment of grade I and II sprains. Good functional results have been reported with both cast immobilization and early controlled mobilization, with no difference in pain, swelling, or stiffness.[33] A course of physical therapy consisting of ROM, strengthening exercises, and proprioceptive retraining is desirable to reverse the effects of immobilization. Return to full activity may not be possible until strength and ROM have returned to near-normal levels. Taping or bracing is helpful at this time to minimize the risk of reinjury. It can take several weeks to months before an athlete with a grade III ligament injury returns to a preinjury level of performance.

Chronic Ligament Injuries

Even after appropriate treatment of an acute medial or lateral ankle ligament injury, chronic instability or pain can result. The etiology of these chronic disorders can be multifactorial and may not be the sole result of a compromised ligamentous restraint. Treatment of chronic ankle instability should be directed toward the specific etiologic factor(s).

Patient History and Physical Examination

Patients with chronic ankle instability often will report a history of repeated ankle sprains. These recurrent sprains are usually of a lesser magnitude than the original ankle injury. Some will report recurrent sprains caused by participating in athletic activities, but others will report episodes of ankle turning during routine activities. Sometimes, just walking on an uneven surface or stepping on something as trivial as a pebble will cause an episode of ankle turning. These episodes of recurrent ankle instability generally do not result in symptoms that are severe enough to require prolonged immobilization or extensive treatment. The frequency of these recurrent episodes is also highly variable, with some patients reporting recurrent sprains almost daily,

whereas others have weeks or months between recurrent episodes of chronic ankle instability.

It is important to determine the severity of the index injury and the severity of subsequent sprains. Equally important is the presence and timing of pain in association with the recurrent sprains. Although some patients report a recurrent sprain followed by a variable degree of pain (sometimes none at all), others report a prodrome of pain before the sprain. Patients may report a paroxysm of pain that causes their ankle to give way, which may be an indication of some disorder other than primary ankle instability.

The physical examination of a patient with a history of chronic ankle pain and instability should be as careful and detailed as the examination of a patient with an acute injury. Attention should be given to every detail, including ROM, strength (especially inversion and eversion strength), and proprioception. Alignment and stability of the ankle in standing and non–weight-bearing positions and a gait evaluation should be performed. Careful palpation about the ankle is needed to determine areas of palpable tenderness. The tendinous and osseous structures around the ankle should be examined to detect other areas of potential injury that were not previously noted.

Imaging Studies

Imaging of the chronically injured ankle should be obtained if recent radiographs (< 6 months old) are not available. Stress radiographs of the affected ankle, when compared with the contralateral side, may be helpful in showing instability that is not readily apparent on routine radiographs.

Other imaging modalities, such as MRI, should be considered for patients whose history, physical examination, and radiographic evaluation indicates the possibility of disorders other than chronic ankle instability. Chronic tendinoplasty (especially of the Achilles or peroneal tendons) can coexist with chronic ankle instability. Other intra-articular pathology can include anterior impingement of the tibiotalar joint, chondral lesions, and osteochondritis dissecans. Successful treatment of chronic ankle instability depends on recognizing and treating any additional pathology.

Treatment

Treatment for the patient with chronic ankle instability may be nonsurgical or surgical depending on several factors, including the age and activity level of the patient, the relative severity of the ankle instability, and the presence of any concomitant injuries. Initially, nonsurgical treatment should be directed toward correction of any functional deficit detected during the physical examination. Successful outcomes depend on restoring lost ROM, strength, and proprioception. The liberal use of physiotherapy is beneficial in helping the injured athlete regain lost function caused by the original injury or through altered function resulting from the injury or treatment. There is no universal agreement regarding which deficits lead to chronic ankle instability. It recently has been shown that mechanical factors, such as inversion laxity and anterior drawer laxity, primarily account for the differences in patients with chronic instability compared with control subjects.[34] However, balance and strength deficits also are present in these patients. Correction of the functional deficits through physical therapy may potentially enable athletes with chronic instability to return to their previous level of performance. Patients should be informed concerning the requirements and duration of participation in a physical therapy program, regardless of whether surgical treatment is needed.

For patients with unresolved instability despite nonsurgical treatment, surgery should be considered. Several surgical procedures have been described for the treatment of lateral ankle instability. At present, reconstruction that preserves ankle anatomy is the preferred treatment for an athlete. A direct repair of the lateral ligamentous structures, such as the Broström procedure, is the treatment of choice.[35] If the preoperative evaluation detects any other pathology (such as an osteochondritis dissecans lesion, a peroneal tendon tear, or anterior ankle impingement), it should be treated at the same time.[36]

Achilles Tendon Injuries

In athletes, the Achilles tendon is the most frequently injured tendon about the ankle. Variable degrees of tendinopathy can occur in the athlete, from tendinosis to complete tendon rupture. The extreme force experienced by the Achilles tendon makes it vulnerable to potential injury in almost every sporting activity, especially in running sports.

Patient History

The history provided by an athlete with pain localized to the Achilles tendon can be an important indicator of the type of pathology involved. Patients with acute tendinopathy will report an insidious onset of pain over a period of a few days to weeks, without a specific inciting traumatic event. Patients often report a rapid increase in weight-bearing activity, especially running, over a short period of time. This type of injury can be more prevalent at the beginning of an athletic season, particularly if the athlete has not maintained a proper level of conditioning during the off-season. The pain associated with Achilles tendinopathy is aggravated by activity and relieved with rest. Refraining from running often results in cessation of pain; however, the pain quickly resumes with a return to activity. Athletes often report improvement with the use of NSAIDs, which are often used before the athlete seeks medical treatment.

Athletes with a complete disruption of the Achilles tendon provide a distinctly different history. A patient with a complete Achilles tendon tear will report feeling or even hearing a "pop" within the tendon. The exact timing of this sentinel event can vary depending on the sport involved. In running sports (such as football and soccer), the athlete may be simply running down the field when the tendon fails. Basketball players will often report the disruption as occurring when running to attempt a rebound shot. Tennis players have reported tendon failure occurring when stretching to return a volley. After the traumatic episode, the athlete is unable to continue play and may have difficulty ambulating without support.

Physical Examination

The physical examination of a patient with Achilles tendinopathy almost always shows some degree of contracture of the gastrocnemius-soleus complex. It is uncertain whether this contracture precedes the tendinopathy or occurs as a result of altered activity caused by the tendinopathy. Other findings include swelling localized to the Achilles tendon, a palpable thickening of the tendon, and fairly discrete tenderness. Although swelling may be generalized, the area of tenderness is distinct. This tenderness is localized to the midsubstance of the Achilles tendon (approximately midway between the myotendinous junction and the insertion of the tendon) or over the insertion of the tendon at the calcaneal tuberosity. The degree of tenderness can vary in severity but is reproducible. Careful palpation about the calcaneus is important to distinguish it from the Achilles tendon insertion as the source of pain. Passive dorsiflexion of the ankle or plantar flexion against resistance also may reproduce the pain. Having the patient perform a repetitive single-stance toe rise is a provocative test that also can cause pain.

The athlete with a complete Achilles tendon tear will have a significant amount of swelling and ecchymosis, depending on the time period between the injury and the examination. The examiner will find marked tenderness at the site of the tear; with careful palpation, a discrete defect within the tendon will be detected.

Imaging Studies

Radiographic evaluation should include lateral and axial radiographs of the calcaneus. These views may show calcification within the midsubstance of the tendon or at the insertion of the tendon, a prominent calcaneal tuberosity (Haglund deformity), or pathology within the calcaneus (such as an intraosseous ganglion or a fracture). If indicated by the physical examination, a complete radiographic examination of the ankle and foot may be appropriate. Additional imaging studies such as MRI may be helpful in evaluating Achilles tendinopathy, especially in patients with long-standing symptoms or in those whose symptoms do not improve with treatment (**Figure 2**). MRI can distinguish between acute or chronic tendinopathy, incomplete or longitudinal tendon tears, or complete tendon tears better than other imaging modalities.

Treatment

Treatment of Achilles tendinopathy should initially consist of cessation of the aggravating activity, the use of NSAIDs at a therapeutic level, and tendon stretching. Physical therapy modalities also can be helpful in the acute phase to alleviate pain and inflammation. A heel lift will provide pain relief during the acute phase. If a patient with Achilles tendinopathy does not improve, a period of immobilization in a removable walking boot for a period of 4 to 6 weeks may break the cycle of inflammation caused by the repetitive stresses of activities of daily living. To maintain cardiovascular fitness, the boot can be removed for low-impact cardiovascular training (such as stationary bicycling, elliptical training, or swimming) if such activities do not exacerbate symptoms. After the immobilization period is completed, the athlete should decrease use of the boot gradually over a period of several days to weeks to allow the tendon to adapt to a gradual increase in weight-bearing stress and to allow time for recovery of bone and muscle mass.

If nonsurgical treatment is unsuccessful, surgical treatment should be considered. MRI is essential (if not obtained previously) to define and localize the source of the pathology. Surgical treatment of chronic Achilles tendinopathy typically consists of débridement of the pathologic tissue, excision of the prominent portion of the calcaneal tuberosity (if it exists), or tendon débridement and repair of an incomplete or longitudinal tear. The FHL tendon is being used with increased frequency to augment the tendon repair or introduce vascularity to the surgical site.[37] However, sacrificing the FHL tendon for adjunctive use with an Achilles tendon repair should be carefully considered when treating an athlete, especially a running athlete.

In athletes with a complete tear of the Achilles tendon, surgical repair provides the best opportunity for athletes to return to their previous level of function. Although long-term benefits versus the risks of surgical repair may be debatable for recreational athletes, surgical repair of the Achilles tendon achieves superior results compared with nonsurgical treatment in athletes.[38] Because numerous techniques have been described for the surgical treatment of the acutely ruptured Achilles tendon, surgeons should select a method that they are comfortable performing.

In patients with a missed or untreated Achilles tendon tear, surgical treatment will always be necessary to provide athletes with the opportunity to return to their previous level of activity. Depending on the length of time from injury to treatment, some type of augmentation may be necessary for the tendon repair or to fill a gap caused by retraction of the proximal tendon stump. The FHL tendon may be used to provide a vascularized graft to fill the gap. The use of the gastrocnemius fascia as a "turn-down" flap also is an accepted alternative.

Postoperative Rehabilitation

The period of immobilization, duration of rehabilitation, and timing of return to athletic activity will depend primarily on the findings at the time of surgery and the surgeon's comfort level with the stability of the

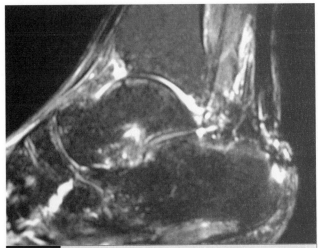

Figure 2 T2-weighted MRI scan showing a subacute insertional tear. (Reproduced from McGarvey WC: Achilles tendon injuries: Acute and chronic, in Richardson EG (ed): Orthopaedic Knowledge Update: Foot and Ankle 3. Rosemont, IL, American Academy of Orthopaedic Surgeons, 2004, pp 91-102.)

repair. Recently, there has been a tendency to decrease the length of the immobilization period and begin physiotherapy earlier following surgery.[39]

Despite modern surgical techniques and advancements in rehabilitation, recovery following repair of a complete Achilles tendon tear is not always predictable. Although an Achilles tendon tear may not end an athlete's career, it often alters the career. It is important for the athlete undergoing surgical treatment of an Achilles tendon tear to thoroughly understand the risks associated with surgical treatment, the duration of rehabilitation following surgery, and the possibility that the pre-injury level of performance will not be achieved. More information on Achilles tendon injuries is available in chapter 11.

Peroneal Tendon Injuries

Injury to the peroneal tendons is probably a more common occurrence than had been previously believed.[29] In the past, it was not uncommon for an injury to one of the peroneal tendons in an athlete to remain undiagnosed for months or years before appropriate treatment was rendered. An understanding of the mechanism of injury leading to acute peroneal tendon injury along with modern imaging modalities has led to significant improvements in patient care.

Patient History

Most athletes with an acute injury to one of the peroneal tendons will report a recent ankle sprain with a usual mechanism of injury of inversion with or without plantar flexion. The accompanying pain, swelling, and ecchymosis are usually attributed solely to the ankle sprain. After the acute symptoms have subsided and

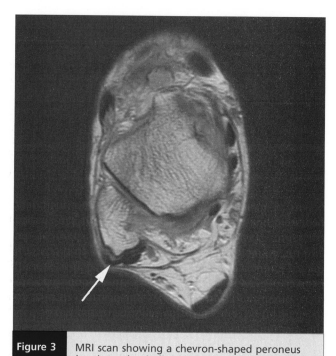

Figure 3 MRI scan showing a chevron-shaped peroneus brevis tendon indicating a tear (*arrow*). (*Reproduced from Ishikawa SN: Imaging of the foot and ankle, in Richardson EG (ed): Orthopaedic Knowledge Update: Foot and Ankle 3. Rosemont, IL, American Academy of Orthopaedic Surgeons, 2004, pp 179-188.*)

hindfoot may elicit pain along the path of the tendons. Circumduction of the ankle can demonstrate subluxation or even frank dislocation of one or both of the peroneal tendons.

Imaging Studies

Radiographic evaluation should include standing images of the ankle and foot. Findings from plain radiographs can be used to rule out fractures of the distal fibula, lateral process of the talus, and anterior process of the calcaneus, all of which can accompany an ankle sprain, and may be helpful in ruling out osteochondral injuries of the talus. Radiographic findings also can be used to rule out chronic conditions (such as degenerative changes in the ankle or subtalar joint) that may have been aggravated by the acute injury.

MRI is usually needed to confirm a tendon tear and to definitively rule out other sources of pathology about the ankle (**Figure 3**). It is important that the radiologist understand the exact nature of the pathology being investigated and the location of the suspected tear. Despite negative MRI findings, an incomplete longitudinal tendon tear can be present. If the index of suspicion for injury remains high following thorough physical and radiographic examinations and the patient remains symptomatic despite appropriate nonsurgical care, surgical exploration of the peroneal tendons should be considered.

Surgical Exploration and Treatment

At the time of surgery, the principal site of tendon exploration will depend on the location of the athlete's pain. If an ankle sprain was the precipitating event that led to symptoms, the exploration site will typically be at or near the inferior border of the fibula where the peroneal tendons turn from their course just posterior to the fibula toward the lateral border of the foot. Although it is important to examine both tendons at this level, the peroneus brevis tendon will almost always be involved. Following surgical repair of the peroneal tendons, immobilization for several weeks is necessary followed by a period of taping or bracing to allow healing of the retinaculum and repaired tendons. A too rapid return to activity can lead to retearing of either of these structures and surgical failure. Outcomes following repair of the peroneal tendons are generally good, with most patients returning to their preinjury level of performance.[40] However, a recent study reported a successful return to sports in only 46% of patients.[41] More information on peroneal tendon injuries is available in chapter 11.

FHL Tendon Injuries

In contrast to the frequency of injuries to the Achilles and peroneal tendons, acute injury to the FHL tendon is relatively rare. Overuse injuries (such as tendinitis) occur more frequently but also are relatively rare. Tendinitis most commonly occurs in dancers because of significant hypertrophy of the FHL muscle and because

athletic ability remains limited, the athlete presents for treatment. A peroneal tendon tear also can result from repetitive stress without a distinct traumatic event.

If treatment was previously provided, the patient may have been treated for tendinitis with varying degrees of success. The athlete will report fairly well localized pain and swelling along the lateral aspect of the ankle. Weakness, despite previous therapy, will be reported. The athlete also may report recurrent ankle sprains since the time of the original injury. Symptom improvement with ankle taping or bracing may occur, but symptoms escalate after external support is discontinued. Although some patients report pain only with athletic participation, others report pain and swelling associated with activities of daily living.

The physical examination may show limited ankle ROM, especially in ankle dorsiflexion and hindfoot eversion. Ankle instability may be shown with the drawer test; however, if the drawer test elicits pain, patient guarding can limit the ability for accurate results. The patient will have well-localized tenderness directly over one or both of the peroneal tendons. With resisted eversion, the peroneal tendons often are visible beneath the skin and can be palpated along a large portion of their course; however, the tendons can be obscured by swelling or synovitis accompanying the tendons. Comparison of the degree of swelling with the opposite ankle will demonstrate a significant side-to-side difference. Resisted eversion or passive inversion of the dancers use the FHL muscle-tendon unit more frequently than most athletes. Dancers with FHL tendinitis generally report an insidious onset of symptoms without a definitive event preceding the onset. Pain is generally increased with activity, especially activity involving the toes (such as en pointe ballet). Pain is localized to the posterior aspect of the ankle and/or the medial aspect of the hindfoot.

Physical Examination

On examination, swelling may be observed along the course of the tendon. When present, swelling usually occurs along the medial aspect of the hindfoot, where it is most superficial. Tenderness along the path of the tendon is also common. It is important to palpate carefully along the entire accessible path of the FHL tendon. Plantar flexion of the hallux against resistance or passive dorsiflexion of the first MTP joint (with the ankle also dorsiflexed) may elicit pain. Actively flexing and extending the first MTP joint also can "trigger" the hallux. It is important to carefully examine the accompanying tendinous structures as they pass in close proximity within the tarsal tunnel. It is essential to perform a thorough neurologic examination to exclude involvement of the posterior tibial nerve.

Imaging Studies

Imaging principles for an athlete with suspected FHL tendinitis are similar to those for other tendon injuries about the ankle. Plain radiographs are initially obtained to rule out any associated bone or joint pathology. Radiographs may show a prominent posterolateral talar process or os trigonum. If an os trigonum is suspected as the cause of symptoms, a lateral radiograph of the ankle in maximum plantar flexion and maximum dorsiflexion may show movement of the os in relationship to the talus. MRI of the FHL tendon is valuable in defining pathology within and around the tendon. The radiologist should be informed regarding the location of the suspected injury. The tortuous route of the FHL tendon makes it challenging to obtain accurate imaging.

Treatment

Most athletes with FHL tendinitis will respond to conservative treatment, including the use of NSAIDs and rest. The use of a removable knee-high walking boot may be appropriate for the resting athlete. If immobilization is necessary, it is important to immobilize the ankle and the MTP joint to minimize excursion of the tendon. The use of other treatment modalities also may be helpful in patients with inflammatory sites that are easily accessible, such as the medial aspect of the hindfoot. If symptoms have abated after an adequate rest period, a gradual return to sports activities is recommended.

For patients who remain symptomatic following nonsurgical treatment, surgery may be necessary. It is essential to carefully examine the patient prior to surgery and to focus the initial surgical exposure at the primary location of symptoms. In the athlete with symptoms localized to the posterior aspect of the ankle or with a symptomatic os trigonum, a posterolateral approach will allow access to the os trigonum and the FHL tendon as it passes from the posterior aspect of the ankle to the medial aspect of the hindfoot. It is important to release the FHL tendon as it passes through the fibro-osseous tunnel along the posterior aspect of the talus. This approach avoids the posterior tibial artery and nerve medially. If a medial approach is predicated by the location of the athlete's symptoms, meticulous dissection is essential to avoid injury to the neurovascular structures that travel adjacent to the tendon.

Surgical findings can vary from tenosynovitis to a longitudinal split within the tendon. Any area of impingement of the tendon (especially posteriorly) must be freed to allow normal excursion of the tendon. The tendon should be carefully inspected to ensure that any fissures within the tendon are recognized and repaired. Some pathology within the tendon may not be apparent on the preoperative MRI scan.

Return to activity after surgery can be achieved fairly quickly if a posterior approach is used. If a medial exposure is used, a period of immobilization is needed to allow healing of the retinaculum.

Bone Injuries

Acute Ankle Fractures

Acute fractures of the ankle in athletes are common, but the prevalence of these injuries varies significantly from sport to sport. The initial traumatic event is almost always recognized and may be captured on video and available for study in those events covered by the media.

Physical Examination

With the prevalence of athletic trainers at practice sessions and team physicians on hand at most sporting events, the initiation of appropriate treatment typically occurs within a matter of minutes. Often, the team physician is afforded the unique opportunity of examining a patient with an acute fracture literally within seconds of the injury and before significant swelling has occurred. Splinting of the affected extremity and the liberal use of ice to control swelling should be started as soon as possible. If significant subluxation or dislocation is present, it should be reduced as soon as possible to minimize the risk of neurologic or vascular compromise.

Imaging Studies

Although actual witnessing of the traumatic event and the opportunity for an immediate physical examination may clearly show the nature or extent of the injury, the need for plain radiography is essential. In the professional sports arena, the availability of routine radiography on-site is almost universal. Plain radiographs and additional studies, if indicated, should be obtained as soon as possible.

Treatment

The ultimate return of athletes to their previous level of sports participation may depend, in part, on the timely initiation of appropriate treatment. For athletes with acute fractures of the ankle, following the principles of anatomic reduction and rigid internal fixation are important for early rehabilitation, which leads to an earlier return to activity. Most athletes with acute ankle fractures who require surgical treatment have excellent bone density that allows stable fracture fixation.

Occult Ankle Fractures

Occult (subacute, overuse, stress) fractures about the ankle are usually more difficult to recognize in the absence of an acute traumatic event or history that is typical for a stress-type fracture (such as a rapid increase in weight-bearing activity or the return to sports following a prolonged period of rest). An athlete with an occult fracture often will report a gradual onset of pain. This pain is typically relieved by rest and aggravated by a return to athletic activity. Many times the patient can ambulate with no pain but will have pain if running is attempted. The athlete may have ankle swelling after a period of standing or walking, which is relieved with overnight rest. As is the case with many chronic athletic injuries, initial treatment may have already been started by an athletic trainer or the patient, with the presumptive diagnosis of some type of overuse syndrome (typically tendinitis).

Physical Examination

Examination of the athlete with a suspected occult fracture must include all the ligamentous and tendinous structures about the ankle to exclude each as a potential source of pain. The ankle may show swelling and erythema, which usually is not well localized. The key to examining a patient with a suspected occult fracture is careful palpation of the osseous structures about the ankle and hindfoot. A comparison with the bony structures on the contralateral side may be helpful. A systematic approach when examining the ankle is important to ensure that no anatomic area is overlooked.

Imaging

Obtaining radiographs of the ankle for a suspected stress-type fracture may be helpful if findings are positive, but they cannot exclude a fracture if findings are negative. A stress fracture about the ankle may become evident after a period of time if it involves the tibia or fibula diaphysis. When present, the appearance of callus aids in the diagnosis. The absence of an abnormality on plain radiographs should be considered in context with the information obtained from the patient history and physical examination.

MRI may be helpful in situations in which symptoms have a relatively short duration. The abnormalities seen on MRIs are the presence of excessive bone edema on T2-weighted or short-tau inversion recovery images. It is imperative for the examining physician to review the actual MRI scans because current radiology criteria do not call for the diagnosis of a fracture in the absence of a visible fracture line. In patients with symptoms of longer duration, a radioisotope bone scan may be more helpful. Although the edema observed on MRI scans will clear within a few weeks, the increased uptake seen with technetium pyrophosphate scans will remain positive for 18 to 24 months.

Treatment

Stress fractures about the ankle are treated by altering the weight-bearing stresses until the injury has healed. Depending on the individual patient and the sports activity involved, treatment may vary from cessation of participation in physical activity, protected ambulation in a walking boot, or not bearing weight on the affected extremity. Unless patient compliance is an issue, immobilization in a cast is rarely indicated. Low-impact activities, such as swimming, bicycling, and elliptical training, can be used to maintain the athlete's level of cardiovascular fitness if such activities do not exacerbate symptoms.

After an adequate period of rest or protected weight bearing, a gradual return to physical activity can begin. It is important for the athlete to avoid returning to full participation in sports activities without a gradual transition from non–weight-bearing activities (or protected weight-bearing activites) to full activity without restriction. Failure to follow these guidelines may result in either a return of symptoms at the original site of injury or a new focus of pain in the same extremity.

Summary

Foot and ankle injuries frequently occur in athletes. A thorough and detailed physical examination along with an awareness of and high index of suspicion for subtle injuries is essential for evaluating an athlete with a foot or ankle injury. Many conditions, such as turf toe, can be treated with rest and activity modification. Surgical treatment may be appropriate in athletes with severe injuries or when nonsurgical treatment does not relieve symptoms.

Annotated References

1. Bowers KD Jr, Martin RB: Turf-toe: A shoe-surface related football injury. *Med Sci Sports* 1976;8:81-83.

2. Clanton TO, Ford JJ: Turf toe injury. *Clin Sports Med* 1994;13:731-741.

3. Coker TP, Arnold JA, Weber DL: Traumatic lesions of the metatarsophalangeal joint of the great toe in athletes. *Am J Sports Med* 1978;6:326-334.

4. Rodeo SA, Warren RF, O'Brien SJ, Pavlov H, Barnes R, Hanks GA: Diastasis of bipartite sesamoids of the first metatarsophalangeal joint. *Foot Ankle* 1993;14: 425-434.

5. Douglas DP, Davidson DM, Robinson JE, Bedi DG: Rupture of the medial collateral ligament of the first metatarsophalangeal joint in a professional soccer player. *J Foot Ankle Surg* 1997;36:388-390.

6. Fabeck LG, Zekhnini C, Farrokh D, Descamps PY, Delincé PE: Traumatic hallux valgus following rupture of the medial collateral ligament of the first metatarsophalangeal joint: A case report. *J Foot Ankle Surg* 2002;41:125-128.

7. Mullis DL, Miller WE: A disabling sports injury of the great toe. *Foot Ankle* 1980;1:22-25.

8. Frey C, Andersen GD, Feder KS: Plantarflexion injury to the metatarsophalangeal joint (sand toe). *Foot Ankle* 1996;17:576-581.

9. Watson TS, Anderson RB, Davis WH: Periarticular injuries to the hallux metatarsophalangeal joint in athletes. *Foot Ankle Clin* 2000;5:687-713.

10. Giannikas AC, Papachristou G, Papavasiliou N, Nikiforidis P, Hartofilakidis-Garofalidis G: Dorsal dislocation of the first metatarsophalangeal joint: Report of 4 cases. *J Bone Joint Surg Br* 1975;57:384-386.

11. Sarafin SK: *Anatomy of the Foot and Ankle: Descriptive, Topographic, Functional.* Philadelphia, PA, JB Lippincott, 1983.

12. Stokes IA, Hutton WC, Stott JR: Forces under the hallux valgus foot before and after surgery. *Clin Orthop Relat Res* 1979;142:64-72.

13. Clanton TO, Butler JE, Eggert A: Injuries to the metatarsophalangeal joint in athletes. *Foot Ankle* 1986;7: 162-176.

14. Graves SC, Prieskorn D, Mann RA: Posttraumatic proximal migration of the first metatarsophalangeal joint sesamoids. *Foot Ankle* 1991;12:117-122.

15. Anderson RB: Turf toe injuries of the hallux metatarsophalangeal joint. *Tech Foot Ankle Surg* 2002;1: 102-111.

16. Pagenstert GI, Valderrabano V, Hintermann B: Medial sesamoid nonunion combined with hallux valgus in athletes: A report of two cases. *Foot Ankle Int* 2006;27: 135-140.

    The authors describe two patients with an insidious onset of sesamoid nonunion and hallux valgus. The patients were treated with open reduction and internal fixation of the sesamoid nonunion, and hallux valgus correction with a modified chevron procedure.

17. Lee S, James WC, Cohen BE, Davis WH, Anderson RB: Evaluation of hallux alignment and functional outcome after isolated tibial sesamoidectomy. *Foot Ankle Int* 2005;26:803-809.

    The authors present the results of 32 patients treated with tibial sesamoidectomy. Eighteen patients resumed all preoperative activities, six had extreme difficulty in tip toe standing, and two had transfer metatarsalgia. In the 14 patients who returned for evaluation, no postoperative hallux alignment changes were identified.

18. Biedert R, Hintermann B: Stress fractures of the medial great toe sesamoids in athletes. *Foot Ankle Int* 2003;24: 137-141.

    The results of six surgical procedures in five athletes with stress fractures of the medial great toe sesamoid are presented. The proximal fragment was excised, and the flexor hallucis brevis defect was repaired. All patients had good to excellent results; one patient had restriction of sports activities.

19. Saxena A, Krisdakumtorn T: Return to activity after sesamoidectomy in athletically active individuals. *Foot Ankle Int* 2003;24:415-419.

    The authors present the results of 10 fibular and 16 tibial sesamoidectomy procedures in 24 patients.

20. Blundell CM, Nicholson P, Blackney MW: Percutaneous screw fixation for fractures of the sesamoid bones of the hallux. *J Bone Joint Surg Br* 2002;84:1138-1141.

21. Brodsky JW, Robinson AN, O'Krause J, Watkins D: Excision and flexor hallucis brevis reconstruction for painful sesamoid fracture and nonunion. *J Bone Joint Surg Br* 2000;82(suppl III):21.

22. Orava S, Hulkko A: Delayed unions and nonunions of stress fractures in athletes. *Am J Sports Med* 1988;16: 378-382.

23. Anderson RB, McBryde AM: Autogenous bone grafting of hallux sesamoid nonunions. *Foot Ankle Int* 1997;18: 293-296.

24. Jahss MH: Traumatic dislocations of the first metatarsophalangeal joint. *Foot Ankle* 1980;1:15-21.

25. Richardson EG: Injuries to the hallucal sesamoids in the athlete. *Foot Ankle* 1987;7:229-244.

26. McBryde AM, Anderson RB: Sesamoid foot problems in the athlete. *Clin Sports Med* 1988;7:51-60.

27. Ozkoç G, Akpinar S, Ozalay M, et al: Hallucal sesamoid osteonecrosis: An overlooked cause of forefoot pain. *J Am Podiatr Med Assoc* 2005;95:277-280.

    Sesamoidectomy was used to treat histopathology confirmed osteonecrosis of two fibular and two tibial sesamoids.

28. Brostroem L: Sprained ankles I: Anatomic lesions in recent sprains. *Acta Chir Scand* 1964;128:483-495.

2: Foot and Ankle Trauma

29. Coughlin MJ, Mann RA, Saltzman CL (eds): *Surgery of the Foot and Ankle*, ed 8. Philadelphia, PA, Mosby, 2007, pp 1451-1520.

     This book is the most recent edition of a classic text on the foot and ankle. Tables of several classification systems are included.

30. Stiell IG, McKnight RD, Greenberg GH, et al: Implementation of the Ottawa ankle rules. *JAMA* 1994;271: 827-832.

31. Stiell I, Wells G, Laupacis A, et al: Multicentre trial to introduce the Ottawa ankle rules for use of radiography in acute ankle injuries. *BMJ* 1995;311:594-597.

32. Bachmann LM, Kolb E, Koller MT, Steurer J, ter Riet G: Accuracy of Ottawa ankle rules to exclude fractures of the ankle and mid-foot: Systemic review. *BMJ* 2003;326(7386):417.

     The authors present a meta-analysis of 27 studies reporting on 15,581 patients.

33. Gerber JP, Williams GN, Scoville CR, Arciero RA, Taylor DC: Persistent disability associated with ankle sprains: A prospective examination of an athletic population. *Foot Ankle Int* 1998;19:653-660.

34. Hubbard TJ, Kramer LC, Denegar CR, Hertel J: Contributing factors to chronic ankle instability. *Foot Ankle Int* 2007;28:343-354.

     Thirty patients with chronic unilateral ankle instability are compared with 30 control individuals.

35. DiGiovanni BF, Partal G, Baumhauer JF: Acute ankle injury and chronic lateral instability in the athlete. *Clin Sports Med* 2004;23:1-19.

     Ankle injuries often occur during sports activities. The lateral ligamentous complex is often injured. A functional ankle rehabilitation program is the mainstay of treatment for patients with acute lateral ligament injuries.

36. DiGiovanni BF, Fraga CJ, Cohen BE, et al: Associated injuries found in chronic lateral ankle instability. *Foot Ankle Int* 2000;21:809-815.

37. Wilcox DK, Bohay DR, Anderson JG: Treatment of chronic Achilles tendon disorders with flexor hallucis longus tendon transfer/augmentation. *Foot Ankle Int* 2000;21:1004-1010.

38. Wong J, Barrass V, Maffulli N: Quantitative review of operative and nonoperative management of Achilles tendon ruptures. *Am J Sports Med* 2002;30:565-575.

     The authors present a review of retrospectively and prospectively collected data from 125 journal articles with data on 5,370 patients.

39. Rettig AC, Liotta FJ, Klootwyk TE, Porter DA, Mieling P: Potential risk of rerupture in primary Achilles tendon repair in athletes younger than 30 years of age. *Am J Sports Med* 2005;33:119-123.

     The authors present a retrospective study of 89 athletes treated with surgical repair of an Achilles tendon rupture.

40. Krause JO, Brodsky JW: Peroneus brevis tendon tears: Pathophysiology, surgical reconstruction, and clinical results. *Foot Ankle Int* 1998;19:271-279.

41. Steel MW, DeOrio JK: Peroneal tendon tears: Return to sports after operative treatment. *Foot Ankle Int* 2007; 28:49-54.

     A retrospective review of 30 patients (average follow-up 31 months) who were surgically treated for a peroneal tendon tear is presented. The authors reported that 46% of patients successfully returned to sports participation.

Chapter 13

Osteochondral Lesions of the Talus: Acute and Chronic

Jeff Feinblatt, MD   Stanley C. Graves, MD

Introduction

Osteochondral lesions of the knee were first described by Konig[1] in 1888, and osteochondral ankle lesions were described by Kappis[2] in 1922. Roden and associates[3] reported on 55 cases of talar osteochondritis dissecans prior to Berndt and Harty's[4] seminal article on transchondral talus fractures in 1959. Synonymous terms in the literature include chip fracture, flake fracture, juvenile osteonecrosis, osteochondral fracture, and osteochondral defect.[5] The term osteochondritis dissecans is typically reserved for a chronic condition with separation of a necrotic bone and overlying cartilage from an ischemic cancellous bed without a history of trauma. The term osteochondral lesion of the talus (OLT) was introduced by Ferkel and Fasulo[6] in 1994.

Berndt and Harty[4] provided insight into the etiology of this lesion with cadaveric studies. Lateral lesions were recreated with inversion and dorsiflexion, whereas medial lesions were created by inversion, plantar flexion, and external rotation of the leg. These investigators also provided a radiographic classification that is still used, although more recent studies have shown a low correlation between radiographic and arthroscopic findings.[7]

Incidence and Clinical Presentation

The talus is the third most common location for osteochondral lesions, following the knee and elbow.[8] An OLT is believed to occur after 2% to 6% of all ankle sprains.[4,9,10] Clinical characteristics include prolonged pain, swelling, and weakness or continued subjective instability after an inversion injury. The incidence of missed or delayed diagnosis for an OLT is reported to be as high as 81%.[11] Bilateral lesions occur in up to 10% of patients.[4,12] The physical examination may reveal tenderness at the level of the ankle joint anteriorly or posteriorly, with or without effusion. It had been believed that most lesions were located anterolaterally (associated with a high rate of trauma) or posteromedially (with a less consistent history of trauma).[8,13,14] In addition, lateral lesions have typically been described as more superficial, whereas medial lesions typically extend deeper into subchondral bone.[15]

The authors of a 2007 study reviewed MRIs from 424 patients with an OLT.[16] A grid dividing the talar dome into three columns and three rows (nine equal zones) was devised. Medial lesions were seen in 62% of patients and lateral lesions in 34%. In contrast to the historically described anterolateral and posteromedial locations, the midtalar dome (equator) was involved in 80% of lesions whereas the anterior third of the talar dome and posterior third were affected much less often (6% and 14% respectively). The most commonly affected location was the medial equator in 53% of cases followed by the lateral equator in 26% of cases. In agreement with previously published reports, lesions in the medial one third of the dome involved significantly more surface area and were deeper than lesions in the lateral one third of the dome. Medial lesions occurred in slightly older patients (44.6 years versus 39.3 years for patients with lateral lesions). No difference in lesion location was noted based on gender.

Etiology and Natural History

Most authors believe trauma is the underlying etiology in most osteochondral talar lesions. These lesions may occur as a single macroscopic event, such as an inversion injury with the foot in dorsiflexion where the superolateral talar dome impacts the articular surface of the fibula, or with the foot in plantar flexion where the posterior edge of the tibial plafond shears off a posteromedial fragment of the talar dome.[4,5] An OLT also may result from continuous microtrauma in excess of the body's reparative capacity. Genetic factors including hypercoagulability, hypoparathyroidism, hyperparathyroidism, and altered lipid metabolism have been proposed as causative factors in atraumatic occurrences.

The natural history of an OLT is difficult to ascertain because of significant selection bias in available studies. In one study, 30 patients with an OLT found on retrospective radiographic review were examined at an average follow-up of 21 years (range, 11 to 31 years) to determine the natural history of the disease.[17] Six of these patients had surgical procedures, and four

2: Foot and Ankle Trauma

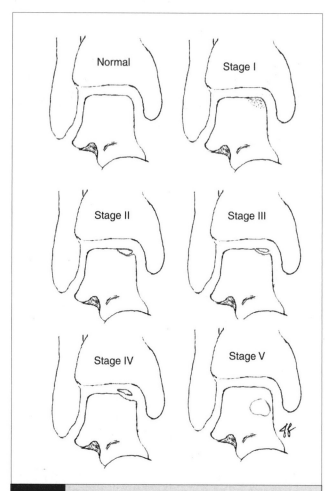

Figure 1 Loomer and associates' modification of the Berndt and Harty radiographic classification of osteochondral lesions of the talus. Stage I: Compression of subchondral bone. Stage II: Partially detached osteochondral fragment. Stage III: Completely detached osteochondral fragment remaining in fragment bed. Stage IV: Displaced osteochondral fragment. Stage V: Presence of cystic component. *(Adapted from Loomer R, Fischer C, Lloyd-Schmidt R, et al: Osteochondral lesions of the talus. Am J Sports Med 1993;21:13-19.)*

of these surgeries were exploratory arthrotomies. Although the presenting symptoms and diagnoses at the time of initial radiography were unknown, there were few changes in the lesion on follow-up radiographs. Six previously undiagnosed and asymptomatic lesions were noted in the contralateral talus on follow-up radiographic examinations. Osteoarthrosis of the ankle was an uncommon outcome, with decreased joint space in only two patients on follow-up radiographs. Subjectively, 53% of outcomes were considered excellent, 27% were good, and 20% were fair.

The authors of a 2006 study reviewed serial MRIs (average follow-up of 13.7 months) of 29 patients who were not surgically treated for OLT.[18] Of these lesion, 45% showed progression based on MRI criteria, 24% had improved, and 31% remained unchanged. Bone marrow edema and subchondral cysts were not reliable indicators of lesion progression. For one patient whose initial MRI showed cysts, the cysts were resolved on follow-up examination. This study was limited by the lack of available clinical information and the inherent selection bias in reviewing patients who had elected not to undergo surgery and may have been minimally symptomatic.

Pathoanatomy

An OLT involves both native hyaline cartilage and the underlying subchondral bone. Although the articular cartilage, once detached, will not spontaneously heal, the chondrocytes continue to receive nutrition from the synovial fluid and remain metabolically active. A recent study has shown that these chondrocytes have the potential to serve as graft for culture and expansion for autologous chondrocyte transplantation (Carticel, Genzyme, Cambridge, MA).[19] Underlying bone may be in a state of compression with surrounding edema as seen on MRI or may be separated from the underlying bed in a state of avascularity. Although not commonly performed, administration of intra-articular gadolinium can improve visualization of a chondral lesion and can assist with assessment of fragment stability and recognition of loose bodies.[20]

Classification

Berndt and Harty's radiographic classification of osteochondral talar lesions is commonly used, although correlation with arthroscopic findings are poor.[7] Loomer and associates[21] modified Berndt and Harty's classification and added stage V to describe lesions with a cystic component (Figure 1). Ferkel and Sgaglione[22] proposed a four-stage classification of the lesions based on CT findings (Figure 2).

In 1989, Anderson and associates[23] developed an MRI classification system for osteochondral talar lesions based on the Berndt and Harty classification system. This system included subchondral cysts as stage IIA. In 1991, Dipaola and associates[24] also proposed an MRI classification system. In 1999, Hepple and associates[25] revised the MRI classification system, subdividing stage 2 based on the presence (stage 2a) or absence (stage 2b) of surrounding edema, believing that the resolution of edema provided evidence of chronicity. Lesions with subchondral cysts were classified as stage 5 (Figure 3). In 2003, Mintz and associates[26] developed an MRI grading system based on Cheng's arthroscopic grading system (Table 1). Other arthroscopic grading systems have been devised by Pritsch and associates[7] and the International Cartilage Repair Society[27] (Table 2).

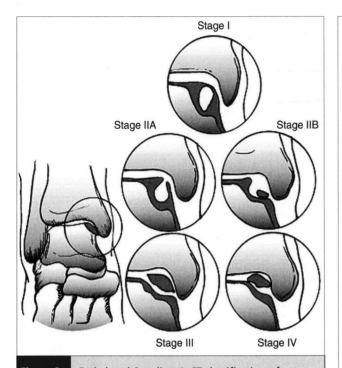

Figure 2 Ferkel and Sgaglione's CT classification of osteochondral lesions of the talus. Stage I: Cystic lesion within the dome of the talus, intact roof on all views. Stage IIA: Cystic lesion with communication to the talar dome surface. Stage IIB: Open articular surface lesion with overlying nondisplaced fragment. Stage III: Nondisplaced lesion with lucency. Stage IV: Displaced fragment.

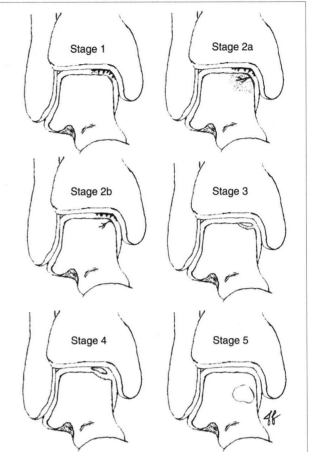

Figure 3 Hepple and associates' MRI classification of osteochondral lesions of the talus. Stage 1: Articular cartilage injury only. Stage 2a: Cartilage injury with bony fracture and surrounding edema. Stage 2b: Cartilage injury with bony fracture without edema. Stage 3: Detached osteochondral fragment remaining in native bed. Stage 4: Detached and displaced osteochondral fragment. Stage 5: Subchondral cyst formation. *(Adapted from Mintz DN, Tashjian GS, Connell DA, Deland JT, O'Malley M, Potter HG: Osteochondral lesions of the talus: A new magnetic resonance grading system with arthroscopic correlation. Arthroscopy 2003;9:353-359.)*

The Pediatric Population

A 2003 study evaluated 24 patients with a mean age of 13 years and 4 months who were diagnosed with an OLT.[28] Lesions were medial in 19 patients (73%), lateral in 5 (19%), and central in 2 (8%). Two patients had bilateral lesions. Eight of 11 ankles treated nonsurgically had good long-term results. Surgical treatment (including drilling, excision, and pinning) was required in 58% of patients. At the most recent clinical examination, complete radiographic healing was seen in six lesions (23%); at final follow-up, 96% showed improvement. Indications for surgery in children are the same as in adults: an unsuccessful course of nonsurgical treatment, displacement of the fragment, increasing severity of the lesion, and decreased potential for fragment revascularization. Earlier surgery is recommended for older children and a longer course of nonsurgical treatment is recommended for young children because of their greater healing potential. A medial malleolar osteotomy is not recommended in skeletally immature patients because of the risk of angular growth deformity.

A review of osteochondral talar lesions in nine adolescent patients with an average age of 14.8 years showed that all lesions but one were Berndt and Harty type III or IV lesions.[29] Débridement and drilling with 0.062 Kirschner wire was performed in all patients. Retrograde drilling was used for medial lesions to avoid physeal injury. At an average follow-up of 12 months, eight patients had no activity limitations and seven were pain free. Three patients underwent additional procedures. The authors believed that surgical outcomes for osteochondral talar lesions in adolescent patients are similar to outcomes in the adult population.

Nonsurgical Treatment

A trial of conservative treatment is appropriate for most lesions with the exception of those with displaced

Table 1

Mintz and Associates' MRI Classification Compared With Cheng's Arthroscopic Staging System for Osteochondral Lesions of the Talus

MRI	Arthroscopic
Grade 0: Normal	Stage A: Smooth, intact but soft
Grade I: Hyperintense but intact cartilage surface	Stage B: Rough surface
Grade II: Fibrillation of fissures not extending to bone	Stage C: Fibrillation or fissuring
Grade III: Flap present or exposed bone	Stage D: Flap present or exposed bone
Grade IV: Loose, nondisplaced fragment	Stage E: Loose, nondisplaced fragment
Grade V: Displaced fragment	Stage F: Displaced fragment

Table 2

International Cartilage Repair Society (ICRS) Arthroscopic Classification of Osteochondritis Dissecans (OCD)

ICRS OCD I	Stable in continuity with softening
ICRS OCD II	Partial discontinuity but stable
ICRS OCD III	Complete discontinuity, but not displaced
ICRS OCD IVA	Displaced fragment, < 10 mm deep lesion
ICRS OCD IVB	Displaced fragment, > 10 mm deep lesion

fragments. Studies have shown that providing a trial of nonsurgical management does not compromise later surgical treatment.[8,14]

A 2003 review of published studies included 14 studies with an aggregate of 201 patients treated nonsurgically.[30] An overall success rate of 45% was reported. Chronic lesions (of > 6 months duration), reviewed in three studies, showed a 56% success rate. In studies using immobilization (duration of 3 weeks to 4 months), 54 of 131 patients (41%) had successful outcomes. The use of rest or activity restrictions alone was reported in seven studies with a 59% success rate.

Preoperative Evaluation and Planning

Based on the lesion present, the goals of surgery may include removal of a loose fragment, securing a larger fragment anatomically, creating an environment for fibrocartilaginous proliferation, or resurfacing with hyaline cartilage. If an OLT is seen on radiographs and is consistent with the patient's symptoms, MRI is recommended. The MRI provides better three-dimensional localization and sizing of the lesion and allows assessment of stability and determination of the presence of a cystic component.

Numerous exposure methods have been described to treat an OLT, including several variations of medial malleolar osteotomies, distal tibial osteotomies, combined anterior and posterior arthrotomies, and transmalleolar and retrograde drilling. Depending on the comfort level of the surgeon, marrow stimulating techniques often can be performed using a 2.7-mm, wide-angle arthroscope.

Surgical Treatment

A 2003 systematic review of 126 published reports of the treatment of osteochondral talar lesions between 1966 and 2000 was an update to a review of the literature performed in 2000.[30,31] Eighty-seven studies were excluded because of inappropriate length of follow-up (< 6 months), improper description or use of a combination of therapies, inclusion of patients younger than 18 years of age, results that could not be interpreted, case reports, and repeat publication. Thirty-nine studies with a total of 879 patients remained for review. The average patient age was 26.9 years, with 65% male patients and 35% female. The lesion was laterally located in 42% of patients and medially located in 58%. Antecedent trauma was noted in 93% of lateral lesions and 61% of medial lesions. No randomized controlled trials had been published at the time of the review. The authors also noted significant heterogeneity in patient characteristics, staging of the defect, duration of follow-up, and outcome measures used in the literature.

In four studies (39 patients) a 38% success rate with open excision alone was reported. One hundred twenty-six patients in 10 studies were treated with excision and curettage. A 63% success rate was reported for open procedures and an 84% success rate for arthroscopic procedures (overall success rate of 76%). Twenty-one studies (272 patients) reported an 86% success rate with excision, curettage, and drilling (84% success rate with open and 87% success rate with arthroscopic procedures).

Two studies (33 patients) reported an 85% success rate with cancellous bone grafting. One study (36 patients) reported a 94% success rate with osteochondral transplantation for defects up to 10 mm. Three studies evaluated fixation of lesions in 11 patients using various implants (all open procedures) with an overall success rate of 73%. One study of 16 patients treated with retrograde drilling reported an 81% success rate.

Cystic Lesions

The etiology of a cystic lesion remains unclear. One theory postulates that synovial fluid under pressure erodes subchondral bone after development of a fissure in the cartilage. The point in the development of an OLT when a cyst occurs remains unknown. A 2006 MRI study included a single patient whose cystic lesion regressed and disappeared without surgical treatment.[18] In general, an OLT with a cystic component is believed to be more difficult to treat; even after bone grafting, a cystic component can remain on follow-up imaging. In one study, various surgical procedures, all without bone grafting, were compared in 20 patients with OLT cysts and 18 without cysts.[32] At 30-month follow-up, no significant difference was seen in American Orthopaedic Foot and Ankle Society (AOFAS) ankle-hindfoot scores between the two groups. Cyst size decreased from 49 mm^2 to 23 mm^2.

Surgical Choices and Results

Primary Repair

Larger lesions with healthy appearing cartilage can be internally stabilized with small headless screws, Kirschner wires, or absorbable pins. Three studies of OLT fixation showed a 73% overall success rate.[30]

Débridement

Commonly used in the knee, chondroplasty can be used to remove a cartilage flap to a stable base. However, débridement alone has the lowest success rate (38%) of any surgical procedure for treating osteochondral talar lesions.[30] The authors of a 2007 study reported on 12 patients treated with repeat arthroscopic débridement after failure of initial débridement at an average of 22 months after the index procedure.[33] At a mean follow-up of 5.9 years, 11 patients were satisfied with their outcome. Mean AOFAS scores had improved from 34.8 to 80.5. Patients with cystic lesions were excluded from the study group because of historically poor results with débridement alone in these lesions.

Microfracture and Drilling

The goals of microfracture and drilling are to promote bleeding and the development of a fibrin clot and subsequent healing response. There are no current pharmacologic methods of inducing expression of type II (hyaline) cartilage; therefore, these methods result in a fibrocartilage covering that is biomechanically inferior to the native hyaline cartilage but has been shown to provide good pain relief in short- and medium-term follow-up studies. Microfracture and drilling cause bleeding by violating subchondral bone. Drilling has the potential complication of causing thermal necrosis. An overall 86% rate of successful outcomes has been reported across 21 studies using excision, curettage, and drilling.[30] Early range-of-motion exercises and partial weight bearing are believed to be important for rapid recovery and are generally recommended.

Autologous Restorative Techniques

The theoretic advantage of these techniques is restoration of a normal hyaline cartilage surface using the patient's own cells, which is achieved using one of two methods. The first method, osteochondral autografting, uses a plug of cartilage and associated subchondral bone that is harvested either locally or from a distal site (usually the ipsilateral knee) and implanted into the prepared OLT defect. If more than a single plug is used, the term mosaicplasty is used.

The second method to restore the patient's own hyaline cartilage is autologous chondrocyte transplantation. In this two-procedure technique, chondrocytes are harvested and cultured. During the second procedure, the cultured chondrocytes are reimplanted under a patch of periosteum. These procedures are typically reserved for lesions larger than 10 mm in diameter or lesions refractory to treatment with other reparative techniques.

Mosaicplasty

In 2003, 63 consecutive patients with osteochondral talar lesions treated with mosaicplasty were reviewed at an average follow-up of 5.8 years.[34] The mean patient age was 25.2 years and the average defect was 1 cm^2 in diameter. The average number of grafts used was three (range, one to seven grafts). The primary donor site was the superior medial edge of the medial femoral condyle. The location and presumed etiology of the lesions was not provided. At final follow-up, using the Hannover scoring system, the author reported 47 excellent results, 11 good, 3 moderate, and 2 poor results. Biopsy at second-look arthroscopy revealed type II collagen and proteoglycans consistent with articular cartilage. The authors concluded that early term and medium-term results of mosaicplasty were encouraging.

Osteochondral Graft Harvest

Most investigators have used osteochondral plugs obtained from the ipsilateral knee. Osteochondral plugs obtained from the medial or lateral talar articular facets have been used to treat small lesions.[35]

Data from a cadaver study demonstrated that patellofemoral contact pressure was lowest along the medial trochlea and decreased distally along the lateral trochlea (the femoral intercondylar notch was not tested).[36] It was recommended that the primary harvest site should be the medial trochlea for grafts 5 mm or smaller and the lateral trochlea just proximal to the sulcus terminalis for larger grafts. These findings are reflective of similar findings by other authors who found the lateral trochlea and proximal medial trochlea were involved in loading at knee flexion angles of 20° to 50°.[37] The authors concluded the distal-medial trochlea and intercondylar notch sites were ideal harvest sites.[37] Other investigators tested the lateral femoral condyle and intercondylar notch and found that no site was free from contact pressure (the medial femoral condyle was not tested).[38]

MRI modeling of the femoral condyles and talar dome, and computer manipulation was used to determine best matched donor (medial and lateral condyles) and recipient sites on the medial talus.[39] The best donor site was determined to be the superolateral femur for any medial talar lesion. The inferolateral femur had more deviation (1.16 mm) than any other donor site when paired with both the anterior and middle talar recipient sites.

Recently, several authors have evaluated the short- and medium-term morbidity associated with osteochondral autograft harvest from the knee.[34,40-43] Currently, there are no long-term follow-up studies available to assess late complications of autograft harvest. Acute complications include infection, hemarthrosis, and patellofemoral pain, with a complication rate ranging from 2% to 36%.[42,44] The harvest location (medial versus lateral femoral condyle versus intercondylar notch) may affect the rate of patellofemoral pain after the autograft harvest, although no studies have specifically examined this issue.

Eleven patients with a completed Lysholm knee score at a mean follow-up of 47 months from time of mosaicplasty for OLT were evaluated.[42] Preoperatively, all knees were normal. At follow-up, the mean Lysholm score was 81 with five excellent, two good, and four poor results. No difference was found between arthroscopic or open methods, total surface area of harvested grafts, or with the number of grafts harvested. Grafts were harvested from the intercondylar notch or lateral femoral condyle proximal to the sulcus terminale. No grafts were obtained from the medial femoral condyle. Knee complications included instability, pain after walking a mile or more, limp, and difficulty with squatting. No patient required an assistive device. The authors hypothesized that if some of the grafts were obtained from the medial trochlea, donor site morbidity may have been reduced.

In a 2003 study, the authors reviewed 831 patients treated with mosaicplasty over a 10-year period for osteochondral defects of various weight-bearing joints.[34] Donor sites were the periphery of both femoral condyles during open harvest and the medial femoral condyle during arthroscopic harvest. Donor site morbidity was reported in 3% of all patients based on postoperative Bandi scores. Knee symptoms resolved within 6 weeks for 95% of the patients and within 1 year for 98% of patients. The authors believed the low rate of knee symptoms was related to appropriate harvest techniques, specifically, using the periphery of both femoral condyles at the level of the patellofemoral joint

during open procedures and using the medial border of the medial femoral condyle during arthroscopic harvest.

In a study of a subset of 63 patients with an OLT (average size of lesion 1.0 cm²) treated using mosaicplasty, the superomedial edge of the medial femoral condyle was the primary donor site, although specific numbers were not provided.[40] Based on the Bandi scoring system, no patient had long-term morbidity at the knee donor site, although two patients reported slight or moderate patellofemoral pain with strenuous activity after 1 year. Five repeat knee arthroscopies were performed with congruent fibrocartilage covering the donor site noted in each case.

In 18 patients who underwent mosaicplasty with harvest from the superomedial margin of the medial femoral condyle, 2 patients (11%) had mild knee symptoms (Kujala patellofemoral scores 85 to 90) without limitations in daily activities. The remaining 16 patients reported no symptoms, with a Kujala patellofemoral score of 95 to 100.[41]

It appears from the small number of studies available that the superolateral femoral condyle allows greater host-graft conformity in medial talar lesions. However, the distal-medial femoral condyle harvest site has less patellofemoral contact pressures, which may help explain the lower knee morbidity rates reported in clinical studies using this site. Relative contraindications to use of the knee as a donor site include existing arthritic changes, patellofemoral symptoms, and limited range of motion.[40]

Autologous Chondrocyte Transplantation

In 1994, Brittberg and associates[45] were the first investigators to report on the transplantation of enzymatically isolated chondrocytes to recreate a viable articular surface. Since that time, the procedure has remained basically unchanged. The authors of a 2006 study reported on 12 consecutive patients with an OLT larger than 1.0 cm² treated with autologous chondrocyte transplantation.[19] Donor cartilage was obtained from the anterior talus, thus eliminating any potential complications associated with violating an intact joint. MRI showed an unfilled defect at 6-month follow-up in all but one patient. At final follow-up (mean, 63 months), seven joints were nearly congruent, four continued to have irregularities at the surface, and one had an incongruent surface with fissures. No second-look procedures were performed. Patients who were involved in competitive sports returned to preoperative levels of play. The mean Hannover score increased from 40.4 points preoperatively to 85.5 points, with seven excellent, four good, and one satisfactory result. Mean AOFAS ankle-hindfoot scores increased from 43.5 points preoperatively to 88.4 points at final follow-up. Other authors reported similar results with 10 patients treated using autologous chondrocyte transplantation.[46] At 4-year follow-up, 9 of 10 patients were pleased or extremely pleased with the result. Biopsies revealed areas of both hyaline and fibrocartilage.

The authors of a 2005 study attempted to further reduce morbidity associated with cartilage harvest.[47] In 16 patients, detached osteochondral fragments from the talus were harvested as a source of chondrocytes and reimplanted after expansion. Chondrocytes harvested from the detached talar fragment were highly viable (99.9%), with a proliferation rate comparable to normal talar chondrocytes. Polymerase chain reaction evaluation revealed that messenger RNA for collagen type II was higher, whereas collagen type I and aggrecans were lower than those in controls (chondrocytes harvested from the knee in seven separate patients). The histologic appearance was hyaline with high concentrations of proteoglycans. Immunohistochemistry showed type II collagen but no type I collagen. No statistical differences in clinical results occurred between the experimental and control group (those treated with graft obtained from the knee). Both groups reported significant increases in AOFAS scores at minimal follow-up of 12 months (range, 12 to 20 months). The authors believed that high cell viability and histologic, histochemical, and immunohistochemical results justify the use of the detached fragment for chondrocyte expansion.

Allograft Transplantation

The use of allografts eliminates the potential for donor site morbidity, is suitable for large lesions, and can be performed in a single procedure, unlike autologous chondrocyte transplantation. However, there is potential for disease transmission as well as immunologic rejection of the foreign graft. One study reported on nine patients with an OLT treated with osteochondral allografts.[48] At an average 11-year follow-up, three cases had been converted to arthrodesis whereas the remaining allografts continued to function.

It has been suggested that fresh allografts be used instead of fresh-frozen allografts because cryopreservation decreases chondrocyte viability.[49] Because marrow elements are the most immunogenic component of the graft, pulsatile lavage should be used to remove as much marrow as possible.

Future Directions

In a study of osteochondral lesions in Thoroughbred horses, it was found that administering oral hyaluronan gel significantly reduced postoperative effusion.[50] Pharmacologic measures will continue to hasten recovery from surgery.

A second-generation technique of chondrocyte transplantation addresses reported complications with Carticel autologous chondrocyte transplantation, including the need to harvest a periosteal patch, the potential associated morbidity, and risk of hypertrophy. In the second-generation technique, a xenograph collagen matrix or an engineered three-dimensional matrix is used to retain the chondrocytes, rather than using a periosteal covering. This and similar techniques are not currently approved by the Food and Drug Administration but are being used in Europe and Australia.

Multiple disciplines including genetic engineering, cellular and molecular biology, pharmacology, and tissue engineering continue to work toward the goal of restoring articular cartilage. Improved three-dimensional scaffolding that allows chondrocytes to mimic the normal zonal characteristics of articular cartilage may improve the longevity of transplanted articular surfaces. Ultimately, manipulation of native signaling molecules may allow a true reparative process to be controlled in vivo.

Summary

Symptomatic osteochondral talar lesions are underdiagnosed after ankle sprains, whereas asymptomatic lesions are incidentally found on radiographic examinations of the ankle. Management of a painful OLT is complex and continues to evolve. In determining appropriate treatment, the surgeon must consider the size and location of the lesion, the presence of cystic or necrotic bone, and the patient's age and physical demands. Although overall success rates are good, methods of treatment will continue to improve with technologic and pharmacologic advancements.

Annotated References

1. Konig F: Über freie Korper in den Gelenken. *Dtsch Z Chir* 1888;27:90.

2. Kappis M: Weitere Beitrange zur traumatisch-mechanischen Entstehung der "spontanen" Knorpelablosungen (sogen. Osteochondritis dissecans). *Dtsch Z Chir* 1922;171:13.

3. Roden S, Tillegard P, Unander-Scharin L: Osteochondritis dissecans and similar lesions of the talus: Report of five cases with special reference to etiology and treatment. *Acta Orthop Scand* 1953;23:51-66.

4. Berndt AL, Harty M: Transchondral fracture of the talus. *J Bone Joint Surg Am* 1959;41:988-1020.

5. Sanders RW, Lindvall E: Fractures and fracture-dislocations of the talus, in Coughlin MJ, Mann RA, Saltzman CL (eds): *Surgery of the Foot and Ankle*, ed 8. St. Louis, MO, Mosby, 2006, p 2121.

   The authors present an excellent review of talar anatomy and traumatic injuries with an emphasis on both acute management and salvage for dislocations and fractures of the talar neck, body, and processes as well as osteochondral defects.

6. Ferkel RD, Fasulo GJ: Arthroscopic treatment of ankle injuries. *Orthop Clin North Am* 1994;25:17-32.

7. Pritsch M, Horoshouski H, Farine I: Arthroscopic treatment of osteochondral lesions of the talus. *J Bone Joint Surg Am* 1986;68:862-865.

8. Alexander AH, Lichtman DM: Surgical treatment of transchondral talar-dome fractures (osteochondritis dissecans): Long-term follow-up. *J Bone Joint Surg Am* 1980;62:646-652.

9. Smith GR, Winquist R, Allan NK, Northrop CH: Subtle transchondral fractures of the talar dome: A radiological perspective. *Radiology* 1977;124:667-673.

10. Van Buecken K, Barrack RL, Alexander AH, Ertl JP: Arthroscopic treatment of transchondral talar dome fractures. *Am J Sports Med* 1989;17:350-356.

11. Ferkel RD, Sgaglione NA, DelPizzo W, et al: Arthroscopic treatment of osteochondral lesions of the talus: Long-term results. *Orthop Trans* 1990;14:172-173.

12. Blevins FT, Steadman JR, Rodrigo JJ, Silliman J: Treatment of articular cartilage defects in athletes: An analysis of functional outcome and lesion appearance. *Orthopedics* 1998;21:761-767.

13. Canale ST, Belding RH: Osteochondral lesions of the talus. *J Bone Joint Surg Am* 1980;62:97-102.

14. Flick AB, Gould N: Osteochondritis dissecans of the talus (transchondral fractures of the talus): Review of the literature and new surgical approach for medial dome lesions. *Foot Ankle* 1985;5:165-185.

15. Bruns J, Rosenbach B, Kahrs J: Etiopathogenetic aspects of medial osteochondrosis dissecans tali. *Sportverletz Sportschaden* 1992;6:43-49.

16. Raikin SM, Elias I, Zoga AC, Morrison WB, Besser MP, Schweitzer ME: Osteochondral lesions of the talus: Localization and morphologic data from 424 patients using a novel anatomical grid scheme. *Foot Ankle Int* 2007;28:154-161.

    The authors reviewed 428 ankles with an OLT imaged with MRI. A grid dividing the talar dome into three columns and three rows (nine equal zones) was devised. The most common location of the lesion was the medial one third and midcoronal one third dome seen in 53% of ankles, followed by the lateral one third and midcoronal one third dome in 26%. Medial one third lesions involved significantly more surface area and were deeper than lateral one third lesions.

17. Bauer M, Jonsson K, Lindén B: Osteochondritis dissecans of the ankle: A 20-year follow-up study. *J Bone Joint Surg Br* 1987;69:93-96.

18. Elias I, Jung JW, Raikin SM, Schweitzer MW, Carrino JA, Morrison WB: Osteochondral lesions of the talus: Change in MRI findings over time in talar lesions without operative intervention and implications for staging systems. *Foot Ankle Int* 2006;27:157-166.

    The authors present a retrospective review of an institu-

tion's MRI records and multiple examination records for patients with an OLT. All surgically treated patients were excluded. Of the remaining 29 patients, 13 lesions (45%) had progressed based on MRI criteria, 7 (24%) had improved, and 9 (31%) remained unchanged. Bone marrow edema and subchondral cysts were not reliable indicators of progression. Level of evidence: IV.

19. Baums MH, Heidrich G, Schultz W, Steckel H, Kahl E, Klinger HM: Autologous chondrocyte transplantation for treating cartilage defects of the talus. *J Bone Joint Surg Am* 2006;88:303-308.

    Twelve patients with an OLT were treated with autologous chondrocyte transplantation. Inclusion criteria included a lesion larger than 1.0 cm², absence of generalized osteoarthritic change, and absence of instability. Donor cartilage was obtained from the anterior talus. Seven excellent, four good, and one satisfactory results were reported at a mean follow-up of 63 months. Level of evidence: IV.

20. Loredo R, Sanders TG: Imaging of osteochondral injuries. *Clin Sports Med* 2001;20:249-278.

21. Loomer R, Fischer C, Lloyd-Schmidt R, et al: Osteochondral lesions of the talus. *Am J Sports Med* 1993;21:13-19.

22. Ferkel RD, Sgaglione NA: *Arthroscopic Surgery: The Foot and Ankle.* Philadelphia, PA, Lippincott-Raven, 1996, pp 145-184.

23. Anderson IF, Crichton KJ, Grattan ST, et al: Osteochondral fractures of the dome of the talus. *J Bone Joint Surg Am* 1989;71:1143-1152.

24. Dipaola JD, Nelson DW, Colville MR: Characterizing osteochondral lesions by magnetic resonance imaging. *Arthroscopy* 1991;7:101-104.

25. Hepple S, Winson IG, Glew D: Osteochondral lesions of the talus: A revised classification. *Foot Ankle Int* 1999;20:789-793.

26. Mintz DN, Tashjian GS, Connell DA, Deland JT, O'Malley M, Potter HG: Osteochondral lesions of the talus: A new magnetic resonance grading system with arthroscopic correlation. *Arthroscopy* 2003;19:353-359.

    A retrospective analysis of concordant MRI and arthroscopic findings in 54 patients with an OLT is presented. MRI correctly identified the correct grade in 83% of the lesions. The remainder of lesions were graded within one grade of actual findings. Grouping lesions into disease-negative (grades 0 to 1) and disease-positive (grades 2 to 5) yielded sensitivity of 95%, specificity of 100%, negative predictive value of 88%, and positive predictive value of 100%. Level of evidence: II.

27. Brittberg M, Winalski CS: Evaluation of cartilage injuries and repair. *J Bone Joint Surg Am* 2003;85:58-69.

    A review of the work and classification systems of the International Cartilage Repair Society and an assessment of articular cartilage repair with MRI and arthroscopy is presented.

28. Letts M, Davidson D, Ahmer A: Osteochondritis dissecans of the talus in children. *J Pediatr Orthop* 2003;23: 617-625.

The authors present a review of 24 patients with an OLT (average age at presentation 13 years). Surgery (drilling, excision, pinning) was eventually needed for 58% of the patients; 96% had improvement. Level of evidence: IV.

29. Benthien RA, Sullivan RJ, Aronow MS: Adolescent osteochondral lesion of the talus: Ankle arthroscopy in pediatric patients. *Foot Ankle Clin* 2002;7:651-667.

30. Verhagen RA, Struijs PA, Bossuyt PM, van Dijk CN: Systematic review of treatment strategies for osteochondral defects of the talar dome. *Foot Ankle Clin* 2003;8: 233-242.

The treatment of patients with an OLT between 1966 and 2000 was systematically reviewed in 126 publications. Eighty-seven studies were excluded because of inappropriate length of follow-up (< 6 months), improper description, the use of a combination of therapies, patients younger than 18 years, noninterpretable results, case reports, and repeat publication of the study. The remaining 39 studies had 879 patients (65% male, 35% female) with a mean age of 26.9 years. The lesion was lateral in 42% and medial in 58%. The lesion was associated with a history of trauma in 76% of patients; 93% had lateral lesions and 61% had medial lesions. Studies were divided and results were reported based on the treatment procedure.

31. Tol JL, Struijs P, Bossuyt PM, et al: Treatment strategies in osteochondral defects of the talar dome: A systematic review. *Foot Ankle Int* 2000;21:119-126.

32. Han SH, Lee JW, Lee DY, Kang ES: Radiographic changes and clinical results of osteochondral defects of the talus with and without subchondral cysts. *Foot Ankle Int* 2006;27:1109-1114.

The authors present a retrospective review of 38 patients with an OLT and compare results of defects without cysts with defects with associated cysts (< 1.5 cm²). All patients were treated using multiple methods, but without bone grafting. At an average follow-up of 30 months, there was no significant difference in postoperative AOFAS ankle-hindfoot score between groups. The authors concluded that surgery without bone grafting provided acceptable clinical results that were not compromised by the presence of a (< 1.5 cm²) cyst. Level of evidence: IV.

33. Savva N, Jabur M, Davies M, Saxby T: Osteochondral lesions of the talus: Results of repeat arthroscopic debridement. *Foot Ankle Int* 2007;28:669-673.

Twelve patients who underwent repeat arthroscopic débridement (without drilling or microfracture) to stable cartilage and viable bone for an OLT are retrospectively reviewed. All patients who required repeat débridement had recurrent symptoms by 6 months after the initial procedure. Patients with cystic lesions were excluded

from the study. At a 5.9-year mean follow-up, 11 patients were satisfied and 1 was dissatisfied with the outcome. Level of evidence: IV.

34. Hangody L, Füles P: Autologous osteochondral mosaicplasty for the treatment of full-thickness defects of weight-bearing joints: Ten years of experimental and clinical experience. *J Bone Joint Surg Am* 2003;85 (suppl 2):25-32.

The authors present a review of 831 patients treated over a 10-year period for lesions in multiple joints. The study included 76 patients treated for an OLT; 94% had good to excellent results as measured by the Hannover ankle evaluation. Donor site morbidity was reported in 3% of all patients. In patients with an OLT, knee symptoms resolved in 95% within 6 weeks. Level of evidence: IV.

35. Sammarco GJ, Makwana NK: Treatment of talar osteochondral lesions using local osteochondral graft. *Foot Ankle Int* 2002;23:693-698.

36. Garretson RB III, Katolik LI, Verma N, Beck PR, Bach BR, Cole BJ: Contact pressure at osteochondral donor sites in the patellofemoral joint. *Am J Sports Med* 2004; 32:967-974.

A cadaver examination of the patellofemoral pressures at common harvest sites for osteochondral plugs is presented.

37. Ahmad CS, Cohen ZA, Levine WN, Ateshian GA, Mow VC: Biomechanical and topographic considerations for autologous osteochondral grafting in the knee. *Am J Sports Med* 2001;29:201-206.

38. Simonian PT, Sussmann PS, Wickiewicz TL, Paletta GA, Warren RF: Contact pressures at osteochondral donor sites in the knee. *Am J Sports Med* 1998;26:491-494.

39. Marymont JV, Shute G, Zhu H, et al: Computerized matching of autologous femoral grafts for the treatment of medial talar osteochondral defects. *Foot Ankle Int* 2005;26:708-712.

The authors present the results of an MRI topographic study of cadaveric femora and tali that used computer reconstructions to determine ideally matched donor (medial and lateral condyles) and recipient sites (anterior, middle, and posterior thirds of the medial talus). The best donor site was determined to be the superolateral femur for any medial talar lesion. The maximal deviation (1.16 mm) was noted between the inferolateral femur and the anterior and middle talar sites. Level of evidence: IV.

40. Hangody L: The mosaicplasty technique for osteochondral lesions of the talus. *Foot Ankle Clin* 2003;8:259-273.

A review of 63 patients (mean age, 25.2 years) with an OLT (mean defect size, 1 cm²) treated with mosaicplasty is presented. The mean follow-up period was 5.8 years and average number of grafts used was three (range, one to seven). Using the Hannover scoring system, 47 excellent, 11 good, 3 moderate, and 2 poor results were re-

2: Foot and Ankle Trauma

ported. Biopsy at second-look arthroscopy showed type II collagen and proteoglycans consistent with articular cartilage. The authors concluded that early term and medium-term results of mosaicplasty are encouraging. Level of evidence: IV.

41. Lee CH, Chao KH, Huang GS, Wu SS: Osteochondral autografts for osteochondritis dissecans of the talus. *Foot Ankle Int* 2003;24:815-822.

   Eighteen patients with Berndt and Harty stage III and IV osteochondral talar lesions were treated with mosaicplasty with autografts harvested from the medial femoral condyle. The authors reported 88.8% excellent results. Level of evidence: IV.

42. Reddy S, Pedowitz DI, Parekh SG, Sennett BJ, Okereke E: The morbidity associated with osteochondral harvest from asymptomatic knees for the treatment of osteochondral lesions of the talus. *Am J Sports Med* 2007;35: 80-85.

   Eleven patients were evaluated with Lysholm knee scores at mean follow-up of 47 months from time of mosaicplasty for an OLT. Preoperatively all knees were normal. Grafts were harvested from the intercondylar notch or lateral femoral condyle proximal to the sulcus terminale. No grafts were obtained from the medial femoral condyle. Knee complications included instability, pain after walking one mile or more, limp, and difficulty with squatting. Level of evidence: IV.

43. Baltzer AW, Arnold JP: Bone-cartilage transplantation from the ipsilateral knee for chondral lesions of the talus. *Arthroscopy* 2005;21:159-166.

   Forty-three patients were treated with osteochondral autograft transfer. Twenty-two patients had an Outerbridge stage III to IV osteochondral lesion, 16 had cartilage defects, and 5 had focal osteoarthritis. In short-term follow-up, 90% of patients who initially were unable to participate in sports activities showed improvement in pain levels and function. Level of evidence: IV.

44. Scranton PE Jr, Frey CC, Feder KS: Outcome of osteochondral autograft transplantation for type-V cystic osteochondral lesions of the talus. *J Bone Joint Surg Br* 2006;88:614-619.

   Fifty patients with an OLT and a cystic defect (type V) were treated with an osteochondral graft from the ipsilateral knee. At a mean follow-up of 36 months, 90% had a good to excellent Karlsson-Peterson Ankle Score and 34% required further surgery. One patient required débridement of the knee; the remaining patients were free of knee symptoms at 3 months. Level of evidence: IV.

45. Brittberg M, Lindahl A, Nilsson A, Ohlsson C, Isaksson O, Peterson L: Treatment of deep cartilage defects in the knee with autologous chondrocyte transplantation. *N Engl J Med* 1994;331:889-895.

46. Whittaker JP, Smith G, Makwana N, et al: Early results of autologous chondrocyte implantation in the talus. *J Bone Joint Surg Br* 2005;87:179-183.

   The authors examined 10 patients with an OLT treated with autologous chondrocyte implantation. The mean area of the treated lesion was 1.95 cm². At 4-year follow-up, 90% of patients were pleased or extremely pleased with their outcome. Biopsy performed in five patients showed hyaline cartilage present in areas of two specimens; the remaining specimens were fibrocartilage. The authors report that autologous chondrocyte implantation shows encouraging results for large contained defects of the talus. Level of evidence: IV.

47. Giannini S, Buda R, Grigolo B, Vannini F, De Franceschi L, Facchini A: The detached osteochondral fragment as a source of cells for autologous chondrocyte implantation (ACI) in the ankle joint. *Osteoarthritis Cartilage* 2005;13:601-607.

   Detached osteochondral fragments from the talus were harvested as a source of chondrocytes for autologous chondrocyte implantation in 20 patients. The chondrocytes were compared morphologically and with molecular markers to chondrocytes harvested from the ipsilateral knee in seven control patients. Chondrocytes harvested from the talus were highly viable (99.9%), with a proliferation rate comparable with normal talar chondrocytes. There were no statistical differences in clinical results between the experimental and control groups. Both groups had significant increases in the AOFAS score at a minimum follow-up of 12 months. Level of evidence: III.

48. Gross AE, Agnidis Z, Hutchinson CR: Osteochondral defects of the talus treated with fresh osteochondral allograft transplantation. *Foot Ankle Int* 2001;22:385-391.

49. Tasto JP, Ostrander R, Bugbee W, Brage M: The diagnosis and management of osteochondral lesions of the talus: Osteochondral allograft update. *Arthroscopy* 2003;19:138-141.

   The authors present a review of the use of allograft to treat an OLT and recommend depleting the marrow elements with pulsatile lavage. Arthroscopic allograft/autograft with platelet-rich plasma is also described. Level of evidence: V.

50. Bergin BJ, Pierce SW, Bramlage LR, Stromberg A: Oral hyaluronan gel reduces post operative tarsocrural effusion in the yearling Thoroughbred. *Equine Vet J* 2006; 38:375-378.

   Compared with placebo control, horses treated with oral hyaluronan gel had significantly less effusion after surgery for osteochondritis dissecans as measured by blinded examiners. Level of evidence: I.

Arthritis

SECTION EDITOR:

SHELDON S. LIN, MD

Chapter 14

Ankle Arthritis

Nicholas A. Abidi, MD   Steven K. Neufeld, MD   Michael E. Brage, MD   Keri A. Reese, MD
Sanjeev Sabharwal, MD   Dror Paley, MD, FRCSC

Introduction

The ankle is a highly congruent joint with a much lower incidence of primary or hereditary osteoarthritis compared with the hip or knee joints.[1-8] The most common etiology of arthritis in the ankle joint is posttraumatic disease. Posttraumatic arthritis is associated with the severity of the ankle fracture pattern, extent of cartilage damage, and nonanatomic reduction of the articular surfaces.[9] Inflammatory arthritides such as rheumatoid arthritis, psoriatic arthritis, and ankylosing spondylitis also can cause ankle arthritis. Hemochromatosis has been linked to primary osteoarthritis.[10]

Cartilage surfaces of the tibiotalar joint differ from those of the knee joint. Tibiotalar joint cartilage has fewer pores than knee articular cartilage, leading to a lower transport rate of solute molecules through the tibiotalar joint surface and possibly contributing to a decrease in susceptibility to osteoarthritis compared with the knee joint.[7] When stressed, ankle cartilage undergoes higher turnover of cartilage matrix material, such as collagen type II and aggrecan molecules, making it more resistant to degradation than knee cartilage.[6]

Posttraumatic ankle arthritis can result from malunion of an ankle fracture. Joint reactive forces of the tibiotalar joint concentrate in particular areas of the joint after fibular shortening, articular surface incongruence, and deltoid ligament rupture.[11,12] Restoration of normal anatomy after traumatic ankle injuries can help re-create normal tibiotalar joint biomechanical forces and lessen the potential of tibiotalar arthritis.

Conservative treatment of ankle arthritis involves the use of anti-inflammatory drugs, orthoses, and intra-articular steroid injections; however, ankle arthritis can be difficult to treat nonsurgically. Surgical treatment of ankle arthritis includes a wide variety of procedures. Traditionally, surgical options for osteoarthritis of the ankle have included joint-sparing procedures, such as arthroscopic or open débridement and realignment osteotomies around the ankle and joint-sacrificing procedures, such as arthrodesis and total joint arthroplasty. Arthrodesis of the ankle is a salvage procedure for patients with advanced osteoarthritis. Ankle arthrodesis is successful at alleviating pain; however, it is associated with long-term sequelae, such as decreased range of motion, infection, nonunion, malunion, and the risk of secondary progressive arthritis in the midfoot and hindfoot.[13] Total ankle arthroplasty is gaining in popularity for the treatment of advanced ankle arthritis, but may not be appropriate for young, active adults because of concerns regarding implant loosening and complications with wound healing.[14-17] Recently, joint distraction arthroplasty (arthrodiastasis) has been advocated as a joint-sparing alternative for young patients with congruent, painful osteoarthritic ankle joints. Other newer treatment modalities, such as subchondral drilling, autologous chondrocyte transplantation, and osteochondral transplantation are being used to treat patients with ankle arthritis. Fresh osteochondral allograft transplantation provides an alternative treatment option for young and active patients with end-stage tibiotalar arthritis.

Patient Evaluation

The initial evaluation of a patient with ankle arthritis consists of the usual elements of patient evaluation that may provide information on the etiology of the disease and potential pitfalls in proposed treatment options. Information should be obtained on possible systemic diseases, confounding medications that could affect treatment, retained hardware from previous surgeries, and the occurrence of previous infections from any surgical procedure. The presence of indolent bacteria, whether *Staphylococcus epidermidis* or methicillin-resistant *Staphylococcus aureus,* also should be determined.

Diabetes mellitus can affect both the peripheral nerves and healing capability if surgery is planned. Diseases affecting macrocirculation and microcirculation of the lower extremity can lead to wound healing complications and increase the rate of nonunion at the surgical site. Patients who smoke have a significantly higher rate of surgical complications related to wound healing and can have a nonunion rate after ankle arthrodesis that is up to 16 times higher than that of nonsmokers.[18] Osteonecrosis of the talus can lead to a nonunion rate of 40% in patients treated with standard arthrodesis techniques.[19]

When obtaining the patient's medical history, it should be determined if a palliative procedure such as ankle arthroscopy will abate symptoms or if a more aggressive surgical procedure is necessary. When a patient presents with anterior ankle joint pain caused by ambulation or stair climbing, anterior decompression of impinging osteophytes will often be necessary. If the patient reports diffuse ankle pain and has severely limited ankle joint motion, ankle arthrodesis may be beneficial.

The physical examination should evaluate the patient's hips, knees, and overall gait. Outcomes after ankle arthrodesis will depend on overall limb alignment and contiguous joint function. Proximal disorders, such as hip or knee arthritis, should be treated with arthroplasty or corrective osteotomy prior to ankle arthrodesis. A neurovascular examination of the affected limb is vital in surgical planning. Patients with diminished circulation may require vascular consultation and a stent or bypass surgery to ensure a successful surgical outcome. To avoid postoperative malunion or Charcot breakdown, patients with peripheral neuropathy require more rigid fixation techniques and longer periods of protected weight bearing and immobilization than patients with normal sensory function.[20,21]

The use of certain medications, such as steroids or cyclooxygenase-2 inhibitors, also can affect wound healing and treatment outcomes.[22] The nature of deleterious effects of prednisone, disease-modifying antirheumatic drugs, and methotrexate on postoperative wound healing and rates of successful ankle arthrodesis is argued.[23] These factors, along with risks and benefits of various treatments, should be considered in preoperative and postoperative treatment plans.

Radiologic documentation of deformity is important for preoperative planning. The degree of deformity may affect the surgical approach or dictate the type of instrumentation used in procedures such as ankle arthrodesis. Weight-bearing radiographs are important for determining tibiotalar joint space narrowing, deformity, and in evaluating the surrounding joints. Arthritis in the subtalar or talonavicular joints may affect the choice of procedure. If weight-bearing radiographs do not show the degree of arthritis in the joints surrounding the talus, MRI may be appropriate for documenting the degree of disease in these joints and for ruling out osteonecrosis of the talus.

Nonsurgical Treatment

Patients with mild arthritis of the ankle joint may benefit from certain conservative modalities to treat pain, prevent progression of disease, and improve overall function. Oral nonsteroidal anti-inflammatory medications can be used to limit ankle joint pain and inflammation. If these medications are administered for long-term use, patients should undergo baseline laboratory testing, including liver function tests, a complete blood count, serum chemistry panel, and urinalysis. These tests should be repeated approximately every 6 months to monitor the patient for renal insufficiency. Periodic corticosteroid injection of the ankle joint may limit inflammation and reduce pain; however, routine injec-

tions may lead to skin discoloration, fat necrosis, and an increase in the potential for local infection.

Bracing of the affected ankle can limit ankle motion and offload forces from the joint, thereby reducing ankle inflammation and pain. Leather and polypropylene gauntlet braces can limit pain while permitting ankle function. The circumferential gauntlet-type leather braces have a high patient acceptance rate because of comfort afforded by the smooth edges of the brace compared with rigid, plastic ankle-foot orthoses. Hinged, double, upright calf-lacing ankle-foot orthoses can offload the tibiotalar joint. Stiff-shank, rocker-bottom soled shoes with cushioned heels can improve patient gait patterns by compensating for the lack of inherent ankle motion. These shoes also may be used in the early postoperative period for isolated tibiotalar joint arthrodesis or on a long-term basis for combined tibiotalocalcaneal arthrodesis. This type of shoe with a 2.5-cm arch lift normalizes the gait pattern in patients with abnormal ankle motion and can reduce strain on the medial collateral ligament.[24]

Ankle Arthrodesis

Ankle arthrodesis remains the gold standard of surgical treatment for improving function and relieving pain in patients with tibiotalar joint arthritis, although the procedure has complications and disadvantages that will be discussed later in this chapter. Significant controversy exists regarding the optimal surgical approach, instrumentation, and postoperative care for patients treated with ankle arthrodesis. To achieve optimal postoperative gait regardless of the surgical technique, the ideal final position for ankle arthrodesis is 5 mm of posterior offset, 5° to 7° of hindfoot valgus, and 10° of external rotation with neutral dorsiflexion.[25]

Arthroscopic Techniques
Arthroscopic ankle arthrodesis has been shown to be a reliable surgical technique for treating patients with minimal ankle deformity.[26-31] When compared with traditional open tibiotalar arthrodesis, patients undergoing arthroscopic and mini-open ankle arthrodesis have reported more rapid arthrodesis (< 8 weeks) compared with patients treated with traditional open methods.[27] These outcomes are believed to result from less tissue stripping and therefore less disruption of the blood supply to the tibiotalar joint during arthroscopic and mini-open ankle arthrodesis. The fibula is usually preserved and crossing compression screws are used for fixation during arthroscopic ankle arthrodesis. Ankle distraction can be achieved by placement of an external fixator or with a noninvasive ankle distraction device. Intraoperative fluoroscopy is generally used to confirm ankle positioning and hardware placement. When significant preoperative deformity is present, ideal positioning may be difficult to achieve with an arthroscopic technique by all but the most skilled and experienced

surgeons. However, acceptable outcomes are generally achieved with arthroscopic arthrodesis.[29,30]

Open Techniques

Because most candidates for ankle arthrodesis have significant posttraumatic deformity, these patients often benefit from open arthrodesis techniques. Open ankle arthrodesis techniques generally allow the surgeon to reduce the tibiotalar joint into a suitable position for arthrodesis. Multiple approaches have been described. The selection of the approach depends on the status of the patient's circulation, the condition of the skin in the area of consideration, and the presence of preexisting hardware. Preparation of the joint surfaces may involve the use of a high-speed burr, osteotomes, a saw, or the use of a power chisel. The burr and saw can theoretically burn bone surfaces and increase the rate of nonunion. Osteotomes and power chisels permit custom sculpting of the tibiotalar joint into an acceptable position that permits coaptation of the joint surfaces while limiting thermal necrosis to bone surfaces.

The classic approach to tibiotalar arthrodesis is a transfibular approach with an accessory medial portal.[32-37] Some techniques involve lateral reattachment of all or a portion of the fibula as a buttress to prevent lateral talar migration. The pattern of débridement can be concave, flat, or chevron.[38]

The pattern of screw placement is controversial. The pattern for transfibular ankle arthrodesis typically consists of crossing or parallel screws with or without a "home-run" screw. Crossing and parallel screws have shown various modes of failure in biomechanical models.[39] The home-run screw is a lag screw that travels from the posterior malleolus into the plantar medial talar neck and head.[40] It encourages neutral dorsiflexion of the tibiotalar joint and mild posterior offset of the talus relative to the tibia. This screw can be placed through the Achilles tendon if necessary. A pattern of multidirectional screw placement will ensure stability and resistance to torque, inversion, and eversion in multiple planes.

Lateral plates have been used to provide fixation that is more rigid than that provided by simple screws alone. Many studies have shown successful arthrodesis with lateral plating.[41-45] Plate application may require a larger area of exposure of the tibiotalar joint and may lead to more soft-tissue stripping. Biomechanical studies have supported the feasibility of using smaller, less invasive plating by demonstrating rigidity comparable or superior to that provided by the crossed-screw techniques. These plating systems incorporate locking techniques, which convert standard plates into a blade-plate construct. Locking plates have more inherent stability than conventional plating, particularly in the presence of comorbidities involving soft metaphyseal bone. Locking the plate distally in the talus permits improved compression across the arthrodesis site when combined with a compression outrigger placed proximally during plate application. Clinical studies with these newer plates are currently underway. Cannulated and noncannulated blade plates and retrograde intramedullary nails have demonstrated clinical efficacy and improved arthrodesis rates in patients undergoing revision arthrodesis and in those with Charcot arthropathy and talar osteonecrosis.[43,45-50]

The anterior approach to the ankle has been used successfully to denude articular cartilage from the tibiotalar joint. Plating of the anterior aspect of the joint uses the Achilles tendon to create a tension-band construct.[51-53] This technique has shown clinical efficacy; however, it is necessary to avoid anterior subluxation of the talus during tibiotalar joint fixation.

The posterior approach to the ankle joint is used when the blood supply or the skin has been compromised in the area used for more traditional approaches to the ankle joint.[46,54,55] The posterior approach to the tibiotalar joint is typically accomplished by splitting the tendon or by a Z-lengthening technique, which permits placement of a posterior blade-plate or a locking plate with locking screws placed into the talus. Care must be taken to avoid injury to neurovascular structures and flexor tendons on the posterior medial aspect of the ankle joint. **Table 1** shows a comparison of various open techniques for tibiotalar arthrodesis.

Autogenous bone graft generated locally or from the proximal tibia has been used to fill gaps that develop in the tibiotalar surfaces during preparation. Randomized, controlled trials have not been performed that compare the efficacy of allograft, autograft, or not using a graft in tibiotalar arthrodesis. Two studies have shown the efficacy of autologous platelet-derived growth factor in tibiofibular arthrodesis.[56,57] Multicenter studies are currently underway that will evaluate the efficacy of recombinant growth factors compared with autologous bone graft in promoting ankle arthrodesis.

Total Ankle Arthroplasty

Total ankle arthroplasty was developed in the 1970s as an alternative treatment to ankle arthrodesis following the success of total hip and knee arthroplasty. Unfortunately, first-generation total ankle replacements were not as successful as implants used in other joint arthroplasties and were associated with numerous complications and failures. Most clinical studies of first-generation implants included few patients and had short follow-up periods. Clinical outcomes were associated with initially promising results; however, longer follow-up showed poor results with varying levels of patient satisfaction.[58] The constrained prosthetic designs (for example, the Imperial College of London Hospital prosthesis, TPR prosthesis [Smith and Richards, Memphis, TN], and the Oregon [Zimmer, Warsaw, IN]) treated the ankle as a hinge joint providing motion in only the sagittal plane. Unacceptably high rates of radiographic loosening (up to 75%) probably resulted from this limited concept of highly constrained

Table 1

Comparison of Various Tibiotalar Arthrodesis Open Techniques

Technique	Suggested Contraindications	Time To Arthrodesis	Advantages	Potential Pitfalls
Mini-Open	Osteonecrosis, severe bone loss, more than 10° varus or valgus, more than 25% anterior talar subluxation	97% at 8 weeks	Minimal soft-tissue stripping, débridement not required for posterior third Suitable as potentially reversible arthrodesis for future ankle arthroplasty	Difficult visualization, screw fixation is percutaneous
Lateral Transfibular	Lateral wound compromise, circulatory compromise	74% to 97% at 12 to 16 weeks	Wide exposure, able to correct significant deformity	Significant soft-tissue stripping, possible lateral drift if the fibular strut is not reattached
Posterior	Posterior wound compromise, typically used for tibiotalocalcaneal arthrodesis with intramedullary rod or blade plate	14.5 weeks	Excellent posterior blood supply if split angiosomes in midline of Achilles tendon	Difficult to easily débride anterior joint and gutters, possible accidental plantar flexion during fixation while prone

prosthetic design and cement fixation. The first generation implants also required removal of excessive bone and implantation in soft metaphyseal bone; subsequent loosening of these prostheses was common. The implant provided initial stability but did not take into account the significant rotational forces acting on the ankle joint. There also was a significant propensity for bearing subluxation that led to severely reduced clinical motion. The unconstrained first-generation prostheses (such as the Newton [Howmedica, Rutherford, NJ], Smith [Dow Corning Wright, Arlington, TN], and New Jersey Low Contact Stress [DePuy, Warsaw, IN] designs) relied on the inherent stability of the ankle ligaments and soft tissue. Once the soft-tissue constraints became lax, subsequent outcomes were poor. Impingement of the periarticular soft tissues caused pain, and multiaxial motion was allowed at the expense of stability.[58,59]

Design Issues and Rationale

Interest in ankle arthroplasty continued with the introduction of second-generation total ankle prostheses because of dissatisfaction with complications of ankle arthrodeses and the desire to maintain motion. Improved prosthetic designs and fixation methods and a better understanding of the indications and contraindications for arthroplasty contributed to this new enthusiasm. Intermediate-term results with second-generation implants and current approaches have been encouraging.

Current designs for ankle prostheses include three components. The bearing (either fixed or mobile) between the surfaces of the tibial and talar components is believed to help absorb the forces passing through the ankle joint. These prostheses typically have a flat tibial component and a talar component with anatomic cur-

vature in the sagittal plane. An advantage of this type of design is that the flat upper surface allows some rotation, which reduces stress at the prosthesis-bone interface. A disadvantage of the design is that the flat geometry does not reproduce the convex-concave articulation of the talus in the tibial mortise.

Design engineers now understand that the intrinsic stability of current total ankle implants must be neither too low nor too high. A prosthetic design with a mobile bearing has a low risk for loosening of the talar and/or tibial component but is susceptible to impingement of the mobile bearing against the malleoli. In contrast, a prosthetic design with a fixed bearing (high inherent stability) has a high propensity for loosening of the talar and/or tibial component or requires tibiotalar fusion and removal of large amounts of bone and ligament. Significant design issues exist regarding the amount of ankle articulation to be resurfaced and the size and geometry of the contact area between the bone and implant. Currently, it is not known if it is better to resurface only the superior tibiotalar articulation or the medial and/or lateral articulation as well.

Designers of total ankle prostheses are gaining a better understanding of physiologic ankle motion, which is characterized by rolling and sliding. Researchers found that the ankle moves "as a complex joint with coupled three-dimensional motions."[60] The talus is wedge shaped with different radii of curvature on the medial and lateral talar domes and anteriorly and posteriorly. The ankle joint axis continuously changes throughout range of motion. The second- and third-generation ankle prostheses should take into account this changing axis of rotation, which results in approximately 12° of axial rotation of the tibia relative to the talus during normal activities.[59] Certain current prosthetic designs,

3: Arthritis

however, do not use a different radius of curvature and may place more stress on the ankle ligaments as they strain to accommodate the prosthesis through its range of motion.[61] Typically, the prostheses have conically shaped talar components that allow the articular surfaces to slide and roll on each other; the ankle ligaments rotate about their origins and insertions on the bones without resistance.[62] Theoretically, this action may place additional stress on posteromedial aspects of the ankle or may cause significant deltoid strain. Longer follow-up periods will determine if this design leads to complications.

The newer generation of implants uses improved osseous integration materials. Most prostheses have ingrowth characteristics that require no cement. Some use a hydroxyapatite coating, an inorganic substance that promotes bone ingrowth, and some have a coating of sintered metal beads, plasma spray metals, or fiber metals. These roughened microsurfaces are added as an external layer on the surface of the prosthesis, leave more bone intact, and achieve fixation through bony ingrowth. Ingrowth can occur into these roughened surfaces.

Most second-generation implants include a mobile bearing between the tibial and talar component. The bearing typically is made of ultra-high molecular weight polyethylene (UHMWPE) and offers the opportunity for greater congruence and, theoretically, less wear. One disadvantage of mobile-bearing prosthetic designs with two articulations is the increased risk for dislocation and small particle disease.[63] A mobile bearing by definition allows backside wear but may be made fully conforming, which greatly reduces contact stresses in the bearing.

Other second-generation prosthetic designs such as the Agility Ankle (DePuy) and Salto prosthesis (Tornier SA, Montbonnot, France) have three components but the UHMWPE meniscus is fixed within the tibial component. Fixed bearings are less likely to break or subluxate. These prostheses offer more constraint with weight bearing because of their matching conformity. A fixed-bearing polyethylene surface may potentially reduce backside wear if there is an effective locking mechanism. A recent study of fixed- and mobile-bearing ankle prostheses showed generation of wear particles similar to that seen in knee arthroplasty.[64]

In general, goals for newer total ankle prosthetic designs include minimizing bone removal, maximizing the surface area for prosthetic support, allowing sufficient polyethylene thickness and conforming geometry, establishing proper balance between constraint and freedom, using a bearing surface that minimizes wear, using a firm locking mechanism for ankles with a fixed bearing, and improving instrumentation to ensure proper alignment of the prosthesis.[61] The clinical goals continue to be pain resolution, restoration of motion, and improved function.

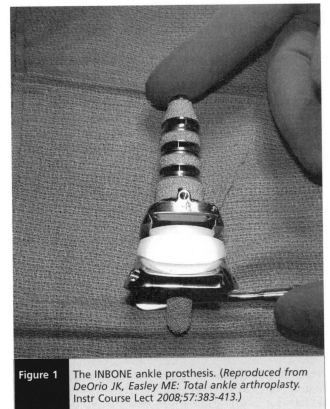

| Figure 1 | The INBONE ankle prosthesis. (*Reproduced from DeOrio JK, Easley ME: Total ankle arthroplasty. Instr Course Lect 2008;57:383-413.*) |

Evolution of Prostheses and Clinical Efficacy

US Food and Drug Administration (FDA)-approved total ankle systems include the Agility total ankle prosthesis, INBONE total ankle system (Wright Medical, Arlington, TN) (**Figure 1**), and the Salto-Talaris prosthesis (Tornier, Stafford, TX). The Eclipse total ankle (Integra, Plainsboro, NJ) received FDA approval in 2006; however, case reports of implantation in the United States are not available. In other countries, many companies such as Baumer, Corin, Endotec, Integra, Eska, Euros, W. Link GmbH and Co, Fournitures Hospitaliers, Protetim, Tornier, Sovereign, and Japan Medical provide alternative ankle systems. These systems may become available in the United States.

Currently available prostheses can be categorized into two-component designs, three-component designs with a mobile bearing, or three-component designs with a fixed bearing. These prostheses differ in materials, fixation techniques, contour of the articulating surfaces, and in the areas covered (some cover the medial or lateral recesses as well as the superior tibiotalar surfaces).

Two-Component Prosthetic Designs

The TNK ankle (Kyocera, Kyoto, Japan) was developed and initially implanted by Takakura in Japan. The original design was composed of a metallic tibial component and polyethylene talar component. The current design is a fixed-bearing, cementless, metallic tibial component on a ceramic hydroxyapatite-coated talar

3: Arthritis

prosthesis. Bony fixation includes a tibial screw. Older designs were marked by loosening and subsidence but the newer prosthesis is reported to have good early results.[65] No long-term follow-up studies are available for this prosthesis.

Mobile-Bearing Three-Component Designs

Mobile-bearing three-component prostheses have a more anatomic design and require less bone resection than the fixed-bearing, three-component designs. There are two metal components—the superior component consists of a flat tibial tray, and the inferior component is an anatomically designed talar dome that sits on top of a resurfaced talus. Both components have a porous backing and rely on biologic fixation. Typically, a mobile polyethylene bearing sits between the two metal components.

The Scandinavian Total Ankle Replacement (STAR; W. Link GmbH and Co, Hamburg, Germany) is currently undergoing FDA trials in the United States. The STAR is a cobalt-chromium prosthesis without hydroxyapatite, with a titanium porous coating. A version of this prosthesis, available in Europe, is made with a dual coating of calcium phosphate that is electrochemically bonded onto a titanium porous coating and applied to the cobalt-chromium prosthesis. The STAR has a flat tibial tray and an anatomically designed talar dome. Between the tray and the dome is a mobile-bearing polyethylene insert with a radiopaque marker. The insert has a flat articulation with the tibial interface and a circular articulation with a central groove at the talar interface. Flexion-extension occurs at the talar-meniscal interface and rotation and sliding occurs at the tibial-meniscal interface. The prosthesis resurfaces the tibiotalar articulation and provides a hemiresurfacing of the two facet areas. The implant has shown promising results in follow-up studies of up to 15 years.[66-68] The STAR has been used in Europe for 20 years but is awaiting approval by the US FDA. A report of 200 cementless STAR implants showed a 5-year survival rate of 92.7%. The most common complications were delayed wound healing and malleolus fracture, which became less common as the operating surgeon gained experience.[69] Other studies had less promising results, with one study reporting a 5-year survival rate of 70%.[70] In a recent prospective study of 200 STAR prostheses, the 5-year survival rate was 93.3% and the 10-year survival rate was 80.3%.[71] Twelve percent of prostheses required revision (20 with fusion and 4 with replacement). A revision rate of 21% at 3.7-year follow-up in 65 patients who had arthroplasty with the STAR was reported in one study,[72] and 7 of 50 STAR prostheses (14%) required revision in another study.[73]

Another mobile-bearing, three-component design, the Buechel-Pappas Low Contact Stress Ankle (Endotec, South Orange, NJ), is not currently approved by the FDA for use in the United States; however, studies conducted in Europe and the United States show good intermediate-term results.[74-77] The implant is made of cobalt-chromium alloy, is porous-coated, and is covered with a beaded, titanium coating for surface ingrowth. It has three components, including a fully conforming polyethylene mobile bearing. The prosthesis resurfaces only the tibiotalar area and not the facets. The tibial component must be implanted through an anterior cortical window, which compromises the cortical integrity proximal to the implant. Despite this requirement, the risk of tibial component subsidence or loosening appears to be offset by the support afforded by the stem. One recent observational study of 93 Buechel-Pappas ankles implanted in patients with inflammatory arthritis (mostly rheumatoid) showed a mean overall 8-year survival rate of 84%.[78] A significantly increased failure rate was found in ankles with a preoperative deformity in the coronal plane and in ankles in which an undersized tibial component had been used. Fifteen prostheses failed because of aseptic loosening. A review of the study by the designers of the Buechel-Pappas ankle showed 88% good to excellent results with a mean 5-year follow-up. Problems with bearing subluxation in the original shallow sulcus design were eliminated in the subsequent deep sulcus prosthetic design. Improvement in talar component fixation was achieved with the addition of two fixation fins. Because delayed wound healing was the most common complication (17.4%), the authors recommended extending the incisions and avoiding constant retraction.[75]

The Hintegra ankle implant (Integra Life Sciences, Plainsboro, NJ) consists of a flat tibial and anatomically shaped (truncated conical, smaller medially than laterally) talar component fitted with screw fixation and a UHMWPE bearing. The tibial component is designed for minimal tibial resection (2 to 3 mm) and screw fixation into the anterior tibial cortex. The talar component consists of a highly polished articular surface, and a medial and lateral surface. There is an anterior shield for placement of two screws. The interface is coated with porous titanium and hydroxyapatite to aid bony ingrowth. Initial results with the Hintegra ankle have been encouraging. In a short-term follow-up study of 116 patients (122 ankles) by the prosthesis designers, 8 ankles required revision.[79] Four ankles were revised because of loosening of at least one component, one because of dislocation of the meniscus, and three for other reasons. At an average follow-up of 18.9 months (range, 1 to 3 years), 84% of patients were satisfied with the procedure. Clinical results were rated as good or excellent in 82% of patients.[79] A recent study showed that the Hintegra ankle allowed increased participation in sports activities in patients with arthritis and that patients who actively participated in sports after an ankle replacement had a higher functional American Orthopaedic Foot and Ankle Society (AOFAS) hindfoot score than did those who were not active in sports. Activities included biking, hiking, swimming, skiing, golfing, and aerobic exercises.[80] No

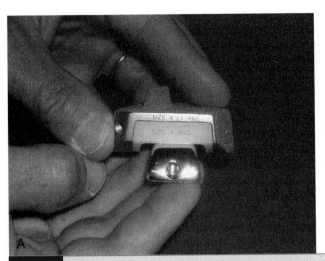 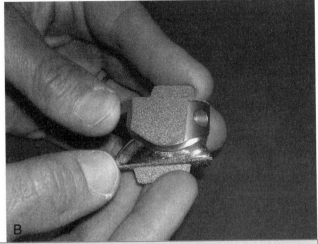

| Figure 2 | The Agility ankle prosthesis. Front view **(A)** and view from the medial side **(B)**. (*Reproduced from DeOrio JK, Easley ME: Total ankle arthroplasty.* Instr Course Lect *2008;57:383-413.*) |

studies in the United States have been reported with this prosthesis.

The Salto ankle prosthesis is a press-fit, hydroxyapatite-coated, mobile-bearing, three-component implant that was designed in France and has been implanted since 1997. The tibial component has a cylindrical stem and a bearing contact surface with a medial edge to control bearing translations. The polyethylene bearing communicates with the congruent surface of the talar component. The original design has a polyethylene implant on the fibula that articulates with the talar cap piece. Preliminary results of this prosthesis have been encouraging, with a 98% implant survival rate of 68 months.[81] A fixed-bearing, three-component modification has been made for use in the United States and recently received FDA approval in 2006.

Fixed-Bearing, Three-Component Prosthetic Designs
A widely used ankle replacement in the United States is the Agility ankle (**Figure 2**). This prosthesis is a semiconstrained, three-component, uncemented implant with a highly congruent talar-polyethylene articulation. The Agility ankle has a talar component made of a porous-coated, cobalt-chromium alloy and a titanium-backed polyethylene tibial component. Studies have shown good early and intermediate results; however, a longer-term follow-up study showed only a 60% survival rate at 11 years (50% of the patients were lost to follow-up).[82,83] The development of periprosthetic lucencies, lysis, and radiographic evidence of component migration and subsidence has caused significant concern. Despite these complications, continued high rates of patient satisfaction have been reported.[82-84] The Agility ankle has a unique design requiring a stable platform achieved by tibiotalar arthrodesis. The medial, lateral, and superior articular surfaces of the ankle also are resurfaced. The Agility ankle absorbs rotational forces by allowing a space between the medial and lateral sides of the talar component resting against the

fixed bearing. The articular surface of the tibial component is larger than that of the talar component; this lack of congruence allows the ankle to slide from side to side, resulting in rotational and sagittal motion. In this unique design, stability of the implant partly relies on a successful fusion of the distal tibiofibular syndesmosis. In a 2- to 12-year follow-up study of the initial 100 patients treated by the designers of the Agility ankle, a 6% revision rate was reported; 93% of the ankles had satisfactory outcomes.[84] Delayed union or nonunion of the syndesmosis is associated with excessive motion, leading to mechanical lysis along the lateral margin of the tibial component as a result of abnormal motion between the tibial component and the lateral malleolus. This radiographic finding ultimately leads to a significant increase in tibial subsidence rates and ballooning osteolysis, with rates reported from 5% to 34%.[82,84-86] Fusion of the syndesmosis is achieved by locally preparing the bone, removing some of the thick cortical bone at the syndesmosis, packing with bone graft, and stabilizing the fusion site with screws. Union is expected by 3 months postoperatively but may be difficult to confirm radiographically. In one report, 41% of patients had a successful syndesmotic fusion after 6 months; nonunion occurred in 8% of patients.[83] A syndesmotic nonunion necessitates revision of the arthrodesis with placement of rigid internal fixation and autograft. A five-hole or six-hole, one-third tubular plate on the fibula allows greater compression and stability across the distal tibiofibular fusion site.[87] Recently, modifications to the Agility ankle have been made including a wider talar component to prevent talar subsidence, and a front-loading polyethylene insert to aid in implantation and revision surgery. Follow-up studies of the newer design have not been published to date.

The Salto-Talaris ankle prosthesis (**Figure 3**) is a fixed-bearing design based on the Salto mobile-bearing ankle prosthesis. The Salto mobile-bearing prosthetic

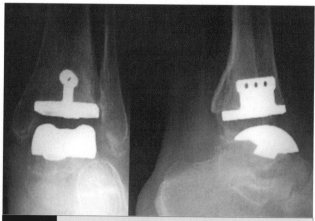

Figure 3 AP (left) and lateral (right) radiographic views of the Salto-Talaris anatomic ankle prosthesis. (*Reproduced from DeOrio JK, Easley ME: Total ankle arthroplasty.* Instr Course Lect *2008;57:383-413.*)

design has been in use in Europe since 1997 with encouraging short-term and midterm results.[81] The fixed-bearing design includes a titanium tibial component with a tibial post, a highly conforming polyethylene articulating insert, and a talar component that resurfaces the anterior/posterior and lateral surfaces. The Salto-Talaris ankle prosthesis was recently approved by the FDA for use in the United States. Its designers publicize that the "mobile tibia concept" instrumentation was developed from the mobile-bearing design that allows accurate tibia component positioning. No long-term studies are available for this prosthesis.

Indications

Total ankle arthroplasty is indicated for patients with severe end-stage primary arthritis, rheumatoid arthritis, or posttraumatic tibiotalar joint arthritis that has been unsuccessfully managed with nonsurgical treatment. Patients with ipsilateral hindfoot (ankle and subtalar) arthritis who also require a triple arthrodesis would benefit from total ankle replacement. Ankle arthroplasty is typically used to treat older patients with lower demands and those with multiple joint osteoarthritis or inflammatory arthropathy to provide relief of unrelenting pain. In patients with rheumatoid arthritis or inflammatory arthropathy, the frequent involvement of the smaller joints of the foot is a concern when considering that ankle fusion will lead to increased stress across those joints; therefore, rheumatoid arthritis is a predictive factor for a better outcome in patients undergoing total ankle arthroplasty.[88] After ankle fusion, the small joints of the foot are needed to compensate for the stiff ankle; therefore, the lack of compensatory small joint motion may make ankle arthroplasty favorable over fusion.[89]

Patients with bilateral ankle disease have poor functional outcome scores after bilateral ankle fusions. This patient population would benefit from ankle replacement in at least one ankle because a mobile ankle im-

proves gait. Careful selection is necessary for patients undergoing ankle arthroplasty. An ideal candidate should have good bone stock, normal overlying skin, normal vascular examination results, no immunosuppression disorders, correct hindfoot-ankle alignment, well-preserved ankle joint motion with sufficient stability, and relatively low physical demands (such as bicycle riding, swimming, walking, golfing).[62,90] Total ankle arthroplasty for middle-aged patients, manual laborers, and those with diabetes or high physical demands is controversial. Younger patients typically want to resume more rigorous activities after total ankle arthroplasty than do older, more sedentary patients; therefore, younger patients should be instructed on the need to restrict some activities after ankle replacement.

Contraindications

Contraindications for total ankle arthroplasty include large areas of talar dome osteonecrosis, absence of muscular function in the lower leg and foot, a Charcot or neuropathic joint, severe coronal plane deformity or malalignment, deficient soft tissues, vascular insufficiency, severe loss of bone stock, and current infection. MRI is optimal for determining the vascularity of the talus. Because most modern prosthetic designs rely on bony ingrowth for stability, an avascular talus is likely to result in failed arthroplasty.

Relative contraindications for total ankle arthroplasty include osteoporosis, which may lead to inadequate component fixation (although cement may be used); significant ligament instability; prior ankle infection; morbid obesity; diabetes, peripheral neuropathy, or poor skin quality. Arthroplasty also is contraindicated in young patients, extremely active patients, or those who perform heavy labor. In these patients, ankle arthrodesis is a better alternative. Relative contraindications also exist for patients with the inability to follow postoperative protocols or those with unrealistic goals or expectations. The use of total ankle arthroplasty in patients who smoke is controversial; cessation of smoking for at least 1 month before surgery may optimize results.

Surgical Considerations

Despite improvements in the newer generation of implants and good intermediate-term results, total ankle arthroplasty remains technically demanding. Complication rates have been high and a steep learning curve exists for surgeons. Studies have shown that with more surgical experience, intraoperative complications decrease and optimal alignment and reliability improve.[91,92]

In one study, 10 intraoperative complications occurred in the first 25 procedures performed, whereas only 2 occurred in the next 25 surgeries.[93] The most common complications of total ankle arthroplasty include delayed wound healing, medial and lateral malleolar fractures, polyethylene bearing wear and osteolysis, component subsidence, instability, bony impingement, and infection. To prevent these complications, surgeons must be familiar with the surgical approach, plan for anatomic variations, and be comfortable with the chosen prosthesis. Authors of a recent study of 306 consecutive Agility total ankle replacements reported that 28% of patients required at least one additional procedure following arthroplasty and also found a below-knee amputation rate of 2.6%.[85] Débridement of heterotopic bone (especially in the gutters), correction of axial malalignment, and component replacement were the most common procedures performed at reoperation. In another study of the STAR prosthesis, periarticular hypertrophic bone formation occurred in 63% of patients at 3.7-year follow-up.[72]

Preoperative CT scans and radiographs may be used to assess the ankle and adjacent joints. Tibial bowing, tibial or fibular malunion, and severe flatfoot deformities make surgery technically more difficult; therefore, these malalignments should be corrected prior to ankle arthroplasty. The talus should be inspected for subchondral cysts that may need treatment with a bone graft prior to arthroplasty. Significant arthritis of the subtalar joint may require this joint to be fused before implanting the ankle prosthesis.

Technique

An anterior incision is typically used for most total ankle arthroplasties. The patient is supine with a bump made of sterile, folded towels placed under the ipsilateral hip. A thigh tourniquet is applied. The incision is made in line with the extensor hallucis longus tendon, starting 15 to 20 cm proximal to the ankle joint. This incision is directly over the interval between the tibial anterior and extensor hallucis longus, with avoidance of the superficial peroneal nerve, which must be retracted and protected. Postoperatively, an injured nerve may produce a painful and debilitating neuroma. If the nerve is accidentally transected, it should be buried away from its superficial location. The soft-tissue envelope surrounding the ankle joint is relatively thin, offering little protection to the implant if a wound occurs. Wound dehiscence has been reported in up to 12% of patients.[86] It is important to be cognizant of excessive retraction during the surgical procedure; the anterior incision should be of adequate length to allow optimal exposure without the need for excessive retraction. Because the deep peroneal nerve and the dorsalis pedis artery cross the midline of the ankle in the deeper part of the anterior incision, they should be retracted and well protected. After the joint is exposed, osteophytes are removed and implantation is performed following the manufacturer's guidelines. Excellent hemostasis should be followed by careful multilayered closure starting at the periosteal-capsular layer.

It also is important to pay attention to the posteromedial soft tissues to avoid injury. The posterior tibial tendon, flexor hallucis longus tendon, and the neurovascular bundle run directly behind the posterior medial aspect of the tibia and can be inadvertently transected during bone resection. These neurovascular structures should be repaired intraoperatively if damage occurs. Making cuts too far medially can fracture the medial malleolus, which also should be repaired intraoperatively.

Pitfalls

Technical pitfalls include malpositioning or incorrectly aligning the implant. Component malposition can include excessive varus or valgus, too much extension or flexion, or placing the components too far anteriorly or posteriorly. Malalignment of the semiconstrained or constrained components can lead to loss of joint conformity and theoretically can increase polyethylene wear. Polyethylene wear and osteolysis are not major complications with current ankle prostheses, although these complications may occur with time. Standards for minimum polyethylene thickness in ankle prostheses have not been determined, but it is accepted that the thickness should be at least 8 mm. Thicker polyethylene may help prevent implant failure, but larger bone cuts may be needed.

Intraoperative Monitoring

Fluoroscopic intraoperative checking of alignment in all planes can prevent malalignment. If the tibial component is placed too far medially, it may lead to a malleolar fracture. If it is positioned too far laterally, the talus is shifted laterally, placing excessive tension on the deltoid ligament, which can lead to varus angulation of the talus. The ankle should not be underdistracted or overdistracted by using components that are too thick or too thin; the prosthesis should be seated on the anterior and posterior cortex of the tibia and talus.[94] Because most current ankle prostheses rely on ligamentous stability, failure to recognize and correct ankle instability will lead to failures and poor outcomes.

Ankle implant range of motion should be considered intraoperatively. A normal ankle moves from approximately 20° of dorsiflexion to 50° of plantar flexion. A range of 24° to 30° of combined motion (dorsiflexion and plantar flexion) is needed for normal walking, 37° is needed for ascending stairs, and 55° is needed for descending stairs.[95] If dorsiflexion is limited, a smaller implant or polyethylene bearing may be needed. A plantar flexion contracture has been shown to increase the peak forces across adjacent joints, which may lead to increased loading and future arthritis; thus, it is recommended that an Achilles tendon lengthening be done intraoperatively if 15° of dorsiflexion cannot be achieved at the time of the surgery.[91] Despite intraoperative findings, preoperative range of motion is a critical factor for determining postoperative ankle range of motion. Patients with good preoperative range of motion maintain or may lose some motion after ankle arthroplasty. Ankle arthroplasty does not typically increase ankle range of motion; however, decreased pain allows the patient to use existing range of motion more effectively.[96]

Other Concerns

Another surgical concern is insufficient débridement of the medial and lateral ankle gutters, which can lead to limited ankle motion and impingement pain. Adequately resecting preexisting osteophytes and removing all bone fragments should be done to prevent painful impingement. If impingement occurs postoperatively, arthroscopic or open resection can be performed.

Intraoperative malleolar fractures may occur from excessive bone resection, from overdistraction with the external fixator in Agility ankle replacement surgery, or during implantation of the final components. One study showed a 20% incidence in malleolar fractures with both the Agility ankle and STAR prostheses.[97] Malleolar fractures can and should be fixed at the time of surgery. Failure to stabilize these fractures will lead to prosthesis instability and poor outcomes. Guide pins from a 3.5- or 4.0-mm cannulated screw set within the medial malleolus can be percutaneously placed just medial to the proposed saw cut to prevent overcutting of the malleolus and possibly avoid fracture. If fracture occurs, a 3.5- or 4.0-mm cannulated screw can be easily placed over the guide pin. A one-third tubular plate also can be provisionally secured to the fibula prior to the malleolar saw cuts to protect against a lateral malleolar fracture. If the fibula is inadvertently cut, the fracture can be stabilized with the plate. In the Agility ankle prosthesis, application of a fibular plate can aid in syndesmotic fusion stabilization.

Deltoid ligament insufficiency is a challenging complication in total ankle arthroplasty. The current second- and third-generation prostheses do not have significant varus-valgus constraint such as is found in some total knee prostheses. The ankle prostheses rely on intact ankle ligaments for stability; therefore, deltoid insufficiency in a total ankle arthroplasty will most likely lead to failure.

The critical importance of bony support was recognized early in total ankle arthroplasty. The bony anatomy of the distal tibia and talus is such that moving farther from the subchondral plate results in a significant decrease in strength and resistance to compression. Resecting more than 4 to 5 mm of bone from either side of the joint may result in tibial or talar component subsidence after surgery.[98] The overall subsidence rates in the Agility ankle at an average follow-up of 4.8 years is 13% for the tibial component and 8% for the talar component.[84] If subsidence occurs on postoperative radiographs and is progressive, it should be treated before complete failure of the implant occurs. Revision surgery can be performed using larger components and supplemental bone graft. Removing too little bone, however, can result in excessive tightness caused by overstuffing the joint with the implants, which will result in decreased postoperative range of motion and ankle pain.

When significant deformity exists, especially coronal plane deformity of greater than 10° to 15°, good outcomes are less predictable. A high rate of prosthesis failure occurs with recurrence of the preoperative deformity.[69,78,99] Patients with significant deformities (> 10° in the coronal plane) and a painful arthritic ankle can undergo ankle arthroplasty if alignment is restored. Options include opening- or closing-wedge osteotomies in the tibia or foot, alone or in combination.[100] If the deformity is severe and arthritis is extensive, pain relief is more reliable with ankle fusion; the deformity can be corrected through the ankle at the time of the arthrodesis.[101]

Immediate Postoperative Complications

After ankle arthroplasty, concern for soft tissues and wound healing is paramount. Casting for 3 to 4 weeks postoperatively ensures wound healing. During the first few postoperative days, the leg should be elevated above the heart to reduce swelling. After the incisions heal, a removable fracture boot that allows motion with partial weight bearing can be used. Full weight bearing can begin at 6 weeks or when signs of bony consolidation are seen. Superficial wound dehiscence can be treated with dressing changes, local wound care, and prophylactic oral antibiotics, whereas deeper dehiscence should be more aggressively treated with either a vacuum-assisted closure device (VAC, Kinetic Concepts, San Antonio, TX) or plastic surgery to provide coverage with a myocutaneous flap.

Management of Failed Ankle Arthroplasty

The first generation of ankle replacements had a high rate of early failures, with reoperation rates as high as 41%.[72] Failure rates have significantly declined with newer prosthetic designs. Factors associated with early failure include wound complications, deep infections, loosening, and malposition of the components.[102] Surgical goals after failed ankle arthroplasty are restoration of alignment, length, stability, and function of the limb. Treatment options for a failed ankle arthroplasty include a revision implant, salvage fusion, or amputation. The choice of procedure depends on the cause of the failure, the surgeon's expertise and experience, and the patient's wishes.

Revision arthroplasty is contraindicated when infection is present. However, two-stage salvage surgery for the failed implant can be attempted. The first stage involves removal of the components and insertion of a methylmethacrylate antibiotic cement spacer. Aggressive débridement is the most important aspect for eliminating the infection because the bone must be free from infection before planning for definitive treatment. Once the infection is cleared, the second stage involves either fusion or amputation.[103]

In the setting of aseptic loosening and no infection, revision of a failed ankle arthroplasty occasionally can be achieved with the use of larger components in a one-stage revision; however, an ankle fusion or extended hindfoot fusion is often necessary. If there is adequate remaining talus for satisfactory screw fixation, tibiotalar arthrodesis is possible. If there is extensive bone destruction, loss, or arthritic involvement of the subtalar joint, tibiotalocalcaneal arthrodesis is recommended.[104] This surgery usually requires the use of a bulk allograft interposition.[103,105,106] Multiple factors must be taken into account, including loss of bone stock in the tibia and talus, and fractures of the malleoli and the soft-tissue envelope. Osteonecrosis of the talus may lead to nonunion and failure of the salvage procedure; amputation often may be the only treatment option.[107]

Subsidence of the ankle implant has been a complication since total ankle arthroplasty was first performed. In early first-generation prosthetic designs, cement fixation and subsequent excessive bony resections commonly led to subsidence. Insufficient bone ingrowth, insufficient bone stock, abnormal loading of the ankle replacement, overstuffing of the joint, and overstressing the joint with high-demand activities or too much weight are common causes of subsidence.[108] Not all subsidence of ankle prostheses requires conversion to fusion. If the original prosthesis was incorrectly inserted, an early revision is often the best option. If the subsidence resulted in substantial bone loss, a custom or revision implant larger than the original implant can be used. Alternatively, bone graft can be used to fill the defect. When allograft is used, the component can be secured to the implant with cement.[108]

Particulate polyethylene debris may cause significant osteolysis. Particles in sufficient numbers incite a chronic inflammatory process, which can lead to osteolysis, aseptic loosening, and eventual loss of implant support. Wear of polyethylene in total ankle arthroplasty has not yet become a major concern, most likely because long-term follow-up studies are not yet available. Early generation implants probably did not survive long enough for polyethylene failure to manifest.[61] In a study of intermediate-term results with the Agility ankle, 15% of the ankles had expansile lysis at an average follow-up of 7.2 years. Over time, four of these ankles showed definite signs of osteolysis progression on serial radiographic examinations.[83]

Progressive and ballooning osteolysis should be treated when recognized because these lesions tend to enlarge, destroy bone, and undermine stable fixation. Treatment includes exchanging the polyethylene component and complete curettage and bone grafting of the lesions. If excessive wear of the polyethylene component is caused by a malaligned implant or a malaligned ankle, mechanical balance must be corrected; revision arthroplasty then can be performed. If severe deformity exists, ankle fusion may be the best option.

Fracture of the polyethylene component has been reported to occur most often in physically active patients.[109] The patient usually reports a sudden catastrophic event that is followed by pain and swelling in the involved ankle. In such instances, the insert should be replaced; this treatment usually results in good outcomes.

In two large studies of arthrodesis for failed ankle arthroplasty, a compression external fixator was used successfully in 81% to 89% of the patients. Good or excellent results were reported in 80% of patients.[107,110] To maintain limb length, intercalated iliac crest bone graft or femoral head allograft can be used, along with retrograde intramedullary tibiotalocalcaneal fusion nails.[105,111-114] Screw fixation alone is insufficient, whereas an intramedullary nail gives firm fixation both distally and proximally and is the method of choice when tibiotalocalcaneal arthrodesis is indicated.[104,107]

Arthrodesis Versus Total Ankle Arthroplasty

For more than 100 years, ankle arthrodesis has been the traditional treatment for severe ankle arthritis. Improved surgical techniques, better fixation methods, and an understanding of appropriate fusion positions have led to its continued use. Although many positive results for ankle arthrodesis are described in the literature, many patients report loss of motion at the ankle joint and prolonged postoperative immobilization. The loss of motion is significant. One study reported a 74% loss of sagittal motion and 70% loss of inversion and eversion in 77% of patients after ankle arthrodesis.[37] Abnormal gait patterns, difficulty in ambulation on inclined surfaces, pain with rigorous activities, and difficulty in running also have been reported after ankle arthrodesis.[101,115] Patients treated with ankle arthrodesis require a long period of immobilization in a cast, are at risk of pseudarthrosis, and have loss of the compensatory mechanisms in the foot that facilitate gait. Recent studies, including gait analyses, have confirmed substantial differences in hindfoot function and gait in patients treated with ankle arthrodesis compared with individuals with healthy ankles. Significant differences between the two groups have been found in cadence and stride length; patients treated with arthrodesis also have shown significantly decreased sagittal, coronal, and transverse range of motion during the stance and swing phases of gait.[116] In one study, patients who had been treated with ankle arthrodesis demonstrated a 16% decrease in gait velocity, a 3% increase in oxygen consumption, and an overall decrease of 10% in gait efficiency when walking barefoot.[117] These alterations in gait and potential complications (particularly nonunion, and in the longer term, degeneration of adjacent joints) have caused some orthopaedic surgeons to question the concept that ankle fusion is the gold standard of treatment for ankle arthritis.[118-120]

Gait analysis studies have shown improved function following total ankle arthroplasty. Postoperatively, patients treated with ankle arthroplasty had a significantly improved external ankle dorsiflexion moment compared with their preoperative status. This finding indicates improved function of the ankle joint.[121] Gait analysis was performed before and after ankle arthroplasty in 12 patients and compared with 12 patients treated with ankle fusion and with a healthy control group of 12 patients.[122] The ankle replacement group had greater movement at the ankle, symmetrical timing of gait, and a restored ground reaction force pattern. In another study, nearly normal gait patterns in terms of knee, ankle, and tarsal joint kinematics were achieved after successful total ankle arthroplasty, despite reduced dorsiflexion in the ankle joint.[123]

If a young patient is treated with ankle arthrodesis, a significant likelihood exists that hindfoot arthritis will develop in the subsequent 10 to 20 years, which may necessitate additional surgeries. An isolated ankle fusion may progress into a pantalar fusion with associated impaired gait and morbidity. Ankle arthroplasty may provide a better option than arthrodesis in many patients because it preserves motion and decreases stresses on the midfoot and subtalar joints.

A recent meta-analysis and systematic review of total ankle arthroplasty and ankle arthrodesis evaluated intermediate- and long-term outcomes.[124] The mean AOFAS hindfoot score for total ankle arthroplasty was 78.2 and for ankle arthrodesis 75.6. Overall, 52% of patients treated with total ankle arthroplasty had excellent results, 30% had good results, 4% had fair results, and 13% had poor results. Of those treated with ankle arthrodesis, 31% had excellent results, 37% had good results, 13% had fair results, and 13% had poor results. The 5- and 10-year implant survival rates were 78% and 77%, respectively. The revision rate for total ankle arthroplasty was 7.4%, with most revisions performed because of loosening or subluxation. The revision rate following ankle arthrodesis was 8.6%, with most revisions performed because of nonunion. Below-knee amputation was necessary in 1% of the patients who had been treated with a total ankle arthroplasty compared with 5% of the patients treated with ankle arthrodesis. Based on these findings, the authors concluded that despite sparse data, the intermediate outcome of total ankle arthroplasty is similar to that of ankle arthrodesis. The authors of a similar meta-analysis concluded that a properly designed randomized trial is needed to compare total ankle arthroplasty to ankle fusion.[125]

In patients with severe varus or valgus deformities, ankle arthrodesis may be a better option. A recent study of ankle arthrodeses in patients with a preoperative coronal plane deformity of at least 20° showed a short-term high level of patient satisfaction and a low rate of nonunion (4%).[101] Interestingly, the patients in this study did not show improved stair-climbing ability but did show a reduced need for walking aids. Osteotomies were used to correct the deformities and rigid internal fixation was used.

Conclusion

Designs for total ankle prostheses are continually evolving. Good results have been reported in older, low-demand, nonobese patients who have endstage osteoarthritis or rheumatoid arthritis. Successful design of total ankle prostheses has proven far more challenging than those used in total hip or total knee arthroplasty because of limitations of bone strength and osseous structure (tibia, talus), and the fragile soft-tissue envelope surrounding the ankle joint. Healing complications also are much more common at the ankle. Forces are large at the ankle but the surface area for support is small, making fixation difficult. The polyethylene component needs to be sufficiently thick to maintain its integrity; however, thicker implants require larger bone resection, which weakens bone support. Most current prosthetic designs involve the use of a three-component fixed- or mobile-bearing polyethylene implant. Outcomes of long-term studies from multicenter, prospective, and randomized clinical trials are needed before definitively concluding that current ankle implants are superior to ankle fusions for all patients with painful ankle arthritis. Currently, most orthopaedic surgeons believe that total ankle arthroplasty should continue to be included in the armamentarium of treatment for selected patients. Considering the current status of ankle fusions and the resulting progressive hindfoot arthritis, cementless ankle prostheses, whether mobile- or fixed-bearing, offer a reasonable treatment alternative in properly selected patients.[13,126]

Joint Distraction Arthroplasty

The use of external fixation for joint distraction arthroplasty has evolved as a viable alternative to arthrodesis and joint arthroplasty for a select group of patients with symptomatic osteoarthritis of the tibiotalar joint and may have a role complementary to the newer joint-preserving modalities. The external fixation technique was first reported for knee and elbow joints in 1975.[127] Encouraging results achieved by using such techniques in young adults with early arthritis of the hip and ankle joints were reported in the 1990s.[128,129]

Rationale

Several mechanisms that affect the clinical success of joint distraction arthroplasty have been proposed. These mechanisms include temporary relief of mechanical stress on the articular cartilage, intermittent changes in intra-articular fluid pressure nourishing the articular cartilage, and transient periarticular osteopenia that diminishes subchondral sclerosis with the consequent decrease in forces on the articular cartilage that allows the chondrocytes of the osteoarthritic cartilage to restore the mechanical integrity of the intercellular matrix. Other possible mechanisms include decreased synovial inflammation, decreased joint reactive forces, stretching of the joint capsule, an effect on capsular nerve endings, and the possibility of a placebo effect from the external fixator.

Irrespective of the affected site, the progression of osteoarthritis is manifested by decreased production and loss of proteoglycans and destruction of the collagen network from the matrix of the hyaline cartilage, with resultant impairment of its mechanical properties. The basis for using joint distraction to treat ankle arthritis is controversial. Some authors have proposed that controlled distraction across the affected joint provides a low-pressure environment that allows the osteoarthritic cartilage to repair itself.[129] The release of mechanical stress on the articular cartilage while maintaining intra-articular intermittent fluid pressure allows reparative activity. Investigators measured intra-articular pressure by using a pressure-sensitive catheter placed into the ankle joint in three patients undergoing joint distraction treatment for arthritis.[130] An increase in the mean intra-articular pressure of 10 kPa during loading and a return to a preloading value of 3 kPa during the unloading response of the gait cycle was noted. In vitro, intermittent hydrostatic compressive force of low physiologic magnitude (0 to 13 kPa at a frequency of 0.33 Hz) stimulated synthesis of proteoglycans of human osteoarthritic cartilage.[131] Production of catabolic cytokines, such as interleukin 1 and tumor necrosis factor-α, decreased when the osteoarthritic chondrocytes were co-cultured with mononuclear cells isolated from the synovial fluid of autopsy specimens with osteoarthritis.[132] Such a response to low levels of pressure was not observed in the chondrocytes harvested from joints without osteoarthritis, suggesting that the chondrocytes in osteoarthritis may have distinct phenotypic characteristics.

Animal Studies

The physiologic environment of a synovial joint is dependent on joint mobility and loading force. It is well established that continuous passive motion has a beneficial biologic effect on the healing of full-thickness articular cartilage defects that penetrate the subchondral bone of knee joints of young rabbits.[133] Several authors have attempted to study the effect of controlled joint distraction on the articular cartilage by using various experimental animal models. When articulated distraction was applied to nonarthritic rabbit knee joints, morphologic changes in the shape and density of the chondrocytes of the superficial and intermediate zones were noted by 3 weeks, with subsequent reduction in the thickness of the articular cartilage along with surface erosions and tidemark irregularity by 9 weeks.[134] The results support the hypothesis that the forces perceived by chondrocytes in weight-bearing joints can dictate their shape, with resultant alterations in cellular biochemistry and matrix metabolism. The authors suggested that further investigation was needed regarding the use of articulated distraction to treat arthritis.

In another study using a canine model with osteoarthritis of the knee induced by transection of the anterior cruciate ligament, researchers evaluated the effect of articulating and nonarticulating circular external fixators on the affected knee joint.[135] Although the improvement in synovial inflammation and proteoglycan synthesis was more noticeable in the group undergoing articulated joint distraction, neither group of animals showed significant improvement in the overall proteoglycan content or in histologic changes in the osteoarthritic knee joints. The authors suggested that

their follow-up was too short and that further improvement in the histologic and biochemical markers of the osteoarthritic cartilage might have been found if the study design allowed a longer follow-up period.

In another study, osteoarthritis of the knee was experimentally induced in adult rabbits using intra-articular papain injections.[136] The authors used a monolateral external fixator to accomplish intra-articular distraction. Based on histologic analysis, no beneficial effect of joint distraction on the osteoarthritic cartilage was shown. The group of rabbits with nonarticulated distraction had more advanced degenerative changes than did the animals undergoing articulated distraction of the knee joint.

In another study, investigators found that a combination of subchondral drilling, joint motion, and distraction by an articulated external fixator promoted repair of a fresh osteochondral defect in an animal model.[137] A full-thickness osteochondral defect was created bilaterally in the weight-bearing area of the medial femoral condyles of adult rabbits. After the defect was drilled, the experimental knee joint was distracted 1.5 mm with the use of an external fixator that allowed knee motion. The contralateral knee joint served as a control with no apparatus. Partial repair with cartilage-like tissue was observed in the joints of the experimental group, whereas destructive changes were observed in the control joints. Although no significant difference was noted in the histologic grading of the articular cartilage between experimental and control knees at 4 weeks, the knees treated with articulated distraction showed significantly better morphology at 8 and 12 weeks than did those in the control group. Results showed that articulated joint distraction may promote repair of osteochondral defects in the weight-bearing joints with cartilage-like tissue. Longer follow-up duration with assessment of the mechanical strength and biomechanical characteristics of the articular cartilage in the distracted joint was not available.

The effects of joint distraction and autologous culture-expanded bone marrow-derived mesenchymal cell transplantation (ACBMT) on the repair characteristics of large, full-thickness, articular cartilage defects in rabbits have been studied.[138] After application of a hinged external fixator, the entire articular cartilage of the tibial plateau along with menisci, cruciate, and collateral ligaments were resected. The animals were divided into four groups. Some of the animals were treated with joint distraction alone, and others were allowed to bear weight without joint distraction. A third group of animals underwent joint distraction along with intra-articular injection of ACBMT and atelocollagen carrier gel; the fourth group received injection of the carrier gel without mesenchymal cells. The regenerated soft tissue was significantly greater in the animals undergoing joint distraction than in those allowed weight bearing without distraction. Compared with "vehicle only" treated animals, the ACBMT group showed superior morphology of the matrix, cell distri-

3: Arthritis

bution, and area of regenerated cartilage. The findings suggest that the repair of large defects of cartilage can be enhanced by joint distraction and intra-articular injection of ACBMT.

Surgical Technique

The technique of joint distraction is based on restoring the joint space with the use of ligamentotaxis across an arthritic joint; by decreasing the intra-articular compressive loads, the damaged hyaline cartilage is allowed to recover. A circular fixator is preferred for ankle joint distraction. Two variations of the frame construct have been described. The traditional construct is an all-wire frame without hinges across the ankle joint that depends on the flexibility of the tensioned wires to allow physiologic changes in intra-articular pressure.[130] More recently, an all-wire or hybrid construct that uses a combination of half pins and wires with articulated hinges across the ankle joint has been used to control distraction while allowing joint mobility.[139,140] Proponents of both types of constructs encourage weight bearing in the frame.

The traditional nonarticulated distraction technique uses a two-ring preassembled external fixator that is mounted on the tibia with all wires tensioned to 1.3 kN.[130] Two olive wires are inserted medially and laterally through the calcaneus at a 30° to 45° angle to each other and are tensioned at 0.9 kN to a half ring around the heel. One wire is inserted through the talar neck and attached to the foot ring to prevent inadvertent distraction across the subtalar joint. Another laterally directed olive wire is inserted through the bases of the first and fourth or fifth metatarsal and tensioned to 0.5 kN over a dorsal half ring over the forefoot that is attached to the hindfoot ring. Proper technique in placement and tensioning of the wires to avoid injury to the adjacent neurovascular structures and preserve the integrity of the subtalar and midfoot joints is essential for a good clinical outcome. The hindfoot construct is connected to the tibial ring via four threaded rods, fixing the ankle in neutral dorsiflexion to allow weight bearing on a plantigrade foot. It is important that the foot ring be positioned cephalad to the plantar surface of the foot to allow weight bearing. Mechanical unloading across the degenerative articular surfaces is achieved by gradually distracting the threaded rods spanning the ankle joint at a rate of 0.5 mm twice per day until a total distraction of 5 mm is confirmed on radiographs of the weight-bearing ankle. During the 3-month treatment period, the radiographic tibiotalar joint distraction of 5 mm is maintained by performing minor adjustments, if needed. Weight bearing as tolerated is allowed within 1 week of surgery; a rocker-bottom soled shoe is used to compensate for the absence of ankle motion during ambulation. The ring fixator is removed after 3 months and weight bearing as tolerated is continued.

The articulated distraction technique (**Figure 4**) involves application of a two-ring fixation block to the tibia with all wires or a combination of wires and half pins.[139,140] A temporary wire simulating the center of rotation of the ankle joint from the tip of the medial malleolus to the tip of the lateral malleolus is then inserted and medial and lateral threaded rods are suspended from the distal tibial ring to the level of the ankle axis wire. Articulated universal hinges are connected to the rods at the level of the axis wire, with the medial hinge located slightly proximal and anterior to the lateral hinge. With the use of short, threaded rods or bolts, the distal ends of the universal hinges are connected to a foot ring that is mounted parallel to the sole of the foot. The foot ring is fixed with two crossed wires in the calcaneus, one talar neck wire, and two wires across the metatarsals. A posterior distraction rod is added and can be removed for range-of-motion exercises. The remaining postoperative regimen and duration of fixator application is similar to that used in traditional fixation protocols.

In a cadaveric study of six ankle specimens, the authors determined the instant axis of rotation of the talocrural joint from three-dimensional kinematic data acquired with an electromagnetic motion-tracking system.[141] By deliberately introducing varying amounts of relative malalignment between the optimal talocrural joint axis and the actual fixator hinge axis, it was possible to measure the corresponding amounts of additional resistance to joint motion. Malpositioning the hinge by 10 mm caused an increase in motion resistance of more than five times that amount. Additional energy evoked by off-axis hinge alignment is transmitted through the ankle joint with either compressive forces to the articular surfaces and/or tensile forces to the constraining ligaments across the tibiotalar joint.

Adjunctive Procedures

Some investigators have advocated an "a la carte" approach, including removal of impinging osteophytes, release of joint contractures, and correction of osseous malalignment before application of a hinged external fixator across the ankle joint[139,142,143] (**Figure 5**). If dorsiflexion is limited by anterior distal tibial or talar neck osteophytes, the osteophytes are resected (**Figures 6** and **7**). If equinus contracture is present, Achilles tendon lengthening or gastrocnemius recession can be performed. If such soft-tissue procedures do not provide sufficient ankle dorsiflexion, a more formal posterior capsular release can be performed (**Figure 8**). Occasionally, tarsal tunnel release is needed to safely bring the ankle into a plantigrade position. Before embarking on joint distraction for posttraumatic ankle arthritis, it is necessary to assess the orientation of the distal tibia based on radiographs centered at the ankle. Frontal and sagittal plane malalignments, especially valgus and recurvatum deformities, often are seen and should be treated with an appropriate supramalleolar osteotomy to realign the tibial plafond. Assessment of compensatory deformities in the hindfoot and possible correction should be performed before ankle joint distraction.

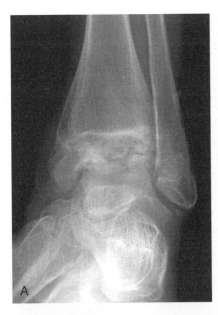
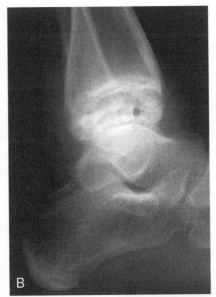
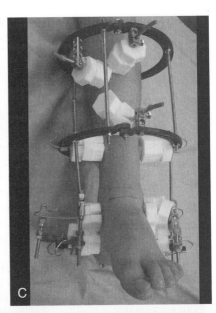

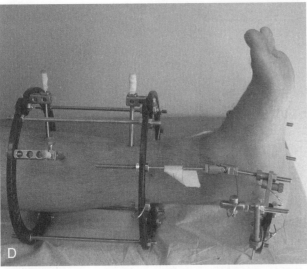
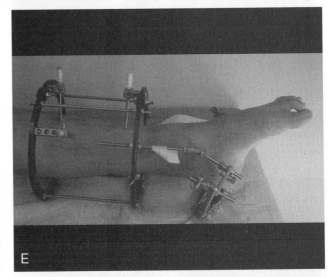

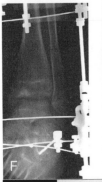
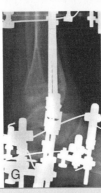
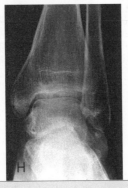
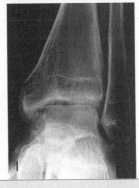
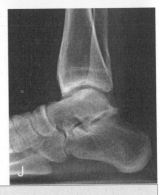

Figure 4 An adolescent patient sustained posttraumatic chondrolysis of the tibiotalar joint. The patient was treated with ankle joint distraction. Standing AP **(A)** and lateral **(B)** radiographic views of the ankle. Clinical photographs of a hinged external fixator **(C)** showing the ability of the patient to actively dorsiflex **(D)** and plantar flex **(E)** the ankle. AP **(F)** and lateral **(G)** radiographic views of the left ankle showing distraction across the tibiotalar joint with the use of a hinged external fixator. Weight-bearing AP **(H)**, mortise **(I)**, and lateral **(J)** radiographic views of the affected ankle 5.5 years after articulated joint distraction. Reconstitution of the joint space and mild subchondral sclerosis of the distal tibia are noted. The patient was asymptomatic and regained full mobility of the ankle joint. *(Reproduced with permission from Sabharwal S, Schwechter EM: Five-year follow-up of ankle joint distraction for post-traumatic chondrolysis in an adolescent: A case report. Foot Ankle Int 2007;28:942-948.)*

3: Arthritis

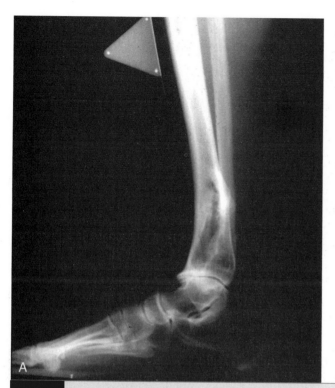
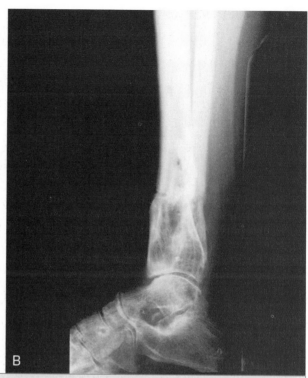

Figure 5 Radiograph showing ankle arthritis with posttraumatic recurvatum deformity **(A)**. Improved anterior coverage and joint space was noted after flexion osteotomy of the distal tibia and débridement of anterior osteophytes **(B)**. Six years after treatment, the patient had no recurrence of pain or further loss of motion. *(Reproduced with permission from Paley D: Ankle and foot considerations, in Paley D:* Principles of Deformity Correction, *ed 1. Berlin, Germany, Springer-Verlag, 2002, p 585.)*

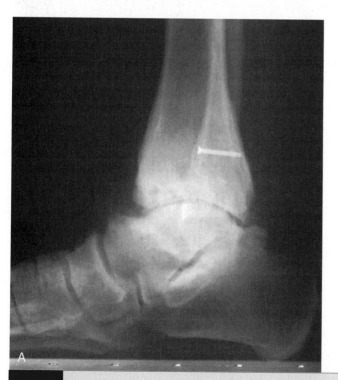
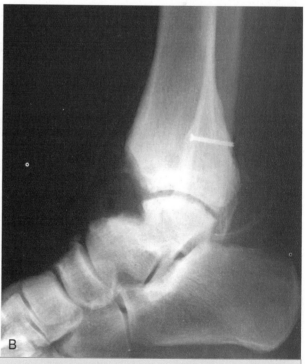

Figure 6 **A,** Anterior and posterior osteophytes limit dorsiflexion and plantar flexion, respectively. **B,** The patient was treated with resection of blocking anterior and posterior distal tibial osteophytes and deepening of the talar neck combined with ankle joint distraction. *(Reproduced with permission from Paley D, Lamm BM: Ankle joint distraction.* Foot Ankle Clin *2005;10:685-698.)*

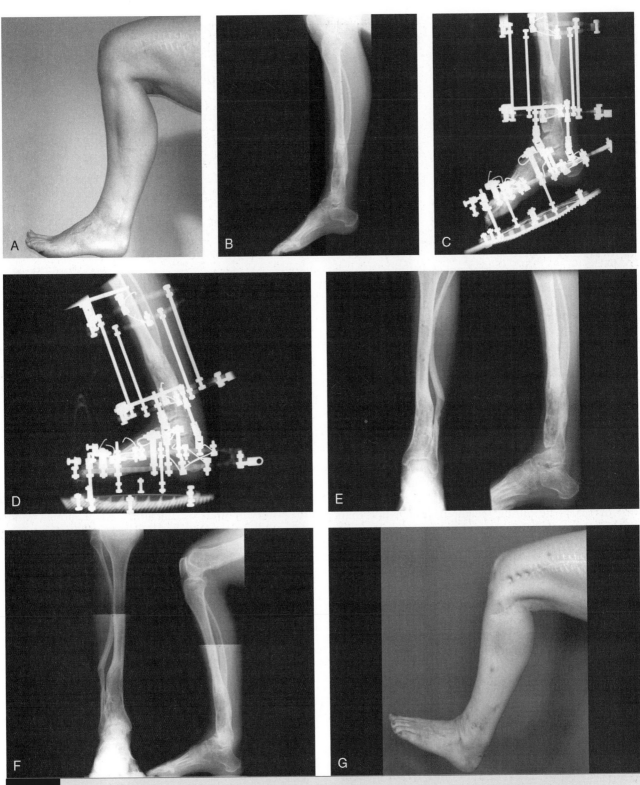

Figure 7   Ankle joint realignment with ankle joint distraction. **A,** Clinical photograph shows tibial recurvatum and maximum ankle dorsiflexion. **B,** Lateral view radiograph shows previous lengthening and recurvatum correction of the distal tibia. Note the anterior ankle osteophytes and ankle joint arthritis. **C,** Lateral radiography shows resection of the anterior ankle osteophyte and hinged ankle distraction of the ankle joint. Note maximum plantar flexion with the hinged ankle distraction. **D,** Lateral radiographic view shows maximum dorsiflexion with the hinged ankle distraction. **E,** AP (left) and lateral (right) radiographs taken immediately after removal of the external fixator show good ankle joint space achieved with distraction. **F,** AP (left) and lateral (right) radiographic views taken at 3-year follow-up show slight narrowing of the ankle joint space. **G,** Clinically, an increase in ankle dorsiflexion was noted with a decrease in pain and resolution of limb-length difference and malalignment. *(Reproduced with permission from Paley D, Lamm BM: Ankle joint distraction.* Foot Ankle Clin *2005;10:685-698.)*

3: Arthritis

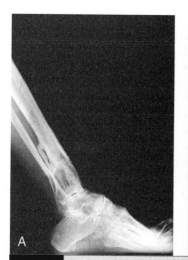
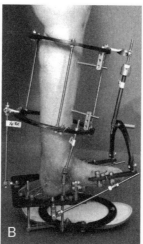
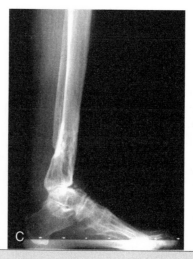
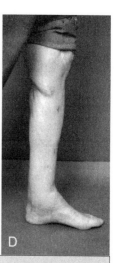

Figure 8 **A,** Preoperative radiograph of the ankle in maximum dorsiflexion showing equinus deformity and narrowing of the ankle joint space. Equinus contracture was corrected with Achilles tendon lengthening, posterior ankle joint capsular release, and gradual soft-tissue distraction. **B,** Hinged ankle joint distraction was performed simultaneously with correction of equinus deformity. Lateral radiographic view **(C)** and clinical photograph **(D)** taken at the 3-year follow-up visit shows a plantigrade foot position. *(Reproduced with permission from Paley D, Lamm BM: Ankle joint distraction.* Foot Ankle Clin *2005;10:685-698.)*

Clinical Studies

Based on the concept that osteoarthritic cartilage undergoes some reparative activity when the damaged cartilage is mechanically unloaded, investigators have reported improved clinical outcome after 3 months of joint distraction of the osteoarthritic ankle with an Ilizarov external fixator. The indications and techniques of ankle joint distraction continue to evolve. The goal of ankle distraction is to unload the damaged articular cartilage during weight bearing while maintaining intermittent pressures of the synovial fluid, thus stimulating the synthesis of proteoglycans and improving the longevity of the osteoarthritic joint. Ankle joint distraction is contraindicated in the presence of active joint infection and substantial loss of bone stock around the ankle. Although the underlying mechanism of pain relief and improved function after ankle joint distraction remains debatable, clinical reports with up to 10 years of follow-up have shown the efficacy of this technique as a joint-preserving procedure in young adults with congruous, painful ankle arthritis. Most clinical reports have come from the same group of investigators who use the traditional nonarticulated Ilizarov frame for ankle joint distraction.[129,130,143-145]

In a multicenter prospective study, 17 young adults with severe traumatic ankle osteoarthritis were evaluated at 1 and 2 years after treatment with nonhinged ankle joint distraction using the Ilizarov all-wire frame.[143] Arthroscopic débridement of osteophytes and intra-articular fibrosis, without surgery on the articular cartilage, was performed in 13 of the 17 patients. Preoperative and follow-up data were graded based on physical and functional impairment, pain, ankle joint mobility, and radiographic appearance of the tibiotalar joint on biplanar standing radiographs. Pin tract infec-

tions were treated with orally administered antibiotics. Broken foot wires were removed in four patients; no other complications were noted. Thirteen of 17 patients (76%) noted significant improvement in functional impairment and pain 1 year after ankle distraction, with a trend for further improvement at the 2-year follow-up visit. The progressive improvement in clinical results over time supports the belief of the study's authors that joint distraction treatment can favorably alter the natural history of ankle osteoarthritis. Ankle mobility and radiographic joint space width was minimally improved but did not reach a statistically significant level. In the remaining four patients, treatment was considered a failure. These patients underwent ankle arthrodesis because of persistent discomfort within 1 year of ankle distraction arthroplasty. Ilizarov joint distraction was noted to be a promising treatment modality for young adults with severe ankle osteoarthritis and was found to be an effective procedure for delaying arthrodesis in most patients.

In a subsequent study by the same group of investigators, 57 patients with severe osteoarthritis at three institutions were enrolled in an open prospective study.[144] Exclusion criteria included intra-articular infection, bilateral ankle osteoarthritis, and psychologic disorders. All patients were adults with a mean age of 44 years (range, 18 to 65 years). Approximately two thirds of the patients were treated with arthroscopic débridement of osteophytes and intra-articular fibrosis. Clinical evaluation showed substantial improvement in pain and functional activity with further improvement over time. Radiographs, which were available for fewer than one half of the patients, were evaluated by blinded observers using digitized radiographic measurements of mean joint space width and subchondral sclerosis. At 1 year postoperatively, joint space width increased 17% with an additional 10% improvement by 3 years after surgery. Similarly, subchondral sclerosis decreased 10% at the 1-year follow-up visit, with an additional 7% improvement by 3 years after surgery. A statistically significant correlation was shown between clinical improvement and radiographic parameters. The persistent decrease in subchondral sclerosis after joint distraction may indicate decreased stiffness of the subchondral bone, thus improving the capacity of the articular cartilage to absorb stress during joint loading. Cartilage repair also protects the subchondral bone from overloading and may be a factor in diminishing subchondral sclerosis.

The same authors evaluated the role of joint distraction in patients undergoing débridement of osteophytes and intra-articular fibrosis.[144] Nine patients underwent joint distraction, which was combined with débridement in seven of the patients, and eight others were treated with débridement alone. At 1-year follow-up, the patients who were treated with joint distraction had significantly better clinical outcomes than those undergoing débridement alone. Three patients who did not have any pain relief after débridement subsequently underwent joint distraction and reported significant clinical benefits. The results suggest that the clinical improvement was likely secondary to the joint distraction and not a result of the débridement procedure.

In a midterm follow-up study, investigators with several years of experience with the Ilizarov technique used joint distraction as disease-modifying therapy for osteoarthritis of the ankle.[145] Twenty-seven young adults with a mean age of 37 years (range, 19 to 55 years) who were being considered for arthrodesis because of symptomatic osteoarthritis of the ankle were treated with joint distraction at one of three western European medical centers using similar surgical techniques and postoperative protocols. Most patients had a history of ankle trauma. At an average follow-up period of 10 years (range, 7 to 15 years), 16 of 22 patients (73%) available for follow-up had improvement in pain and functional scores, with minimal improvement in ankle joint mobility. Radiographic data were not available. The authors were unable to identify any specific preoperative patient characteristics that would predict a successful outcome after joint distraction arthroplasty. Despite impressive clinical outcomes for most patients, no second-look surgeries were performed to assess the nature and extent of intra-articular cartilage repair after ankle joint distraction.

In a 2007 study, a successful outcome after articulated joint distraction in an adolescent with advanced posttraumatic chondrolysis of the ankle joint was reported.[140] At 5.5-year follow-up, acceptable radiographic and clinical outcomes had been achieved in the young symptomatic patient who had limited surgical options.

Conclusion

Few joint-preserving alternatives exist for a patient who has ankle arthritis that is refractory to conservative measures.[146] Distraction arthroplasty has been proposed as one of the treatment options for the patient for whom arthrodesis or joint arthroplasty is not appropriate. Unlike arthrodesis and arthroplasty, joint distraction preserves bone stock around the ankle. Potential drawbacks of joint distraction include pin tract infections, the inconvenience of wearing a bulky external fixator, and the need for a surgeon familiar with the instrumentation and technique of external fixation.

Although the mechanism of action remains unknown, reports presented by several researchers support the potential beneficial effects achieved with joint distraction in patients with advanced osteoarthritis of the ankle. Studies published to date suggest that the effects may persist for years and improve with time during the first several years after treatment. The data suggest that joint distraction arthroplasty may be a viable alternative to arthrodesis and replacement arthroplasty for the treatment of a congruent, painful, mobile, and arthritic ankle joint in a young patient. Additional laboratory studies are needed to understand the biochemical and biomechanical effects of distraction arthroplasty. Prospective clinical studies from other centers also are needed to validate the results of ankle joint distraction and to compare the outcomes of treatment with articulated and nonarticulated constructs. Based on preliminary animal studies, the role of joint distraction as an adjunct to other joint-preserving techniques, such as subchondral drilling and autologous chondrocyte transplantation, is encouraging but requires further investigation, including high-level clinical trials.

Allograft Replacement

Fresh allografts have been used successfully in the knee and recently are playing a more important role in the treatment of end-stage tibiotalar arthritis in selected patients. Osteochondral allografts provide a congruent articular surface and relieve pain. Structural allografting differs from ankle arthroplasty because it maintains the bone stock of the ankle. This procedure also lessens secondary degeneration of the surrounding joints that occurs after ankle arthrodesis.

The unique characteristics of the osseous and chondral tissue components allow successful transplantation. Unlike fresh-frozen allografts, research using fresh allografts has shown that chondrocytes can survive transplantation. Approximately 70% of chondrocytes are viable after 28 days in storage media.[147] The subchondral bone provides support and fixation of the chondral surfaces and is slowly replaced by host bone by the process of creeping substitution. During the time of revascularization, the graft is at risk of collapse.

3: Arthritis

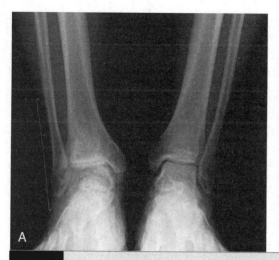
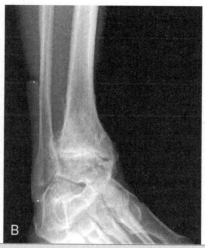
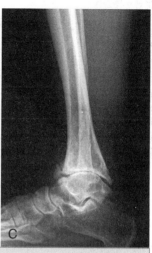

Figure 9 Preoperative AP **(A)**, mortise **(B)**, and lateral **(C)** radiographs should be obtained before ankle reconstruction with fresh osteochondral allografts.

Preoperative Patient Assessment

History and Physical Examination

When planning surgery with an allograft procedure for tibiotalar arthritis, the patient's age and lifestyle should be considered because the allograft procedure is most beneficial for young, active patients. A thorough orthopaedic history and physical examination are needed; other causes of hindfoot pain should be excluded. Tests for ligamentous instability, malalignment, and other deformities of the foot and ankle, such as equinus contracture, should be performed. Varus or valgus alignment deformity, if present, may need to be corrected at the time of surgery to prevent unnecessary forces across the allograft.[148] Contraindications for ankle reconstruction using fresh osteochondral allografts are diminished peripheral pulses, varus or valgus malalignment of the tibiotalar joint of more than 10°, large cystic lesions, ankle joint instability, and obesity.

Imaging

Preoperative weight-bearing radiographs of the ankle should include AP, mortise, and lateral views (**Figure 9**). When indicated, stress radiographs should be obtained to help diagnose instability. Ankle instability is indicated by an anterior translation between the talus and tibia of 3 to 5 mm greater than that of the contralateral ankle.[149] Talar tilt is measured on stress radiographs with the ankle internally rotated 30°. A difference in tilt greater than 15° compared with the contralateral ankle also is indicative of instability.[13] CT and MRI can be useful for evaluating the bony architecture and diagnosing cystic lesions of the tibia or talus.

Preoperative Planning

The mediolateral width of the host talus measured 0.5 cm below the talar dome on the AP weight-bearing ankle radiograph is used to determine the size of the allografts. Size-matched osteochondral allografts are then obtained from a regional tissue bank.

Because fresh allografts have living chondrocytes, they offer an advantage compared with frozen allografts, which have few or no living chondrocytes. Fresh allografts are harvested within 24 hours of the donor's death and require approximately 21 days for disease testing. Graft specimens are cultured and tested for antibodies to human immunodeficiency virus, hepatitis, and syphilis. Allografts are placed in sterile bags, immersed in a culture medium containing 1 g/L of cephalothin and 10 mg/L of gentamicin, and are stored at 4°C until use. Fresh allografts should be implanted within 28 days of procurement.[15]

Although no documented transmission of disease has occurred using allograft replacement in the tibiotalar joint, all patients should be counseled concerning risks, which are similar to those of homologous blood transfusion. No tissue or blood-type matching is necessary because immunologic response to unmatched allografts has no proven clinical significance.[15]

Surgical Technique

The patient is positioned supine on a radiolucent operating table. A standard anterior approach to the ankle is used between the tibialis anterior and extensor hallucis longus tendon. The neurovascular bundle is retracted laterally and dissection is carried through the joint capsule to expose the distal tibia and talus.

Débridement and Distraction of the Ankle Joint

Prior to inflating the tourniquet, a unilateral external fixator is applied to the leg medially with half pins in the talar neck and calcaneus, and two half pins in the tibia (**Figure 10**). The position of the external fixator is locked and the external fixator is removed. The tourniquet is inflated and the ankle joint is entered through the standard anterior approach; débridement of the joint is performed with osteotomes and rongeurs (**Figure 11**). The external fixator then is applied again to distract the joint symmetrically approximately 1 cm.

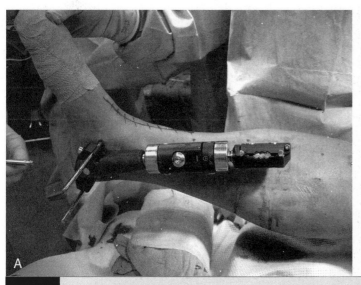
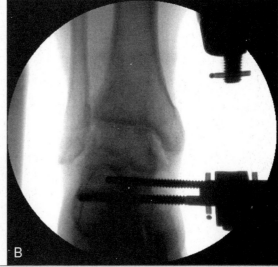

Figure 10 A unilateral external fixator is applied to the leg medially **(A)** and placement is checked with fluoroscopy **(B)**.

Tibial and Talar Cuts

The ankle joint is inspected and the surgeon decides if bipolar tibiotalar or hemijoint resurfacing will be used. The ankle radiographs are templated and a corresponding Agility Ankle (Depuy, Warsaw, IN) arthroplasty jig, which is used to increase the precision of the cuts, is pinned into place over the anterior ankle (**Figure 12, A**). Placement and size are confirmed with intraoperative fluoroscopy (**Figure 12, B**).

Using a blunt reciprocating saw, the tibial plafond and talar dome are resected to a 7- to 10-mm depth (**Figure 13**). A 3- to 4-mm articular portion of the medial malleolus also is removed. Extreme care is needed because the posterior tibial neurovascular bundle lies in close proximity to the posteromedial corner of the ankle joint. On the lateral aspect of the tibial cut, contact with the fibula is avoided to maintain full preservation.

Allograft Preparation and Cuts

The Agility Ankle cutting block for cutting the donor graft tibia is one size larger than the block used on the recipient's native tibia. The cutting block or jig is manually placed onto the tibial allograft, proper fit is confirmed with fluoroscopy, and the allograft is cut with an oscillating saw (**Figure 14**). The talus graft then is cut freehand using as an oscillating saw. The cut is made at the interface between the anterior neck and cartilage (**Figure 15**). Both grafts are lavaged to remove immunogenic marrow elements. The graft are articulated on the back table (**Figure 16**).

Placement and Fixation of the Grafts

With the ankle in plantar flexion, the grafts are seated into the recipient mortise (**Figure 17**). The external fixator is removed and the ankle is moved through a range of motion to confirm stability. Imaging is used to confirm that the grafts have complete apposition to the host bone and that the anatomy of the tibiotalar joint

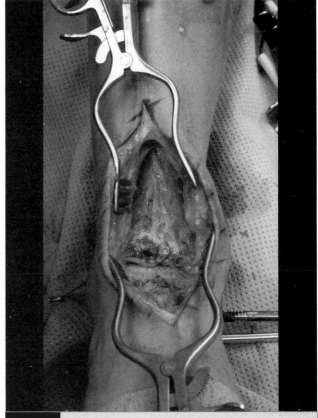

Figure 11 Photograph showing the anterior approach with the removal of osteophytes.

has been restored. Two parallel 3.0-mm cannulated screws are placed into each graft for additional fixation. The screws are placed from the anterior portion of the tibial graft while aiming superiorly and posteriorly. Two fixation screws are placed on the anterior portion of the talar graft through the most anterior

3: Arthritis

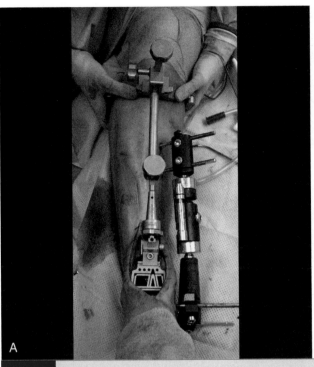
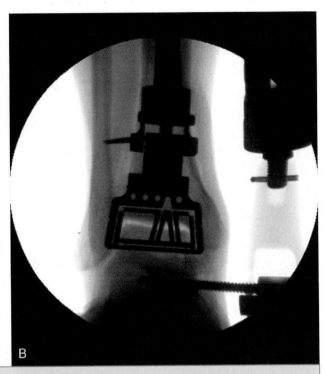

Figure 12 The ankle arthroplasty jig is placed over the anterior leg/ankle (**A**) and the position is confirmed with fluoroscopy (**B**).

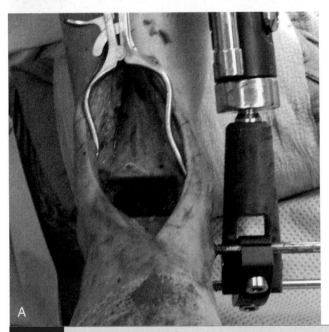
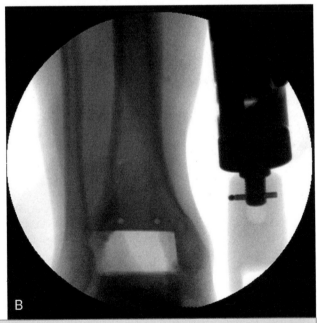

Figure 13 **A,** Photograph showing the resected plafond and talus. **B,** Fluoroscopic image of the native tibia and talus after resection.

portion of the articular cartilage and countersunk into subchondral bone (**Figure 18**). The patient is then tested for equinus contracture and, if present, a gastrocnemius recession or percutaneous Achilles tendon lengthening is performed. The patient should have at least 10° of ankle dorsiflexion at the end of the procedure.

Closure and Postoperative Care
Copious irrigation and routine wound closure of the ankle is performed, and the ankle is placed in a bulky cotton splint with the ankle in dorsiflexion. Standard perioperative antibiotics and medication for pain control are administered. Range-of-motion exercises are started when the wound is healed, approximately 10

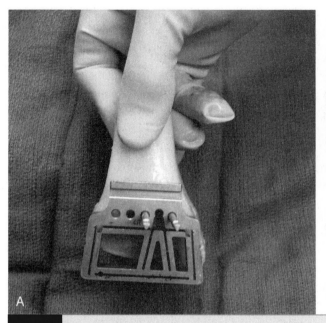

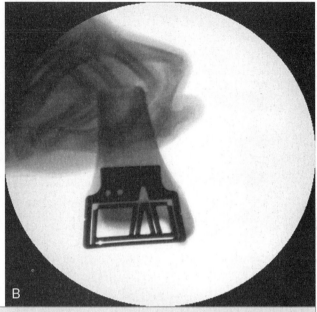

Figure 14 **A,** Placement of ankle cutting jig on the tibia allograft. **B,** Placement of the jig is confirmed with fluoroscopy.

days postoperatively. Patients are instructed not to bear weight for 3 months, after which weight bearing is allowed as tolerated (**Figure 19**).

Complications

Complications of reconstructive ankle surgery using allografts include intraoperative fractures, graft failure, and nerve damage. Extreme care is needed when making cuts to avoid fractures to the lateral and medial malleolus. The use of cutting jigs improves the precision of cuts and decreases the risk of graft failure from improperly cut grafts. Care must be taken to prevent damage to the posterior tibial neurovascular bundle at the posteromedial corner of the ankle joint. If the graft fails, the patient can be treated using a repeat allograft procedure or with conversion to arthrodesis or total ankle arthroplasty.

Study Results

In one study, investigators reported on the long-term outcomes of seven patients treated with total ankle replacement using fresh allografts.[14] At 12-year follow-up, four of seven patients had good or excellent results. Two patients (two ankles) had revision surgery with arthrodesis; their complications appeared to be related to technical difficulties, such as allograft size matching. The use of cutting blocks and better methods for precise size matching of the allografts has reduced the number of technical errors.

The authors of another study reported on nine patients treated with fresh allografts for osteochondral lesions of the talus.[150] Six of nine patients had successful procedures and the allografts remained in situ with a mean survival of 11 years. Fragmentation and collapse

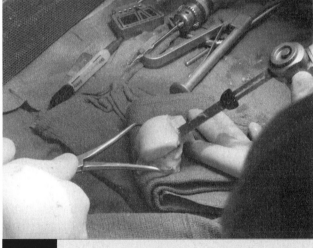

Figure 15 The talus allograft is cut freehand on the back table.

of the grafts occurred in three patients who were then treated with arthrodeses.[150]

In a 2005 study, 11 patients were treated with fresh osteochondral allograft transplantation of the tibiotalar joint.[15] At a minimum follow-up of 2 years, successful outcomes were reported in 6 of the 11 patients. Three of the five patients in whom the allograft failed underwent successful repeat allografting, one patient was treated with ankle arthroplasty, and one patient chose not to have further surgery. Complications included one intraoperative fibula fracture and one superficial wound infection. The investigators concluded that graft collapse was more likely to occur if graft thickness was less than 7 mm.[15]

3: Arthritis

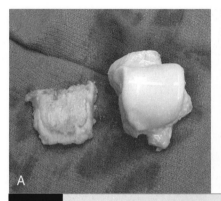
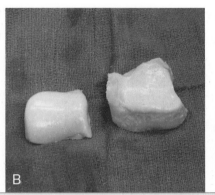
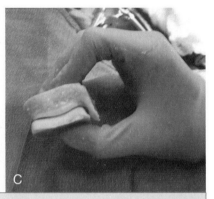

Figure 16 **A,** Native talus and allograft talus on the back table. **B,** Cut tibia and talar allografts on the back table. **C,** Grafts articulated on the back table.

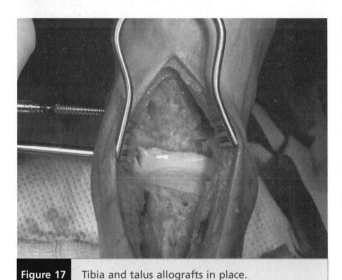

Figure 17 Tibia and talus allografts in place.

The Role of the Immune System

Many studies have indicated that the human immune system most likely plays a role in the success or failure of fresh osteochondral allograft transplantation. In animal studies, mismatched allografts have higher resorption rates, more inflammation, and less incorporation. [151]

In a 2008 study, rats received tibia (fresh or frozen) syngeneic or allogeneic cortical segments.[151] The rat strains were identical except for the major histocompatibility complex. Frozen allografts had less biologic activity and fewer areas of normal osteocyte density. The frozen allografts also showed less bone bridging. The fresh allogeneic grafts had less blood flow and ultimately less bone bridging, mineral content, and torsional strength compared with the fresh syngeneic allografts. Ultimately, the fresh allogeneic grafts had higher resorption rates compared with the fresh syngeneic grafts.

Another study used several cytotoxic drugs and evaluated their effect on distal femoral allografts to test the suppression of the immune system.[152] The tested drugs included single-dose cyclophosphamide, double-dose cyclophosphamide, azathioprine/steroids for 4 weeks, cyclosporin (25 mg/kg/day for 14 days), cyclosporin (15 mg/kg/day for 28 days), and 1,200 rads total lymphoid irradiation. At 6 weeks, antibody response was suppressed more than 50% in the groups treated with cyclosporin and irradiation. The group treated with azathioprine had the least immune response inhibition.

Because of an increase in antibody response at 6 weeks in the group treated with cyclophosphamide, it was concluded that sensitized lymphocytes were not able to make clones of antibodies until the activity of the cytotoxic drug was no longer available. The antibody response in the group treated with cyclosporin for 14 days increased at 12 weeks, leading the authors to conclude that antigens persist for more than 2 weeks from the time of implantation. In the group treated with cyclosporin for 28 days, antibody production was inhibited for more than 3 months. This result may indicate that antigens are not viable for 4 weeks after implantation.[152]

Cytotoxic drugs have some adverse effects. There was a significant increase in the death rate and in the number of leukopenic rats in the double-dose cyclophosphamide group. The rats treated with cyclosporin for 4 weeks had increased kidney toxicity and a higher death rate. The irradiated rats had such high levels of leukopenia that the treatment was considered too toxic and was discontinued.[152]

There are few available studies on the immune response to fresh osteochondral allograft implantation in humans. One study used MRI to evaluate fresh osteochondral allograft implantation in the knee.[153] Antibody-positive and antibody-negative patients were compared. Using serial nonenhanced MRIs, the antibody-positive and antibody-negative groups were evaluated for factors including host marrow edema, graft-host interface, graft marrow signal intensity grade, cyst formation, graft cartilage integrity, graft contour, and effusion. The antibody-positive patients had significantly greater host marrow edema, graft-host interface thickness, and graft marrow signal intensity grade compared with the

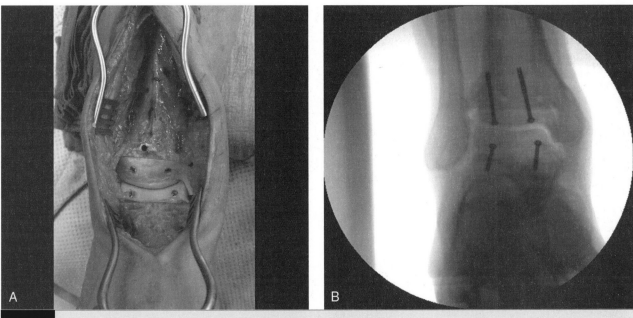

Figure 18 **A,** The tibia and talus allografts are secured with screws. **B,** Mortise intraoperative fluoroscopic view of screw fixation of the tibia and talus allografts.

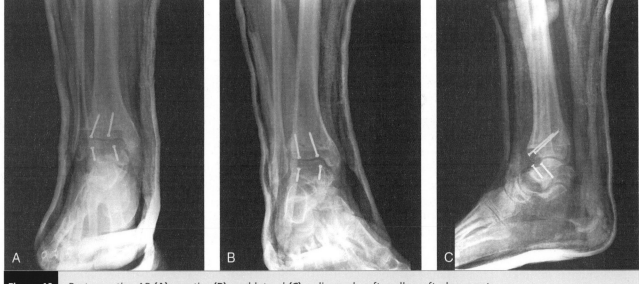

Figure 19 Postoperative AP **(A)**, mortise **(B)**, and lateral **(C)** radiographs after allograft placement.

antibody-negative group. Other factors were not significantly different between the two groups. These changes in the subchondral bone may cause failure of allografts in antibody-positive patients.

Another study in humans measured chondrocyte viability using confocal microscopy of fresh allograft transplants in the human knee.[154] Tissue samples were taken from patients with failed fresh osteochondral allograft transplantations at the time of revision surgery. Chondrocyte viability and anabolic activity, glycosaminoglycan content, and cartilage integrity were analyzed. Although all specimens had some type of cartilage degeneration (such as fibrillation or complete break-

down), chondrocyte viability averaged 82% in the specimens. Histologic analysis of the subchondral bone showed osteonecrosis in 8 of 25 specimens. This study shows long-term chondrocyte viability in fresh osteochondral allografts.

Although it is clear that the immune system plays a role in fresh osteochondral allograft implantation, there is currently no immunologic matching of grafts prior to implantation. No human studies have been published to indicate that tissue matching will increase the survival rate of these grafts. The time needed for this matching would most likely make the use of such grafts exorbitantly expensive.

3: Arthritis

Because the immune response is probably directed toward the osseous portion of these allografts, pulse lavage is used to rid the bone of immunogenic elements. Irradiation and freezing the allografts reduces the viability of cartilage cells. Cytotoxic drugs may increase the rate of graft incorporation; however, patients and physicians would have to consider the adverse effects of such drugs. Further study is needed to delineate the immune response and explore possible methods to decrease graft failure.

Salvage Techniques

After failure of osteochondral allograft transplantation, several salvage techniques are available. Depending on the cause of the allograft failure and the alignment of the ankle, revision with fresh osteochondral allografting can be performed. If the patient is a candidate, total ankle arthroplasty can be performed. Ankle arthrodesis also can be used as a salvage technique. Usually, a femoral head allograft is used for bone stock and to prevent shortening of the limb.

Conclusion

Although the ultimate success of total ankle allograft reconstruction has yet to be determined, revision rates are similar to those of younger patients treated with total ankle arthroplasty. For young patients with end-stage tibiotalar arthritis who do not want to accept the functional limitations of ankle arthrodesis, fresh osteochondral allografting is an attractive alternative to arthrodeses or arthroplasty procedures.

Summary

The ankle is a highly congruent joint that is susceptible to altered biomechanics. Ankle arthritis, although not as common as arthritis of the hip and knee, can be debilitating for patients. There are many pathologic conditions that can lead to ankle arthritis; however, the common causes of degenerative changes in the ankle are trauma and abnormal ankle mechanics. Successful treatment of patients with ankle arthritis requires an understanding of ankle biomechanics along with a thorough patient medical history, physical examination, and imaging studies. Both nonsurgical and surgical treatments may be appropriate depending on the patient's age, functional expectations, comorbidities, and the stage of the arthritis. Surgical options include arthrodesis, total ankle arthroplasty, and newer treatment modalities such as joint distraction arthroplasty and the use of allograft replacement.

Annotated References

1. Svoboda SJ, McHale K, Belkoff SM, Cohen KS, Klemme WR: The effects of tibial malrotation on the biomechanics of the tibiotalar joint. *Foot Ankle Int* 2002;23:102-106.

2. Huch K, Kuettner KE, Dieppe P: Osteoarthritis in ankle and knee joints. *Semin Arthritis Rheum* 1997;26:667-674.

3. Kang Y, Koepp H, Cole AA, Kuettner KE, Homandberg GA: Cultured human ankle and knee cartilage differ in susceptibility to damage mediated by fibronectin fragments. *J Orthop Res* 1998;16:551-556.

4. Chubinskaya S, Kuettner KE, Cole AA: Expression of matrix metalloproteinases in normal and damaged articular cartilage from human knee and ankle joints. *Lab Invest* 1999;79:1669-1677.

5. Cole AA, Margulis A, Kuettner KE: Distinguishing ankle and knee articular cartilage. *Foot Ankle Clin* 2003; 8:305-316.

   Degenerative changes in the talar and femoral distal cartilage of 2,000 tissue donors were examined and graded based on the appearance of articular cartilage and osteophyte formation. The rate of degeneration was much slower in the talar cartilage than the distal femoral cartilage. The rate of degeneration was more severe in males and correlated with the patient's weight.

6. Aurich M, Squires GR, Reiner A, et al: Differential matrix degradation and turnover in early cartilage lesions of human knee and ankle joints. *Arthritis Rheum* 2005; 52:112-119.

   This study was conducted to compare matrix turnover and degradation after injury to talar and knee cartilage. The authors reported an increase in collagen synthesis and aggrecan turnover in ankle lesions when compared with knee lesions. The results indicated an emphasis on matrix assembly in early ankle cartilage lesions, whereas there is degradation in early knee lesions.

7. Fetter NL, Leddy HA, Guilak F, Nunley JA: Composition and transport properties of human ankle and knee cartilage. *J Orthop Res* 2006;24:211-219.

   This study showed that ankle cartilage has a higher proteoglycan content and a trend toward lower water content than knee cartilage. This finding suggests that ankle cartilage has a smaller effective pore size than knee cartilage. These findings provide further support for the hypothesis that the transport properties of cartilage may play a role in the differences in the incidence of osteoarthritis in these joints by altering the concentration of growth factors to which the chondrocytes are exposed.

8. Patwari P, Cheng DM, Cole AA, Kuettner KE, Grodzinsky AJ: Analysis of the relationship between peak stress and proteoglycan loss following injurious compression of human post-mortem knee and ankle cartilage. *Biomech Model Mechanobiol* 2007;6:83-89.

   Human cartilage disk explants from the ankle and knee were subjected to peak stress forces in a compression model. Damage to knee cartilage disks after peak stress was reported in 36% of specimens, whereas damage to ankle cartilage disks was reported in 6% of specimens. Ankle cartilage appears to be more resilient to peak stress compression forces than knee cartilage.

9. Thomas RH, Daniels TR: Current concepts review: Ankle arthritis. *J Bone Joint Surg Am* 2003;85:923-936.

    The authors present a comprehensive review of the pathophysiology and epidemiology of ankle arthritis. Nonsurgical and surgical treatment options also are discussed.

10. Carroll GJ: Primary osteoarthritis in the ankle joint is associated with finger metacarpophalangeal osteoarthritis and the H63D mutation in the HFE gene: Evidence for a hemochromatosis-like polyarticular osteoarthritis phenotype. *J Clin Rheumatol* 2006;12:109-113.

    A strong and statistically significant association was observed between *HFE* gene mutations and primary osteoarthritis in the ankle joint. The frequent presence of second-third metacarpophalangeal joint osteoarthritis in these patients suggests the existence of a type 2 polyarticular osteoarthritis phenotype that closely resembles the arthropathy of hereditary hemochromatosis and which appears to be clinically differentiable from type 1 osteoarthritis or nodal generalized osteoarthritis. *HFE* gene mutations may be a marker for the type 2 polyarticular osteoarthritis phenotype and a clue to osteoarthritis pathogenesis.

11. Curtis MJ, Michelson JD, Urquhart MW, Byank RP, Jinnah RH: Tibiotalar contact and fibular malunion in ankle fractures: A cadaver study. *Acta Orthop Scand* 1992;63:326-329.

12. Yoshimine F: Effects of fibular malunion on contact area and stress distribution at the ankle with six simulated loading conditions. *Nippon Seikeigeka Gakkai Zasshi* 1995;69:460-469.

13. Coester LM, Saltzman CL, Leupold J, Pontarelli W: Long-term results following ankle arthrodesis for post-traumatic arthritis. *J Bone Joint Surg Am* 2001;83-A: 219-228.

14. Kim CW, Jamali A, Tontz W, Convery R, Brage M, Bugbee W: Treatment of post-traumatic ankle arthrosis with bipolar tibiotalar osteochondral shell allografts. *Foot Ankle Int* 2002;23:1091-1102.

15. Meehan R, McFarlin S, Bugbee W, Brage M: Fresh ankle osteochondral allograft transplantation for tibiotalar joint arthritis. *Foot Ankle Int* 2005;26:793-802.

    Patients with diseased articular cartilage of the ankle were treated with fresh tibiotalar allograft transplantation.

16. Tontz WL, Bugbee WD, Brage ME: Use of allografts in the management of ankle arthritis. *Foot Ankle Clin* 2003;8:361-373.

    The authors report on 12 patients treated with fresh osteochondral allografts for ankle arthritis.

17. Kitaoka HB, Patzer GL, Ilstrup DM, Wallrichs SL: Survivorship analysis of the Mayo total ankle arthroplasty. *J Bone Joint Surg Am* 1994;76:974-979.

18. Cobb TK, Gabrielsen TA, Campbell DC II, Wallrichs SL, Ilstrup DM: Cigarette smoking and nonunion after ankle arthrodesis. *Foot Ankle Int* 1994;15:64-67.

19. Frey C, Halikus NM, Vu-Rose T, Ebramzadeh E: A review of ankle arthrodesis: Predisposing factors to nonunion. *Foot Ankle Int* 1994;15:581-584.

20. Stuart MJ, Morrey BF: Arthrodesis of the diabetic neuropathic ankle joint. *Clin Orthop Relat Res* 1990;253: 209-211.

21. Dalla Paola L, Volpe A, Varotto D, et al: Use of a retrograde nail for ankle arthrodesis in Charcot neuroarthropathy: A limb salvage procedure. *Foot Ankle Int* 2007; 28:967-970.

    Eighteen diabetic patients with a history of ankle Charcot arthropathy were treated with tibiotalocalcaneal arthrodesis with retrograde nail fixation. A cast was used to prevent weight bearing in all patients for 3 months, followed by 3 months of partial weight bearing in a cast. Three patients required proximal screw removal because of screw prominence beneath the skin. At follow-up, solid arthrodesis was achieved in 14 patients and a stable fibrous union was reported in 4 patients.

22. Hill K, Berlet GC, Philbin TM, Lee TH: The role of cyclooxygenase-2 inhibition in foot and ankle arthrodesis. *Foot Ankle Clin* 2005;10:729-742.

    This review article of basic science animal model data and clinical studies outlines the physiology and pathophysiology of the cyclooxygenase-2 (COX-2) enzyme in prostaglandin metabolism. Evidence from basic science studies exists regarding the deleterious effects of COX-2 inhibitors on fracture healing and spinal arthrodesis in rat studies with medication administration and gene knockout models. No decrease in hindfoot or ankle arthrodesis rates has been reported in case control studies of human patients who were perioperatively treated with COX-2 inhibitors. Short-term COX-2 inhibitor use in this patient population does not appear to be detrimental.

23. Cracchiolo A III, Cimino WR, Lian G: Arthrodesis of the ankle in patients who have rheumatoid arthritis. *J Bone Joint Surg Am* 1992;74:903-909.

24. Sirveaux F, Beyaert C, Paysant J, Molé D, André JM: Increasing shoe instep improves gait dynamics in patients with a tibiotalar arthrodesis. *Clin Orthop Relat Res* 2006;442:204-209.

    An instep of 20 to 25 mm was shown to shift ground reaction forces closer to the metatarsal heads. This stimulates more normal ground reaction forces and reduces the maximal foot and tibial dorsiflexion angles.

25. Buck P, Morrey BF, Chao EY: The optimum position of arthrodesis of the ankle: A gait study of the knee and ankle. *J Bone Joint Surg Am* 1987;69:1052-1062.

26. Schneider D: Arthroscopic ankle fusion. *Arthrosc Video J* 1983;3.

27. Myerson MS, Quill G: Ankle arthrodesis: A comparison

3: Arthritis

of an arthroscopic and an open method of treatment. *Clin Orthop Relat Res* 1991;268:84-95.

28. Dent CM, Patil M, Fairclough JA: Arthroscopic ankle arthrodesis. *J Bone Joint Surg Br* 1993;75:830-832.

29. Glick JM, Morgan CD, Myerson MS, Sampson TG, Mann JA: Ankle arthrodesis using an arthroscopic method: Long-term follow-up of 34 cases. *Arthroscopy* 1996;12:428-434.

30. Tasto JP, Frey C, Laimans P, Morgan CD, Mason RJ, Stone JW: Arthroscopic ankle arthrodesis. *Instr Course Lect* 2000;49:259-280.

31. Zvijac JE, Lemak L, Schurhoff MR, Hechtman KS, Uribe JW: Analysis of arthroscopically assisted arthrodesis. *Arthroscopy* 2002;18:70-75.

32. Morrey BF, Wiedeman GP Jr: Complications and long-term results of ankle arthrodeses following trauma. *J Bone Joint Surg Am* 1980;62:777-784.

33. Kirkpatrick JS, Goldner JL, Goldner RD: Revision arthrodesis for tibiotalar pseudarthrosis with fibular onlay-inlay graft and internal screw fixation. *Clin Orthop Relat Res* 1991;268:29-36.

34. Mann RA, Van Manen JW, Wapner K, Martin J: Ankle fusion. *Clin Orthop Relat Res* 1991;268:49-55.

35. Papa JA, Myerson MS: Pantalar and tibiotalocalcaneal arthrodesis for post-traumatic osteoarthrosis of the ankle and hindfoot. *J Bone Joint Surg Am* 1992;74:1042-1049.

36. Wang GJ, Shen WJ, McLaughlin RE, Stamp WG: Transfibular compression arthrodesis of the ankle joint. *Clin Orthop Relat Res* 1993;289:223-227.

37. Mann RA, Rongstad KM: Arthrodesis of the ankle: A critical analysis. *Foot Ankle Int* 1998;19:3-9.

38. Kopp FJ, Banks MA, Marcus RE: Clinical outcome of tibiotalar arthrodesis utilizing the chevron technique. *Foot Ankle Int* 2004;25:225-230.

    The authors evaluated the results of patients treated with tibiotalar arthrodesis with the chevron fusion technique with cross screws. The Mazur scores averaged 72.8 of 90. The most common reason for unsatisfactory postoperative results was postoperative subtalar arthrosis that had been noted on preoperative studies. A 93% rate of clinical and radiographic union was reported and 90% of patients were satisfied with their surgical outcomes.

39. Friedman RL, Glisson RR, Nunley JA II: A biomechanical comparative analysis of two techniques for tibiotalar arthrodesis. *Foot Ankle Int* 1994;15:301-305.

40. Holt ES, Hansen ST, Mayo KA, Sangeorzan BJ: Ankle arthrodesis using internal screw fixation. *Clin Orthop Relat Res* 1991;268:21-28.

41. Scranton PE Jr, Fu FH, Brown TD: Ankle arthrodesis: A comparative clinical and biomechanical evaluation. *Clin Orthop Relat Res* 1980;151:234-243.

42. Scranton PE Jr: Use of internal compression in arthrodesis of the ankle. *J Bone Joint Surg Am* 1985;67:550-555.

43. Sowa DT, Krackow KA: Ankle fusion: A new technique of internal fixation using a compression blade plate. *Foot Ankle* 1989;9:232-240.

44. Braly WG, Baker JK, Tullos HS: Arthrodesis of the ankle with lateral plating. *Foot Ankle Int* 1994;15:649-653.

45. Morgan SJ, Thordarson DB, Shepherd LE: Salvage of tibial pilon fractures using fusion of the ankle with a 90 degrees cannulated blade-plate: A preliminary report. *Foot Ankle Int* 1999;20:375-378.

46. Gruen GS, Mears DC: Arthrodesis of the ankle and subtalar joints. *Clin Orthop Relat Res* 1991;268:15-20.

47. Alvarez RG, Barbour TM, Perkins TD: Tibiocalcaneal arthrodesis for nonbraceable neuropathic ankle deformity. *Foot Ankle Int* 1994;15:354-359.

48. Myerson MS, Alvarez RG, Lam PW: Tibiocalcaneal arthrodesis for the management of severe ankle and hindfoot deformities. *Foot Ankle Int* 2000;21:643-650.

49. Nasson S, Shuff C, Palmer D, et al: Biomechanical comparison of ankle arthrodesis techniques: Crossed screws vs. blade plate. *Foot Ankle Int* 2001;22:575-580.

50. Alfahd U, Roth SE, Stephen D, Whyne CM: Biomechanical comparison of intramedullary nail and blade plate fixation for tibiotalocalcaneal arthrodesis. *J Orthop Trauma* 2005;19:703-708.

    Seven pairs of fresh frozen cadaver specimens were instrumented with a lateral cannulated blade plate or a retrograde intramedullary nail simulating tibiotalocalcaneal arthrodesis. The cadavers were tested with plantar/dorsiflexion and inversion/eversion. Maximum displacements were measured in these planes. No significant differences were reported in three of the loading configurations. A small but significant reduction in internal rotation was found in the blade plate construct when compared with the retrograde nailed construct.

51. Mears DC, Gordon RG, Kann SE, Kann JN: Ankle arthrodesis with an anterior tension plate. *Clin Orthop Relat Res* 1991;268:70-77.

52. Kakarala G, Rajan DT: Comparative study of ankle arthrodesis using cross screw fixation versus anterior contoured plate plus cross screw fixation. *Acta Orthop Belg* 2006;72:716-721.

    This study used AOFAS scoring to compare the clinical outcome of a group of patients treated with ankle arthrodesis with cross fixation alone to a group of patients treated with ankle arthrodesis with cross screws

3: Arthritis

and an anterior contoured locking plate. The two groups had similar AOFAS outcome scoring at follow-up; however, there were two nonunions in the group treated with cross screw fixation only that required revision with an anterior contoured plate and cross screw fixation.

53. Tarkin IS, Mormino MA, Clare MP, Haider H, Walling AK, Sanders RW: Anterior plate supplementation increases ankle arthrodesis construct rigidity. *Foot Ankle Int* 2007;28:219-223.

Cadaver models of ankle arthrodeses were created with three screws alone and with three screws and anterior plating. The anterior plate construct was reported to have an increased stiffness of 3.5 in the sagittal mode, 1.9 in the coronal mode, and 1.4 in the torsional mode. Anterior plate supplementation increased construct rigidity and decreased micromotion at the ankle fusion interface.

54. Hammit MD, Hobgood ER, Tarquinio TA: Midline posterior approach to the ankle and hindfoot. *Foot Ankle Int* 2006;27:711-715.

The authors of this retrospective study evaluated wound healing in patients who had ankle surgery through a midline posterior approach. This approach provides dissection between angiosomes, which should preserve the blood supply to skin flaps. No incidences of full-thickness skin flap necrosis were reported using this approach.

55. Ritter M, Nickisch F, DiGiovanni C: Technique tip: Posterior blade plate for salvage of failed total ankle arthroplasty. *Foot Ankle Int* 2006;27:303-304.

This technique paper describes the posterior approach for tibiotalocalcaneal ankle arthrodesis in a patient with a failed total ankle arthroplasty and compromised anterior skin. The authors emphasize the need for precontouring the plate to decrease tourniquet time.

56. Barrow CR, Pomeroy GC: Enhancement of syndesmotic fusion rates in total ankle arthroplasty with the use of autologous platelet concentrate. *Foot Ankle Int* 2005;26:458-461.

When compared with historic controls (62% fusion rate), the addition of an autologous platelet concentrate improved syndesmotic fusion rates to 100%.

57. Coetzee JC, Pomeroy GC, Watts JD, Barrow C: The use of autologous concentrated growth factors to promote syndesmosis fusion in the Agility total ankle replacement: A preliminary study. *Foot Ankle Int* 2005;26:840-846.

Autologous concentrated growth factors reduced syndesmotic nonunion rates from 27% to 6%. Autologous growth factors appear to make a significant positive difference in the syndesmotic union rate in total ankle replacements using the Agility Ankle.

58. Neufeld SK, Lee TH: Total ankle arthroplasty: Indications, results and biomechanical rationale. *Am J Orthop* 2000;29:593-602.

59. Lewis G: Biomechanics of and research challenges in uncemented total ankle replacement. *Clin Orthop Relat Res* 2004;424:89-97.

The authors describe 13 design requirements, including kinematics, kinetics, and stability for future ankle prosthetic designs. Characteristics of three second-generation designs are described and seven future research areas are discussed.

60. Michelson JD, Schmidt GR, Mizel MS: Kinematics of a total arthroplasty of the ankle: Comparison to normal ankle motion. *Foot Ankle Int* 2000;21:278-284.

61. Gill LH: Challenges in total ankle arthroplasty. *Foot Ankle Int* 2004;25:195-207.

The author describes difficulties encountered in performing total ankle arthroplasty, including wound healing and prosthetic design challenges.

62. Hintermann B, Valderrabano V: Total ankle replacement. *Foot Ankle Clin* 2003;8:375-405.

This article reviews the available literature on total ankle replacements, includes a discussion of current designs, and presents recommendations for future studies.

63. Lecomte AR, Singh SK, Fitzgerald B, Weissman BN: Small joint arthroplasty. *Semin Musculoskelet Radiol* 2006;10:64-78.

The types of joint replacement, clinical efficacy, and expected radiographic appearances are reviewed for small upper and lower extremity joints. Potential complications and their radiographic appearances are presented.

64. Kobayashi A, Minoda Y, Kadoya Y, Ohashi H, Takaoka K, Saltzman CL: Ankle arthroplasties generate wear particles similar to knee arthroplasties. *Clin Orthop Relat Res* 2004;424:69-72.

This study examined and compared the size, shape, and concentration of polyethylene particles in synovial fluid with total ankle arthroplasties and established posterior-stabilized total knee arthroplasties.

65. Takakura Y, Tanaka Y, Kumai T, Sugimoto K, Ohgushi H: Ankle arthroplasty using three generations of metal and ceramic prostheses. *Clin Orthop Relat Res* 2004;424:130-136.

The authors report on their study of metal and ceramic prostheses. Overall results for patients with osteoarthritis and rheumatoid arthritis are discussed.

66. Anderson T, Montgomery F, Carlsson A: Uncemented STAR total ankle prostheses: Three to eight-year follow-up of fifty-one consecutive ankles. *J Bone Joint Surg Am* 2003;85-A:1321-1329.

The authors present a review of the intermediate-term results of 51 consecutive STAR arthroplasties and conclude that this prosthesis may be a realistic alternative to arthrodesis provided that the components are correctly sized and positioned. The authors noted that the risks of loosening and failure were higher than after total hip or total knee replacement.

67. Natens P, Dereymaeker G, Abbara M, Matricali G: Early results after four years experience with the S.T.A.R. uncemented total ankle prosthesis. *Acta Orthop Belg* 2003;69:49-58.

In this study, the authors evaluate the results of 26 uncemented, hydroxyapatite-coated STAR prostheses, all implanted between January 1996 and December 1999, with an average follow-up of 15.8 months. No major complications occurred and there were no revision surgeries.

68. Lodhi Y, McKenna J, Herron M, Stephens MM: Total ankle replacement. *Ir Med J* 2004;97:104-105.

Twenty-nine patients were treated over a 4-year period by a single surgeon using 30 STAR prostheses. The intermediate-term results showed 90% of patients had excellent and good functional outcomes in a mixed osteoarthritic and rheumatoid population.

69. Wood PL, Deakin S: Total ankle replacement: The results in 200 ankles. *J Bone Joint Surg Br* 2003;85:334-341.

The authors review 200 cementless, mobile-bearing STAR prostheses.

70. Anderson T, Montgomery F, Carlsson A: Uncemented STAR total ankle prostheses. *J Bone Joint Surg Am* 2004;86-A:103-111.

This article presents the results of a follow-up study by the authors of their previous review of 51 consecutive STAR prostheses. The median Kofoed score increased from 39 points before the surgery to 70 points at the time of the follow-up examination. The estimated 5-year survival rate, with revision for any reason as the end point, was 0.70.

71. Wood PL, Prem H, Sutton C: Total ankle replacement: Medium-term results in 200 Scandinavian Total Ankle Replacements. *J Bone Joint Surg Br* 2008;90:605-609.

The authors describe the medium-term results of a prospective study of 200 total ankle replacements at a single center using the STAR. Anterior subluxation of the talus was corrected in most patients and anatomic alignment was restored.

72. Valderrabano V, Hintermann B, Dick W: Scandinavian total ankle replacement: A 3.7-year average followup of 65 patients. *Clin Orthop Relat Res* 2004;424:47-56.

The purpose of this study was to determine the midterm results of 68 total ankle replacements with the STAR prosthesis. The authors' early experience with the STAR was encouraging; however, they found more complications and potential complications than had been previously reported.

73. Hintermann B: Short- and mid-term results with the STAR total ankle prosthesis. *Orthopade* 1999;28:792-803.

74. San Giovanni TP, Keblish DJ, Thomas WH, Wilson MG: Eight-year results of a minimally constrained total ankle arthroplasty. *Foot Ankle Int* 2006;27:418-426.

The authors investigated the efficacy and safety of 31 Buechel-Pappas total ankle prostheses in a select, low-demand patient population. They reported that improvements in prosthetic design, such as cementless fixation and decreased constraint, appeared to make arthroplasty a more predictable procedure. The authors were encouraged by the intermediate-term results.

75. Buechel FF Sr, Buechel FF Jr, Pappas MJ: Twenty-year evaluation of cementless mobile-bearing total ankle replacements. *Clin Orthop Relat Res* 2004;424:19-26.

Two consecutive studies of patients who had cementless, porous-coated, congruent-contact, mobile-bearing, total ankle replacements were evaluated during a 20-year period. The 12-year overall survivorship for the deep-sulcus prosthetic design was 92%.

76. Buechel FF Sr, Buechel FF Jr, Pappas MJ: Ten-year evaluation of cementless Buechel-Pappas meniscal bearing total ankle replacement. *Foot Ankle Int* 2003;24:462-472.

A porous-coated, cementless, congruent-contact, three-piece, meniscal-bearing, total ankle prosthesis was developed and used clinically during a 2- to 10-year period for patients with disabling ankle arthritis. The designers reported that cumulative survivorship using an end point of revision of any component for any reason was 93.5% at 10 years.

77. Ali MS, Higgins GA, Mohamed M: Intermediate results of Buechel Pappas unconstrained uncemented total ankle replacement for osteoarthritis. *J Foot Ankle Surg* 2007;46:16-20.

The authors present functional and radiologic results after implantation of 35 uncemented Buechel-Pappas ankles with an average follow-up period of 5 years.

78. Doets HC, Brand R, Nelissen RG: Total ankle arthroplasty in inflammatory joint disease with use of two mobile-bearing designs. *J Bone Joint Surg Am* 2006;88:1272-1284.

This study focuses exclusively on patients with the diagnosis of inflammatory joint disease and provides a detailed analysis of the risk factors for failure of cementless, mobile-bearing, total ankle arthroplasty in these patients.

79. Hintermann B, Valderrabano V, Dereymaeker G, Dick W: The HINTEGRA ankle: Rationale and short-term results of 122 consecutive ankles. *Clin Orthop Relat Res* 2004;424:57-68.

The designers of the Hintegra ankle report on their short-term results in a consecutive series of 116 patients (122 ankles).

80. Valderrabano V, Pagenstert G, Horisberger M, Knupp M, Hintermann B: Sports and recreation activity of ankle arthritis patients before and after total ankle replacement. *Am J Sports Med* 2006;34:993-999.

The authors report a significant correlation between sports activity and AOFAS hindfoot scores in patients after total ankle replacement using the Salto prosthesis. Level of evidence: IV.

3: Arthritis

81. Bonnin M, Judet T, Colombier JA, Buscayret F, Graveleau N, Piriou P: Midterm results of the Salto Total Ankle Prosthesis. *Clin Orthop Relat Res* 2004;424:6-18.

The authors report on 93 Salto total ankle prostheses with a mean follow-up of 35 months. Results were encouraging.

82. Kopp FJ, Patel MM, Deland JT, O'Malley MJ: Total ankle arthroplasty with the Agility prosthesis: Clinical and radiographic evaluation. *Foot Ankle Int* 2006;27:97-103.

The authors report on intermediate-term clinical and radiographic results of 40 Agility ankle arthroplasties. Radiographic follow-up commonly showed periprosthetic lucency, lysis, and component migration or subsidence; however, this did not appear to adversely affect the intermediate-term clinical outcomes.

83. Knecht SI, Estin M, Callaghan JJ, et al: The Agility total ankle arthroplasty: Seven- to sixteen-year follow-up. *J Bone Joint Surg Am* 2004;86-A:1161-1171.

The authors present the follow-up results on their earlier intermediate-term results with the early version of 132 Agility ankles.

84. Pyevich MT, Saltzman CL, Callaghan JJ, Alvine FG: Total ankle arthroplasty: A unique design. Two to twelve-year follow-up. *J Bone Joint Surg Am* 1998;80:1410-1420.

85. Spirt AA, Assal M, Hansen ST Jr: Complications and failure after total ankle arthroplasty. *J Bone Joint Surg Am* 2004;86-A:1172-1178.

The authors describe complications, revision rates, and failures after primary total ankle arthroplasties. Level of evidence: IV.

86. Saltzman CL, Amendola A, Anderson R, et al: Surgeon training and complications in total ankle arthroplasty. *Foot Ankle Int* 2003;24:514-518.

This study assessed the problems encountered by surgeons initially using ankle arthroplasty. Three groups were studied: surgeons who were trained by observing the surgeon/inventor (group I); those who completed a structured, hands-on surgical training course (group II); and those who were trained during a 1-year foot and ankle fellowship (group III).

87. Jung HG, Nicholson JJ, Parker B, Myerson MJ: Radiographic and biomechanical support for fibular plating of the agility total ankle. *Clin Orthop Relat Res* 2004;424:118-124.

Radiographs for 40 consecutive ankles treated with the Agility Total Ankle system with two syndesmotic scans were compared with the radiographs of 40 subsequent consecutive total ankle replacements with an added fibular plate.

88. Hurowitz EJ, Gould JS, Fleisig GS, Fowler R: Outcome analysis of agility total ankle replacement with prior adjunctive procedures: Two to six year followup. *Foot Ankle Int* 2007;28:308-312.

The authors present a retrospective case review of 65 Agility total ankle replacements to more closely identify factors that may be predictive of a favorable outcome, including a comparison of outcome measures between patients who had preoperative corrective procedures and those who did not.

89. Su EP, Kahn B, Figgie MP: Total ankle replacement in patients with rheumatoid arthritis. *Clin Orthop Relat Res* 2004;424:32-38.

The authors report on a study of patients with rheumatoid arthritis treated with a second-generation total ankle prosthesis. Results showed that it can provide reliable relief of pain and good functional results at intermediate-term follow-up.

90. Clare MP, Sanders RW: Preoperative considerations in ankle replacement surgery. *Foot Ankle Clin* 2002;7:709-720.

91. Raikin SM, Myerson MS: Avoiding and managing complications of the Agility Total Ankle Replacement system. *Orthopedics* 2006;29:930-938.

The authors discuss common pitfalls with the implantation process of the Agility ankle and the diagnosis and treatment of complications occurring intraoperatively and in the intermediate- and longer-term postoperative period. Recommendations on avoiding complications are presented.

92. Haskell A, Mann RA: Perioperative complication rate of total ankle replacement is reduced by surgeon experience. *Foot Ankle Int* 2004;25:283-289.

Ten surgeons completed retrospective chart and radiographic reviews of their first 10 patients as well as 10 subsequent patients using the STAR prosthesis. This study showed a decrease in the rate of perioperative adverse events that was commensurate with surgeon experience with the STAR prosthesis.

93. Myerson MS, Mroczek K: Perioperative complications of total ankle arthroplasty. *Foot Ankle Int* 2003;24:17-21.

A retrospective radiographic and chart review was performed for the initial 50 patients who underwent total ankle arthroplasty with the Agility ankle. The study focused on the perioperative complications of nerve or tendon lacerations, intraoperative fractures, acute deep infections, wound complications, and component positioning.

94. Conti SF, Wong YS: Complications of total ankle replacement. *Clin Orthop Relat Res* 2001;391:105-114.

95. Murray MP, Drought AB, Kory RC: Walking patterns of normal men. *J Bone Joint Surg Am* 1964;46:335-360.

96. Coetzee JC, Castro MD: Accurate measurement of ankle range of motion after total ankle arthroplasty. *Clin Orthop Relat Res* 2004;424:27-31.

A protocol was developed to accurately measure the true tibiotalar and midfoot motion before and after an

3: Arthritis

ankle replacement. The authors report that this protocol results in true measurements of ankle and midfoot motion. They recommend that those measurements be used when reporting results of ankle replacements.

97. McGarvey WC, Clanton TO, Lunz D: Malleolar fracture after total ankle arthroplasty: A comparison of two designs. *Clin Orthop Relat Res* 2004;424:104-110.

To determine the clinical relevance of malleolar fracture with the two most commonly used ankle prostheses in the United States, the authors retrospectively compared the first 20 STAR arthroplasties with the first 25 Agility total ankle arthroplasties performed by two surgeons.

98. Hvid I, Rasmussen O, Jensen NC, Nielsen S: Trabecular bone strength profiles at the ankle joint. *Clin Orthop Relat Res* 1985;199:306-312.

99. Haskell A, Mann RA: Ankle arthroplasty with preoperative coronal plane deformity: Short-term results. *Clin Orthop Relat Res* 2004;424:98-103.

This study tests the hypotheses that preoperative coronal plane malalignment and incongruence of the ankle can be corrected and maintained for 2 years with total ankle replacement and that factors can be identified that place ankles at risk for progressive edge loading.

100. Swords MP, Nemec S: Osteotomy for salvage of the arthritic ankle. *Foot Ankle Clin* 2007;12:1-13.

The authors discuss osteotomies and how they can play an important role in reestablishing normal alignment, potentially decreasing the rate of wear progression on articular surfaces, and decreasing pain, which may allow more time before arthrodesis or arthroplasty are needed.

101. Smith R, Wood PL: Arthrodesis of the ankle in the presence of a large deformity in the coronal plane. *J Bone Joint Surg Br* 2007;89:615-619.

A consecutive series of 25 ankles with osteoarthritis of the ankle and severe varus or valgus deformity were treated by open arthrodesis. The authors believe that in this group of patients, open arthrodesis as opposed to ankle replacement or arthroscopic arthrodesis continues to be the treatment of choice.

102. Stamatis ED, Myerson MS: How to avoid specific complications of total ankle replacement. *Foot Ankle Clin* 2002;7:765-789.

103. Kotnis R, Pasapula C, Anwar F, Cooke PH, Sharp RJ: The management of failed ankle replacement. *J Bone Joint Surg Br* 2006;88:1039-1047.

The authors report on salvage surgery for failed ankle replacements. They conclude that after either a one-stage or two-stage procedure, a hindfoot fusion appears to be preferable to revision total ankle replacement.

104. Hopgood P, Kumar R, Wood PL: Ankle arthrodesis for failed total ankle replacement. *J Bone Joint Surg Br* 2006;88:1032-1038.

The authors reported on 23 failed total ankle replacements that were converted to arthrodeses. An intramedullary nail was used when significant bone loss was present. Arthrodesis of the tibiotalar joint alone using compression screws was generally possible in patients with osteoarthritis because the destruction of the body of the talus was less extensive.

105. Neufeld SK, Uribe J, Myerson MS: Use of structural allograft to compensate for bone loss in arthrodesis of the foot and ankle. *Foot Ankle Clin* 2002;7:1-17.

106. Wapner KL: Salvage of failed and infected total ankle replacements with fusion. *Instr Course Lect* 2002;51: 153-157.

107. Kitaoka HB, Romness DW: Arthrodesis for failed ankle arthroplasty. *J Arthroplasty* 1992;7:277-284.

108. Coughlin MJ, Mann RA, Saltzman CL (eds): *Surgery of the Foot and Ankle*, ed 8. St. Louis, MO, Mosby, 2006.

Treatments for ankle arthritis are discussed in chapter 17 of this textbook.

109. Wood PL: Experience with the STAR ankle arthroplasty at Wrightington Hospital, UK. *Foot Ankle Clin* 2002;7:755-764.

110. Carlsson AS, Montgomery F, Besjakov J: Arthrodesis of the ankle secondary to replacement. *Foot Ankle Int* 1998;19:240-245.

111. Myerson MS, Neufeld SK, Uribe J: Fresh-frozen structural allografts in the foot and ankle. *J Bone Joint Surg Am* 2005;87:113-120.

The authors reviewed the results of using structural, fresh-frozen, femoral head allografts in foot and ankle procedures and showed that the grafts may be used successfully with a relatively low complication rate in patients with risk factors for less satisfactory bone healing.

112. Groth HE, Fitch HF: Salvage procedures for complications of total ankle arthroplasty. *Clin Orthop Relat Res* 1987;224:244-250.

113. Johl C, Kircher J, Pohlmann K, Jansson V: Management of failed total ankle replacement with a retrograde short femoral nail: A case report. *J Orthop Trauma* 2006;20:60-65.

A case report of arthrodesis of the ankle joint after failed total ankle replacement using intramedullary fixation is presented. The authors believe that advantages include early mobilization and weight bearing provided by the stability of the fixation.

114. Anderson T, Linder L, Rydholm U, Montgomery F, Besjakov J, Carlsson A: Tibio-talocalcaneal arthrodesis as a primary procedure using a retrograde intramedullary nail: A retrospective study of 26 patients with rheumatoid arthritis. *Acta Orthop* 2005;76:580-587.

3: Arthritis

The authors retrospectively reviewed 25 ankles after tibiotalocalcaneal arthrodesis performed because of rheumatoid arthritis. They concluded that tibiotalocalcaneal arthrodesis with a retrograde intramedullary nail results in a high rate of healing and patient satisfaction as well as relatively few complications.

115. Mazur JM, Schwartz E, Simon S: Ankle arthrodesis: Long-term follow-up with gait analysis. *J Bone Joint Surg Am* 1979;61:964-975.

116. Thomas R, Daniels TR, Parker K: Gait analysis and functional outcomes following ankle arthrodesis for isolated ankle arthritis. *J Bone Joint Surg Am* 2006;88: 526-535.

The authors compare the intermediate-term clinical results for a group of patients in whom an ankle arthrodesis had been performed using modern surgical techniques with findings for a group of healthy gender- and age-matched control subjects. They concluded that an ankle fusion will help relieve pain and improve overall function; however, it is a salvage procedure that will cause persistent alterations in gait with a potential for deterioration caused by the development of ipsilateral hindfoot arthritis.

117. Waters RL, Barnes G, Husserl T, Silver L, Liss R: Comparable energy expenditure after arthrodesis of the hip and ankle. *J Bone Joint Surg Am* 1988;70: 1032-1037.

118. Muir DC, Amendola A, Saltzman CL: Long-term outcome of ankle arthrodesis. *Foot Ankle Clin* 2002;7: 703-708.

119. Trouillier H, Hansel L, Schaff P, Rosemeyer B, Refior HJ: Long-term results after ankle arthrodesis: Clinical, radiological, gait analytical aspects. *Foot Ankle Int* 2002;23:1081-1090.

120. Sheridan BD, Robinson DE, Hubble MJ, Winson IG: Ankle arthrodesis and its relationship to ipsilateral arthritis of the hind- and mid-foot. *J Bone Joint Surg Br* 2006;88:206-207.

The authors reviewed the preoperative radiographs of 70 patients with osteoarthritis of the ankle treated with 71 ankle arthrodesis procedures. Sixty-eight patients showed preexisting arthritis in either the hindfoot or midfoot, with the subtalar joint the most commonly affected. Ipsilateral hindfoot and midfoot arthritis is almost universally present in patients with arthritis of the ankle requiring arthrodesis. The authors suggest that such changes may not be a consequence of arthrodesis.

121. Dyrby C, Chou LB, Andriacchi TP, Mann RA: Functional evaluation of the Scandinavian Total Ankle Replacement. *Foot Ankle Int* 2004;25:377-381.

The authors evaluated the function of the ankle joint during walking before and after arthroplasty with the STAR prosthesis. Patients treated with arthroplasty showed reduced range of motion at the ankle compared with the control group; however, the moment in arthroplasty patients was increased, indicating improved function of the ankle joint.

122. Piriou P, Culpan P, Mullins M, Cardon JN, Pozzi D, Judet T: Ankle replacement versus arthrodesis: A comparative gait analysis study. *Foot Ankle Int* 2008;29: 3-9.

Gait analysis was performed before and after ankle arthroplasty in 12 patients and compared with 12 patients treated with ankle fusion and with a healthy control group of 12 patients. Ankle arthrodesis resulted in a faster gait with a longer step length compared with ankle replacement. The ankle replacement group had greater movement at the ankle, symmetrical timing of gait, and a restored ground reaction force pattern.

123. Doets HC, van Middelkoop M, Houdijk H, Nelissen RG, Veeger HE: Gait analysis after successful mobile bearing total ankle replacement. *Foot Ankle Int* 2007; 28:313-322.

The gait of 10 patients who underwent an uneventful, unilateral, mobile-bearing total ankle replacement was compared with that of 10 control subjects. The authors concluded that the groups had a nearly normal gait pattern in terms of joint kinematics of the knee, ankle, and foot after uneventful mobile-bearing total ankle replacement. The ground reaction forces and the electromyogram activity, however, did not fully normalize in the arthroplasty group.

124. Haddad SL, Coetzee JC, Estok R, Fahrbach K, Banel D, Nalysnyk L: Intermediate and long-term outcomes of total ankle arthroplasty and ankle arthrodesis: A systematic review of the literature. *J Bone Joint Surg Am* 2007;89:1899-1905.

The purpose of this study was to determine whether there are sufficient objective cumulative data in the literature to compare total ankle arthroplasty and ankle arthrodesis. After a systematic review of the literature, the authors concluded that the intermediate outcome of total ankle arthroplasty appears to be similar to that of ankle arthrodesis; however, data were sparse. Level of evidence: IV.

125. Stengel D, Bauwens K, Ekkernkamp A, Cramer J: Efficacy of total ankle replacement with meniscal-bearing devices: A systematic review and meta-analysis. *Arch Orthop Trauma Surg* 2005;125:109-119.

A systematic meta-analysis of studies exploring the efficacy of three-component total ankle prostheses was conducted. The authors concluded that ankle arthroplasty improves pain and joint mobility in endstage ankle arthritis but its performance in comparison with the current reference standard (ankle fusion) remains to be defined in a properly designed randomized trial.

126. Buchner M, Sabo D: Ankle fusion attributable to posttraumatic arthrosis: A long-term followup of 48 patients. *Clin Orthop Relat Res* 2003;406 :155-164.

This study justifies the value of ankle fusion as a surgical treatment option in patients with end-stage arthrosis in the ankle, provided that precise intraoperative positioning of the arthrodesis and the importance of the subtalar joint are given due consideration.

127. Volkov MV, Oganesian OV: Restoration of function in the knee and elbow with a hinge-distractor appara-

3: Arthritis

tus. *J Bone Joint Surg Am* 1975;57:591-600.

128. Aldegheri R, Trivella G, Saleh M: Articulated distraction of the hip: Conservative surgery for arthritis in young patients. *Clin Orthop Relat Res* 1994;301:94-101.

129. van Roermund PM, Lafeber FP: Joint distraction as treatment for ankle osteoarthritis. *Instr Course Lect* 1999;48:249-254.

130. van Valburg AA, van Roermund PM, Lammens J, et al: Can Ilizarov joint distraction delay the need for an arthrodesis of the ankle? A preliminary report. *J Bone Joint Surg Br* 1995;77:720-725.

131. Lafeber F, Veldhuijzen JP, Vanroy JL, Huber-Bruning O, Bijlsma JW: Intermittent hydrostatic compressive force stimulates exclusively the proteoglycan synthesis of osteoarthritic human cartilage. *Br J Rheumatol* 1992;31:437-442.

132. van Valburg AA, van Roy HL, Lafeber FP, Bijlsma JW: Beneficial effects of intermittent fluid pressure of low physiological magnitude on cartilage and inflammation in osteoarthritis: An in vitro study. *J Rheumatol* 1998;25:515-520.

133. Salter RB, Simmonds DF, Malcolm BW, Rumble EJ, MacMichael D, Clements ND: The biological effect of continuous passive motion on the healing of full-thickness defects in articular cartilage: An experimental investigation in the rabbit. *J Bone Joint Surg Am* 1980;62:1232-1251.

134. Hung SC, Nakamura K, Shiro R, Tanaka K, Kawahara H, Kurokawa T: Effects of continuous distraction on cartilage in a moving joint: An investigation on adult rabbits. *J Orthop Res* 1997;15:381-390.

135. van Valburg AA, van Roermund PM, Marijnissen AC, et al: Joint distraction in treatment of osteoarthritis (II): Effects on cartilage in a canine model. *Osteoarthritis Cartilage* 2000;8:1-8.

136. Karadam B, Karatosun V, Murat N, Ozkal S, Gunal I: No beneficial effects of joint distraction on early microscopical changes in osteoarthrotic knees: A study in rabbits. *Acta Orthop* 2005;76:95-98.

Osteoarthrosis was induced by intra-articular papain injection into rabbit knees. Joint distraction did not have any beneficial effect on the osteoarthrotic cartilage; animals undergoing nonarticulated distraction had worse results. Level of evidence: II.

137. Kajiwara R, Ishida O, Kawasaki K, Adachi N, Yasunaga Y, Ochi M: Effective repair of a fresh osteochondral defect in the rabbit knee joint by articulated joint distraction following subchondral drilling. *J Orthop Res* 2005;23:909-915.

A combination of subchondral drilling, joint motion, and distraction by an articulated external fixator promoted repair of a fresh osteochondral defect in the weight-bearing area of the rabbit knee joint. Although 4 weeks of distraction was not a long enough period to repair the defect, distraction for 8 and 12 weeks resulted in good outcomes. Level of evidence: III.

138. Yanai T, Ishii T, Chang F, Ochiai N: Repair of large full-thickness articular cartilage defects in the rabbit: The effects of joint distraction and autologous bone-marrow-derived mesenchymal cell transplantation. *J Bone Joint Surg Br* 2005;87:721-729.

Using a rabbit knee model, investigators found that repair of large cartilaginous defects can be enhanced by joint distraction, especially when accompanied by ACBMT along with collagen gel. Level of evidence: II.

139. Paley D, Lamm BM: Ankle joint distraction. *Foot Ankle Clin* 2005;10:685-698.

In this review article, the authors outline in detail the technique of articulated joint distraction for the ankle joint and suggest an "a la carte" approach to treating ankle arthritis. Level of evidence: III.

140. Sabharwal S, Schwechter EM: Five-year followup of ankle joint distraction for post-traumatic chondrolysis in an adolescent: A case report. *Foot Ankle Int* 2007;28:942-948.

Articulated joint distraction was used to successfully treat an adolescent with severe posttraumatic aseptic chondrolysis of the ankle joint with satisfactory clinical and radiographic outcomes at 5.5-year follow-up. Level of evidence: IV.

141. Bottlang M, Marsh JL, Brown TD: Articulated external fixation of the ankle: Minimizing motion resistance by accurate axis alignment. *J Biomech* 1999;32:63-70.

142. Chiodo CP, McGarvey W: Joint distraction for the treatment of ankle osteoarthritis. *Foot Ankle Clin* 2004;9:541-553.

The authors present an overview of the rationale, surgical technique, clinical results, and pitfalls of joint distraction for ankle arthritis. Level of evidence: III.

143. van Valburg AA, van Roermund PM, Marijnissen AC, et al: Joint distraction in treatment of osteoarthritis: A two-year follow-up of the ankle. *Osteoarthritis Cartilage* 1999;7:474-479.

144. Marijnissen AC, Van Roermund PM, Van Melkebeek J, et al: Clinical benefit of joint distraction in the treatment of severe osteoarthritis of the ankle: Proof of concept in an open prospective study and in a randomized controlled study. *Arthritis Rheum* 2002;46:2893-2902.

145. Ploegmakers JJ, van Roermund PM, van Melkebeek J, et al: Prolonged clinical benefit from joint distraction in the treatment of ankle osteoarthritis. *Osteoarthritis Cartilage* 2005;13:582-588.

Based on an average 10-year follow-up (range, 7 to 15 years) after joint distraction, 16 of 22 patients (73%) had improvement in pain and functional scores, with minimal improvement in ankle joint mobility. Patient factors indicating nonresponse to this form of surgical treatment are unknown. Level of evidence: III.

146. Morse KR, Flemister AS, Baumhauer JF, DiGiovanni BF: Distraction arthroplasty. *Foot Ankle Clin* 2007;12: 29-39.

The authors present an up-to-date review article on the history, basic science, and surgical techniques of distraction arthroplasty of the ankle. The clinical results of various studies are detailed. Level of evidence: III.

147. Williams SK, Amiel D, Ball ST, et al: Prolonged storage effects on the articular cartilage of fresh human osteochondral allografts. *J Bone Joint Surg Am* 2003;85: 2111-2120.

The authors examined the changes in human allograft cartilage as a function of storage for different lengths of time. Cell viability and density were determined by confocal microscopy. Metabolic activity and biomechanical properties also were measured. It was concluded that the cartilage matrix is preserved for 28 days; however, there is a decrease in cartilage viability and metabolic activity after 14 days.

148. Reider B: *The Orthopaedic Physical Exam.* Philadelphia, PA, Elsevier, Inc, 2005.

The authors describe current physical examination techniques for the evaluation of foot and ankle pathology.

149. Coughlin MJ, Mann RA: *Surgery of the Foot and Ankle.* St Louis, MO, Mosby, 1999.

150. Gross AE, Agnidis Z, Hutchison CR: Osteochondral defects of the talus treated with fresh osteochondral allograft transplantation. *Foot Ankle Int* 2001;22:385-391.

151. Reikeras O, Shegarfi H, Naper C, Reinholt FP, Rolstad B: Impact of MHC mismatch and freezing on bone graft incorporation: An experimental study in rats. *J Orthop Res* 2008;26:925-931.

The authors studied the syngeneic and allogeneic tibia cortical allografts in rats. The fresh allogeneic grafts had less blood flow and ultimately less bone bridging, mineral content, and torsional strength compared with fresh syngeneic allograft.

152. Rodrigo JJ, Schnaser AM, Reynolds HM Jr, et al: Inhibition of the immune response to experimental fresh osteoarticular allografts. *Clin Orthop Relat Res* 1989; 243:235-253.

153. Sirlin CB, Brossmann J, Boutin RD, et al: Shell osteochondral allografts of the knee: Comparison of MR imaging findings and immunologic responses. *Radiology* 2001;219:35-43.

154. Williams SK, Amiel D, Ball ST, et al: Analysis of cartilage tissue on a cellular level in fresh osteochondral allograft retrievals. *Am J Sports Med* 2007;35:2022-2032.

This study shows long-term chondrocyte viability in fresh osteochondral allografts.

Chapter 15

Hindfoot Osteoarthritis and Fusion

*Adolph S. Flemister Jr, MD

Introduction

Approximately one half of the elderly population of the United States is estimated to have some form of arthritis involving the foot or ankle, with osteoarthritis (OA) the most common type.[1] Hindfoot OA is a frequent sequelae of fractures and dislocations but also may be primarily degenerative in nature (**Figure 1**). Regardless of the etiology, hindfoot OA can be a painful and disabling condition. If significant deformity is present, patients will experience pain and difficulty with shoe wear, which can lead to skin irritation and breakdown.

Anatomy and Biomechanics

The hindfoot consists of the talonavicular, subtalar, and calcaneocuboid joints. These joints work together in a complex manner and are mainly responsible for inversion and eversion movements that allow the hindfoot to accommodate ambulation on uneven ground. During the normal gait cycle, coupled movements of the hindfoot with the tibia allow the foot to lock the transverse tarsal joint at heel rise, creating a rigid lever for push off, and to unlock the transverse tarsal joint at heel strike, allowing the foot to act as a shock absorber. Arthritic conditions of the hindfoot limit the foot's ability to invert and evert and thereby disrupt normal gait mechanics, leading to significant dysfunction.

History and Physical Examination

Patients with symptomatic hindfoot arthritis report pain, swelling, and stiffness of the foot. Patients often describe ankle pain, but will localize this pain to the sinus tarsi or areas distal to the medial and lateral malleoli. This pain is often aggravated by ambulating on uneven ground. The physical examination begins with a careful analysis of barefoot walking, with the physician noting gait disturbances and the position of the foot during stance. On barefoot weight bearing, the overall alignment of the limb from the knees to the toes should

be assessed. Foot position must be evaluated for the presence of excessive hindfoot varus or valgus, which lead to forefoot pronation and supination. Any areas of swelling and tenderness should be recorded. The joints of the hindfoot and midfoot should be assessed for mobility and to determine if deformities are flexible or fixed. The flexibility of the cavus hindfoot can be further determined using the Coleman block test.[2] Motion of the hindfoot is often difficult to quantify and should be compared with the uninvolved contralateral limb. Active and passive ankle motion and the presence of Achilles tendon or isolated gastrocnemius tightness should be evaluated.[3] A detailed neurovascular examination also should be performed to determine weakness in any muscle of the foot or ankle, loss of sensation, and the presence or absence of pulses. Patients without palpable pulses must be further evaluated with vascular studies, especially if surgery is considered.

Imaging

Weight-bearing radiographs are essential to accurately assess alignment and the degree of degenerative changes in the joints. AP, oblique, and lateral radiographs of the foot are routinely obtained. Weight-bearing ankle studies are necessary to evaluate tibiotalar joint asymmetry, loose bodies, and other manifestations of ankle pathology that may present as hindfoot arthritis. CT may be helpful to evaluate rigid deformities; however, because these scans are usually non–weight-bearing studies, they are less helpful in evaluating flexible deformities. MRI may be used to evaluate more subtle arthritic changes, but is not routinely needed.

Nonsurgical Treatment

A variety of braces, shoe wear modifications, and orthotic devices are used in the treatment of hindfoot OA.[4] These devices act as mechanical aids to limit painful joint motion, accommodate rigid deformity, help correct flexible deformity, and relieve pressure from sensitive areas. Such devices may be used to provide temporary treatment for patients who wish to delay surgery for medical or personal reasons or as definitive treatment in those who are not candidates for or wish to avoid surgical treatment.

*Adolph S. Flemister Jr, MD or the department with which he is affiliated has received research or institutional support from Aircast and Biomedics.

3: Arthritis

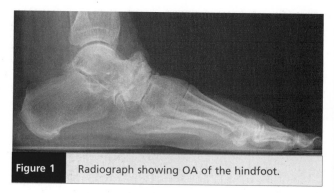

Figure 1 Radiograph showing OA of the hindfoot.

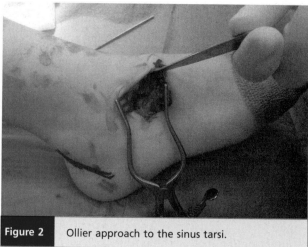

Figure 2 Ollier approach to the sinus tarsi.

Ankle-foot orthoses (AFOs) are made in a variety of designs and from a variety of materials. Regardless of the type of design or material used, the primary goal of these devices is to control hindfoot motion and alignment. A solid AFO made of lightweight polypropylene has traditionally been used to treat patients with ankle and hindfoot arthritis. This type of AFO typically extends from the toes to just below the knee and provides rigid control to both the ankle and hindfoot. Because these devices tend to be bulky and uncomfortable with long-term use, lower profile devices such as the Arizona AFO (Ernesto Castro, Mesa, AZ) have been developed.[5]

Devices worn within the shoe, such as the University of California Biomechanics Laboratory orthosis, are used to correct flexible hindfoot deformity and limit painful hindfoot motion. However, because these devices are made from rigid polypropylene, they tend to put pressure on bony prominences and may be poorly tolerated by some patients. Such devices are contraindicated in patients with rigid deformities and peripheral neuropathy.

Surgical Treatment

Arthrodesis of the involved joints remains the treatment of choice for symptomatic hindfoot arthritis in patients who have not been successfully treated with bracing or do not choose to wear a brace.

Fusing all three joints of the triple joint complex is controversial if only one or two joints are primarily involved. Arthrodesis of one joint of the triple joint complex tends to limit the motion of the other two joints; arthrodesis of the talonavicular joint has the greatest effect on the remaining joints.[6] Arthrodesis of the talonavicular joint results in approximately a 90% loss of subtalar and calcaneocuboid joint motion, whereas arthrodesis of the subtalar joint limits talonavicular joint motion by 75% and calcaneocuboid motion by 55%. Isolated arthrodesis of the calcaneocuboid joint will result in the least loss of motion to the hindfoot, with the talonavicular joint maintaining 67% of its motion and the subtalar joint 92% of its motion. The clinical benefit of retaining maximal motion of the hindfoot complex is unknown, although it may theoretically mini-

mize the long-term complication of contiguous joint arthritis.

Subtalar Arthrodesis

Isolated subtalar arthrodesis is indicated for a variety of conditions including nontraumatic arthritis, posttraumatic arthritis, deformity secondary to posterior tibial tendon dysfunction, and residual talocalcaneal coalition. Surgical techniques for isolated subtalar arthrodesis vary depending on the pathologic findings. In situ arthrodeses are performed when correction of deformity is not required. Most in situ arthrodeses are performed with the patient supine or in the lateral decubitus position using a lateral approach.[7] Typically, either a longitudinal incision or a transverse Ollier incision is used (**Figure 2**). One or two lag screws may be used depending on the surgeon's preference. Regardless of the surgical technique, final heel alignment should be neutral to slightly valgus.

Subtalar arthritis associated with a calcaneal fracture malunion is challenging to treat. To variable degrees, these malunions leave the hindfoot shortened, widened, and malaligned (**Figure 3**). In addition to painful subtalar arthritis, the residual deformity results in lateral calcaneofibular impingement associated with lateral wall "blowout" and anterior tibiotalar impingement caused by loss of talar declination and subsidence of the talus into the fractured calcaneus. Successful treatment of these calcaneal malunions requires subtalar arthrodesis and restoration of the height, width, and alignment of the hindfoot. A lateral wall exostectomy will relieve only lateral impingement. If the patient has acceptable ankle dorsiflexion without anterior impingement, an in situ subtalar fusion may be performed (**Figure 4**). When anterior impingement is present, restoration of talar declination with subtalar distraction bone block arthrodesis is needed. This procedure requires that a bone block graft be placed in the subtalar posterior facet followed by placement of position screws to hold the graft in place. If hindfoot malalignment (usually varus malalignment) is present, an osteotomy of the calcaneal tuberosity is needed. Treatment protocols

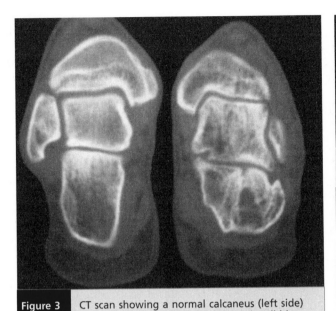

Figure 3 CT scan showing a normal calcaneus (left side) and calcaneal malunion with lateral wall blow-out and subtalar arthritis (right side).

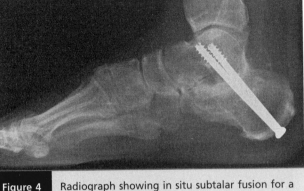

Figure 4 Radiograph showing in situ subtalar fusion for a calcaneal malunion.

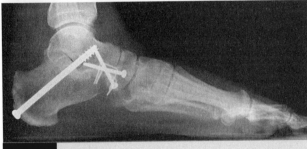

Figure 5 Radiograph showing triple arthrodesis of the hindfoot with internal fixation.

that address all aspects of the calcaneal malunion are effective in relieving pain and restoring function.[8]

Following subtalar arthrodesis, most patients have some degree of residual pain and dysfunction regardless of the indication for the procedure or the technique used.[9-11] Worse outcomes occur in patients with diabetes mellitus and those claiming workers' compensation benefits.[10] Union rates ranging from 86% to 95% have been reported in large studies.[8-10] Factors associated with higher rates of nonunion include older patient age, smoking, and the presence of avascular bone in the posterior facet.

Arthroscopic Subtalar Arthrodesis

Arthroscopically assisted in situ subtalar arthrodesis may be performed in patients with minimal or no deformity.[12,13] The patient may be supine, prone, or in the lateral decubitus position. In the supine and lateral decubitus positions, anterolateral portals and a posterolateral portal are commonly used. If the patient is prone, one posteromedial and either one or two posterolateral portals are used to denude the posterior talocalcaneal facet. Bone grafting may be performed percutaneously and screws are used for fixation. Union rates and clinical outcomes are comparable to those achieved with open arthrodesis. No major neurovascular complications have been described.

Triple Arthrodesis

Triple arthrodesis of the hindfoot may be performed using various combinations of screws, staples, and plates (**Figure 5**). Restoration of a plantigrade foot with a sightly valgus heel is essential for a successful outcome. In the long term, most patients have persistent pain with ambulation on uneven ground and during recreational activities. Compensatory OA of the sur-

rounding joints of the midfoot and ankle is common.[14] Despite these progressive complications, overall patient satisfaction is high.

Talonavicular and Calcaneocuboid Arthrodesis

Isolated talonavicular arthrodesis is indicated for arthritis confined to that joint or in some patients with severe abduction deformity associated with acquired adult flatfoot deformity.[15,16] If osteonecrosis of the navicular is present, degenerative changes also will be present at the naviculocuneiform joints. Fusion should include the naviculocuneiform and the talonavicular joint (**Figure 6**). High fusion rates can be achieved with the use of internal fixation; successful clinical outcomes have been reported. As is the situation in other hindfoot fusions, progressive OA of the surrounding foot and ankle is likely to occur.

Isolated arthrodesis of the calcaneocuboid joint is most commonly performed as a distraction bone block procedure to correct severe abduction deformity associated with acquired adult flatfoot.[17,18] In this operation, a wedge of bone is placed in a denuded calcaneocuboid joint in an effort to restore coverage of the talonavicular joint (**Figure 7**). This procedure is most often combined with medial-sided procedures, such as transfer of the flexor digitorum longus tendon to the navicular or fusion of an unstable first tarsometatarsal articulation. Although successful clinical outcomes are possible, some patients may experience prolonged lateral foot pain. Nonunion rates are high and hardware removal is

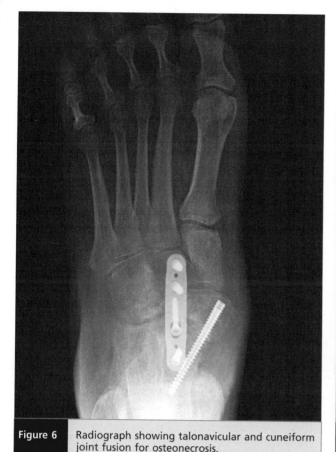

Figure 6 Radiograph showing talonavicular and cuneiform joint fusion for osteonecrosis.

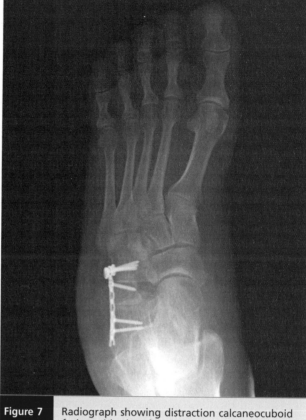

Figure 7 Radiograph showing distraction calcaneocuboid fusion with plate fixation.

frequently required. Union rates can be improved with the use of plate fixation versus fixation with screws only.

External Fixation in Hindfoot Arthrodesis

Circular and hybrid external fixation provide alternative techniques to achieve hindfoot arthrodesis and offer the advantage of gradual correction of complex deformity, thereby minimizing soft-tissue complications.[19] Circular fixators also allow lengthening with fusion. This type of fixation is indicated in patients with complex hindfoot deformities, soft-tissue compromise, significant shortening, and infection. High union rates can be achieved in patients with most types of pin site complications. Because of the complex nature of these procedures, they should be performed only by surgeons with experience in these techniques.

Supplemental Adjuncts of Hindfoot Arthrodeses

The need for supplemental bone grafting for hindfoot arthrodeses is controversial. Because nonunion can be a devastating complication, many surgeons routinely use some type of supplemental bone graft, even in primary hindfoot fusions. Graft material from the proximal or distal tibia and calcaneus are alternative donor sites to the iliac crest. Major wound complications from these

sites are rare, with minor incisional hypersensitivity or numbness the most common complications.[20,21]

Multiple alternatives to autologous bone graft have been suggested to avoid potential donor site morbidity and enhance union rates. In small studies, freeze-dried, cancellous allograft bone; demineralized bone matrix; and coralline hydroxyapatite have shown fusion rates similar to autografts.[11,22,23] Large prospective studies comparing autograft with these types of bone graft substitutes are needed.

Platelet-rich plasma, derived from autologous blood, is an abundant source of growth factors believed to enhance bone healing.[24] In a complex mechanism, platelet degranulation leads to release of growth factors, which stimulate stem cell lines and eventually enhance bone healing. Use in the hindfoot has been suggested for certain patients with risk factors for nonunion such as smoking and diabetes mellitus. Platelet-rich plasma may be used alone or combined with autograft or allograft.

Contractures of the Gastrocnemius-Soleus Complex

Contractures of the gastrocnemius-soleus complex may develop in many patients with hindfoot OA, especially if a flatfoot deformity is present.[25] It is important to distinguish isolated gastrocnemius tightness from a combined gastrocnemius-soleus (Achilles) contracture. Patients with isolated gastrocnemius tightness exhibit decreased ankle dorsiflexion with the knee extended, whereas those with an Achilles contracture have decreased ankle dorsiflexion with the knee held in both flexion and extension. Patients with an isolated gastrocnemius contracture can be treated with a release of the gastrocnemius. Patients with a combined Achilles contracture require open or percutaneous lengthening of the tendon.

Postoperative Course and Evaluation

Postoperative care following hindfoot arthrodesis varies among surgeons. Most protocols involve an 8- to 12-week period with non–weight-bearing restrictions and a similar period of cast wear. In general, patients are allowed to bear weight when there is radiographic evidence of healing. However, evaluation using plain radiographs tends to provide an overestimation of the amount of fusion; CT scans provide more reliable evaluation.[26]

Summary

Hindfoot OA is a common disorder that can be challenging to treat. Currently, there are no joint-sparing procedures for the patient with hindfoot arthritis who is unresponsive to conservative measures. Hindfoot arthrodeses, although considered salvage procedures, remain the gold standard for treating this often painful and disabling condition. Improvement in arthrodesis techniques focuses on increasing the rate of fusion and decreasing the time to fusion. Arthroscopic techniques offer the potential to achieve these goals by minimizing soft-tissue damage. The use of newer nonautologous bone graft materials may eliminate donor site morbidity while enhancing the rates of fusion and recovery.

Annotated References

1. Lawrence RC, Helmick CG, Arnett FC, et al: Estimates of the prevalence of arthritis and selected musculoskeletal disorders in the United States. *Arthritis Rheum* 1998;41:778-799.

2. Younger AS, Hansen ST Jr: Adult cavovarus foot. *J Am Acad Orthop Surg* 2005;13:302-315.

   The authors review the diagnosis and management of all aspects of the cavovarus foot including fusion for arthritic joints. An emphasis is placed on soft-tissue balancing and restoring a plantigrade foot.

3. Digiovanni CW, Kuo R, Tejweni N, et al: Isolated gastrocnemius tightness. *J Bone Joint Surg Am* 2002;84:962-970.

4. Cohen BE: Orthotic and pedorthic management of the arthritic foot and ankle. *Foot Ankle Clin* 1999;4:293-302.

5. Augustin JF, Lin SS, Berberian WS, et al: Nonoperative treatment of adult acquired flat foot with the Arizona brace. *Foot Ankle Clin* 2003;8:491-502.

   The design of the Arizona brace, a custom molded AFO, and its indications for use are described. The use of this brace to control hindfoot deformity is specifically discussed.

6. Astion DJ, Deland JT, Otis JC, et al: Motion of the hindfoot after simulated arthrodesis. *J Bone Joint Surg Am* 1997;79:241-246.

7. Greisberg J, Sangeorzan B: Hindfoot arthrodesis. *J Am Acad Orthop Surg* 2007;15:65-71.

   The authors review indications, contraindications, and surgical technique for hindfoot arthrodesis. A detailed discussion of medial and lateral approaches and fixation methods is provided. Alternative arthrodesis techniques are discussed.

8. Clare MP, Lee WE, Sanders RW: Intermediate to long-term results of a treatment protocol for calcaneal fracture malunions. *J Bone Joint Surg Am* 2005;87:963-973.

   The authors present a retrospective study of 45 feet treated for calcaneal malunions following nonsurgical treatment. Using a protocol designed to restore anatomic alignment, a plantigrade foot was achieved in all 45 feet and union in 93%. Level of evidence: IV.

9. Davies MB, Rosenfeld PF, Stavrou P, et al: A comprehensive review of subtalar arthrodesis. *Foot Ankle Int* 2007;28:295-297.

   A retrospective review of 95 isolated subtalar fusions, most using a single screw and local bone graft, is presented. A 95% union rate was achieved with 93% of patients having a good or fair outcome. Level of evidence: IV.

10. Chahal J, Stephen DJ, Bulmer B, et al: Factors associated with outcome after subtalar arthrodesis. *J Orthop Trauma* 2006;20:555-561.

    In this retrospective review of 88 patients, smokers were 3.8 times more likely to have a nonunion after subtalar arthrodesis. In general, patients with subtalar arthrodeses had significantly worse functional outcomes compared with normative populations. The worst outcomes occurred in patients with diabetes and those receiving workers' compensation. Level of evidence: III.

11. Easley ME, Trinka HJ, Schon LC, et al: Isolated subtalar arthrodesis. *J Bone Joint Surg Am* 2000;82:613-624.

12. Amendola A, Lee KB, Saltzman CL, et al: Technique and early experience with posterior arthroscopic subtalar arthrodesis. *Foot Ankle Int* 2007;28:298-302.

    Eleven arthroscopic fusions in 10 patients were retrospectively evaluated. All patients had minimal or no deformity. There was one nonunion and 9 of 10 patients were satisfied with the procedure. Level of evidence: IV.

13. Glanzmann MC, Sanhueza-Hernandez R: Arthroscopic subtalar arthrodesis for symptomatic osteoarthritis of the hindfoot: A prospective study of 41 cases. *Foot Ankle Int* 2007;28:2-7.

This retrospective review evaluated 37 patients treated with arthroscopic subtalar arthrodesis. Union was achieved in all 37 patients. Level of evidence: IV.

14. Smith RW, Shen W, Dewitt S, Reischl SF: Triple arthrodesis in adults with non-paralytic disease: A minimum ten-year follow-up study. *J Bone Joint Surg Am* 2004; 86:2707-2713.

The authors present a retrospective review of 31 feet treated for hindfoot OA with triple arthrodesis and followed for an average of 14 years. Most patients were satisfied with the procedure; however, 59% experienced pain with moderate activity and 74% had difficulty ambulating on uneven ground.

15. Castro MD: Arthrodesis of the navicular. *Foot Ankle Clin* 2004;9:73-83.

A comprehensive review of the management of OA of the talonavicular-cuneiform complex is presented. Indications and techniques for isolated fusion are outlined.

16. Chen CH, Huang PJ, Chen TB, et al: Isolated talonavicular arthrodesis for talonavicular arthritis. *Foot Ankle Int* 2001;22:633-636.

17. van der Krans A, Louwerens JW, Anderson P: Adult acquired flatfoot deformity treated by calcaneocuboid distraction arthrodesis, posterior tibial tendon augmentation, and percutaneous Achilles lengthening: A prospective outcome study of 20 patients. *Acta Orthop* 2006;77:156-163.

In this retrospective study, 10 of 20 patients had medial column fusions for flatfoot deformity. Seventeen patients had complete relief of pain and nonunion occurred in two. These procedures resulted in significant radiographic improvement of the flatfoot deformity. Level of evidence: IV.

18. Toolan BC, Sangeorzan BJ, Hansen ST: Complex reconstruction for the treatment of dorsolateral peritalar subluxation of the foot: Early results after distraction arthrodesis of the calcaneocuboid joint in conjunction with stabilization of, and transfer of the flexor digitorum tendon to the midfoot to treat acquired pes planovalgus in adults. *J Bone Joint Surg Am* 1999;81: 1545-1560.

19. McGarvey WC: The use of external fixation in arthrodesis and salvage of the foot and ankle. *Foot Ankle Clin* 2002;7:147-173.

20. Raikin SM, Brislin K: Local bone graft harvested from the distal tibia or calcaneus for surgery of the foot and ankle. *Foot Ankle Int* 2005;26:449-453.

Bone graft was harvested from the distal tibia in 70 patients and calcaneus in 44 patients. No major complications were identified. Ten patients had minor complications such as local numbness or initial incisional hypersensitivity. Level of evidence: IV.

21. Geideman W, Early JS, Brodsky J: Clinical results of harvesting autogenous cancellous graft from ipsilateral proximal tibia for use in foot and ankle surgery. *Foot Ankle Int* 2004;25:451-455.

The authors retrospectively evaluated 155 patients treated with foot and ankle surgeries including hindfoot fusions with bone graft harvest from the proximal tibia. An adequate amount of graft was available in all surgeries and donor site complications were minimal. Level of evidence: IV.

22. Coughlin MJ, Grimes JS, Kennedy MP: Coralline hydroxyapatite bone graft substitute in hindfoot surgery. *Foot Ankle Int* 2006;27:19-22.

Coralline hydroxyapatite bone graft substitute was used in 10 patients undergoing hindfoot fusion. One patient had a nonunion of the talonavicular joint. Graft material remained visible on radiographs at 6-year follow-up. Level of evidence: IV.

23. Thordarson DB, Kuehn S: Use of demineralized bone matrix in ankle/hindfoot fusion. *Foot Ankle Int* 2003; 24:557-560.

Sixty-three patients underwent ankle or hindfoot fusion using a demineralized bone matrix compound. Primary union was achieved in 89% of patients. Level of evidence: IV.

24. Liporace FA, Bibbo C, Azad V, et al: Bioadjuvants for complex ankle and hindfoot reconstruction. *Foot Ankle Clin* 2007;12:75-106.

This review article discusses the use of multiple bioadjuvant therapies available to aid in achieving union in foot and ankle surgery. The clinical applications of platelet-rich plasma are presented in detail.

25. Digiovanni CW, Langer P: The role of isolated gastrocnemius and combined Achilles contractures in the flatfoot. *Foot Ankle Clin* 2007;12:363-379.

The diagnosis and management of isolated gastrocnemius and combined Achilles contractures in patients with flatfoot deformities are discussed.

26. Coughlin MJ, Grimes JS, Traughber PD, et al: Comparison of radiographs and CT scans in the prospective evaluation of hindfoot arthrodesis. *Foot Ankle Int* 2006;27:780-787.

The authors compared plain radiographs and CT scans of patients following hindfoot fusions. Studies were performed at 6 weeks, 12 weeks, and 6 months. Progressive fusion was noted at each interval; however, physicians using plain radiographs tended to overestimate the amount of fusion compared with those using CT scans.

Chapter 16

Midfoot and Forefoot Arthritis and Hallux Rigidus

Wayne S. Berberian, MD, MBA   Robert G. Najarian, MD

Introduction

Midfoot and forefoot arthrosis are relatively common clinical disorders treated by foot and ankle specialists. Symptoms are often mild and can be managed by a variety of nonsurgical modalities. As the disease progresses, involvement of the metatarsophalangeal (MTP) joints, midfoot joints, or the transverse longitudinal arch of the foot can lead to disabling symptoms and a loss of function requiring more advanced treatment. This chapter examines midfoot and forefoot arthritis including clinical presentations, pathophysiology, and various treatment options. Common inflammatory arthritides that affect the midfoot and forefoot and hallux rigidus, a common pathologic disorder of the first ray, will be discussed. More information on hallux rigidus can be found in chapter 20.

Midfoot Arthritis

Anatomy and Biomechanics

The midfoot is composed of three distinct articular compartments that form the basis of a columnar division of the foot: the medial, containing the first metatarsal cuneiform (MTC) joint; the central, containing the second and third MTC joints and the intercuneiform joints; and the lateral compartment, containing the cuboid fourth and fifth metatarsal joints. A strong soft-tissue envelope consisting of complex ligamentous connections of dorsal, plantar, and interosseous ligaments provides stability to the midfoot. The three cuneiform joints and cuboid form the transverse arch with the apex at the third MTC articulation.

Midfoot motion has been measured as approximately 10° in the sagittal plane and in supination-pronation at the cubometatarsal joints, and considerably less (0.6° to 3.5°) at the MTC joints. First MTC joint motion averages 4.37° in the sagittal plane. Motion occurs at the naviculocuneiform articulation, but decreases from medial to lateral. The second metatarsal has the least motion, and the third metatarsal has slightly more motion than the second; these two articulations are the most likely sources of painful arthritis. The fourth and fifth metatarsals have more motion in the sagittal and horizontal planes; however, the cubometatarsal articulation is the least likely to be symptomatic even with radiographic evidence of arthritis.

The second metatarsal base is recessed 1 to 4 mm between the medial and lateral cuneiforms. The Lisfranc ligament, a strong oblique interosseous ligament between the second metatarsal base and the medial cuneiform, is the largest in the tarsometatarsal (TMT) complex. The Lisfranc ligament is approximately 8 to 10 mm long and 5 to 6 mm thick. A separate plantar ligament, connecting the medial cuneiform to the second and third metatarsal bases, is the strongest ligament and provides additional stability. Bony and ligamentous structures of the second metatarsal joint provide primary stabilization of the midfoot. The first MTC joint is stabilized during weight bearing primarily by its plantar ligament.

Pathophysiology

Midfoot arthritis can be caused by primary osteoarthrosis, rheumatoid disease, or can be secondary to trauma (such as a Lisfranc fracture-dislocation). As the inflammatory, traumatic, or degenerative process ensues, continued stress is placed across the intercuneiform and MTC joints, causing increased deterioration of these articulations. Osteoarthritis, characterized by destruction of the articular cartilage, joint surface erosion, and periarticular osteophytes, disturbs the complex architectural relationships of the small joints and articulations of the midfoot. As a result, weight bearing places increased stress on the longitudinal arch, leading to pain, a pes planus deformity, and difficulty with ambulation. Bony prominences on the dorsal aspect of the midfoot, which occur as a result of the degenerative process, make it difficult to wear shoes. Continued deterioration of the midfoot leads to altered biomechanics including instability of the MTC joint, osteophyte formation, and a progressive pronation, dorsiflexion, and abduction deformity of the midfoot.

Incidence and Etiology

Arthrosis of the midfoot and the TMT complex occurs as primary degenerative arthrosis and also as a post-

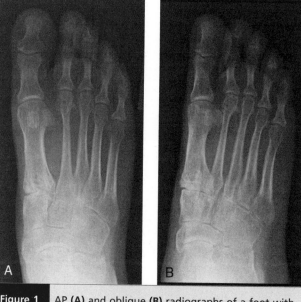

Figure 1   AP **(A)** and oblique **(B)** radiographs of a foot with posttraumatic midfoot arthritis show joint-space narrowing, subchondral sclerosis, and cysts.

Clinical Presentation

The evaluation of patients who present with foot pain begins with a detailed history and physical examination. Pain is the most common presenting symptom of patients with midfoot arthritis and is described as a deep, aching pain that is worse with weight bearing. A bony prominence may be present dorsally at the apex of the arch and can cause local pressure symptoms with shoe wear, resulting in an additional source of pain. Neuritic pain that radiates to the hallux and first webspace can occur secondary to irritation of the deep peroneal, medial dorsal cutaneous branch of the superficial peroneal or saphenous nerve against osteophytes. Pain also can be elicited with extension of the toes; this pain is likely secondary to inflammation of the extensor tendons, which are aggravated by the bony prominence. As the disease process progresses, continued collapse of the arch ensues and a pronated, dorsiflexed, abduction deformity occurs. This deformity further complicates wearing shoes and causes continued pain and pressure against bony prominences.

With the patient standing, both feet are examined to determine the degree and location of the deformity. Both feet are then examined with the patient sitting to determine the passive and active range of motion of the ankle and midfoot, to assess the flexibility of any deformity, and to determine the presence of heel cord contracture. Neurovascular and skin status are assessed. Transverse plane alignment of the metatarsal heads is determined while the patient is sitting. The midfoot also can be stressed with a pronation-abduction maneuver. Each MTC joint should be carefully palpated medially to laterally. When evaluating arthritis at the MTC joint, it is always important to maintain a high index of suspicion for Charcot arthropathy, which can affect the midfoot in patients with neuropathy.

The radiographic evaluation of midfoot arthritis begins with standing AP, lateral, and oblique radiographs of both feet for comparison. The third lateral MTC cuneiform joint absorbs most of the stress during the stance phase and is the most likely area to show the earliest clinical and radiographic signs of osteoarthritis. Joint-space narrowing, osteophytes, subchondral sclerosis, and cysts occur in the later stages of osteoarthritis (**Figure 1**). In patients with significant deformity whose midfoot arthritis is difficult to quantify on plain radiographs, bone scans and/or CT with three-dimensional reconstructions can often be useful, especially for preoperative planning. MRI provides no additional information regarding the extent of arthritic changes and bony erosion and is not routinely used in the evaluation of midfoot arthritis. If the clinical diagnosis remains unclear after repeated examinations, selective injection of lidocaine into the TMT joints under fluoroscopic guidance may be helpful. Pain relief in the fourth and fifth TMT joints has been shown to be a prognostic indicator of the potential success of resection arthroplasty of the lateral column.[2]

traumatic disorder. Studies have shown that patients with primary degenerative arthritis of the TMT complex tend to be older (60 years versus 40 years) and have more extensive arthrosis with greater deformity compared with patients with posttraumatic arthritis. Primary degenerative arthrosis can affect only one joint and may cause no deformity. A recent study of the etiology of midfoot arthrosis examined the role of anatomic factors in the evolution of the degenerative process.[1] The authors compared the relative length of the metatarsals in patients with idiopathic arthrosis of the midfoot with metatarsal length in a group of control patients without arthrosis. Patients with midfoot arthrosis had a different ratio of first to second metatarsal length than did a similarly age-matched cohort without midfoot arthrosis. These patients had a relatively short first metatarsal, a relatively long second metatarsal, or both conditions when compared with a control group without midfoot arthrosis. This finding supports the theory that midfoot arthrosis has a mechanical and/or anatomic etiology. Dorsal osteophyte formation is typically present with severe involvement, but also can be present with isolated joint involvement. It may cause pain with shoe wear or nerve impingement symptoms secondary to compression of the peroneal nerve branches. Posttraumatic arthrosis of the TMT joint complex is prevalent despite advances in the diagnosis and treatment of TMT joint injuries. It can occur following even subtle injuries to the TMT complex. Posttraumatic arthritis is associated with persistent malalignment, collapse of the medial longitudinal arch, and significant articular injury.

Nonsurgical Treatment

The goal of treatment of midfoot arthrosis is to decrease motion across the midfoot and relieve pressure from bony prominences. Nonsurgical treatment modalities include anti-inflammatory medications, shoe modifications, and bracing. Padding and/or skip lacing can decrease pressure from dorsal osteophytes. A shoe with a rocker-bottom sole with or without stiffening provided by an extended steel shank or full-length carbon fiber insert can provide relief. A fixed angle, ankle-foot orthosis is an effective treatment modality that will decrease sagittal plane motion and partially unload the involved joints while providing cushioning, support for the longitudinal arch, and pressure relief for the metatarsal head.

Surgical Treatment

When nonsurgical management fails to provide symptom relief, four main surgical options should be considered in the treatment of midfoot arthritis. The simplest method of surgical treatment involves resection of problematic osteophytes; however, this option may not improve the patient's symptoms. In situ arthrodesis usually involves fusion of the involved midfoot joints, most often the second and third MTC articulations. The first MTC joint is involved less often, and the fourth and fifth cubometatarsal articulation is the least often involved. In situ arthrodesis should be considered only in patients with arthrosis and normal weight-bearing alignment. A variety of internal fixation methods have been described including Kirschner wires (4.0 mm) and/or screws (3.5-mm to 4.5-mm cortical or partially threaded screws), screw fixation without bone graft, and dowel peg iliac crest bone graft with or without screw fixation[3,4] (**Figure 2**). Plate fixation also has been advocated; both medial plating and plantar plating have been popularized. A recent study examined the use of a dorsal, modified, calcaneal plate for extensive midfoot arthrodesis in patients with midfoot arthritis. In patients with involvement of more than four joints, a low-profile dorsally placed calcaneal plate without extensive plantar or medial foot dissection was used. Fusion rates of 95% were achieved in patients with midfoot arthrosis ranging from primary osteoarthrosis to Charcot arthropathy.[5]

Most patients who present for treatment of midfoot arthritis exhibit some degree of deformity. In these patients, arthrodesis must be combined with corrective osteotomies to restore alignment in the sagittal, frontal, and transverse planes and to reconstruct the longitudinal arch. Medial and plantar closing wedge osteotomies will correct the abduction and plantar flexion deformities. Muscle tendon balancing may be required in addition to realignment arthrodesis to completely correct the deformity. Studies have shown that peroneus brevis lengthening or release, peroneus brevis to peroneus longus transfer, posterior tibial tendon reconstruction, and Achilles tendon lengthening or gastrocnemius recession can be used to correct deformities secondary to midfoot

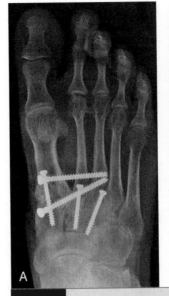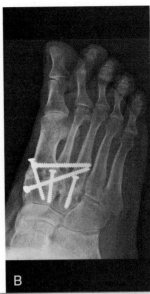

Figure 2   Postoperative AP **(A)** and oblique **(B)** radiographs of the patient shown in Figure 1 who was treated with arthrodesis of the first, second, and third TMT joints. Cannulated screws were used for fixation.

arthritis. If radiographic signs of disease are evident in the intercuneiform complex, these articulations should be included in the fusion. Bone graft, either local autograft or allograft, can be used to improve the fusion rate.

Osteoarthrosis of the TMT joint complex can present with varying degrees of deformity and joint erosion. A recent retrospective study evaluated the spectrum of surgical treatments and clinical outcomes for atraumatic osteoarthrosis of the TMT joints.[6] The authors evaluated 59 patients (67 feet) with atraumatic TMT joint osteoarthritis treated with TMT fusion. Four subtypes were identified based on associated foot deformities: pes planovalgus, hallux valgus, in situ without deformities, and rocker-bottom deformity. Rocker-bottom deformity was corrected with a plantar medial closing wedge resection. A medial sliding calcaneal osteotomy was performed for pes planovalgus deformity. In patients with TMT osteoarthritis with severe pes planovalgus, a lateral column lengthening with medial sliding calcaneal osteotomy was performed; triple arthrodesis was used to treat rigid pes planovalgus. TMT arthritis with hallux valgus deformity was corrected with first TMT joint arthrodesis. American Orthopaedic Foot and Ankle Society (AOFAS) and Medical Outcomes Study 36-Item Short Form scores improved postoperatively. Based on the Foot Function Index, patients reported a high rate of satisfaction (86%); the pes planovalgus group showed significant radiographic improvement. The authors concluded that when classifying feet with atraumatic TMT osteoarthritis into four main categories based on associated deformities, appropriate concurrent procedures can be done

3: Arthritis

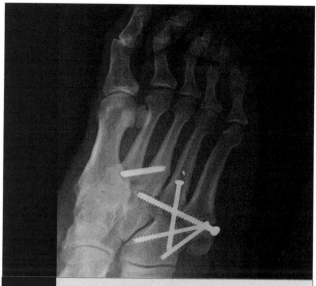

| Figure 3 | Symptoms at the fourth and fifth TMT joints developed in a patient with posttraumatic arthritis who had been previously treated with arthrodesis of the first, second, and third TMT joints. Arthrodesis was extended to include the lateral column. |

resulting in a high rate of satisfaction and improved functional outcomes.

Maintaining mobility of the fourth and fifth TMT joints for ambulation is important in arthrodesis of the midfoot; therefore, fusion of the lateral column is seldom recommended to avoid an extremely rigid midfoot. In patients with a neuropathic foot who need additional stability, it may be necessary to perform arthrodesis of the lateral column joints. In a 2003 retrospective study, 22 feet were treated with complete midfoot arthrodesis (including the lateral column) as part of corrective surgery for a neuropathic rocker-bottom deformity and 6 normosensate feet with painful arthritis involving the lateral joints were treated with arthrodesis of the fourth and fifth TMT joints[7] (Figure 3). A comparison of average preoperative and postoperative scores showed that functional incapacity from lateral midfoot pathology decreased, overall pain scores improved, pain scores in the arthritic subgroup decreased, and the modified overall AOFAS midfoot score improved despite arthrodesis of the lateral column in nonneuropathic feet. Arthroplasty is an alternative procedure to treat lateral column osteoarthritis. A recent retrospective study evaluated eight patients who underwent débridement of the fourth and fifth TMT joints and resection of the base of the lateral two metatarsals with collagen tendon interposition.[2] At a mean follow-up of 25 months, 75% of patients reported satisfactory results with the procedure.

Patients with extensive midfoot arthritis involving the medial and central columns and the naviculocuneiform joint with extension into the cuboid articulations are often treated nonsurgically with an ankle-foot orthosis with forefoot extension or steel shank shoe or boot. If surgical treatment is planned, internal fixation with inlay bone grafting (rectangular slot of bone from the talus to the involved cuneiform bones or metatarsal bases) or interpositional bone grafting should be performed.

Surgical Complications

Early complications associated with the surgical treatment of midfoot arthritis include impaired wound healing, nonunion, malunion, nerve injury, neuroma formation, metatarsalgia, and sesamoid pain. Late complications often involve prominent and bothersome hardware and progressive arthritis of adjacent joints.

Forefoot Arthritis and Hallux Rigidus

Anatomy and Biomechanics

Forefoot arthritis involves degenerative changes of the first MTP joint and the interphalangeal (IP) joints. The first MTP joint is cam shaped and characterized by a convex metatarsal head and concave proximal phalangeal base. Stout medial and lateral collateral ligaments, a metatarsosesamoid suspensory ligament, and a thick plantar plate provide stability to the joint, while musculotendinous structures power the hallux and provide motion at the first MTP joint.

Two sesamoids lie in the articular sulci beneath the first metatarsal head and are embedded within the two tendon slips of the flexor hallucis brevis. The sesamoids protect the metatarsal head and the flexor hallucis longus tendon, distribute load transmission to the medial forefoot, and increase the flexor strength to the hallux. Strong ligamentous attachments stabilize the sesamoids, restricting their motion to approximately 72°.

Incidence and Etiology

Hallux rigidus can be considered a form of degenerative arthrosis affecting the first MTP joint. A broader definition also includes a rarer form of this condition, characterized by the presence of an osteochondral lesion. Its etiology has been associated with causes such as acute traumatic events, repetitive microtrauma, poorly fitting shoe wear, and predisposing anatomic variations of the foot.[8]

A 2006 retrospective cohort study of 1,592 patients over a 13-year period showed an association between increased hindfoot valgus and the subsequent development of osteoarthritis of the first MTP joint.[9] After adjusting for confounding variables, the authors noted that first MTP joint osteoarthritis was 23% more likely to develop in individuals with positive hindfoot valgus than in individuals with normal hindfoot alignment.[9]

Pathophysiology

Arthrosis affecting the first metatarsal head in hallux rigidus begins at the dorsolateral aspect of the joint. It

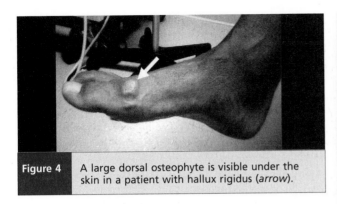

Figure 4 A large dorsal osteophyte is visible under the skin in a patient with hallux rigidus (*arrow*).

is associated with formation of a dorsal osteophyte and joint synovitis. Pathologic specimens taken from patients undergoing surgery for hallux rigidus are uniformly consistent with osteoarthritis.[10]

Clinical Presentation

Symptoms associated with hallux rigidus include pain at the first MTP joint or over the dorsal bony prominence on the first metatarsal head, joint stiffness, joint locking, intolerance to shoe wear, and an everted gait. Physical examination may show palpable or visible dorsal osteophytes, tenderness to palpation, and limited passive range of motion with pain at the extremes or even throughout the entire arc (Figure 4). A late finding is altered gait characterized by supination of the forefoot and resultant transfer lesions beneath the lesser metatarsal heads.

Early radiographic evaluation of the foot shows dorsal and lateral osteophyte formation and subchondral sclerosis (Figure 5). An ossicle may be present at the dorsal margin of the base of the proximal phalanx. Progression of the disease can result in joint-space narrowing and a widened, flattened first metatarsal head (Figure 6). The degree of joint-space narrowing is best evaluated on an internal oblique view because the AP view may overestimate the severity of the disease. Advanced imaging studies are rarely necessary, except if there is suspicion of an osteochondral lesion in a patient with juvenile hallux rigidus. An MRI will confirm the presence of such a lesion.

Hallux rigidus may be misdiagnosed as hallux valgus, gout, or rheumatoid arthritis. Although hallux valgus may coexist with hallux rigidus, this circumstance is relatively uncommon. In a retrospective cohort study of 110 patients, 12% had a hallux valgus angle of more than 15° and a first-second intermetatarsal angle of more than 9°, and only two patients had concurrent symptomatic hallux rigidus and hallux valgus.[8] A thorough history and physical examination should distinguish these diagnoses, especially on the basis of tenderness and pain over the medial eminence rather than over the dorsum of the joint. Acute gout has an episodic presentation with a different radiographic appearance characterized by periarticular erosions. Rheumatoid arthritis commonly presents in the forefoot and should be considered if there is early pain at the first

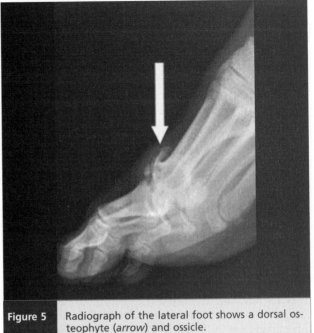

Figure 5 Radiograph of the lateral foot shows a dorsal osteophyte (*arrow*) and ossicle.

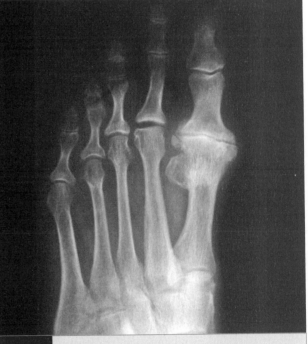

Figure 6 Radiograph of the foot of a patient with severe hallux rigidus. There is marked narrowing of the joint with widening and flattening of the first metatarsal head. Note the incidental flattening of the second metatarsal head resulting from previous Freiberg infraction.

MTP joint without other clinical or radiographic signs. As rheumatoid arthritis progresses, its presentation may be more easily distinguished from that of hallux rigidus because of the presence of hallux valgus deformity and claw toes, as well as radiographic signs of

3: Arthritis

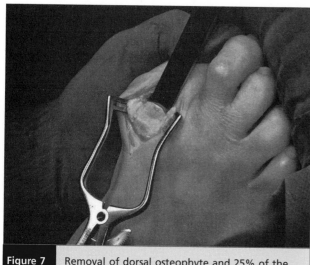

Figure 7 Removal of dorsal osteophyte and 25% of the first metatarsal head during cheilectomy.

concentric joint-space narrowing and the absence of osteophytes.

A grading system that encompasses clinical and radiographic criteria has been proposed as a method to stage the severity of hallux rigidus.[10] Information on this classification system for hallux rigidus is available in chapter 20.

Nonsurgical Treatment

Nonsurgical treatment of hallux rigidus focuses on restricting joint motion to decrease dorsal impingement and secondary synovial inflammation, as well as eliminating pressure over large osteophytes. Techniques that have been used to achieve these goals include taping of the hallux, commercially available orthotic insoles, custom-molded carbon-fiber insoles with a Morton extension, and extra-depth shoes to relieve pressure over large dorsal osteophytes.

Pharmacologic treatment includes the use of oral nonsteroidal anti-inflammatory drugs, intra-articular corticosteroid injections, and intra-articular injections of sodium hyaluronate. One randomized, prospective, single-blinded study evaluated 37 patients with hallux rigidus who were administered either a single intra-articular injection of triamcinolone acetate (a corticosteroid) or a single intra-articular injection of sodium hyaluronate.[11] Twenty feet in each group were compared over a 3-month period with respect to joint pain, AOFAS scores, use of analgesics, and global assessment by the patient and investigator. AOFAS scores at all follow-up visits up to 3 months were significantly better in the sodium hyaluronate group; however, at 1 year after treatment, 46.6% of the patients treated with sodium hyaluronate and 52.9% of patients treated with triamcinolone acetate required surgery because of continued pain and reduced function.

Surgical Treatment

The form of surgical treatment that is chosen depends on the grade and extent of disease, age and activity level of the patient, and the preference and experience of the treating physician. Surgical goals include relief of painful dorsal impingement, relief of pressure over large osteophytes, and lessening of associated secondary synovitis. In patients with symptoms resulting from an osteochondral lesion, débridement and/or drilling of the lesion is advised. In those patients with severe arthrosis at the MTP joint, arthrodesis or arthroplasty has been used to relieve symptoms.

Débridement and Drilling

Osteochondral lesions of the first metatarsal head may mimic the clinical presentation of arthrosis-induced hallux rigidus. These lesions may present acutely or subacutely and are best detected with MRI. Osteophytes or restricted motion may not be present. Dorsal lesions can be treated with dorsal cheilectomy, effectively removing the lesion along with the dorsal aspect of the metatarsal head. Central or plantar lesions are more challenging to treat surgically. Débridement of the chondral flap, with drilling or microfracture technique, may be performed through an open or arthroscopic approach. A recent report described osteoarticular transfer (OATS procedure) used for central lesions of the first metatarsal head. Osteochondral plugs were harvested from the dorsal metatarsal head before performing cheilectomy. No outcome studies are presently available for this procedure.[12]

Cheilectomy

In patients with hallux rigidus of mild to moderate severity, dorsal cheilectomy is the recommended surgical option. In this technique, the dorsal and lateral osteophytes along with approximately 25% of the articular surface of the first metatarsal head are resected through a dorsal approach (Figure 7). This procedure decreases the mechanical impingement of the proximal phalanx on the dorsal osteophyte of the first metatarsal head and removes most or the entire arthritic portion of the joint. Intraoperative passive dorsiflexion should increase to at least 70°.

Moberg Osteotomy

Another surgical technique used in the treatment of hallux rigidus of mild to moderate severity is the dorsal closing wedge osteotomy of the base of the proximal phalanx. In this osteotomy procedure, a portion of the plantar flexion arc is converted into dorsiflexion to create a more functional range of motion for the hallux. This osteotomy has been performed with and without adjunctive dorsal cheilectomy.

Arthrodesis

In those patients with severe hallux rigidus, arthrodesis is the most commonly used procedure with the most extensive supportive literature. By fusing the first MTP joint, arthritic symptoms associated with motion can be eliminated. The full extent of drawbacks to this procedure related to function and gait are yet unknown. One prospective study evaluated gait parameters in 23 patients with hallux rigidus before and after undergoing first MTP arthrodesis.[13] Improvements were noted postoperatively in propulsive power, weight-bearing function of the foot, and stability during gait. However, another study evaluated nine patients who had undergone first MTP arthrodesis and compared the surgical limb with the contralateral limb using kinematic and kinetic gait analysis.[14] Data indicated that the surgical side exhibited a significantly shorter step length with some loss in ankle plantar flexion at toe-off and reduced ankle torque and ankle power at push-off.

Optimal position for arthrodesis of the hallux is approximately 10° to 20° of valgus, 10° to 15° of dorsiflexion with respect to the first metatarsal, or 20° to 30° of dorsiflexion with respect to the plantar aspect of the foot, with rotation equal to the other toes. Because metatarsal declination angles and intermetatarsal angles differ between individuals, optimal angles for arthrodesis may differ as well. Accuracy of the angles used may be more significant than previously believed. A recent study used computer modeling to develop a three-dimensional finite element model of the first ray. Modeling of first MTP arthrodesis showed that a 1° change in dorsiflexion and valgus fixation angles introduced approximated changes in peak hallux pressure of 95 kPa and 22 kPa, respectively.[15]

Many techniques for first MTP arthrodesis have been proposed. These techniques vary according to the method of joint preparation and the type of implant used for fixation. Using a synthetic bone model, five commonly used techniques were compared in a biomechanical study.[16] The most stable technique used a combination of machined conical reaming with an oblique interfragmentary 3.5-mm lag screw and a four-hole dorsal miniplate. This construct was more than two times stronger than an oblique lag screw alone. The two weakest techniques used either a dorsal plate without a lag screw or fixation with Kirschner wires.

Another biomechanical study using a cadaveric model compared crossed 4.0-mm interfragmentary screw fixation with 6.5-mm intramedullary screw fixation.[17] The intramedullary screw was placed through the plantar aspect of the first metatarsal and engaged the intramedullary canal of the proximal phalanx. Cantilever bending was performed. Fixation provided by the intramedullary screw was stiffer and stronger than that provided by the crossed compression screws.

A prospective study reported on 49 patients treated with first MTP joint arthrodesis with a minimum follow-up of 1-year.[18] Dome-shaped reamers with crossed lag screws and a low-profile, contoured, titanium plate were used. The union rate was 92% with 4% of patients requiring revision surgery. Patient satisfaction was reported as 96%. A smaller prospective study using similar methods of joint preparation and

fixation supports these encouraging results.[19]

An alternative method of fixation using parallel 3.5-mm screws was retrospectively reviewed in 60 feet.[20] Screws were introduced through the dorsum of the first metatarsal to engage the plantar cortex of the proximal phalanx. No nonunions were reported and 94% of patients stated that they would have the surgery again.

Another method of fixation had worse results in a retrospective review of 95 consecutive patients.[21] Arthrodesis using a 2.4-mm lag screw and six-hole dorsal plate from the Synthes modular hand set (Synthes USA, Paoli, PA) was performed on 107 feet. Nonunion and mechanical failure occurred in 13% of the arthrodeses. It was concluded that these implants are not sufficiently strong for this application.

Soft-Tissue Arthroplasty

Resection arthroplasty is an alternative to arthrodesis that is used to treat severe hallux rigidus. The Keller procedure consists of excision of the base of the proximal phalanx and may be used to treat elderly patients and those with minimal ambulatory requirements. Sequelae to the procedure may include cock-up hallux deformity, transfer metatarsalgia, weak push-off strength, and shortening of the hallux. In an effort to minimize the incidence of these complications, modifications to the Keller arthroplasty have been proposed. A retrospective review of 18 patients who underwent 21 interposition arthroplasties reports outcomes with one such modification.[22] The procedure included dorsal cheilectomy, resection of 10% of the base of the proximal phalanx to retain the insertion of the flexor hallucis brevis, and interposition of the capsule and extensor hallucis brevis. At a mean follow-up of 38 months, there was an average 37° postoperative increase in joint motion, a complication rate of 6%, and 17 of 18 patients reported that they would have the procedure again.

A recent report describes a modified procedure that consists of a metatarsal cheilectomy combined with an oblique resection of the phalangeal base, thus preserving the attachment of the flexor hallucis brevis.[23] The dorsal joint capsule is interposed in the joint and sutured to the plantar soft tissues. This procedure purports to preserve length and avoid cock-up deformity, although outcome studies are not yet available.

Joint Implant Arthroplasty

Joint implant arthroplasty used for hallux rigidus is a controversial method of treatment. Silicone implant arthroplasty, used in the past, has frequently resulted in prosthetic failure, silicone synovitis, and osteolysis (**Figure 8**). Implant arthroplasty or hemiarthroplasty, using metal prostheses created from titanium or cobalt chrome, is now being performed. Several reports with midterm follow-up are now available. The results of titanium hemiarthroplasty were reported in a retrospective review of 10 patients with a minimum 2.5-year follow-up.[24] All patients improved and were satisfied

3: Arthritis

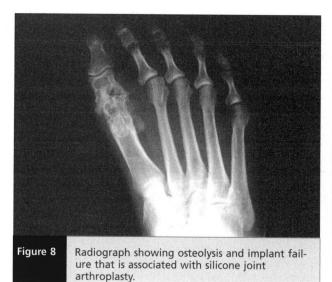

Figure 8   Radiograph showing osteolysis and implant failure that is associated with silicone joint arthroplasty.

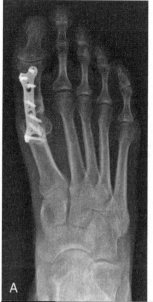
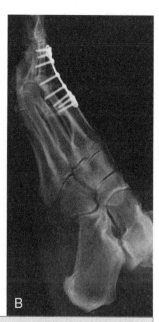

Figure 9   AP **(A)** and lateral **(B)** radiographs of a foot treated with salvage surgery after a failed titanium hemiarthroplasty. The patient had significant shortening of the first ray and required arthrodesis with an interpositional tricortical autograft.

with their outcome in the first 5 years after surgery, but subsidence and lucency in all patients and a painful fracture in one patient brought long-term implant survival into question. The authors concluded that the ultimate longevity of the implant and its long-term functionality are questionable.

Another retrospective review compared long-term clinical and radiographic outcomes of cobalt-chromium hemiarthroplasty to those of arthrodesis performed with screws.[25] Twenty-one hemiarthroplasties and 27 arthrodeses were performed in 46 patients. At the time of final follow-up for each group, satisfaction ratings were superior for the patients who were treated with arthrodesis. Failure occurred in 24% of the hemiarthroplasties, with four subsequently converted to arthrodesis. Eight of the feet with a surviving hemiprosthesis showed evidence of plantar cutout of the prosthetic stem on final follow-up radiographs. The authors concluded that arthrodesis is more predictable than metallic hemiarthroplasty for alleviating symptoms and restoring function in patients with severe hallux rigidus. A randomized prospective study that evaluated 77 feet with hallux rigidus supports this finding.[26] The study compared arthrodesis with total replacement arthroplasty using a titanium and cobalt-chromium prosthesis. Both the phalanx and metatarsal were resurfaced in the arthroplasty group. All arthrodeses united with few complications; in contrast, 6 of the 39 joint prostheses had to be removed because of loosening of the phalangeal component. In the remaining 33 prostheses, the range of motion gained was poor. The cost ratio was 2:1 in favor of arthrodesis; 40% of the patients stated that they would not undergo arthroplasty again.

Salvage Procedures

Failed reconstructive surgery of the first MTP joint presents a challenge for the treating physician. Resection arthroplasty may result in flail toe or cock-up toe defor-

mity, and the first ray is often significantly shortened. Implant arthroplasty may lead to shortening, perhaps involving both the metatarsal and phalanx, and osteolysis surrounding the prosthesis may magnify the deleterious nature of this complication. Reconstructive salvage surgery may involve arthrodesis of the joint; restoration of length with an intercalary structural autograft or allograft may be necessary to avoid transfer metatarsalgia (**Figure 9**). In a retrospective review of patients with failed Keller resection arthroplasty, 29 feet underwent first MTP joint arthrodesis and 21 feet underwent repeat Keller arthroplasty or isolated soft-tissue release.[27] In the arthrodesis group, significant shortening of the first ray was balanced by shortening of the lesser metatarsals rather than by insertion of a bone block at the arthrodesis site. Repeat arthrodesis was performed in five feet because of malposition or pseudarthrosis. In the soft-tissue reconstruction group, AOFAS scores were inferior and most patients were dissatisfied with their outcome. Valgus deviation and cock-up deformity had recurred in most feet at the time of final follow-up. Arthrodesis was recommended for salvage of failed Keller arthroplasty because of the higher rate of patient satisfaction and better clinical results.

A prospective study of arthrodesis performed for failed Keller arthroplasty in 22 feet with a minimum 24-month follow-up showed positive outcomes.[28] Seven feet had intercalary tricortical bone grafts to restore length. Overall, 72% of feet were pain free at final follow-up and 28% had mild, occasional pain. Pedobarographic analysis showed a significant improvement in parameters, with a more physiologic loading

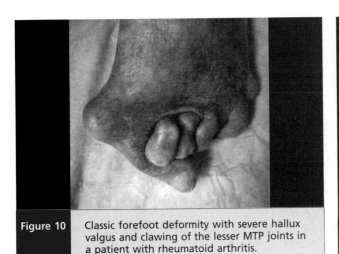

Figure 10 | Classic forefoot deformity with severe hallux valgus and clawing of the lesser MTP joints in a patient with rheumatoid arthritis.

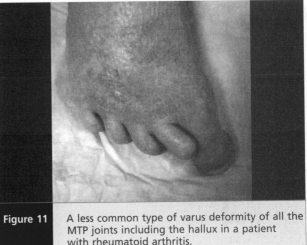

Figure 11 | A less common type of varus deformity of all the MTP joints including the hallux in a patient with rheumatoid arthritis.

pattern occurring under the hallux and metatarsal heads. The procedure was recommended as a safe and reliable technique that resulted in a marked reduction of pain, functional gains, and high rates of patient satisfaction.

Degenerative Arthrosis at Other Forefoot Sites

Degenerative arthrosis can occur at the IP joint of the hallux and can occur in conjunction with hallux rigidus of the MTP joint. A higher incidence of IP arthritis occurs in patients who had previously undergone arthrodesis for hallux rigidus. Other common etiologies of IP joint arthropathy are trauma and psoriasis. Nonsurgical treatment of this condition includes insole modifications to limit joint motion. If this treatment fails, IP joint arthrodesis of the hallux may be performed, usually with an intramedullary screw placed using a distal approach. A retrospective evaluation of seven feet treated with simultaneous arthrodesis of the MTP and IP joints of the ipsilateral hallux revealed adequate resolution of pain and the ability to wear nonprescription shoes.[29] Participation in athletic activities was limited, but there was no interference with moderately demanding daily activities.

Arthrosis at other sites in the forefoot, such as the MTP and IP joints of the lesser toes and the sesamoid-metatarsal articulations, is comparatively rare. Arthrosis at these sites may result from trauma, although late-stage Freiberg infraction can lead to MTP joint degeneration. If nonsurgical treatment fails, lesser toe IP joint arthrosis can be treated with excisional arthroplasty or arthrodesis, whereas MTP arthrosis may require joint débridement.

Inflammatory Arthritides of the Forefoot

Rheumatoid Arthritis

Rheumatoid arthritis is a systemic inflammatory disease that often affects the foot. The pathophysiology consists of an inflammatory synovitis modulated by the patient's immune system, resulting in the destruction of soft-tissue restraints and articular cartilage. The forefoot is commonly involved and is the initial site of involvement in 16% of patients. One study used MRI scans of both the hand and foot to detect early radiographic signs of this autoimmune disorder.[30] MRI scans of the forefeet detected synovitis and bone edema in patients with early rheumatoid arthritis in whom MRI scans of the finger joints were normal. This finding may allow earlier detection of autoimmune disorders and will permit earlier decisions regarding appropriate medications and treatments.

Rheumatoid arthritis occurs in 0.5% to 1% of the population, with the peak incidence occurring in women from 30 to 50 years of age. Although the most commonly affected region in the foot is the MTP joints, the hindfoot joints are often involved as well. Midfoot and ankle involvement is relatively rare. Forefoot disease classically takes the form of a severe hallux valgus deformity (**Figure 10**), but various other hallux deformities have been described, including hallux varus (**Figure 11**). Lesser toe deformities often involve clawing, with dorsal displacement of the MTP joints that may progress to subluxation or dislocation. This constellation of deformities leads to painful metatarsalgia and joint pain that is most symptomatic with weight-bearing activities and produces difficulties with gait. In a cross-sectional, descriptive study of 22 patients with preoperative rheumatoid arthritis and 25 control patients, a 15-camera motion analysis system was used to obtain data on multisegmental gait kinematics.[31] The group with rheumatoid arthritis showed prolonged stance time, shortened stride length, increased cadence, and a mean walking speed that was 80% of that of the control group.

Nonsurgical treatments including shoe wear modification, orthotic insoles, and administration of appropriate medications can be used for patients with early, mildly symptomatic disease. A rheumatologist or internist should be consulted for medical management.

3: Arthritis

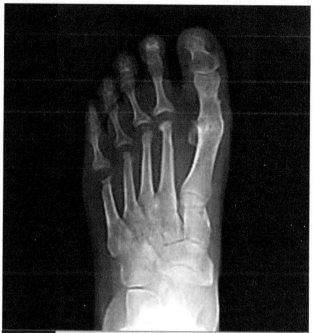

Figure 12 Radiograph of the foot of a patient with rheumatoid arthritis after first MTP arthrodesis, resection of the lesser metatarsal heads, and subsequent removal of hardware.

Surgery is indicated for symptomatic patients with more advanced disease. Forefoot reconstruction usually consists of excision arthroplasty of the lesser metatarsal heads, often combined with arthrodesis of the first MTP joint (**Figure 12**). The efficacy of this procedure is supported by a long-term follow-up study.[32]

Another retrospective review was performed on 13 feet in 8 patients treated with isolated resection of the lesser metatarsal heads with an attempt to preserve the hallux MTP joint.[33] Osteotomies of the hallux were performed in 9 feet; a valgus deformity or inflammatory erosions subsequently developed in 11 feet, with a mean time to failure of 24 months. It was concluded that a surgical procedure that does not involve fusion of the hallux MTP joint will be unsuccessful in most patients who have a well-preserved hallux MTP joint with minimal or no deformity, but who have severe lesser toe involvement.

Controversy exists concerning the best procedure for treating a first MTP joint affected by rheumatoid arthritis. An alternative to arthrodesis was investigated in a retrospective review with an average 5.5-year follow-up.[34] Thirty-seven consecutive forefoot arthroplasties were performed in 20 patients using a technique involving resection of all five metatarsal heads. At final follow-up, the AOFAS forefoot score was 64.5, the average hallux valgus angle was 22.3°, and no revision surgery was needed. It was concluded that resection of all five metatarsal heads in patients with metatarsalgia and hallux valgus associated with rheumatoid arthritis

can be a safe procedure that provides reasonable, if rarely complete, relief of symptoms. These results are supported by another retrospective study in which 26 patients (39 feet) that underwent first through fifth metatarsal head resection were examined clinically and radiographically at a mean follow-up of 5.3 years.[35] Results showed that 18% of patients were satisfied with the procedure and 78% were satisfied but with reservations.

A retrospective review of 138 feet in 79 patients who underwent rheumatoid forefoot reconstruction compared feet treated with resection arthroplasty of the first MTP joint with those that had a stable first MTP joint by means of either arthrodesis or no surgery.[36] All patients underwent resection of the lesser MTP joints. Results showed that maintenance of a stable first MTP joint had advantages over resection arthroplasty in terms of cosmesis, distribution of forefoot pressures, and patient satisfaction. However, a potential confounding factor was the disparity in length of follow-up between the two groups.

A 2005 prospective randomized study evaluated outcomes in 31 patients who underwent resection of the lesser metatarsal heads and extensor tenotomy, combined with either arthrodesis or resection of the first metatarsal head.[37] At a mean follow-up of 36 months, there was no significant difference between the two groups in terms of median subjective satisfaction score and Foot Function Index measures, no difference in the patients' willingness to have the procedure again, and no recurrences of prominences or tenderness under the forefoot in either group. In a follow-up study, 29 of these patients were reexamined at a mean of 72 months using the Foot Function Index, plantar pressure analysis, and gait analysis.[38] Cadence was higher and the stance phase shorter in the arthrodesis group, but no statistically significant difference was found in patient satisfaction or mean pressure. It was concluded that resection of the first metatarsal head may be an equally good option as arthrodesis in reconstruction of the rheumatoid forefoot.

Seronegative Arthritides and Crystal Deposition Diseases

Other inflammatory arthritides that may affect the forefoot include psoriatic arthritis, systemic lupus erythematosus, Reiter syndrome, and ankylosing spondylitis. Of these, psoriatic arthritis is the most common, with the IP joint of the hallux being most vulnerable. Swelling of the toes, also known as sausage digits, are characteristic of both psoriatic arthritis and Reiter syndrome.

Crystal deposition diseases also can affect the foot, with long-term gouty arthropathy occasionally leading to severe arthritis of the hallux MTP joint. Pseudogout has a milder clinical presentation and only rarely occurs in the forefoot.

Summary

Midfoot and forefoot arthritis has a variable etiology, location, and level of severity. Treatment depends on these diverse factors as well as the patient's activity level and expectations. With the evolution of better measurement tools and outcome studies, surgical algorithms can be refined and improved to provide the most efficacious care.

Annotated References

1. Davitt JS, Kadel N, Sangeorzan BJ, Hansen ST Jr, Holt SK, Donaldson-Fletcher E: An association between functional second metatarsal length and midfoot arthrosis. *J Bone Joint Surg Am* 2005;87:795-800.

   Nine patients (15 feet) treated with arthrodesis of the first, second, and third TMT joints for primary osteoarthrosis were compared with a control group consisting of individuals with normal feet and with the uninjured feet of patients who had an acute traumatic injury to the hindfoot. Patients with midfoot arthrosis had a different ratio of the first to second metatarsal length than did a similarly aged cohort without arthrosis, suggesting that midfoot arthrosis may have a mechanical etiology. Level of evidence: III.

2. Berlet GC, Anderson RB: Tendon arthroplasty for basal fourth and fifth metatarsal arthritis. *Foot Ankle Int* 2002;23:440-446.

3. Lin SS, Bono CM, Treuting R, Shereff MJ: Limited intertarsal arthrodesis using bone grafting and pin fixation. *Foot Ankle Int* 2000;21:742-748.

4. Sizensky JA: Forefoot and midfoot arthritis: What's new in surgical management? *Curr Opin Orthop* 2004;15: 55-61.

   The author provides an overview of the recent trends in the surgical management of midfoot and forefoot arthritis and hallux rigidus. Recent studies of surgical treatment options for hallux rigidus and various degrees of midfoot and forefoot arthritis are highlighted.

5. Suh JS, Amendola A, Lee KB, Wasserman L, Saltzman CL: Dorsal modified calcaneal plate for extensive midfoot arthrodesis. *Foot Ankle Int* 2005;26:503-509.

   A retrospective review of nine patients with diagnoses ranging from primary osteoarthrosis to Charcot arthropathy that underwent midfoot arthrodesis with a dorsal calcaneal plate is presented. Ninety-five percent of joints were fused within 4 months of surgery. Postoperative complications included nonunion with broken screws in one patient; three wound complications were successfully treated with local dressing changes. High patient satisfaction was reported.

6. Jung HG, Myerson MS, Schon LC: Spectrum of operative treatments and clinical outcomes for atraumatic osteoarthritis of the tarsometatarsal joints. *Foot Ankle Int* 2007;28:482-489.

   Four main subtypes of atraumatic osteoarthritis of the TMT joints were identified based on associated foot deformities. When patients with atraumatic TMT arthrosis are categorized into these subtypes, appropriate concurrent procedures can be used to achieve high patient satisfaction and improved functional scores. Pes planovalgus feet, in particular, may benefit from concurrent procedures with improved radiographic measures.

7. Raikin SM, Schon LC: Arthrodesis of the fourth and fifth tarsometatarsal joints of the midfoot. *Foot Ankle Int* 2003;24:584-590.

   In this retrospective review, 23 patients (28 feet) with arthrodesis of the fourth and fifth TMT joints were evaluated at a minimum 2-year follow-up. Twenty-two procedures were performed on neuropathic rocker-bottom feet and six on normosensate feet with painful arthritis. A comparison of preoperative and postoperative scores showed a decrease in functional incapacity from lateral midfoot pathology and an improvement in overall pain scores and AOFAS midfoot scores.

8. Coughlin MJ, Shurnas PS: Hallux rigidus: Demographics, etiology, and radiographic assessment. *Foot Ankle Int* 2003;24:731-743.

   A retrospective cohort of patients who had undergone surgery for hallux rigidus over a 19-year period showed a positive association with hallux valgus interphalangeus, a flat or chevron shaped metatarsal head, female gender, and a positive family history in bilateral cases, and no association with metatarsus primus elevatus, first ray hypermobility, increased first metatarsal length, Achilles or gastrocnemius tendon tightness, abnormal foot posture, symptomatic hallux valgus, adolescent onset, shoe wear, or occupation.

9. Mahiquez MY, Wilder FV, Stephens HM: Positive hindfoot valgus and osteoarthritis of the first metatarsophalangeal joint. *Foot Ankle Int* 2006;27:1055-1059.

   The authors evaluated 1,592 individuals who were free of first MTP joint osteoarthritis of either the left or right foot, or both, at baseline. Subjects were grouped according to the absence or presence of either left or right hindfoot valgus. Over the 13-year study period, it was noted that first MTP joint osteoarthritis was 23% more likely to develop in individuals with positive hindfoot valgus than in individuals with normal hindfoot alignment.

10. Coughlin MJ, Shurnas PS: Hallux rigidus: Grading and long-term results of operative treatment. *J Bone Joint Surg Am* 2003;85:2072-2088.

    A grading system that encompasses both clinical and radiographic criteria was applied retrospectively to a cohort of patients who underwent either cheilectomy or first MTP arthrodesis. This grading scale appeared to be reliable because it correctly predicted a successful outcome in 108 of 110 patients. It accurately predicted a fair or poor outcome in patients with grade 4 hallux rigidus treated with cheilectomy, rather than arthrodesis. Level of evidence: IV.

11. Pons M, Alvarez F, Solana J, Viladot R, Varela L: Sodium hyaluronate in the treatment of hallux rigidus: A

3: Arthritis

single-blind, randomized study. *Foot Ankle Int* 2007;28: 38-42.

The authors of this randomized, prospective, single-blinded study evaluated patients with hallux rigidus who were treated with either a single intra-articular injection of triamcinolone acetate or sodium hyaluronate. AOFAS scores at all follow-up visits (up to 3 months) were better in the the group treated with sodium hyaluronate; however, at 1 year after injection, approximately 50% of patients in both groups required surgery.

12. Title CI, Zaret D, Means KR, Vogtman J, Miller SD: First metatarsal head OATS technique: An approach to cartilage damage. *Foot Ankle Int* 2006;27:1000-1002.

The authors present a case study describing the osteoarticular transfer technique for central lesions of the metatarsal head.

13. Brodsky JW, Baum BS, Pollo FE, Mehta H: Prospective gait analysis in patients with first metatarsophalangeal joint arthrodesis for hallux rigidus. *Foot Ankle Int* 2007;28:162-165.

Gait parameters in 23 patients with hallux rigidus before and after first MTP arthrodesis were evaluated in this prospective study. Improvements were noted post-operatively in propulsive power, weight-bearing function of the foot, and stability during gait.

14. DeFrino PF, Brodsky JW, Pollo FE, Crenshaw SJ, Beischer AD: First metatarsophalangeal arthrodesis: A clinical, pedobarographic and gait analysis study. *Foot Ankle Int* 2002;23:496-502.

15. Budhabhatti SP, Erdemir A, Petre M, Sferra J, Donley B, Cavanagh PR: Finite element modeling of the first ray of the foot: A tool for the design of interventions. *J Biomech Eng* 2007;129:750.

This study used a computational modeling approach to develop a three-dimensional finite element model of the first ray. First MTP arthrodesis was modeled. The authors concluded that a 1° change in dorsiflexion and valgus fixation angles introduced approximated changes in peak hallux pressure of 95 kPa and 22 kPa, respectively.

16. Politi J, John H, Njus G, Bennett GL, Kay DB: First metatarsal-phalangeal joint arthrodesis: A biomechanical assessment of stability. *Foot Ankle Int* 2003;24:332-337.

The authors of this biomechanical study compared five commonly used techniques for first MTP arthrodesis using a synthetic bone model. It was concluded that the most stable technique was the combination of machined conical reaming with an oblique interfragmentary 3.5-mm lag screw and a four-hole dorsal miniplate.

17. Molloy S, Burkhart BG, Jasper LE, Solan MC, Campbell JT, Belkoff SM: Biomechanical comparison of two fixation methods for first metatarsophalangeal joint arthrodesis. *Foot Ankle Int* 2003;24:169-171.

Crossed 4.0-mm interfragmentary screw fixation was biomechanically compared with 6.5-mm intramedullary screw fixation in a cadaveric model. Fixation provided

by the intramedullary screw was stiffer and stronger than that from the crossed compression screws.

18. Goucher NR, Coughlin MJ: Hallux metatarsophalangeal joint arthrodesis using dome-shaped reamers and dorsal plate fixation: A prospective study. *Foot Ankle Int* 2006;27:869-876.

The authors of this prospective study reported on 49 patients treated with hallux MTP arthrodesis with a minimum 1-year follow-up. The authors used dome-shaped reamers with crossed lag screws and a low-profile, contoured, titanium plate. Outcome measures showed a union rate of 92%, a revision rate of only 4%, and a patient satisfaction rate of 96%.

19. Flavin R, Stephens MM: Arthrodesis of the first metatarsophalangeal joint using a dorsal titanium contoured plate. *Foot Ankle Int* 2004;25:783-787.

Positive outcomes for hallux MTP arthrodesis using a lag screw and dorsal contoured plate were shown in this prospective study.

20. Brodsky JW, Passmore RN, Pollo FE, Shabat S: Functional outcome of arthrodesis of the first metatarsophalangeal joint using parallel screw fixation. *Foot Ankle Int* 2005;26:140-146.

In this retrospective study on hallux MTP fusion, parallel screws were introduced through the dorsum of the first metatarsal to engage the plantar cortex of the proximal phalanx. Results showed no nonunions; 94% of patients stated that they would have the surgery again.

21. Bennett GL, Kay DB, Sabatta J: First metatarsophalangeal joint arthrodesis: An evaluation of hardware failure. *Foot Ankle Int* 2005;26:593-596.

The authors present a retrospective review of 95 consecutive patients who underwent hallux MTP arthrodesis using a 2.4-mm lag screw and a six-hole dorsal plate from the Synthes modular hand set. Nonunion and failure of hardware occurred in 13% of the arthrodeses.

22. Kennedy JG, Chow FY, Dines J, Gardner M, Bohne WH: Outcomes after interposition arthroplasty for treatment of hallux rigidus. *Clin Orthop Relat Res* 2006;445:210-215.

The authors present a retrospective review of 21 interposition arthroplasties with dorsal cheilectomy, resection of the base of the proximal phalanx, and capsular interposition. At a mean follow-up of 38 months, results showed an increase in joint motion and a complication rate of 6%. Most patients stated that they would have the procedure again.

23. Mroczek KJ, Miller SD: The modified oblique Keller procedure: A technique for dorsal approach interposition arthroplasty sparing the flexor tendons. *Foot Ankle Int* 2003;24:521-522.

This case study describes the oblique Keller procedure for interpositional arthroplasty.

24. Konkel KF, Menger AG: Mid-term results of titanium hemi-great toe implants. *Foot Ankle Int* 2006;27:922-929.

A retrospective review of 10 patients who underwent titanium hemiarthroplasty of the hallux MTP joint is presented. All patients improved and reported satisfaction with the procedure in the first 5 years after surgery; however, subsidence and lucency in all patients and a painful fracture in one patient made long-term implant survival questionable.

25. Raikin SM, Ahmad J, Pour AE, Abidi N: Comparison of arthrodesis and metallic hemiarthroplasty of the hallux metatarsophalangeal joint. *J Bone Joint Surg Am* 2007;89:1979-1985.

This retrospective review compared long-term outcomes of hemiarthroplasty with those of arthrodesis. Satisfaction ratings were superior for the patients who were treated with arthrodesis. Twenty-four percent of the hemiarthroplasties failed, four were subsequently converted to arthrodesis, and eight feet in which the hemiprosthesis survived showed evidence of plantar cutout of the prosthetic stem on final follow-up radiographs. Level of evidence: III.

26. Gibson JN, Thomson CE: Arthrodesis or total replacement arthroplasty for hallux rigidus: A randomized controlled trial. *Foot Ankle Int* 2005;26:680-690.

Arthrodesis was compared with total replacement arthroplasty in 77 feet with hallux rigidus in this randomized prospective study. All arthrodeses united with few complications; in contrast, 6 of the 39 joint prostheses required removal. In the patients with the remaining 33 prostheses, gains in range of motion were poor; 40% of the patients stated that they would not undergo arthroplasty again.

27. Machacek F Jr, Easley ME, Gruber F, Ritschl P, Trnka HJ: Salvage of a failed Keller resection arthroplasty. *J Bone Joint Surg Am* 2004;86:1131-1138.

The authors present the results of a retrospective study of patients with failed Keller resection arthroplasty. First MTP joint arthrodesis was performed in 29 feet, and 21 feet underwent repeat Keller arthroplasty or isolated soft-tissue release. The authors recommended arthrodesis for salvage of failed Keller arthroplasty because of a higher rate of patient satisfaction and better clinical results. Level of evidence: III-2.

28. Vienne P, Sukthankar A, Favre P, Werner CM, Baumer A, Zingg PO: Metatarsophalangeal joint arthrodesis after failed Keller-Brandes procedure. *Foot Ankle Int* 2006;27:894-901.

This prospective study of arthrodesis performed for failed Keller arthroplasty in 22 feet with a minimum 24-month follow-up revealed positive outcomes. Overall, 72% of feet were pain free at final follow-up and 28% had mild, occasional pain. Pedobarographic analysis showed a significant improvement in parameters.

29. Mizel MS, Alvarez RG, Fink BR, Temple HT: Ipsilateral arthrodesis of the metatarsophalangeal and interphalangeal joints of the hallux. *Foot Ankle Int* 2006;27: 804-807.

A retrospective evaluation of seven feet that had undergone simultaneous arthrodesis of the MTP and IP joints of the ipsilateral hallux revealed adequate resolution of pain and the ability to wear nonprescription shoes. Limitations in athletic activities were noted, but there was no interference with moderately demanding daily activities.

30. Ostendorf B, Scherer A, Modder U, Schneider M: Diagnostic value of magnetic resonance imaging of the forefeet in early rheumatoid arthritis when findings on imaging of the metacarpophalangeal joints of the hands remain normal. *Arthritis Rheum* 2004;50:2094-2102.

The authors used MRI scans of both the hand and foot to detect early radiographic signs of rheumatoid arthritis. They concluded that MRI scans of the forefeet detected synovitis and bone edema in patients with early rheumatoid arthritis in whom MRI scans of the finger joints were normal. Such scanning may allow an earlier decision to begin appropriate medications and treatments.

31. Khazzam M, Long JT, Marks RM, Harris GF: Kinematic changes of the foot and ankle in patients with systemic rheumatoid arthritis and forefoot deformity. *J Orthop Res* 2007;25:319-329.

The authors present the findings of a cross-sectional, descriptive study of 22 preoperative patients with rheumatoid arthritis and 25 control patients. A 15-camera motion analysis system was used to obtain data on multisegmental gait kinematics. The group with rheumatoid arthritis showed prolonged stance time, shortened stride length, increased cadence, and a mean walking speed that was 80% of that of the control group.

32. Coughlin MJ: Rheumatoid forefoot reconstruction: A long-term follow-up study. *J Bone Joint Surg Am* 2000; 82:322-341.

33. Thordarson DB, Aval S, Krieger L: Failure of hallux MP preservation surgery for rheumatoid arthritis. *Foot Ankle Int* 2002;23:486-490.

34. Thomas S, Kinninmonth AW, Kumar CS: Long-term results of the modified Hoffman procedure in the rheumatoid forefoot. *J Bone Joint Surg Am* 2005;87:748-752.

A retrospective review of 37 consecutive forefoot arthroplasties using a technique involving resection of all five metatarsal heads is presented. At an average 5.5-year follow-up, the AOFAS forefoot score was 64.5, the average hallux valgus angle was 22.3°, and there were no revisions.

35. Reize P, Ina Leichtle C, Leichtle UG, Schanbacher J: Long-term results after metatarsal head resection in the treatment of rheumatoid arthritis. *Foot Ankle Int* 2006; 27:586-590.

In this retrospective study, 26 patients (39 feet) that underwent first through fifth metatarsal head resection were examined clinically and radiographically at a mean 5.3-year follow-up. Results showed that 18% of patients were satisfied with the procedure and 78% were satisfied with reservations.

36. Mulcahy D, Daniels TR, Lau JT, Boyle E, Bogoch E: Rheumatoid forefoot deformity: A comparison study of

3: Arthritis

2 functional methods of reconstruction. *J Rheumatol* 2003;30:1440-1450.

This retrospective review of 138 feet in 79 patients who underwent rheumatoid forefoot reconstruction compared feet treated with resection arthroplasty of the first MTP joint with those that had a stable first MTP joint by means of either arthrodesis or no surgery. All patients underwent resection of the lesser MTP joints. The group with a stable first MTP joint showed advantages in terms of cosmesis, distribution of forefoot pressures, and patient satisfaction compared with the group with resection arthroplasty.

37. Grondal L, Hedstrom M, Stark A: Arthrodesis compared to Mayo resection of the first metatarsophalangeal joint in total rheumatoid forefoot reconstruction. *Foot Ankle Int* 2005;26:135-139.

The authors present the findings of a prospective randomized trial of 31 patients with rheumatoid arthritis who underwent resection of the lesser metatarsal heads and extensor tenotomy, combined with either arthrode-sis or resection of the first metatarsal head. After a mean follow-up of 36 months, there was no significant difference in outcomes between the two groups.

38. Grondal L, Brostrom E, Wretenberg P, Stark A: Arthrodesis versus Mayo resection: The management of the first metatarsophalangeal joint in reconstruction of the rheumatoid forefoot. *J Bone Joint Surg Br* 2006;88:914-919.

The authors evaluated 29 patients with rheumatoid arthritis who underwent resection of the lesser metatarsal heads and extensor tenotomy combined with either arthrodesis or resection of the first metatarsal head. Patients were reexamined at a mean of 72 months using the Foot Function Index, plantar pressure analysis, and gait analysis. Cadence was higher and the stance phase shorter in the arthrodesis group, but no statistically significant difference was found in patient satisfaction or mean pressure.

Chapter 17

Adult Acquired Flatfoot Deformity and Posterior Tibial Tendon Dysfunction

Richard G. Alvarez, MD   *Julian Price, MD, ATC   Andrew Marini, DPT, ATC, MS
Norman S. Turner, MD   Harold B. Kitaoka, MD

Introduction

Adult acquired flatfoot deformity (AAFD) is a common and potentially debilitating foot and ankle condition. Posterior tibial tendon dysfunction (PTTD), which occurs when the tendon is elongated or torn, is the most common cause of AAFD. Loss of PTTD function and pathologic changes in the spring ligament cause subsequent loss of the medial arch and malalignment of the hindfoot. The etiology of PTTD includes inflammatory, degenerative, and traumatic conditions. Inflammatory arthropathy often occurs in younger patients (30 to 40 years of age), whereas degenerative disease often occurs in older patients (50 to 60 years of age). Treatment is based on the severity of the symptoms and the stage of the disease.

Original reports of PTTD date from 1936, when a patient with tenosynovitis of the posterior tibial tendon sheath was described.[1] From the mid-1950s through the mid-1970s, case reports of spontaneous ruptures and degenerative and inflammatory processes of the posterior tibial tendon appeared in the literature.[2-4] With evolving knowledge, the term posterior tibial tendon dysfunction was created to describe the condition.

Anatomy and Pathophysiology

The posterior tibial tendon originates from the posterior tibia, interosseous membrane, and posterior fibula. The tendon courses posterior to the medial malleolus and makes a sharp turn to insert onto the navicular tuberosity, with several arms extending to structures including the cuneiforms and the metatarsal bases. The proximal portion of the tendon is supplied with blood

by the mesotenon, which terminates 1 to 1.5 cm distal to the medial malleolus. The sole blood supply of the distal tendon is from periosteal vessels from its respective osseous insertions.

In patients with AAFD, pathologic changes develop in the posterior tibial tendon, spring ligament, and portions of the deltoid ligament.[5] The posterior tibial tendon is the primary dynamic stabilizer of the arch. In AAFD, changes occur in both the molecular composite of matrix collagens and the structural organization of the tendon.[6] These changes are believed to occur secondary to microtrauma in a hypervascular zone located in the retromalleolar region. Dye studies have confirmed the concept of a watershed area of hypovascularity, which correlates with the common site of pathology[7] (**Figure 1**). Recent cadaver studies using direct observation under a light microscope have challenged the validity of the findings made with intra-arterial injection dye techniques regarding the presence of a hypovascular zone in the tendon.[8]

The spring ligament (calcaneal navicular ligament) has two components, the superior medial and the inferior calcaneonavicular ligament. The superior medial

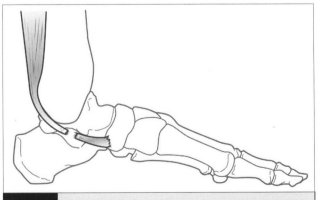

Figure 1   Frey watershed area of the posterior tibial tendon. The area of hypovascularity is from the medial malleolus to 1 to 1.5 cm distally.

*Julian Price, MD, ATC or the department with which he is affiliated has received miscellaneous nonincome support, commercially derived honoraria, or other nonresearch-related funding from Synthes Spine.

3: Arthritis

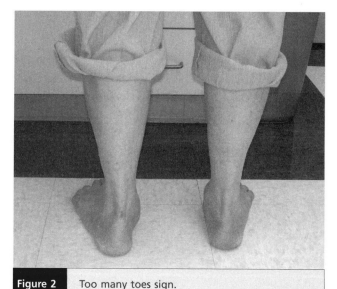

Figure 2 Too many toes sign.

calcaneonavicular ligament is located medial to the head of the talus and combines with the deltoid ligament.[9] This portion of the ligament is susceptible to stress during midstance and leads to the pathologic changes in AAFD.

The primary function of the posterior tibial tendon is adduction, inversion, and plantar flexion of the transverse tarsal, subtalar, and tibiotalar joints, respectively. More specifically, the posterior tibial tendon is the primary initiator of inversion as the ankle is plantar flexed. Adduction of the midfoot provides a rigid lever for transition from midstance to the propulsion phases of gait. These functions provide a biomechanical advantage in preparing the gastrocnemius-soleus complex for toe-off. The peroneal brevis is the primary antagonist of the posterior tibialis. Because the excursion of the posterior tibial tendon is only 2 cm, any degenerative lengthening or rupture significantly impairs the function of the tendon. As posterior tibial tendon function diminishes, the peroneal brevis becomes unopposed, which ultimately leads to attenuation of the spring ligament.[10] These findings were confirmed in a 2005 study of 31 patients with PTTD that used MRI to show that 74% of all patients with PTTD had tears of the superomedial spring ligament and 39% had tears of the inferomedial spring ligament; no significant pathology in these ligaments was found in age-matched controls without PTTD.[11] Progressive loss of the medial longitudinal arch occurs with failure of the spring ligament, plantar aponeurosis, deltoid ligament, talocalcaneal ligament, long and short plantar ligaments, and medial calcaneocuboid ligament. As collapse of these supporting structures progresses, hindfoot valgus and plantar flexion of the talar head develops with progressive heel cord contracture. Stresses on the talonavicular joint lead to stretching of the overlying capsule, resulting in transverse tarsal abduction and the associated "too many toes sign"[12] (**Figure 2**).

Etiology

Many factors are associated with PTTD (**Table 1**). Although acute ruptures of the tendon may occur, PTTD usually results from a progressive degenerative process.[13] Elastic properties of the tendon decrease and collagen composition and orientation change. These changes are reflected by myxoid degeneration and increased mucin content seen in histologic specimens of patients with PTTD.[14] Intraoperative findings confirm the tendon pathology, often showing dull, yellow, tendon composition (versus the shiny, white appearance of normal tendon) and the presence of longitudinal tears. Inflammatory arthropathies are associated with PTTD, although there is seldom an isolated tendinopathy. Traumatic ruptures occur with or without underlying degenerative or inflammatory changes. Because intratendinous steroid injections can lead to iatrogenic tendon tears, steroid injections should be avoided in the area of the posterior tibial tendon.

Classification

Staging of PTTD was originally described by Johnson and Strom[15] and later modified by Myerson[16] (**Table 2**). Staging is based on clinical findings and guides both nonsurgical and surgical treatment. MRI grading has been proposed, but its usefulness has not yet been proven.[17] Surgical classification of PTTD is based on intraoperative findings.

Patients with stage I PTTD have medial foot and ankle pain, with or without swelling. Tenosynovitis contributes significantly to stage I disease, although the tendon has normal function and length. Patients can perform single-support heel raises (SSHRs) but repetitive SSHRs may cause pain. The hindfoot is flexible. Patients with stage II PTTD are unable to or have significant difficulty performing SSHRs; however, the hindfoot remains flexible (the valgus heel inverts on double-support heel raises [DSHRs]). Manual muscle testing will show posterior tibial tendon weakness. A recent study has suggested the need for subclassification of stage II disease.[18] Stage IIA is characterized by medial (mild) pain only and stage IIB is characterized by the development of lateral (severe) pain. These classifications guide proposed surgical management. Stage III disease is characterized by the development of a rigid hindfoot as the hindfoot becomes stiffer with arthritic changes over time. The patient cannot perform SSHRs, and the heel remains in valgus during DSHRs. Stage IV disease is stage III disease with tibiotalar involvement. Typically, the talus angulates into valgus because of deltoid incompetency; subfibular impingement on the calcaneus occurs because of the severity of the hindfoot valgus.

The original Johnson and Strom classification of PTTD was recently modified to make treatment decisions more rational.[15,16] Although the new system is somewhat cumbersome, it aids the orthopaedic surgeon in clinically applying the various treatment modalities

Table 1

Etiology of Posterior Tibial Tendon Dysfunction

Trauma (direct)
  Laceration
  Steroid injection

Trauma (indirect)
  Ankle fracture
  Ankle sprain
  Avulsion navicular bone
  Tendon dislocation

Structural
  Accessory navicular
  Tarsal coalition
  Flexible flatfoot

Anatomic
  Osteophyte at medial malleolus
  Shallow groove

Inflammatory
  Rheumatoid arthritis
  Rheumatoid variant (seronegative arthritis)
  Seronegative spondyloarthropathy
  Ankylosing spondylitis
  Psoriatic arthritis
  Reactive arthritis

Other
  Pigmented villonodular synovitis

Associated factors
  Obesity
  Diabetes
  Hypertension
  Female sex
  Overuse
  Athletic participation

Table 2

Clinical Staging of Posterior Tibial Tendon Dysfunction

Stage I	Pain over posterior tibialis with no deformity
Stage II	Deformity is flexible A. Medial pain only B. Lateral pain
Stage III	Deformity is not flexible
Stage IV	Deformity is not flexible and changes at the ankle

necessary to correct or treat the specific anatomic pathology. The Bluman, Title, and Myerson classification system for PTTD[19] is shown in **Table 3**.

Clinical Presentation

Patients with PTTD typically present with a gradual onset of medial foot and ankle pain.[20] Prolonged activity and ambulation on uneven surfaces aggravate symptoms. It is important to determine pain-free ambulatory distance and type of shoe wear. Shoes should be checked for abnormal wear patterns. Obesity, hypertension, diabetes, inflammatory arthropathy, steroid use, and traumatic injuries are associated with PTTD and should be documented.[21,22] In very late stage disease, lateral pain may occur from subfibular impingement.

Examination and Testing

The appearance of the foot is based on the severity of the disease. In early stages, the symptomatic foot will have a normal appearance and mild flatfoot deformity. Typically, the examination will show swelling and fullness distal to the medial malleolus. Patients will have tenderness to palpation along the posteromedial border of the tibia. Absence of a palpable tendon indicates tendon rupture. Pain at the navicular insertion may be absent in patients with long-standing rupture. Collapse of the medial arch, heel valgus, and forefoot abduction occur in later stages of the disease.

A reverse Coleman block testing (placing the block medially) and subtalar motion testing are essential parts of the examination. Flexibility of the hindfoot will guide both the classification and treatment of PTTD.[15,16] Heel cord, midfoot, and forefoot motion must be assessed. With the patient seated, the foot is held in plantar flexion, eversion, and abduction while resistance to inversion is provided. This maneuver isolates the posterior tibial tendon and eliminates synergistic effects of the tibialis anterior. Testing with SSHRs and DSHRs are hallmarks of the examination. Significant difficulty in performing (stage I) or inability to perform (stage II or above) SSHRs is sensitive for PTTD. Delayed inversion of the heel on the symptomatic side with the DSHR is found in late stage I and early stage II PTTD. Care must be taken to ensure that the patient keeps the knees in full extension and body weight centered over the feet. Failure of the valgus heel to invert on DSHRs signifies a rigid hindfoot (**Figure 3**).

Testing for the Hintermann first metatarsal rise sign (**Figure 4, A**) and the Hubscher maneuver (**Figure 4, B**) also are recommended for PTTD.[23] Although the first metatarsal rise test was originally described with the patient standing and fully bearing weight, the test is now performed with the patient sitting on the edge of the examination table with knees flexed 90° and the feet on the floor or a footstool to provide partial weight bearing. As the examiner inverts the heel or externally rotates the leg, the first metatarsal will rise off the surface of the stool or floor, indicating PTTD. When the ligaments are intact, the first metatarsal remains on the surface of the stool or the floor, indicating the integrity of the short and long plantar ligaments.

The Hubscher maneuver is performed with the patient in a relaxed stance. When the great toe is passively

3: Arthritis

Table 3

Blumen, Title, and Myerson Clinical Classification System for Posterior Tibial Tendon Dysfunction

Stage	Substage	Characteristic Clinical Findings	Radiographic Findings	Treatment
I	A: Inflammatory disease	Normal anatomy, tender PTT	Normal	NSAIDs, immobilization, ice, orthoses, tenosynovectomy, treat specific systemic disease
	B: Partial tear	Normal anatomy, tender PTT	Normal	Same as A
	C: Partial tear with mild HF valgus	Slight HF valgus, tender PTT	Slight HF valgus	Same as A
II	A1: HF valgus with flexible FF varus	Flexible HF valgus, flexible FF varus ± tender PTT	HF valgus, Meary's line disrupted, calcaneal pitch lost	Orthoses, medial slide calcaneal osteotomy, Strayer or Achilles tendon lengthening, FDL transfer (if deformity corrects only with ankle PF)
	A2: HF valgus with rigid FF varus	Flexible HF valgus, rigid FF varus ± tender PTT	Same as A1	Same as A1, Cotton osteotomy
	B: FF abduction	Same as A1 and A2 with FF abduction	HF valgus, talonavicular uncovering, FF abduction	Medial slide calcaneal osteotomy, lateral column lengthening, Strayer or Achilles tendon lengthening, FDL transfer
	C: Medial ray instability	Flexible HF valgus, fixed FF varus, medial column instability, first ray dorsiflexion with HF correction, sinus tarsi pain	HF valgus, first TMT joint plantar gaping	Medial slide calcaneal osteotomy, FDL transfer, Cotton osteotomy or first TMT joint fusion
III	A: rigid HF valgus	Rigid HF valgus, sinus tarsi pain	Decreased subtalar joint space, angle of Gissane sclerosis	Triple arthrodesis, custom AFO if not surgical candidate
	B: FF abduction	Same as IIIA, FF abduction	Same as IIIA, FF abduction	Triple arthrodesis with lateral column lengthening, custom AFO if not surgical candidate
IV	A: Rigid HF valgus, flexible ankle valgus, deltoid ligament insufficiency, minimal ankle arthritis	Flexible tibiotalar valgus	Tibiotalar valgus, HF valgus	Correct HF valgus, reconstruct deltoid ligament
	B: Significant ankle arthritis, with or without rigid ankle valgus	Rigid tibiotalar valgus	Tibiotalar valgus, HF valgus	Pantalar fusion or TTC fusion

AFO = ankle-foot orthosis, HF = hindfoot, FDL = flexor digitorum longus, FF = forefoot, NSAIDs = nonsteroidal anti-inflammatory drugs, PF = plantar flexion, PTT = posterior tibial tendon, TAL = tendon Achilles lengthening, TMT = tarsometatarsal, TTC = tibiotalocalcaneal. (Table adapted from Bluman EM, Title CI, Myerson MS: Posterior tibial tendon rupture: A refined classification system. *Foot Ankle Clin* 2007;12:233-249.)

dorsiflexed, a 1:1 elevation of the arch and external rotation of the tibia through the Hicks windlass mechanism occurs. If this 1:1 motion is not present, integrity of the ligaments coupling the foot to the leg is lost.

Imaging

Weight-bearing radiographs of the foot and ankle should be obtained to determine the severity of the de-formity, the presence of hindfoot arthritis, and the absence of other causes of AAFD, such as neuropathic arthropathy, severe midfoot arthritis, or rheumatoid arthritis.[12] (Figure 5). An AP radiograph of the foot will show abduction of the talonavicular joint or an abnormal talonavicular coverage angle. A lateral radiograph will show a decrease in the distance from the floor to the inferior aspect of the medial cuneiform and a decrease in the lateral talometatarsal angle. In patients

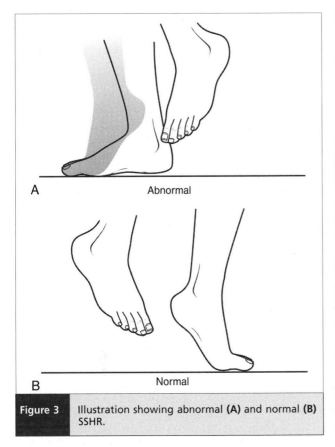

Figure 3 Illustration showing abnormal (A) and normal (B) SSHR.

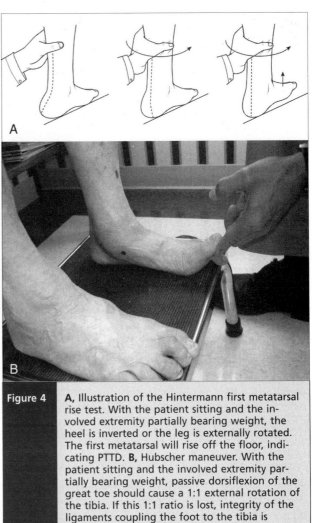

Figure 4 A, Illustration of the Hintermann first metatarsal rise test. With the patient sitting and the involved extremity partially bearing weight, the heel is inverted or the leg is externally rotated. The first metatarsal will rise off the floor, indicating PTTD. B, Hubscher maneuver. With the patient sitting and the involved extremity partially bearing weight, passive dorsiflexion of the great toe should cause a 1:1 external rotation of the tibia. If this 1:1 ratio is lost, integrity of the ligaments coupling the foot to the tibia is compromised.

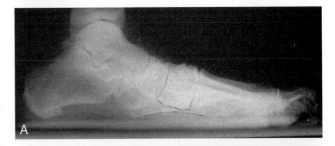

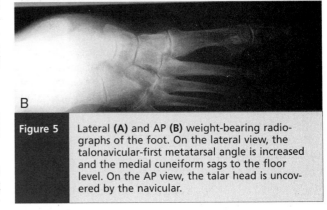

Figure 5 Lateral (A) and AP (B) weight-bearing radiographs of the foot. On the lateral view, the talonavicular-first metatarsal angle is increased and the medial cuneiform sags to the floor level. On the AP view, the talar head is uncovered by the navicular.

with severe deformity, AP views of the ankle may show subluxation or dislocation of the talonavicular joint, degenerative arthritis in the hindfoot, impingement between the lateral malleolus and calcaneus, along with a decrease in the height of the arch. Changes to the tibiotalar joint are seen on the mortise view of the ankle in late stages of disease. MRI, although highly sensitive and specific, is most valuable in diagnosing early disease.[24] Because patient positioning affects results, specific MRI protocols have been developed.[25] Plain radiographs and clinical examination usually provide sufficient evidence in early and later disease stages, and MRI is usually unnecessary for diagnosing PTTD. In a retrospective review of patients with PTTD who were evaluated with ultrasound, a positive correlation between preoperative ultrasound and surgical findings was established.[26] As with other diagnoses, ultrasound is highly operator dependent; a knowledgeable radiologist also is needed to interpret results. Recent prospective data indicate higher sensitivity and specificity for MRI versus ultrasound in identifying PTTD.[27] CT is of little value because of the accuracy of MRI.

Nonsurgical Treatment

Goals

The goal of orthotic treatment is to bring the floor up to the foot, effectively restoring the arch and stabilizing the hindfoot.[28] The flexibility of the hindfoot deter-

3: Arthritis

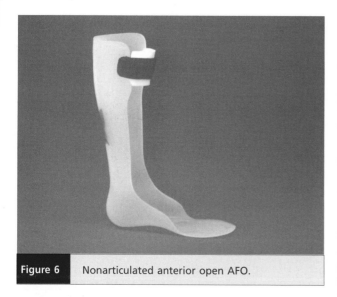

| Figure 6 | Nonarticulated anterior open AFO. |

mines the type of orthosis needed. Rehabilitation and home exercise programs attempt to increase endurance and decrease pain with daily activity through global ankle strengthening and stretching. In general, a trial of conservative treatment is attempted before surgical intervention. The goals of nonsurgical treatment are pain control, maintenance of a flexible hindfoot and forefoot, and prevention of the need for surgery.

Immobilization

Early disease, especially tenosynovitis, can be treated with 6 to 8 weeks of immobilization, activity modification, muscle strengthening exercises, and anti-inflammatory medications; however, the posterior tendon or any tendon in the ankle or foot should never be injected with steroids because of the significant risk of tendon rupture. A short leg walking cast or fracture boot is used for immobilization and patients are encouraged to bear weight in the immobilization device. Immobilization also can help prevent acute flare-ups in patients with chronic disease.

Orthoses and Bracing

Prior to 1996, nonsurgical management of PTTD was either largely ignored or only briefly mentioned in the literature because surgical treatment was preferred.[13,29] In a 1996 study of 49 patients treated with the University of California Biomechanics Laboratory (UCBL) orthosis for stage II PTTD and a molded ankle-foot orthosis (AFO) for stage III PTTD, 67% of patients had good to excellent results[30] (**Figure 6**). The authors determined bracing was most effective in less active, elderly patients. The goal of bracing is to maintain the initial deformity and prevent progression.[31] The UCBL orthosis requires a flexible hindfoot (stage II disease) and is molded with the heel in the neutral position.[32] In cadaver biomechanical studies, the UCBL orthosis most closely restored arch and hindfoot kinematics, followed by a molded AFO. The Arizona AFO (Custom Foot-

wear, Mesa, AZ) restored midfoot height but had no statistically significant effect on hindfoot alignment.[33] Commercial ankle braces did not restore arch or hindfoot kinematics.

The Arizona brace is a custom-fitted leather and polypropylene AFO that extends from the midshaft tibia to the metatarsal heads. In a 2003 prospective study, 19 of 21 patients (90%) with stage I, II, or III PTTD treated with the Arizona brace had good to excellent results.[34] The two patients with worse results had stage III PTTD. The authors concluded that treatment with the Arizona brace effectively relieved symptoms and prevented or delayed the need for surgery.

A 2005 study showed global weakness in all four muscle quadrants of the ankle (posterior tibialis, peroneus brevis/peroneus longus, anterior tibialis, and gastrocnemius-soleus complex) in patients with stage I and II disease.[35] Patients were treated with a short, articulated, posterior-opening AFO followed by a three-fourths length thermoplastic elastomer TPE foot orthosis (with a high medial trim line) and physical therapy (**Figure 7**); 83% of patients had excellent and good outcomes. The desire of patients to avoid the 8- to 12-month period needed to recover from surgery influenced the 89% rate of patient satisfaction with this nonsurgical protocol. The AFO used in this study was subsequently modified to eliminate the solid instep piece, leading to a more user-friendly device;[36] however, the solid instep strap had provided more stability to the midfoot and forefoot by decreasing twisting motions of the device.

The goal of using an AFO and a muscle rehabilitation program is to decrease pain. The patient may be satisfied with an AFO or may choose to be fitted for a foot orthosis. Both the UCBL orthosis and three-fourths length TPE foot orthosis with a high trim line and medial post have been recommended. In patients with early stage PTTD, a foot orthosis with a muscle rehabilitation program may provide sufficient treatment.

For patients with stage I and mild stage II disease, a medial post foot orthosis supports the arch and prevents heel valgus. The UCBL orthosis or a similarly designed three-fourths length TPE foot orthosis with a high medial trim line and medial post can be incorporated into cushioned walking and running shoe wear.

Unlike flexible hindfoot deformity, the rigid hindfoot needs some form of custom-molded AFO to accommodate the fixed (stage III) deformity.[37] A short, articulating AFO with posterior cutout and an instep piece for asymptomatic patients is recommended. In a cadaver study, it was reported that transection of the deltoid ligament and talocalcaneal bifurcate ligament will disconnect the foot from the tibia.[38] There is loss of the normal transfer of rotation movement of the inverting calcaneus to externally rotate the tibia. The best method of recapturing this coupling of the leg and the foot is probably with an AFO. In late stage III disease, a rigid nonarticulating AFO provides the most support

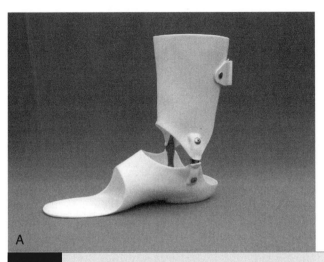

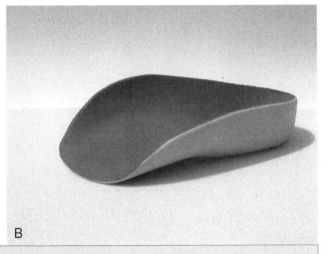

| Figure 7 | Short articulated posterior open AFO with an instep piece **(A)** and a TPE three-fourths length foot orthosis with high medial trim line **(B)**. |

and decreases excursion of the posterior tibial tendon by avoiding push-off and planter flexion.[39] A nonarticulating rigid AFO also provides support to the arthritic tibiotalar joint in patients with stage IV disease.[40]

For early signs and symptoms of PTTD and in instances when a foot orthosis does not provide adequate support, over-the-counter orthoses have increased in popularity. AirLift by AirCast (DJO, LLC, Vista, CA) provides comfort and stability with an ankle segment and an adjustable air support in the arch (**Figure 8**). A good supportive shoe (such as a running shoe) is important to achieve maximal benefit.

Physical Therapy

Physical therapists and orthopaedic surgeons who may have limited experience with the foot and ankle may be unfamiliar with rehabilitation protocols for patients with PTTD. A patient can exhibit a tendinous dysfunction, a mechanical dysfunction, or both. It is important to determine the system that is most involved, how to prevent the injury from worsening, and to ascertain if nonsurgical treatment is appropriate. The physical therapist should obtain baseline and ongoing data to document the need for continued physical therapy. In the absence of documented gains (verbally or graphically), the therapist must stop therapy and refer the patient back to the orthopaedic surgeon for treatment.

Prior to 1997, the role of physical therapy in PTTD was rarely mentioned in the literature, with no published guidelines for rehabilitating patients with PTTD. Over the past 14 years, a nonsurgical physical therapy protocol has been developed. The original protocol for patients with stage I or II disease consisted of four phases. Patients performed sole-to-sole exercises in the pretreatment phase, with the exercises increasing in frequency and duration over a 2-week period (**Figure 9**). In phase I of the protocol, the patient was evaluated and provided with educational material. An isokinetic strength evaluation was performed and the patient re-

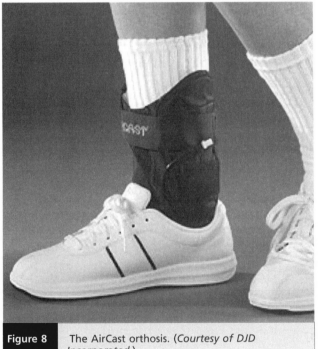

| Figure 8 | The AirCast orthosis. (*Courtesy of DJD Incorporated.*) |

ceived instructions for performing a global ankle home exercise program. Phase II, a period consisting of two to six physical therapy sessions, focused on strengthening, with KinCom 57500 isokinetic training and weight-bearing exercises, including toe walking. Phase III therapy included a repeat strength assessment and four additional sessions with phase II activities performed at greater intensity.

The revised protocol begins with patient evaluation by the orthopaedic surgeon. PTTD rehabilitation is initiated by determining whether an AFO or foot orthosis is needed. A posterior opening short articulated AFO is indicated for patients with a history of pain of more

3: Arthritis

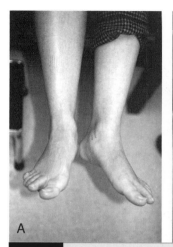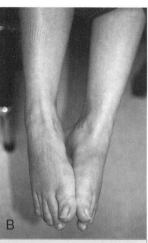

Figure 9 Photographs of a patient performing the sole-to-sole exercise. With the patient sitting or lying down and the heels touching **(A)**, the patient actively places the soles of the feet together with ankles in equinus **(B)**. This also is a good method for the examiner to compare the injured tendon to the contralateral side by palpating each simultaneously.

than 3 months' duration, inability to perform SSHRs, and inability to ambulate more than one block without pain. A three-fourths length TPE foot orthosis is indicated for patients with pain of less than 3 months' duration, ability to perform SSHRs, and ability to ambulate one block with little or no pain. Education is provided on appropriate shoe wear. Instruction in the proper method of sole-to-sole exercises is provided, emphasizing the need to keep the heels together and the ankles in equinus to isolate the posterior tibialis muscle. The patient begins by performing four sets (100 repetitions; one set equals 25 repetitions) of the exercise daily and increases to 12 sets by day 10. As it becomes easier for the patient to perform the exercise, sets are combined (one set equals 50 repetitions and the patient performs six sets; one set equals 100 repetitions and the patient performs three sets; one set equals 300 repetitions and the patient performs two sets).

After the initial stage, physical therapy begins with a modification of the sole-to-sole exercises. The patient is instructed to perform active range-of-motion exercises in which inversion and supination of bilateral feet is performed at a pace of one repetition per second up to 200 to 300 repetitions throughout the day. The patient avoids weight-bearing and impact exercises until discharged from physical therapy. The second physical therapy visit includes isokinetic testing (following the protocol set by the manufacturer for testing inversion and eversion). Range-of-motion testing should include a total excursion between 12° and 30°. Tests should be performed concentrically and eccentrically if the isokinetic device allows. Three to four maximal repetitions into inversion and eversion bilaterally are needed. The uninvolved and involved lower extremity should be compared. The patient is then instructed in using Thera-Band (Hygenic, Akron, OH) resistive band exercises for inversion and eversion, either sitting in a chair or long sitting on the floor. Repetitions of the exercise are performed slowly at a pace of one repetition every 1 to 2 seconds, with a gradual increase to 200 consecutive repetitions in one session daily with frequent rest periods as needed. The program begins with exercises using a yellow or red Thera-Band. The patient is instructed to apply ice to the foot and ankle at home. Modalities of choice may be used by the physical therapist.

The third through fifth physical therapy sessions comprise the next stage of treatment, which begins at least 2 days after the second session. The patient performs a workout on the isokinetic equipment with the same range-of-motion exercises as previously described. Workouts will consist of 200 repetitions (frequent rest permitted) into inversion and repeated into eversion. This workout includes 200 repetitions at 30° and 60° for both inversion and eversion. If the patient cannot perform the full 200 repetitions, the number of repetitions is accelerated at each session as tolerated. The goal is to perform a total of 800 repetitions. If the equipment has the ability to reduce and increase starting and minimal force limits, this tool is advantageous in documenting daily strength gains and measuring progress. The force limit is increased 1 to 2 lb per visit as tolerated. Progression to the use of a blue Thera-Band should be achieved as tolerated.

A biomechanical ankle platform system also is used based on the manufacturer's recommendations. With a level I ball under the board, exercise is started with 2.5 lb per peg and increased to 10 lb per peg, as tolerated. Patients with smaller feet may find the heavier weights difficult to use. Approximately 100 repetitions are performed in a clockwise and counterclockwise manner. The pegs should be rotated about the board every 20 to 30 repetitions. DSHRs are started, with the patient working up to 50 repetitions. SSHRs are initiated as tolerated and can be performed leaning into a table with the arms supporting body weight. The patient should avoid flexing the knee on the involved side when performing DSHRs or SSHRs. When these goals are achieved, the patient progresses to toe ambulation. Independent toe ambulation may require the patient to lean into a table or use a walker. Some older patients or those with grade II or III tears may never ambulate with total independence. Modalities of choice should be incorporated. Manual mobilization and/or stretching is indicated for the Achilles and peroneal tendons. Ice is applied as the final treatment of the day.

The sixth therapy session begins with an isokinetic retest. The minimal goal for nonathletic patients should be approximately 70% of the measurement on the uninvolved side with a goal of 90% to 100% for an athletic patient. If progress is not evident, the patient is not benefiting from the physical therapy and should be reevaluated by the surgeon for other treatment. Progress

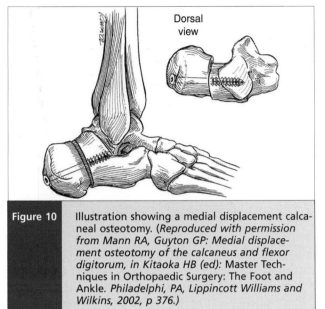

Figure 10 Illustration showing a medial displacement calcaneal osteotomy. (*Reproduced with permission from Mann RA, Guyton GP: Medial displacement osteotomy of the calcaneus and flexor digitorum, in Kitaoka HB (ed): Master Techniques in Orthopaedic Surgery: The Foot and Ankle. Philadelphi, PA, Lippincott Williams and Wilkins, 2002, p 376.*)

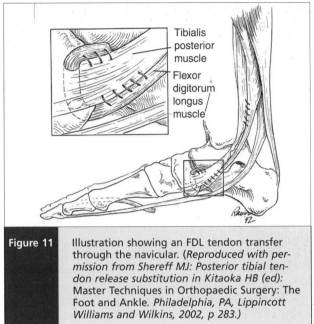

Figure 11 Illustration showing an FDL tendon transfer through the navicular. (*Reproduced with permission from Shereff MJ: Posterior tibial tendon release substitution in Kitaoka HB (ed): Master Techniques in Orthopaedic Surgery: The Foot and Ankle. Philadelphia, PA, Lippincott Williams and Wilkins, 2002, p 283.*)

is determined by verbal feedback from the patient and documented improvements in percentages of muscle strength compared with baseline recordings. Improvement without meeting required goals does not warrant continuation of physical therapy.

If the patient is improving, the remainder of the therapy sessions (up to 18 sessions) should continue with the described protocols for sessions three to five, with isokinetic retesting every three to four visits. If progress is continuing at the 18th session but goals have not been achieved, the patient should continue with a home exercise program with retests every 3 to 4 months to monitor progress. Some patients do not reach the established objective goals but still report improvement. Subjective improvement and independence in activities of daily living are important for patient satisfaction.

Surgical Treatment

Surgical treatment of AAFD resulting from PTTD is reserved for patients in whom nonsurgical treatment has failed to provide sufficient pain relief. A variety of surgical options and procedures have been developed to treat patients with various stages of PTTD. These options allow the treating physician to choose the treatment plan that is the least invasive and is most likely to decrease pain and improve function.

Stage I PTTD

Stage I PTTD rarely requires surgical treatment. Patients are usually managed with a period of immobilization in a cast or boot, followed by a rehabilitation program and the use of an orthotic device. Surgical débridement of tenosynovitis and repair of longitudinal tears have been reported when nonsurgical protocols are unsuccessful and no significant deformity is present.

In one study, 14 of 19 patients were pain-free after débridement of the tenosynovitis and 16 were able to perform SSHRs.[41] In a 2003 study, the authors described débridement of the tendon in eight athletes followed by immobilization for 4 weeks.[42] All patients were able to return to sports activities, with one patient experiencing occasional pain during participation.

Stages II and III PTTD

The best surgical option for patients with stage II PTTD is controversial. Triple arthrodesis has been the primary treatment, but concerns exist regarding postoperative stiffness and adjacent joint pain. Other surgical options that do not involve extensive arthrodeses include soft-tissue reconstruction, bony procedures, or a combination of both. Direct repair of the tendon is rarely performed as the primary procedure. Soft-tissue reconstruction consists of augmenting the diseased posterior tibial tendon. The flexor digitorum longus (FDL) tendon is usually used because of its proximity to the posterior tibial tendon and minimal functional loss. The flexor hallucis longus (FHL) tendon has been advocated by some surgeons because it is usually larger and stronger than the FDL.[43] The transfer of the peroneus brevis to balance the foot in patients with a small or incompetent FDL tendon has been recommended.[44] Other authors recommend a split anterior tibial tendon transfer.[45] These tendon transfers can reduce pain and provide stabilization without fusion, but may not provide lasting improvement in arch alignment. Other soft tissues, such as the spring ligament, also may be repaired to provide static stabilization of the arch.[46] Achilles tendon lengthening or gastrocnemius resection may be performed as adjunctive surgery with posterior tibial tendon reconstruction to treat the equinus deformity.

3: Arthritis

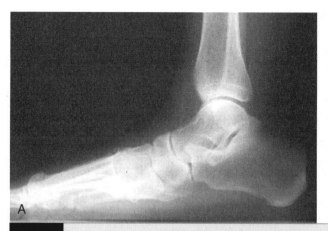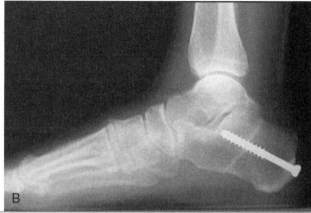

| Figure 12 | Radiographs of the foot of a patient with PTTD and flatfoot before **(A)** and after **(B)** medial displacement calcaneal osteotomy with FDL tendon transfer and Achilles tendon lengthening. The patient had good clinical results. Note the improved arch alignment. |

Bony procedures have been developed with the goal of correcting hindfoot valgus, forefoot abduction, and arch height. Medial displacement calcaneal osteotomy is performed to reduce hindfoot valgus and is usually combined with FDL tendon transfer (**Figures 10 and 11**). Lateral column lengthening with an opening wedge osteotomy through the anterior calcaneus or through the calcaneocuboid joint via distraction arthrodesis can improve forefoot abduction deformity and preserve some hindfoot mobility. Procedures to stabilize the medial column through arthrodesis or osteotomy designed to plantar flex the forefoot have been described. Limited hindfoot arthrodesis is applicable in selected patients, such as those with failed PTTD surgeries, inflammatory arthropathy, degenerative arthritis, obesity, or severe stiffness in which the deformity cannot be corrected through joint-sparing procedures.

The literature has many reports of the results of posterior tibial tendon reconstruction and medial displacement calcaneal osteotomies (**Figure 12**). With high levels of patient satisfaction, medial displacement calcaneal osteotomy has been recommended for less severe, flexible, flatfoot deformities.[18,47-49] However, radiographic results have not always correlated with clinical results. Gait analysis has shown significant improvement in cadence, stride length, and push-off.[50] Biomechanical studies have shown that calcaneal displacement osteotomy improves the peak pressure under the first and second metatarsal heads, but increases the pressure in the lateral forefoot.[51] The authors of a 2005 study compared patients in whom the posterior tibial tendon was removed during tendon transfer with calcaneal osteotomy with those in whom the tendon was retained; no clinical difference in functional scores was found at 1-year follow-up.[52] The Cobb procedure involves a split anterior tibial tendon transfer through the first cuneiform to the posterior tibial tendon insertion. Because good or excellent results were obtained in 21 of 22 patients, the authors concluded that the Cobb procedure was an acceptable alternative to other procedures for supple PTTD.[45]

Lateral column lengthening of the calcaneus corrects the forefoot abduction deformity of the foot by adducting and plantar flexing the midfoot around the talar head.[53] This procedure can be done through the neck of the calcaneus or the calcaneocuboid joint. Both in vivo and in vitro studies have shown improvement in arch alignment. The results of lateral column lengthening with posterior tibial tendon reconstruction are satisfactory.[54] In one study, 27 feet were treated with lateral column lengthening.[55] Ten patients had lateral column lengthening through the neck of the calcaneus with tricortical iliac crest bone graft, and 17 patients had lengthening though the calcaneocuboid joint. Improvement in radiographic and functional outcomes was observed, with no statistical significance between the groups. However, relatively high complication rates have been reported, including nonunion, lateral foot pain, graft failure, development of calcaneocuboid arthritis, and prominent hardware. In another study of 28 feet, the authors reported on a double calcaneal osteotomy with a medial displacement osteotomy and lateral column lengthening as a method of reconstruction in stage II PTTD.[56] At intermediate follow-up, satisfactory clinical results were found along with marked improvement in radiographic appearance. Both tricortical iliac crest autograft and allograft have been used for lengthening procedures. A prospective randomized study reported equal union rates in groups treated with allograft and autograft; however, the group treated with allograft had less morbidity and allograft was less costly because there was no need to harvest the iliac crest.[57]

Subtalar arthroereisis uses an implant placed in the sinus tarsi to limit pronation. This procedure usually is combined with soft-tissue reconstruction. In a 2003 study of 21 patients with stage II PTTD treated with tendon repair or reconstruction with the FDL or FHL followed by arthroereisis, satisfactory results were reported in 17 patients.[58] The implant was removed in two patients because of pain and two patients were lost

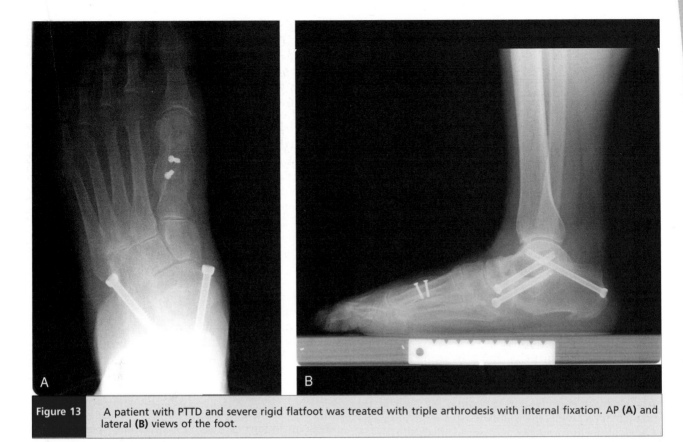

Figure 13 A patient with PTTD and severe rigid flatfoot was treated with triple arthrodesis with internal fixation. AP **(A)** and lateral **(B)** views of the foot.

to follow-up. The authors believed that the procedure was an acceptable alternative to osteotomy or arthrodesis.[58] In another study of this procedure, 18 of 23 patients had satisfactory clinical outcomes, but implant removal was needed for 11 patients because of pain.[59]

Hindfoot arthrodesis is recommended for patients with rigid deformities (stage 3) or for patients with flexible deformities who are obese, elderly, have low physical demands, or have inflammatory or degenerative arthritis. It is also applicable for patients who had unsuccessful hindfoot reconstruction surgery. Arthrodesis is often performed at the calcaneocuboid or subtalar joint. Other options, such as arthrodesis of the talonavicular joint or double arthrodesis at the talonavicular and calcaneocuboid joints, can be used. Triple arthrodesis is recommended for patients with severe deformity and arthritis.

Isolated subtalar arthrodesis can be performed when a patient has a fixed deformity of the subtalar joint with a flexible forefoot. One study of 21 feet treated with isolated subtalar arthrodesis showed 16 good or excellent results and significantly improved alignment.[60] In another study of 17 patients, isolated subtalar arthrodesis was combined with an FDL tendon transfer and repair of the spring ligament. The authors believed that adding soft-tissue reconstruction to the fusion improved the correction. All patients progressed to union with improvement in radiographic and clinical scores comparable with other joint-sparing procedures.[61]

Other surgical options, such as talonavicular arthrodesis, have been recommended in patients with PTTD with no evidence of adjacent joint arthritis; however, a higher nonunion rate has been observed compared with other types of hindfoot arthrodeses. The author of one study reported on isolated talonavicular arthrodesis for AAFD in 27 patients, of which 24 had good or excellent results; nonunion occurred in 1 patient.[62] Double arthrodesis involving talonavicular and calcaneocuboid joints has been recommended for patients with a flexible deformity and no evidence of subtalar joint pain or arthritic changes. This procedure eliminates the range of motion of the subtalar joint. The authors of another study reported the results of 24 patients treated with double arthrodesis with an average follow-up of 56 months; the study included 16 patients with adult AAFD.[63] Two thirds of these patients had good or excellent results. Nonunion occurred in four joints at the talonavicular level. In another study, 12 of 16 patients had good or excellent results with double arthrodesis.[64] There was one asymptomatic nonunion at the talonavicular level.

Triple arthrodesis is recommended for patients with PTTD and associated arthritis, rigid deformity that cannot be passively corrected, and failed reconstructions (**Figure 13**). The goal of this surgery is to realign the hindfoot into approximately 5° of valgus and correct the transverse tarsal joints into a neutral alignment. Triple arthrodesis usually results in satisfactory outcomes; however, the potential for adjacent joint

3. Arthritis

pain or arthritis must be recognized. After successful triple arthrodesis, many patients with PTTD and severe flatfoot with calcaneofibular impingement continue to have aching in the lateral ankle area from the preexisting degenerative changes. Long-term results of 67 triple arthrodeses, performed in 64 patients with various diagnoses, showed that 33% of patients had degenerative ankle changes at 25 years and all patients had such changes at 44 years. However, the radiographic appearance of the ankle joint did not correlate with symptoms.[65]

Stage IV PTTD

Patients with stage IV PTTD have long-standing deformity and symptoms that result in valgus deformity and arthritic changes in the ankle. These patients usually have limited motion of the hindfoot and ankle. Surgical options include triple arthrodesis with or without medial ankle ligament reconstruction if the ankle joint is malaligned in valgus but not severely arthritic. By realigning and reconstructing the hindfoot, it is possible to preserve ankle motion. In other instances, when the ankle joint is not functional and salvageable, tibiotalocalcaneal arthrodesis, or, rarely, pantalar arthrodesis, may be performed. When performing tibiotalocalcaneal arthrodesis, it is preferable to realign the arch at the subtalar level with the talonavicular and calcaneocuboid joints positioned close to neutral. If there is marked rigidity of the entire hindfoot, pantalar arthrodesis is sometimes performed to create a plantigrade foot. After pantalar arthrodesis, ankle and foot stiffness is more obvious. It is important that the patient understands the limitations of this procedure. Triple arthrodesis followed by ankle replacement has the theoretic advantage of preserving ankle motion and improving function; however, study results of this treatment protocol are not available.

Complications of PTTD Surgery

Complications in patients undergoing reconstruction for PTTD are not uncommon and include infection, wound healing difficulties, nerve injury, nonunion, malunion, overcorrection, undercorrection, progression of arthritis, painful hardware, and other medical complications such as deep venous thrombosis. Risks are procedure-specific, but patients with diabetes or those who had previous surgery have an increased risk of complications. Infections can be minimized with appropriate preoperative antibiotics, proper skin preparation, and meticulous surgical technique. Wound complications occur more often in patients with diabetes or severe deformities, those treated with systemic corticosteroid, or those who use nicotine products. Nonunion is rare after medial displacement calcaneal osteotomy but is more common after lateral column lengthening and arthrodesis procedures. Patients who use nicotine products, take corticosteroids, have diabetes, or are un-

able to comply with the non–weight-bearing requirement in the early postoperative period are at higher risk of nonunion. Careful surgical technique decreases the risk of undercorrection or overcorrection, but certain procedures such as isolated tendon repair or reconstruction often are associated with recurrent or residual deformity. The risk of deep venous thrombosis is low after foot and ankle surgery, but prophylaxis could be considered in patients with a history of deep venous thrombosis or when prolonged immobilization is expected.[3] Prominent and painful hardware occasionally is observed and removal of hardware is performed when appropriate. Sural nerve entrapment resulting from lateral hindfoot incisions can be minimized with proper planning of the incision, careful dissection, and protection of the nerve.

Summary

PTTD is a common cause of medial ankle pain and should be considered in the differential diagnosis in traumatic and atraumatic presentations. Patient history, physical examination, and plain radiography are usually sufficient for making a diagnosis. MRI is seldom needed. Treatment is guided by the clinical stage and flexibility of the deformity. A trial of nonsurgical treatment, including activity modification, nonsteroidal anti-inflammatory drugs, bracing, and physical therapy, is justified for most patients. Nonsurgical outcomes are promising in patients with earlier stages of the disorder. Steroid injections have no role in the treatment of PTTD.

If adequate symptomatic relief is not achieved, surgery should be considered. There are multiple options for surgical management; the treatment decision is based on factors such as flexibility and magnitude of the foot deformity, patient comorbidities, age, and functional goals of the patient. The purpose of treatment is to improve pain and function. Recovery can be prolonged after surgical treatment, but most patients are satisfied with the outcome. No single surgical technique is applicable for all patients with PTTD.

Annotated References

1. Kulowski J: General discussion and report of one case involving the posterior tibial tendon. *J Missouri State Med Assn* 1936;33:135-137.

2. Fowler AW: Tibialis posterior syndrome. *J Bone Joint Surg Br* 1955;37:520.

3. Kettelkamp DB, Alexander HH: Spontaneous rupture of the posterior tibial tendon. *J Bone Joint Surg Am* 1969; 51:759-764.

4. Evans D: Calcaneo-valgus deformity. *J Bone Joint Surg Br* 1975;57:270-278.

5. Van Boerum DH, Sangeorzan BJ: Biomechanics and pathophysiology of flatfoot. *Foot Ankle Clin* 2003;8:419-430.

6. Goncalves-Neto J, Witzel SS, Teodoro WR, Carvalho-Júnior AE, Fernandes TD, Yoshinari HH: Changes in collagen matrix composition in human posterior tibial tendon dysfunction. *Joint Bone Spine* 2002;69:189-194.

7. Frey C, Shereff M, Greenidge N: Vascularity of the posterior tibial tendon. *J Bone Joint Surg Am* 1990;72:884-888.

8. Prado MP, de Carvalho Jr AE, Rodrigues CJ, Fernandes TD, Morreira Mendes AA, Salomao O: Vascular density of the posterior tibial tendon: A cadaver study. *Foot Ankle Int* 2006;27:628-631.

    Histologic specimens from 80 cadavers were stained in Masson's trichrome and used to verify vascular density using microscopic analysis. No decreased vascular density was seen in the midportion of the tendon as had been previously reported in the literature.

9. Davis WH, Sobel M, DiCarlo EF, et al: Gross histological, and microvascular anatomy and biomechanical testing of the spring ligament complex. *Foot Ankle Int* 1996;17:95-102.

10. Mizel MS, Temple HT, Scranton PE Jr, et al: Role of the peroneal tendons in the production of the deformed foot with posterior tibial tendon deficiency. *Foot Ankle Int* 1999;20:285-289.

11. Deland JT, de Asla RJ, Sung I, Ernberg LA, Potter HG: Posterior tibial tendon insufficiency: Which ligaments are involved? *Foot Ankle Int* 2005;26:427-435.

    The authors present the results of an observational study using MRI to identify a pattern of ligament failure in a series of 31 consecutive patients diagnosed with PTTD compared with an age-matched control group. The superomedial and inferomedial calcaneonavicular sections of the spring ligament and the talocalcaneal interosseous ligament were the most severely involved. The authors suggest that treatment should protect against the progressive failure of these ligaments.

12. Beals TC, Pomeroy GC, Manoli A II: Posterior tibial tendon insufficiency: Diagnosis and treatment. *J Am Acad Orthop Surg* 1999;7:112-118.

13. Jahss MH: Spontaneous rupture of the tibialis posterior tendon: Clinical findings, tenographic studies, and a new technique of repair. *Foot Ankle* 1982;3:158-166.

14. Mosier SM, Lucas DR, Pomeroy G, Manoli A II: Pathology of the posterior tibial tendon in posterior tibial tendon insufficiency. *Foot Ankle Int* 1998;19:520-524.

15. Johnson KA, Strom DE: Tibialis posterior tendon dysfunction. *Clin Orthop Relat Res* 1989;239:196-206.

16. Myerson MS: Adult acquired flatfoot deformity. *J Bone Joint Surg Am* 1996;78:780-790.

17. Conti S, Michelson J, Jahss M: Clinical significance of magnetic resonance imaging in preoperative planning for reconstruction of posterior tibial tendon rupture. *Foot Ankle* 1992;13:208-214.

18. Vora AM, Tien TR, Parks BG, Schon LC: Correction of moderate and severe acquired flatfoot deformity with medializing calcaneal osteotomy and flexor digitorum longus transfer. *J Bone Joint Surg Am* 2006;88:1726-1734.

    Mild and severe flatfoot deformity of cadaveric specimens was created followed by surgical correction with and without subtalar arthroereisis. Specimens were cyclically loaded at all stages and radiographic and pedobarographic measurements taken. Addition of arthroereisis corrected radiographic measurements in severe deformity versus osteotomy and tendon transfer alone. The group with severe flatfoot deformity was undercorrected. Level of evidence: III.

19. Bluman EM, Title CI, Myerson MS: Posterior tibial tendon rupture: A refined classification system. *Foot Ankle Clin* 2007;12:233-249.

    A four-stage classification system of PTTD with substages for each stage is described. This system improves the orthopaedic surgeon's awareness of the etiologies associated with adult acquired flatfoot. Characteristic clinical findings, radiographic findings, and suggested treatment for each stage of PTTD help in treatment planning.

20. Mizel MS, Hecht PJ, Marymont MD, Temple HT: Evaluation and treatment of chronic ankle pain. *Instr Course Lect* 2004;53:311-321.

    The etiology and treatment of the most common causes of chronic ankle pain, including PTTD, are reviewed.

21. Holmes GB, Mann RA: Possible epidemiological factors associated with rupture of the posterior tibial tendon. *Foot Ankle* 1992;13:70-79.

22. Pinney SJ, Lin SS: Current concept review: Acquired adult flatfoot deformity. *Foot Ankle Int* 2006;27:66-75.

    The authors present a comprehensive review of AAFD specifically focusing on anatomy, biomechanics, clinical manifestations, and treatment.

23. Hintermann B, Gachter A: The first metatarsal rise sign: A simple sensitive sign of tibialis posterior tendon dysfunction. *Foot Ankle Int* 1996;17:236-241.

24. Rosenberg ZS, Cheung Y, Jahss MH, Noto AM, Norman A, Leeds NE: Rupture of posterior tibial tendon: CT and MR imaging with surgical correlation. *Radiology* 1988;169:229-235.

25. Feighan J, Towers J, Conti M: The use of magnetic resonance imaging in posterior tibial tendon dysfunction. *Clin Orthop Relat Res* 1999;365:23-58.

26. Miller SD, Marnix VH, Boruta PM, Wu KK, Katcherian DA: Ultrasound in the diagnosis of posterior tibial tendon pathology. *Foot Ankle Int* 1996;17:555-558.

3: Arthritis

27. Perry MB, Premkumar A, Venzon DJ, Shawker TH, Gerber LH: Ultrasound, magnetic resonance imaging, and posterior tibialis dysfunction. *Clin Orthop Relat Res* 2003;408:225-231.

Using MRI and ultrasound, the authors prospectively evaluated 31 patients with clinically diagnosed PTTD. MRI was found to be more sensitive in identifying posterior tendon tears versus either clinical examination or ultrasound testing.

28. Elftman NW: Nonsurgical treatment of adult acquired flat foot deformity. *Foot Ankle Clin* 2003;8:473-489.

The author presents a review of the pathology, presentation, and nonsurgical treatments of PTTD, specifically concentrating on various orthotic and bracing techniques.

29. Frey CC, Shereff MJ: Tendon injuries about the ankle in athletes. *Clin Sports Med* 1988;7:103-118.

30. Chao W, Wapner KL, Lee TH, Adams J, Hecht PJ: Nonoperative management of posterior tibial tendon dysfunction. *Foot Ankle Int* 1996;17:736-741.

31. Lin SS, Lee TH, Chao W, Wapner KL: Nonoperative treatment of patients with posterior tibial tendonitis. *Foot Ankle Clin* 1996;1:261-277.

32. Sferra JJ, Rosenberg GA: Nonoperative treatment of posterior tibial tendon pathology. *Foot Ankle Clin* 1997;2:261-273.

33. Imhauser CW, Abidi NA, Frankel DZ, Gavin K, Siegler S: Biomechanical evaluation of the efficacy of external stabilizers in the conservative treatment of acquired flatfoot deformity. *Foot Ankle Int* 2002;23:727-737.

34. Augustin JF, Lin SS, Berberian WS, Johnson JE: Nonoperative treatment of adult acquired flat foot with the Arizona brace. *Foot Ankle Clin* 2003;8:491-502.

In this prospective study, 21 patients with clinically diagnosed PTTD were treated with the Arizona brace. Over a 2-year period, 90% of patients showed significant improvement of symptoms, with 100% of those with stage I or II disease showing improvement. The authors concluded that the Arizona brace was a viable nonsurgical treatment for PTTD.

35. Alvarez RG, Marini A, Schmitt C, Saltzman CL: Stage I and II posterior tibial tendon dysfunction treated by a structured nonoperative protocol: An orthosis and exercise program. *Foot Ankle Int* 2006;27:2-8.

In this prospective study, 47 patients received nonsurgical treatment for stage I and II PTTD. The treatment protocol included bracing, a monitored physical therapy program, and a home exercise program. The authors reported that 83% of patients had successful subjective and functional outcomes with an 89% patient satisfaction rate.

36. Marzano R: Orthotic considerations and footwear modifications following fusion techniques. *Foot Ankle Surg* 2002;1:46-49.

37. Wapner KL, Chao W: Nonoperative treatment of posterior tibial tendon dysfunction. *Clin Orthop Relat Res* 1999;365:39-45.

38. Hintermann B, Nigg BM, Summer C, Cole GK: The movement transfer between calcaneus and tibia, in vitro. *Clin Biomech* 1994;9:349-355.

39. Noll KH: The use of orthotic devices in adult acquired flatfoot deformity. *Foot Ankle Clin* 2001;6:25-36.

40. Pomeroy GC, Pike RH, Beals TC, Manoli A II: Acquired flatfoot in adults due to dysfunction of the posterior tibial tendon. *J Bone Joint Surg Am* 1999;81:1173-1182.

41. Teasdall RD, Johnson KA: Surgical treatment of stage I posterior tibial tendon dysfunction. *Foot Ankle Int* 1994;15:646-648.

42. McCormack AP, Varner KE, Marymont JV: Surgical treatment for posterior tibial tendonitis in young competitive athletes. *Foot Ankle Int* 2003;24:535-538.

The authors present a retrospective review of eight competitive athletes treated with surgical débridement for PTTD. Seven of the eight athletes returned to full participation in sports activities without difficulty. Level of evidence: IV.

43. Sammarco GJ, Hockenbury RT: Treatment of stage II posterior tibial tendon dysfunction with flexor hallucis longus tendon transfer and medial displacement calcaneal osteotomy. *Foot Ankle Int* 2001;22:305-312.

44. Song SJ, Deland JT: Outcome following addition of peroneus brevis tendon transfer in treatment of acquired posterior tibial tendon insufficiency. *Foot Ankle Int* 2001;22:301-304.

45. Knupp M, Hintermann B: The Cobb procedure for treatment of acquired flatfoot deformity associated with stage II insufficiency of the posterior tibial tendon. *Foot Ankle Int* 2007;28:416-421.

46. Gazdag AR, Cracchiolo A III: Rupture of the posterior tibial tendon: Evaluation of injury of the spring ligament and clinical assessment of tendon transfer and ligament repair. *J Bone Joint Surg Am* 1997;79:675-681.

47. Wacker JT, Hennessey MS, Saxby TS: Calcaneal osteotomy and transfer of the flexor digitorum longus for stage II dysfunction of the tibialis posterior: Three to five year results. *J Bone Joint Surg Br* 2002;84:54-58.

48. Myerson MS, Badekas A, Schon LC: Treatment of stage II posterior tibial tendon deficiency with flexor digitorum longus tendon transfer and calcaneal osteotomy. *Foot Ankle Int* 2004;25:445-450.

This retrospective review of 129 patients with stage II PTTD treated with FDL tendon transfer and medial displacement calcaneal osteotomy with a mean follow-up of 5.2 years showed significant improvement in radiographic and clinical parameters. Level of evidence: IV.

49. Myerson MS: Adult acquired flatfoot deformity: Treatment of dysfunction of the posterior tibial tendon. *J Bone Joint Surg Am* 1996;78:780-792.

50. Brodsky JW: Preliminary gait analysis results after posterior tibial tendon reconstruction: A prospective study. *Foot Ankle Int* 2004;25:96-100.

   The author presents the results of a prospective study on the preoperative and 1-year postoperative gait analysis of 12 consecutive patients with stage II PTTD who underwent FDL transfer with calcaneal osteotomy. The authors found statistically significant improvement in gait function. Level of evidence: II.

51. Hadfield MH, Snyder JW, Liacouras PC, Owen JR, Wayne JS, Adelaar RS: Effects of medializing calcaneal osteotomy on Achilles tendon lengthening and plantar foot pressures. *Foot Ankle Int* 2003;24:523-529.

   Fourteen fresh-frozen cadaver legs were used to evaluate the effect of medial displacement calcaneal osteotomy on Achilles tendon length and plantar pressures. The authors noted a decrease in plantar pressures in the first and second metatarsophalangeal region. Level of evidence: II.

52. Rosenfeld PF, Dick J, Saxby TS: The response of the flexor digitorum longus and posterior tibial muscles to tendon transfer and calcaneal osteotomy for stage II posterior tibial tendon dysfunction. *Foot Ankle Int* 2005;26:671-674.

   The authors of this prospective study used MRI to evaluate the posterior tibial and FDL muscles in patients who had the posterior tibial muscle excised or retained with FDL transfer and calcaneal osteotomy. Level of evidence: II.

53. Dumontier TA, Falicov A, Mosca V, Sangeorzan B: Calcaneal lengthening: Investigation of the deformity correction in a cadaveric flatfoot model. *Foot Ankle Int* 2005;26:166-170.

   This cadaveric study examined the effect of Evan's procedure on three-dimensional CT of the hindfoot and noted adduction and plantar flexion of the midfoot relative to the hindfoot. Level of evidence: II.

54. Jarde O, Abiraad G, Gabrion A, Vernois J, Massy S: Triple arthrodesis in the management of acquired flatfoot deformity in the adult secondary to posterior tibial tendon dysfunction: A retrospective study of 20 cases. *Acta Orthop Belg* 2002;68:56-62.

55. Thomas RL, Wells BC, Garrison RL, Prada SA: Preliminary results comparing two methods of lateral column lengthening. *Foot Ankle Int* 2001;22:107-119.

56. Moseir-LaClair S, Pomeroy G, Manoli A II: Intermediate follow-up on the double osteotomy and tendon transfer procedure for stage II posterior tibial tendon insufficiency. *Foot Ankle Int* 2001;22:283-291.

57. Dolan CM, Henning JA, Anderson JG, Bohay DR, Kornmesser MJ, Endres TJ: Randomized prospective study comparing tri-cortical iliac crest autograft to allograft in the lateral column lengthening component for operative correction of adult acquired flatfoot deformity. *Foot Ankle Int* 2007;28:8-12.

   The authors of this randomized prospective study compared 18 patients with AAFD treated with lateral column lengthening with an allograft to 15 patients treated with autograft. The union rates were equal for both groups. Level of evidence: II.

58. Viladot R, Pons M, Alvarez F, Omaña J: Subtalar arthroereisis for posterior tibial tendon dysfunction: A preliminary report. *Foot Ankle Int* 2003;24:600-606.

   A retrospective review of 19 patients treated with subtalar arthroereisis for stage II PTTD is presented. At a mean follow-up of 27 months, satisfactory results were reported in 17 patients. The arthroereisis screw was removed in two patients. Level of evidence: IV.

59. Needleman RL: A surgical approach for flexible flatfeet in adults including a subtalar arthroereisis with MBA sinus tarsi implant. *Foot Ankle Int* 2006;27:9-18.

   In this study of arthroereisis sinus tarsi implants in 28 feet (23 patients), 78% of patients reported favorable outcomes; however, 39% of implants were removed because of pain. Level of evidence: IV.

60. Kitaoka HB, Patzer GL: Subtalar arthrodesis for posterior tibial tendon dysfunction and pes planus. *Clin Orthop Relat Res* 1997;345:187-194.

61. Johnson JE, Cohen BE, DiGiovanni BF, Lamdan R: Subtalar arthrodesis with flexor digitorum longus tendon transfer and spring ligament repair for treatment of posterior tibial tendon insufficiency. *Foot Ankle Int* 2000;21:722-729.

62. Harper MC: Talonavicular arthrodesis for the acquired flatfoot in the adult. *Clin Orthop Relat Res* 1999;365:65-68.

63. Mann RA, Beaman DN: Double arthrodesis in the adult. *Clin Orthop Relat Res* 1999;365:74-80.

64. Clain MR, Baxter DE: Simultaneous calcaneocuboid and talonavicular fusion: Long-term follow-up study. *J Bone Joint Surg Br* 1994;76:133-136.

65. Saltzman CL, Fehrle MJ, Cooper RR, Spencer EC, Ponseti IV: Triple arthrodesis: Twenty-five and forty-four year average follow up of the same patients. *J Bone Joint Surg Am* 1999;81:1391-1402.

The Forefoot

Section Editor:

Ruth L. Thomas, MD

Chapter 18

Hallux Valgus

Loretta B. Chou, MD   Alexis A. Dieter, MD   James Aronson, MD   Derek M. Kelly, MD

Introduction

Hallux valgus is a common forefoot deformity that occurs in adults, adolescents, and younger children; however, its etiology is complex and not yet fully understood. The diagnosis of hallux valgus, or bunion, can be made when there is lateral deviation of the proximal phalanx of the great toe with an increased hallux valgus angle (HVA), increased first-second intermetatarsal angle (IMA_{1-2}), pronation of the hallux, and a prominent medial eminence.[1] The deformity as well as the symptoms can be mild, moderate, or severe (**Figure 1**).

Adult Hallux Valgus

Etiology and Pathoanatomy

The direct cause of hallux valgus is still debated but it is hypothesized that the disorder results from a multifactorial process involving both intrinsic and extrinsic factors. The steps involved in the pathogenesis of hallux valgus are well described.[2,3] The development of hallux valgus involves the interaction of both reactive ground forces and dynamic muscular forces. Repetitive valgus force with weight-bearing activity results in valgus deformity at the first metatarsophalangeal (MTP) joint with the proximal phalanx moving laterally. The first metatarsal head drifts into varus alignment. The capsule of the first MTP joint becomes attenuated on the medial side and the ridge separating the medial and lateral sesamoids is worn down. The sesamoids become displaced in the area where the medial sesamoid can lie plantar to the first metatarsal head in the area of the ridge, and the lateral sesamoid is displaced into the first intermetatarsal space. In patients with a chronic deformity, the lateral structures contract and add to the deforming forces pulling the hallux laterally. The most important lateral structures are the lateral joint capsule and the adductor tendon. The resultant alteration of normal alignment leads to an imbalance of the forces on the hallux and medial deviation of the first metatarsal head. The hallux assumes a more dorsiflexed and pronated position, thereby increasing the weight-bearing pressure on the second and possibly third metatarsal heads. With severe hallux valgus, a claw toe deformity can develop in the second toe and the joint may subluxate or dislocate.

Ill-fitting shoes, particularly those with high heels and a narrow toe box, have long been implicated as a contributing extrinsic factor in the development of hallux valgus in adults. The authors of a study comparing unshod and shod individuals in the Chinese population concluded that footwear constricts the naturally mobile and flexible foot, causing alterations leading to static deformities such as hallux valgus.[4] The increased incidence of hallux valgus in shod populations has been demonstrated in the literature, and it is hypothesized that the significantly increased prevalence of hallux valgus deformity among women is strongly influenced by their use of constrictive footwear.[2,3,5]

Multiple intrinsic factors have been proposed that may contribute to the development of hallux valgus. These factors include genetic predisposition, hypermobility of the first tarsometatarsal joint, pes planus, and the shape of the first metatarsal head. In a 2007 study

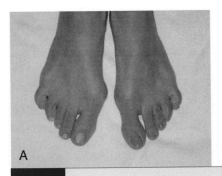
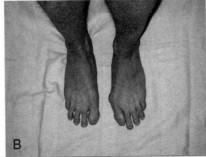
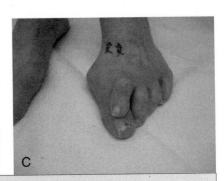

Figure 1   Clinical photographs of painful hallux valgus deformities. **A,** Mild deformity. **B,** Moderate deformity. **C,** Severe deformity that affects the second toe (crossover toe deformity).

of 108 patients with a diagnosis of moderate to severe hallux valgus, 84% of the patients reported a positive family history of the disorder, and of those with a positive history, most patients (64.5%) were younger than 30 years of age.[5] A statistically significant association between bilateral deformity and family history ($P <$ 0.01) also was reported, supporting the hypothesis that inheritance plays a role in the development of hallux valgus.

Hypermobility of the first tarsometatarsal joint has been implicated as an important etiologic factor. Although a definitive method of measurement is still not accepted, multiple investigations support a correlation between increased mobility of the first ray and hallux valgus.[6-11] Hypermobility of the first tarsometatarsal joint is believed to cause hallux valgus by increasing the IMA_{1-2} or by contributing to pes planus. However, the role of this hypermobility (if any) in hallux valgus is controversial because of the lack of prospective data and uncertainty regarding the specific mechanism of action. Interestingly, one study of painful versus painless hallux valgus found that increased mobility of the first ray showed a statistically significant association with the clinical report of pain.[8]

Pes planus is also proposed as a factor associated with the development of hallux valgus. Pes planus is believed to lead to increased forefoot abduction, thus placing a nonphysiologic load on the plantar medial aspect of the great toe, causing hallux valgus; however, this association is controversial and no definitive conclusions can be made at this time.[2]

The shape of the first metatarsal head may be a factor in the development of this deformity. Because a round-shaped first metatarsal head may be less stable than a square-shaped head, a patient with the rounded head may have a greater risk of developing hallux valgus. In one study, 71% of the participants had a curved articular surface.[5] However, because the incidence of individuals with a curved first metatarsal head in the general population is not known, this hypothesis remains an observation.

Clinical Presentation and Evaluation

Patients generally present with reports of pain, difficulties with footwear, and skin irritation, which can be severe with ulceration or infection.[5] The evaluation should include information on the patient's occupation, sport activities, and footwear. Activity level should be assessed and any limitations caused by the deformity and associated symptoms should be determined.[2]

The physical examination begins with an inspection of the feet with the patient standing. Hallux valgus deformity is worse with weight bearing (lesser toe disorders also become more pronounced with weight bearing).[3] Inspection of the plantar aspect of the foot may show callosities under the lesser metatarsal heads (transfer lesions). Palpation for tenderness of the medial eminence and under the second metatarsal head should be performed. Foot and ankle range of motion

is then tested. The motion of the first MTP joint and the first tarsometatarsal joint are compared to the contralateral side, and any limitation is noted. This comparison allows determination of normal values for a particular patient because normal values for the general population are not defined.[2,10] In evaluating first tarsometatarsal hypermobility, the joint is taken through a range of motion in the sagittal and transverse planes.[12,13] It is helpful to test passive range of motion of the first MTP joint while manually correcting the hallux valgus deformity. The resulting motion can be predictive of the range of motion that will be present following surgical correction of the deformity.

The patient's vascular and neurologic statuses are then evaluated to complete the physical examination. Surgery should be avoided in the absence of adequate vascular inflow. Noninvasive vascular testing or consultation with a vascular surgeon is warranted in patients with symptomatic peripheral vascular disease. Because neurologic disorders can adversely affect wound or bone healing, patients with these disorders should be treated nonsurgically.

Radiographic Examination

The hallux is unique and complex because of the sesamoid mechanism. Evaluation of hallux valgus deformity requires weight-bearing AP and lateral radiographs of the foot, a non–weight-bearing oblique view, and a special sesamoid view (axial view of the forefoot) (Figure 2). On the AP view, the HVA, the IMA_{1-2}, and the distal metatarsal articular angle (DMAA) can be measured[2,3,5] (Figure 3). The HVA is measured by drawing lines through the longitudinal axis of the first metatarsal and proximal phalanx. The normal value is less than 15°. The IMA_{1-2} is created by the bisection of the longitudinal axes drawn through the first and second metatarsals. This angle is normally less than 9° and it measures the degree of metatarsus primus varus. The DMAA is measured by the angle of the articular surface of the first metatarsal and the longitudinal axis of the first metatarsal. The normal value of the DMAA is less than 10°. However, the measurement of this angle has high interobserver and intraobserver variability.[14] In contrast, the reliability is excellent for HVA and IMA measurements.[15-17] Using measurements of the HVA and IMA_{1-2}, the severity of hallux valgus can be classified as a mild deformity (HVA < 30°; IMA_{1-2} < 13°), a moderate deformity (HVA = 30° to 40°; IMA_{1-2} = 14° to 20°), or a severe deformity (HVA > 40°; IMA_{1-2} > 20°).[3,5] The longitudinal angulation between the proximal phalanx and the distal phalanx also should be measured. If there is significant lateral deviation, hallux valgus interphalangeus is present.[3] Evaluation of the total deformity should include the location of the sesamoids in relationship to the first metatarsal head, the congruency of the first MTP joint, the size of the medial eminence, and notation of any characteristics of degenerative arthritis.

A congruent joint is present when the articular surface between the first metatarsal head and proximal

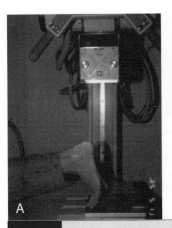
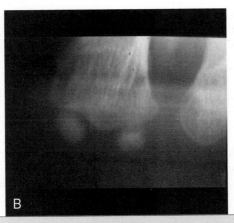
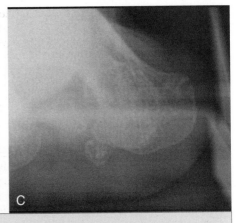

Figure 2   **A,** The sesamoids' position in relation to the metatarsal head is best seen with an axial view of the forefoot. **B,** The sesamoids are normally positioned on either side of the metatarsal crista. With hallux valgus deformity, the sesamoids can be displaced so laterally that the fibular sesamoid eventually rests adjacent to the lateral metatarsal head and the crista can disappear from erosion. **C,** Lateral displacement of the sesamoids in severe hallux valgus.

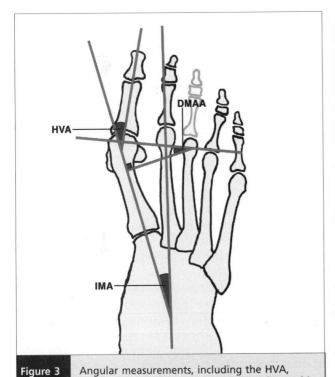

Figure 3   Angular measurements, including the HVA, IMA$_{1-2}$, and DMAA, are used in the radiographic evaluation of a hallux valgus deformity.

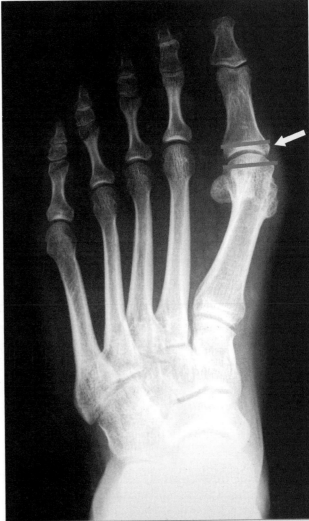

Figure 4   AP weight-bearing radiograph showing a mild hallux valgus deformity and a congruent joint. Note that the articular surface of the base of the proximal phalanx matches that of the metatarsal head (*arrow*).

phalanx are concentrically aligned (the proximal phalanx does not subluxate or deviate laterally from the metatarsal head) (**Figure 4**). The valgus deformity is caused by the lateral tilt of the articular surface.[18,19] A surgical procedure to correct the hallux valgus deformity must not change this congruency or alignment because pain or arthritis may result.

An incongruent joint occurs when the proximal phalanx subluxates or deviates laterally on the first metatarsal head[2] (**Figure 5**). Although the degree of subluxation varies with each patient, instability of the joint

4: The Forefoot

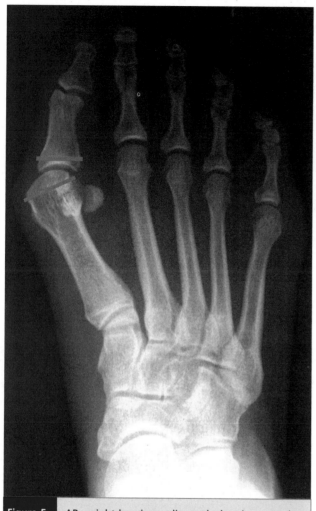

Figure 5 | AP weight-bearing radiograph showing a moderate hallux valgus deformity and an incongruent joint. The MTP joint is deviated so that the articular surface of the base of the proximal phalanx subluxates laterally to the metatarsal head.

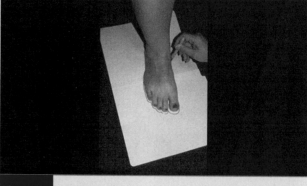

Figure 6 | Outlining the patient's foot and then placing the shoe on top of the outline allows a quick assessment of shoe fit.

can progress with time if the condition is untreated. The surgical procedure to correct this deformity must realign the joint to proper congruency.

The first MTP joint must be evaluated for arthritis. Radiographic findings include loss of joint space, subchondral sclerosis, cysts, and osteophytes. Arthritis will affect the treatment plan as well as the outcome. A bunionectomy will likely lead to unsatisfactory results because the arthritic symptoms may worsen. Patients with arthritis may require arthrodesis.

Nonsurgical Treatment

Patient education is the most important component in treatment of hallux valgus. Nonsurgical management includes the use of sufficiently wide footwear to accommodate the deformity. This concept can be illustrated by having the patient stand while the foot is outlined (**Figure 6**); the outline of the foot is then compared with an outline of the patient's shoe. Shoes with soft leather

uppers and extra width and depth can alleviate pressure and painful symptoms in many patients.[3] The shoe can be further modified with a bunion press to relieve the area of pressure directly over the medial eminence. Padding also can be beneficial and can include over-the-counter foot remedies such as pads, donuts, and toe sleeves. Custom foot orthoses are unlikely to be effective for alleviating the symptoms of hallux valgus, but often are successful in treating metatarsalgia from a transfer lesion under the lesser metatarsal heads.[20]

Surgical Treatment

Surgical treatment is indicated when conservative measures have failed. Failure is characterized by continued pain, limitations of normal daily activities, and inability to wear standard footwear. Surgical treatment should not be undertaken simply for cosmesis. The patient's expectations and results of physical and radiographic examinations are important components in determining the appropriate surgical option.

More than 100 surgical procedures have been described for the treatment of hallux valgus. In developing a surgical plan, the congruency of the first MTP joint is determined. The surgical procedure should not disturb a congruent joint but an incongruent joint must be corrected to normal alignment. Generally, mild deformities may be treated with distal osteotomies, whereas proximal procedures, arthrodesis, or combined osteotomies are used for patients with more severe deformities.[21]

For adults with mild deformities and a congruent joint, a distal chevron osteotomy is a reliable procedure and will retain the congruency of the joint. Moderate to severe deformities with an incongruent first MTP joint can be treated with a distal soft-tissue procedure and proximal osteotomy. HVA deformities greater than 45° may best be treated with arthrodesis. Although less commonly performed, Keller resection arthroplasty may be appropriate for an elderly patient with limited functional expectations who may be at risk for other injuries with limited postoperative weight bearing.[21,22]

Distal Correction

A simple bunionectomy is resection of the exostosis or medial eminence. It is generally not recommended to treat hallux valgus because of the high recurrence rate and poor patient satisfaction. Instead, the modified McBride procedure and distal chevron osteotomy are commonly performed.[21] The modified McBride procedure, usually performed as an adjunct to a bony procedure, involves a medial capsulotomy with imbrication, excision of the medial eminence, and release of the contracted deforming structures (the adductor tendon, lateral capsule, and transverse metatarsal ligament). This procedure allows realignment of an incongruent joint to congruency.

The distal chevron osteotomy is a V-shaped cut of the first metatarsal head. The capital fragment is translated laterally 4 to 6 mm, internally fixed with a Kirschner wire or screw, and the medial joint capsule is plicated. This osteotomy is effective in treating mild to moderate bunion deformity with a congruent joint. Previously, a lateral release was believed to increase the risks of osteonecrosis, but recent studies have shown no increased incidence of first metatarsal head osteonecrosis if soft-tissue stripping of the metatarsal head is minimized.[23] A closing wedge osteotomy based medially can be added to the chevron cut to correct an increased DMAA. This procedure is known as a biplanar chevron osteotomy. A postoperative dressing is used to hold the hallux in the corrected alignment. Complications for distal osteotomies include recurrence, incomplete correction, or osteonecrosis of the capital fragment.

Proximal Correction

Typically, a proximal osteotomy is performed in conjunction with a distal soft-tissue procedure to correct moderate to severe hallux valgus deformity. The distal soft-tissue procedure (modified McBride) will realign the incongruent joint, whereas the proximal osteotomy will correct the increased HVA and IMA_{1-2}. Many first metatarsal osteotomies have shown good surgical outcomes and high rates of patient satisfaction. These procedures include the proximal crescentic osteotomy, proximal chevron osteotomy, the proximal oblique (Ludloff) osteotomy, scarf osteotomy, lateral closing wedge proximal osteotomy, and the medial opening wedge proximal osteotomy[3,21] (Figure 7). Possible complications include considerable shortening of the first metatarsal and dorsiflexion malunion. The proximal crescentic osteotomy can provide good correction of deformity; however, a significant risk of dorsiflexion malunion has been reported.[24,25] The medial opening wedge proximal first metatarsal osteotomy is believed to maintain length in the first metatarsal and offers an interesting alternative when the first metatarsal is relatively short compared with the second metatarsal.[21] Other complications include recurrence of the deformity, hallux varus, and nonunion.

The proximal chevron osteotomy, the proximal crescentic osteotomy, and the long oblique osteotomy have demonstrated superior load-to-failure characteristics with screw fixation as opposed to Kirschner wire or staple fixation.[26] Postoperative management includes a compression dressing to hold the hallux in correct alignment and weight bearing in a postoperative shoe (with a stiff sole and straps to accommodate the dressing and swelling) until radiographic union at approximately 8 weeks.

Arthrodesis

Arthrodesis of the first MTP joint is indicated for arthritis of this joint. A dorsal incision allows good exposure and bony cuts can be made with a sagittal saw or with ball-and-socket–type reamers. The method of internal fixation depends on the bone quality. A combination of lag screws and dorsal plate may be used. Postoperative progressive weight bearing is allowed in a postoperative shoe or removable walking boot until radiographic healing is evident (at approximately 12 weeks). If nonunion occurs, it can be treated with continued protective weight bearing and observation or revision surgery. Malunion is less likely if rigid internal fixation is obtained.

Arthrodesis between the base of the first and second metatarsals and the first metatarsocuneiform joint is known as the Lapidus procedure. This procedure has been used in patients with hypermobility of the first tarsometatarsal joint, especially if the patient has generalized ligamentous laxity.[3] A 2007 study of 103 patients with moderate to severe deformities treated with a proximal osteotomy and distal soft-tissue procedure found that first ray mobility was reduced to normal following bunion deformity correction without the need for arthrodesis of the first metatarsocuneiform joint.[6] This procedure also has been proposed as an effective salvage procedure for hallux valgus recurrence; however, there is insufficient evidence available at this time to make a definitive recommendation.[21]

Proximal Phalanx Osteotomy

In a patient with hallux valgus interphalangeus, an Akin osteotomy will correct this lateral deviation. This osteotomy can be used as an adjunct to a distal or proximal osteotomy to further improve the amount of bunion correction. The incision is an extension distally from the first MTP joint. A medial closing wedge osteotomy is made near the base of the proximal phalanx and held with a Kirschner wire, small screw, or staple.

Double and Triple Osteotomy

Combined osteotomy procedures are performed for more severe or complex deformities. A double osteotomy procedure including a proximal first metatarsal osteotomy or medial opening wedge osteotomy of the first cuneiform (Cotton procedure) to correct a large IMA combined with a distal medial closing wedge osteotomy for the first metatarsal (Reverdin osteotomy) to reduce the DMAA has been used successfully.[21] Additionally, the Cotton procedure can be combined with

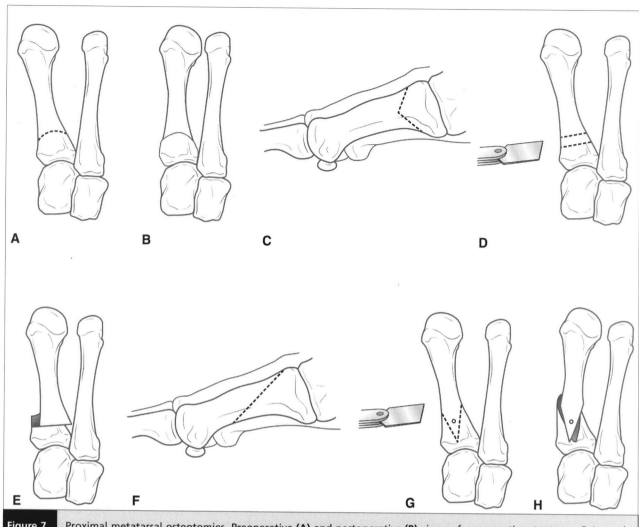

Figure 7 Proximal metatarsal osteotomies. Preoperative **(A)** and postoperative **(B)** views of a crescentic osteotomy. **C,** Lateral view of a proximal chevron osteotomy. AP views before **(D)** and after **(E)** a proximal chevron osteotomy. **F,** Lateral view of an oblique (Ludloff) osteotomy. AP views before **(G)** and after **(H)** an oblique (Ludloff) osteotomy. *(Adapted from Campbell JT: Hallux valgus: Adult and juvenile, in Cohen BE, Donley BG, Johnson JE, Murphy GA, McHale KA, Thordarson DB (eds): Orthopaedic Knowledge Update: Foot and Ankle 3. Rosemont, IL, American Academy of Orthopaedic Surgeons, 2004, pp 3-15.)*

a double osteotomy or a proximal first metatarsal osteotomy and Reverdin osteotomy to enable further correction of the IMA in a triple osteotomy procedure.[18]

Juvenile and Adolescent Hallux Valgus

Introduction
Hallux valgus in children differs from the adult deformity in several ways. In children, the deformity is not related to long-term wear of shoes with a narrow toe box, and children and parents usually are more concerned with cosmetic issues than are adults with the condition. Recurrence of hallux valgus commonly occurs after less aggressive surgical reconstructions in children. Children frequently have associated disorders, such as contracture of the gastrocnemius-soleus muscle-tendon unit, metatarsus adductus, splayfoot, flatfoot, and ligamentous laxity. Children can present with hallux valgus as an isolated deformity or as part of a systemic condition, such as Down syndrome, cerebral palsy, Marfan skewfoot, or Charcot-Marie-Tooth hereditary peripheral neuropathy. Hallux valgus with a flatfoot should not be confused with a painful, peroneal spastic flatfoot that is associated with tarsal coalition in children 10 to 14 years of age.

Pathoanatomy
Like adult hallux valgus, this deformity in children is often associated with metatarsus primus varus, contracture of the adductor hallucis, pronation of the great toe, and subluxation of the lateral sesamoid and proximal phalanx base. At surgery, the abductor hallucis tendon is commonly displaced plantarward and the articular surface of the uncovered metatarsal head is

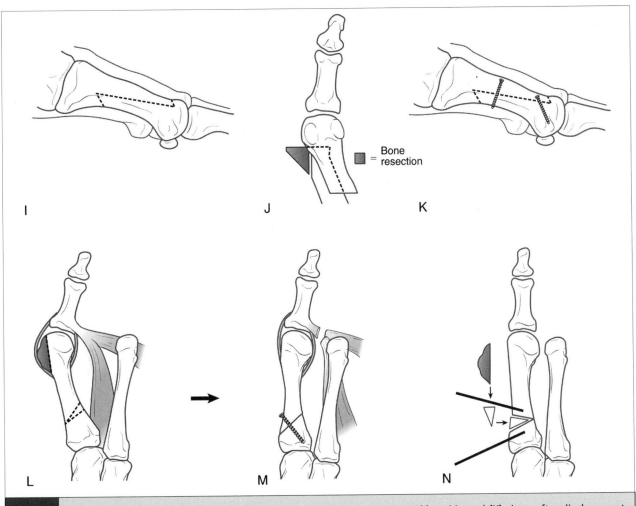

Figure 7 (Cont.) Proximal metatarsal osteotomies. **I,** Lateral view of scarf osteotomy. AP **(J)** and lateral **(K)** views after displacement with fixation. Preoperative AP view **(L)** and postoperative AP view **(M)** of a closing wedge osteotomy with fixation. **N,** AP view of an opening wedge osteotomy using the medial eminence for bone wedge.

eroded medially adjacent to the sulcus (in more severe deformities with surgical indications). Guidelines for the diagnosis of hallux valgus include an IMA of greater than 9° and a HVA greater than 15° on standing AP radiographs. The DMAA is more difficult to measure in children. There may be a familial predisposition to the deformity in children who have a parent or grandparent with hallux valgus.

The age at presentation in children often determines severity and symptoms of the deformity. Juvenile hallux valgus occurs in children between 2 and 10 years of age (prepubertal), is rarely painful, and is less severe radiographically than the adolescent deformity. Adolescent hallux valgus is more likely to progress, more severe radiographically, and often leads to the formation of painful bunions. Infantile hallux valgus (in children younger than 2 years) is rare.

Etiology

A genetic predisposition for both adult and juvenile hallux valgus is likely. Some researchers have found an autosomal dominant inheritance with incomplete penetrance for hallux valgus deformity.[27] Multiple anatomic factors can play a significant role in the development of juvenile hallux valgus; however, no single constellation of deformities occurs in all patients. The entire foot should be examined carefully for coexisting conditions. Pes planus with or without heel cord contracture can place a lateral force on the hallux. The effect of this condition is compounded in patients with general ligamentous laxity. First metatarsal pronation may be present or may develop over time. Residual metatarsus adductus present from birth or acquired metatarsus primus varus may contribute to the abnormal forces generated across the first MTP joint. The orientation of the medial cuneiform-first metatarsal joint or the first metatarsal physis may produce worsening metatarsus primus varus. Metatarsal length also may be an important factor. Metatarsal protrusion distance is a radiographic measure of the length of the first metatarsal relative to the second metatarsal. A positive metatarsal protrusion distance, which indicates a long first meta-

4: The Forefoot

tarsal, has been shown to be a good predictor of juvenile hallux valgus.[28] Hallux valgus interphalangeus also may be present.

In patients with certain systemic conditions, hallux valgus can be related to repetitive lateral impact moments on the great toe, such as in patients with cerebral palsy spastic diplegia or those with Down syndrome, from a combination of tight heel cord, equinovalgus, and external rotation of the feet with a wide-based gait.

Nonsurgical Treatment

Nonsurgical treatment is often appropriate for children with isolated juvenile hallux valgus because the deformity is rarely symptomatic and primary concern comes from the patient's parents. When obtaining the patient history, parents may try to control the child's responses and even exaggerate symptoms to procure surgical treatment. The situation may be further complicated by previous financial and time investments in orthotics and prescribed footwear. Management options should consider the child's expectations and concerns. It may be difficult to differentiate the child's concerns from those of the parents, so skill and experience is mandatory in obtaining an accurate history. The child and family should be carefully educated about the natural history of hallux valgus, which is not always progressive and may never cause pain. Risks of surgery including recurrence, stiffness, scar formation, and painful neuroma should be emphasized to differentiate cosmetic concerns from true pain symptoms. In patients without pain, simple reassurance and education is sufficient treatment. Arch supports for flat feet or other more specific orthoses designed for hallux valgus have not been shown to alter the natural history of the deformity. Shoes with a wide toe box and shoes with soft leather uppers are the simplest, most affordable methods to alleviate symptoms. Passive stretching of tight heel cords also can be helpful. Activity modification and nonsteroidal anti-inflammatory drugs can alleviate symptoms, but usually are not realistic options for active children and do not provide a long-term solution.

Annual or biannual examinations with repeat standing radiographs can convince the family that the deformity is nonprogressive. If the deformity progresses, true symptoms can be assessed and the older child can participate in treatment decisions.

Surgical Treatment

Decision Making

Once the decision to proceed with surgery is made, careful planning is needed. Complications are common in adolescent hallux valgus surgery. Although successful surgical correction can be achieved, patients and families should be counseled about the risks of recurrent deformity, overcorrection, transfer metatarsalgia, osteonecrosis, scarring, stiffness, and infection. The patient and family also should be advised that after radiographic correction of the bunion, the clinical appearance of the foot may be cosmetically unsatisfactory

because of residual or recurrent deformity and scar formation. Some loss in range of motion at the MTP joint is common and can impair running or jumping activities or may limit the selection of shoe wear (such as preventing the wearing of shoes with high heels).

Because many corrective techniques involve a period of immobilization, limited weight bearing, and footwear modification, the patient should be assessed for the ability and willingness to comply with postoperative restrictions and limitations. The presence of an open physis should be noted. Although lateral hemi-epiphyseodesis has been described for treatment of metatarsus primus varus in patients with juvenile hallux valgus, it has rarely been successful unless performed in a young child (younger than 8 years of age). Osteotomies of the first metatarsal can be performed with an open physis at the proximal base; however, the surgical exposure, osteotomy, and fixation must remain distal to the open physis.

In patients with bilateral deformity, surgical correction initially should be performed on one foot, to be sure that the patient and family are pleased with the outcome. The operated foot should be fully rehabilitated before proceeding with surgery on the contralateral side. Usually an interval of at least 6 to 12 months between surgeries is appropriate.

Preoperative Assessment

The goal of hallux valgus surgery is a painless joint that is stable, congruent, and has adequate correction of the deformity. With multiple surgical options, careful planning should determine the most appropriate surgical treatment. A detailed history should rule out systemic etiologies. It is important to establish rapport and understanding with the family. Physical examination of the foot can rule out tarsal coalition, contractures (heel cord, adductor hallucis), and determine the location of pain (often passive correction of the hallux valgus causes pain at the medial MTP joint, indicating erosion of the hyaline cartilage). The preoperative MTP arc of motion (dorsiflexion and plantar flexion) should be obtained as a baseline measurement. Pronation of the hallux is easily visualized and usually associated with subluxation of the abductor hallucis tendon to the plantar surface. Preoperative radiographs should be assessed for MTP joint congruency, HVA, IMA, DMAA, and metatarsal protrusion distance. These measurements localize the sites of deformity and surgical correction. The magnitude of these measurements also provide the magnitude for corrective osteotomies, especially when a double, first metatarsal osteotomy is performed.[29]

The most common deformity in adolescent hallux valgus requiring surgical correction is a congruent MTP joint with a moderate to severe HVA and IMA, with or without hypermobility of the first MTP and first metatarsal-cuneiform joints. However, other deformities may be present and the degree of deformity is quite variable. Although some osteotomies provide greater correction of the HVA, others are more suited for cor-

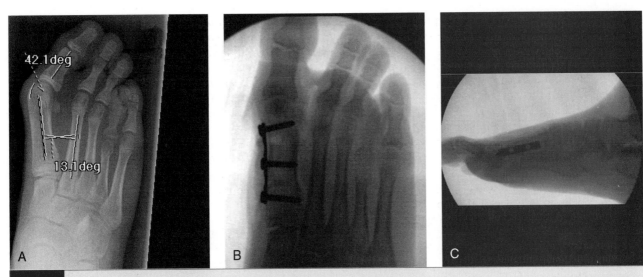

Figure 8 **A,** Preoperative AP measurements on a standing radiograph are used for planning the osteotomy. **B,** Postoperative AP simulated weight-bearing view taken in the operating room. **C,** Postoperative lateral view.

rection of a high IMA. The surgeon should be familiar with the risks and limitations of each procedure.

To guide surgery, MTP joint congruence should be determined by evaluating preoperative radiographs. Congruent joints can be maintained by multiple osteotomies to achieve correction. Soft-tissue procedures such as the modified McBride procedure can transform a congruent joint into a noncongruent joint and should be avoided unless incongruence already exists. With a mild deformity (IMA < 13°; HVA < 30°) and a congruent MTP joint, a distal osteotomy is often sufficient to obtain correction.[30-34] Moderate deformities (IMA = 14° to 18°; HVA = 30° to 40°) may benefit from the addition of a proximal phalangeal osteotomy, a proximal metatarsal osteotomy, or treatment by a primary double first metatarsal osteotomy. Patients with larger deformities (IMA > 18°; HVA > 40°) more typically require a double first metatarsal osteotomy (**Figure 8**). With larger deformities, MTP joint incongruence is more likely and a soft-tissue procedure (adductor release) also may be needed. The double first metatarsal osteotomy includes a distal, medially based, closing wedge osteotomy to correct the high HVA and DMAA, and a proximal, medially based, opening wedge osteotomy to correct the high IMA while maintaining baseline length of the first metatarsal (**Figures 9 and 10**). This osteotomy was originally stabilized with one or two axial Steinmann pins (Peterson procedure) crossing both the interphalangeal and MTP joints, but newer techniques have incorporated plate and screw fixation with good results.[29,35,36] A laterally based, closing wedge osteotomy has been described to correct a high IMA, but can often result in a shortened first metatarsal and transfer metatarsalgia.[37]

Surgical correction of incongruent joints should begin with a distal soft-tissue procedure. The modified McBride procedure achieves mixed results in patients with adolescent hallux valgus, but can often augment

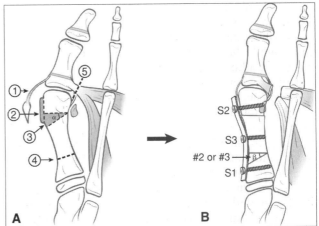

Figure 9 **A,** Illustration showing the AP view of a modified double osteotomy. (1) Distally based osteoperiosteal flap. (2) Bunionectomy at sulcus. (3) Distal closing wedge equal to HVA. (4) Proximal opening wedge. (5) Adductor tenotomy. **B,** AP view of a modified, double osteotomy showing proximal, opening wedge equal to IMA using bone from areas 2 or 3 in part A. Order of screw placement: S1 (leave loose to allow the distal osteoperiosteal flap to be rotated under the plate), S2, and then S3.

an osteotomy in an incongruent joint.[38-40] For mild, incongruent adolescent hallux valgus (IMA < 13°; HVA < 30°), a distal chevron osteotomy with a modified McBride procedure can achieve excellent correction. Larger incongruent hallux valgus deformities typically require multiple osteotomies, such as a double first metatarsal osteotomy or proximal and Akin osteotomies.[40]

Ligamentous laxity of the first metatarsal-medial cuneiform joint often occurs in adolescent hallux valgus and is difficult to treat. Medially based opening wedge

4: The Forefoot

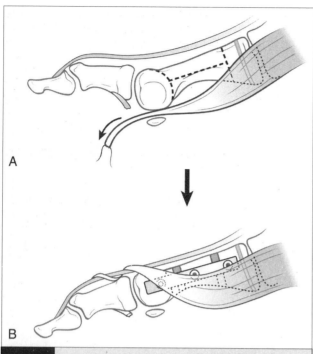

Figure 10 **A,** Illustration showing the lateral view of a modified double osteotomy. The subluxated abductor hallucis tendon is tagged distally for later transfer and the muscle is dissected proximally. The periosteal incision includes the distally based capsule to allow an osteoperiosteal flap; the proximal physis is avoided if open. Dashed line shows the incision of the periosteum on the metatarsal. **B,** Lateral view of the modified double osteotomy shows internal fixation with a minifragment, five-hole plate, and 3.5-mm screws. The abductor hallucis transfer to the extensor hallucis longus covers the plate.

osteotomies for the first metatarsal or medial cuneiform joint can correct the malalignment, but joint laxity can lead to recurrence over time. In this situation, a Lapidus procedure can stabilize the joint, but a joint-sacrificing procedure in children should be used with caution.

Complications

Recurrence is common after bunion correction in adolescents. Inadequate correction or the selection of an improper procedure can increase the risk of this complication. A soft-tissue procedure alone is often inadequate in a growing child and the recurrence rate for hallux valgus is high.[40] Overcorrection also can result in hallux varus and a poor level of patient satisfaction. This complication is more common with overaggressive proximal osteotomies. Transfer metatarsalgia results from shortening of the first metatarsal and is more common in procedures such as the Mitchell or proximal closing wedge osteotomy in which bone is removed and not replaced. The distal chevron and Peterson double osteotomies produce less shortening. Nonunion can

occur from inadequate bone fixation or poor patient compliance with postoperative weight-bearing restrictions. Alternatively, implant complications such as failure or prominence can necessitate repeat surgical intervention. Osteonecrosis is more common with distal osteotomies in combination with aggressive lateral soft-tissue release; care should be taken to preserve soft-tissue attachments to the metatarsal head and to prevent a too distal osteotomy when this combination is used. Loss of MTP joint motion can accompany aggressive soft-tissue procedures when the medial capsule is overly plicated.

Summary

Weight-bearing radiographs are essential for preoperative planning of bunion treatment. In adults, a mild bunion with a congruent joint generally can be treated with a distal osteotomy, such as a chevron osteotomy. A proximal osteotomy is needed to correct a moderate deformity. Arthrodesis is usually appropriate for a severe bunion or for a joint with arthritis.

Hallux valgus deformities and bunions in children are different from those in adults. The etiology of the bunion must be defined, ruling out systemic and associated factors. True symptoms must be determined. The decision for surgery should be made only after multiple discussions with the patient and family and radiographic proof of a progressing deformity. The choice of surgical procedure should include both soft-tissue and bony options with every attempt to completely correct the deformity and decrease the high risk of recurrence.

Annotated References

1. Coughlin MJ: Hallux valgus. *J Bone Joint Surg Am* 1996;78:932-966.

2. Easley ME, Trnka HJ: Current concepts review: Hallux valgus part 1: Pathomechanics, clinical assessment, and nonoperative management. *Foot Ankle Int* 2007;28: 654-659.

   The authors provide a summary of the background, etiology, pathomechanics, typical clinical presentation, and nonsurgical treatment of hallux valgus. The etiology of the deformity is still unclear, but is related to repetitive loading of the hallux. Nonsurgical treatment can improve symptoms, and many bunions are asymptomatic.

3. Robinson AH, Limbers JP: Modern concepts in the treatment of hallux valgus. *J Bone Joint Surg Br* 2005; 87:1038-1045.

   In this review article, the authors examine important factors in choosing the most appropriate technique for proper treatment of hallux valgus.

4. Sim-Fook L, Hodgson A: A comparison of foot forms among the non-shoe and shoe-wearing Chinese population. *J Bone Joint Surg Am* 1958;40:1058-1062.

5. Coughlin MJ, Jones CP: Hallux valgus: Demographics, etiology, and radiographic assessment. *Foot Ankle Int* 2007;28:759-777.

    The authors report on the demographics, etiology, and radiographic findings associated with moderate and severe hallux valgus in patients older than 20 years of age treated surgically over a 33-month period in a single surgeon's practice. Level of evidence: IV.

6. Coughlin MJ, Jones CP: Hallux valgus and first ray mobility: A prospective study. *J Bone Joint Surg Am* 2007; 89:1887-1898.

    This prospective study evaluates the efficacy of proximal crescentic osteotomy and distal soft-tissue repair of the first MTP joint for the surgical treatment of hallux valgus in adult patients with moderate or severe subluxated deformities. First ray mobility was decreased to a normal level without the need for arthrodesis of the metatarsocuneiform joint. Level of evidence: IV.

7. Glasoe WM, Allen MK, Saltzman CL: First ray dorsal mobility in relation to hallux valgus deformity and first intermetatarsal angle. *Foot Ankle Int* 2001;22:98-101.

8. Ito H, Shimizu A, Miyamoto T, Katsura Y, Tanaka K: Clinical significance of increased mobility in the sagittal plane in patients with hallux valgus. *Foot Ankle Int* 1999;20:29-32.

9. Klaue K, Hansen ST, Masquelet AC: Clinical, quantitative assessment of first tarsometatarsal mobility in the sagittal plane and its relation to hallux valgus deformity. *Foot Ankle Int* 1994;15:9-13.

10. Lee KT, Young K: Measurement of first-ray mobility in normal vs. hallux valgus patients. *Foot Ankle Int* 2001; 22:960-964.

11. Myerson MS, Badekas A: Hypermobility of the first ray. *Foot Ankle Clin* 2000;5:469-484.

12. Voellmicke KV, Deland JT: Manual examination technique to assess dorsal instability of the first ray. *Foot Ankle Int* 2002;23:1040-1041.

13. Faber FW, Kleinrensink GJ, Verhoog MW, et al: Mobility of the first tarsometatarsal joint in relation to hallux valgus deformity: Anatomical and biomechanical aspects. *Foot Ankle Int* 1999;20:651-656.

14. Coughlin MJ, Freund E: The reliability of angular measurements in hallux valgus deformities. *Foot Ankle Int* 2001;22:369-379.

15. Hardy RH, Clapham JC: Observations on hallux valgus: Based on a controlled series. *J Bone Joint Surg Br* 1951;33:376-391.

16. Saltzman CL, Brandser EA, Berbaum KS, et al: Reliability of standard foot radiographic measurements. *Foot Ankle Int* 1994;15:661-665.

17. Steel MW III, Johnson KA, DeWitz MA, Ilstrup DM: Radiographic measurements of the normal adult foot. *Foot Ankle* 1980;1:151-158.

18. Coughlin MJ, Carlson RE: Treatment of hallux valgus with an increased distal metatarsal articular angle: Evaluation of double and triple first ray osteotomies. *Foot Ankle Int* 1999;20:762-770.

19. Lau JT, Daniels TR: Effect of increasing distal medial closing wedge metatarsal osteotomies on the distal metatarsal articular angle. *Foot Ankle Int* 1999;20:771-776.

20. Torkki M, Malmivaara A, Seitsalo S, Hoikka V, Laippala P, Paavolainen P: Surgery versus orthosis versus watchful waiting for hallux valgus: A randomized controlled trial. *JAMA* 2001;285:2474-2480.

21. Easley ME, Trnka HJ: Current concepts review: Hallux valgus part II: Operative treatment. *Foot Ankle Int* 2007;28:748-758.

    The authors review surgical treatment methods and potential complications in the management of hallux valgus. Distal chevron osteotomy is effective for mild bunions and arthrodesis for severe deformity.

22. Schneider W, Knahr K: Keller procedure and chevron osteotomy in hallux valgus: Five-year results of different surgical philosophies in comparable collectives. *Foot Ankle Int* 2002;23:321-329.

23. Resch S, Stenstrom A, Gustafson T: Circulatory disturbance of the first metatarsal head after Chevron osteotomy as shown by bone scintigraphy. *Foot Ankle* 1992; 13:137-142.

24. Mann RA, Rudicel S, Graves SC: Repair of hallux valgus with a distal soft-tissue procedure and proximal metatarsal osteotomy: A long-term follow-up. *J Bone Joint Surg Am* 1992;74:124-129.

25. Markbreiter LA, Thompson FM: Proximal metatarsal osteotomy in hallux valgus correction: A comparison of crescentic and chevron procedures. *Foot Ankle Int* 1997;18:71-76.

26. Lian GJ, Markolf K, Cracchiolo A III: Strength of fixation constructs for basilar osteotomies of the first metatarsal. *Foot Ankle* 1992;13:509-514.

27. Pique-Vidal C, Sole MT, Antich J: Hallux valgus inheritance: Pedigree research in 350 patients with bunion deformity. *J Foot Ankle Surg* 2007;46:149-154.

    Three-generation pedigree charts were constructed on 350 probands with painful hallux valgus. Ninety percent of the patients had at least one affected family member. Close evaluation of the pedigrees revealed an inheritance pattern compatible with autosomal domi-

4: The Forefoot

nant inheritance with incomplete penetrance.

28. McCluney JG, Tinley P: Radiographic measurements of patients with juvenile hallux valgus compared with age-matched controls: A cohort investigation. *J Foot Ankle Surg* 2006;45:161-167.

The authors of this radiographic cohort study compared a group of weight-bearing radiographs of patients with juvenile hallux valgus (HVA > 15°) with radiographs from age-matched controls. Multiple radiographic measures were studies including first metatarsal protrusion distance, metatarsus primus adductus angle, metatarsus adductus, first metatarsal cuneiform angle, calcaneal inclination angle, and talocalcaneal angle. Metatarsal protrusion distance had an accuracy of 93.4% in predicting juvenile hallux valgus. A positive metatarsal protrusion distance was believed to be a significant component of juvenile hallux valgus.

29. Aronson J, Nguyen LL, Aronson EA: Early results of the modified Peterson bunion procedure for adolescent hallux valgus. *J Pediatr Orthop* 2001;21:65-69.

30. McDonald MG, Stevens DB: Modified Mitchell bunionectomy for management of adolescent hallux valgus. *Clin Orthop Relat Res* 1996;332:163-169.

31. Weiner BK, Weiner DS, Mirkopulos N: Mitchell osteotomy for adolescent hallux valgus. *J Pediatr Orthop* 1997;17:781-784.

32. Karbowski A, Schwitalle M, Eckardt A, Heine J: Long-term results after Mitchell osteotomy in children and adolescents with hallux valgus. *Acta Orthop Belg* 1998; 64:263-268.

33. Willemen L, Kohler R, Metaizeau J: Surgical treatment of hallux valgus in children and adolescents: 46 cases treated with the Mitchell technique. *Rev Chir Orthop Reparatrice Appar Mot* 2000;86:54-62.

34. Talab YA: Hallux valgus in children: A 5-14-year follow-up study of 30 feet treated with a modified Mitchell osteotomy. *Acta Orthop Scand* 2002;73:195-198.

35. Peterson HA, Newman SR: Adolescent bunion deformity treated with double osteotomy and longitudinal pin fixation of the first ray. *J Pediatr Orthop* 1993;13: 80-84.

36. Johnson AE, Georgopoulos G, Erickson MA, Eilert R: Treatment of adolescent hallux valgus with the first metatarsal double osteotomy: The Denver experience. *J Pediatr Orthop* 2004;24:358-362.

The functional clinical outcomes of nine patients (14 feet) treated with a first metatarsal double osteotomy for severe adolescent hallux valgus are described in this case study. Follow-up was more than 2 years. Radiographic data and function outcomes as measured by the American Orthopaedic Foot and Ankle Society Hallux Metatarsophalangeal-Interphalangeal scale and duPont Bunion Ratio Scale are presented. Radiographic deformity improved by 21.54° for HVA and 9.25° for IMA. Good to excellent results were reported in 90% of patients; two complications occurred.

37. Zembsch A, Trnka HJ, Mühlbauer M, Ritschl P, Salzer M: Long-term results of basal wedge osteotomy in metatarsus primus varus in the young patient. *Z Orthop Ihre Grenzgeb* 1998;136:243-249.

38. Schwitalle M, Karbowski A, Eckardt A: Hallux valgus in young patients: Long-term results after McBride operation. *Arch Orthop Trauma Surg* 1997;116:412-414.

39. Schwitalle M, Karbowski A, Eckardt A: Hallux valgus in young patients: Comparison of soft-tissue realignment and metatarsal osteotomy. *Eur J Pediatr Surg* 1998;8:42-46.

40. Senaris-Rodriguez J, Martinez-Serrano A, Rodriguez-Durantez JA, Sotelo-Martinez J, Gonzalez-Lopez JL: Surgical treatment for bunions in adolescents. *J Pediatr Orthop B* 1998;7:210-216.

Chapter 19
Hallux Varus

Naomi N. Shields, MD

Introduction

Hallux varus is the varus positioning of the hallux (great toe) relative to the first metatarsal that creates both a cosmetic and functional deformity. This deformity occurs in all age groups ranging from children with congenital hallux varus to older patients with post-traumatic or surgical deformities. Many hallux varus deformities are mild and require no surgical intervention. Various methods of surgical realignment are possible to correct both flexible and arthritic deformities.

Anatomy

The relevant anatomy of the first metatarsophalangeal (MTP) joint can be divided into bony architecture, ligamentous capsular structures, and muscular tendon attachments. When balanced, the hallux is generally neutrally aligned relative to the first metatarsal. The shape of the first metatarsal head (flat versus round), the size of the medial sagittal groove, and the sesamoid crista are aspects of the bony architecture affecting MTP stability. The lateral capsule and lateral ligaments limit varus positioning. The adductor hallucis and the flexor hallucis brevis (lateral) are important muscular dynamic stabilizers. With an intrinsic minus position, the hallux develops a hallux varus deformity.

Pathogenesis and Incidence

The etiology of a hallux varus deformity can be congenital, idiopathic (Figure 1), or can occur secondary to trauma or after hallux valgus surgery.[1-7] The most common etiology is overcorrection during hallux valgus surgery with overrelease of the lateral capsular structures, excessive metatarsal head resection lateral to the medial sagittal groove (the medial eminence), overplication of the medial capsule, excision of the lateral sesamoid, or overcorrection of metatarsal varus with a metatarsal osteotomy or first metatarsal-tarsal arthrodesis (Figure 2). The incidence of hallux varus after hallux valgus surgery is between 2% and 24%.[1,6,8] Proximal metatarsal osteotomies, such as the Ludloff osteotomy, can be powerful reducers of the intermetatarsal (IM) angle; caution should be used to prevent overreduction of the IM angle.[9]

Physical and Radiographic Examination

The evaluation of a hallux varus deformity begins with a good patient history. It should be determined when the deformity was first noticed; how the deformity affects the patient (for example, cosmetically or in the choice of shoe wear); the presence and location of pain; prior treatments and surgeries, if any; and functional limitations caused by the deformity (such as occupational or recreational limitations). If the patient had prior surgery to treat hallux valgus, the surgical record may be helpful for planning revision surgery.

The examination should include observation of the foot with the patient in a standing position and during ambulation. Many patients will externally rotate or supinate the foot, walking on the lateral border to avoid toe-off if the first MTP joint is painful or has limited motion. It is important to evaluate existing deformities throughout the foot and to determine if they are fixed or supple. Often the hallux interphalangeal (IP) joint will be flexed and the MTP joint extended. The extensor hallucis longus tendon may be medially displaced, creating a "bowstring" dynamic deformity (Figure 3). The medial or tibial sesamoid also may be medially displaced. Range of motion of the first MTP and IP joints should be assessed. Reducibility of the deformity must be determined and the range of motion in the reduced position evaluated. Callus locations should be noted. The remainder of the forefoot, especially the second

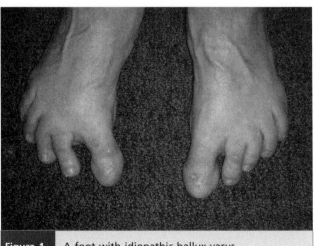

Figure 1 A foot with idiopathic hallux varus.

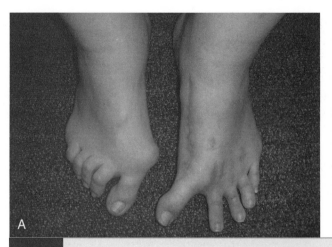 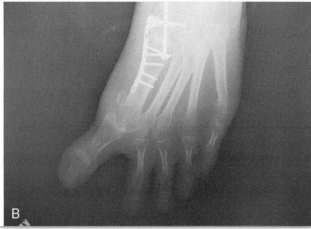

Figure 2 Photograph **(A)** and radiograph **(B)** of the foot of a patient with hallux varus caused by overcorrection of the first metatarsal-tarsal joint.

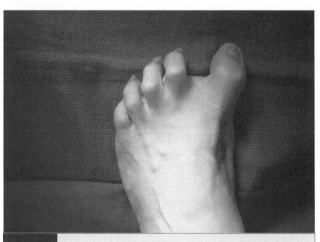

Figure 3 Dynamic hallux varus deformity with IP flexion toe.

and third MTP joints, should be assessed for stability. Metatarsus adductus or adduction of the lesser toes should be determined. Neurovascular assessment also is needed to assess the risks of further surgery.

Radiographic evaluation consists of weight-bearing AP and lateral views of the foot, non–weight-bearing oblique views, and if possible, a sesamoid axial view. The hallux varus angle, the first-second IM angle, MTP joint extension, IP joint flexion, and the degree of arthrosis at the MTP, IP, and sesamoid-metatarsal joints should be evaluated. It also is necessary to determine if both sesamoids are present and the location of the sesamoids relative to the metatarsal head.

At the completion of the evaluation, the physician should have a good understanding of the patient's current symptoms and expectations regarding function, shoe wear, and occupational and recreational activities. The physician should know if the deformity is fixed or flexible and the degree of arthrosis present. The deformity can then be classified and a treatment plan can be created. Discussing nonsurgical and surgical treatment options and expected outcomes will help achieve optimal long-term satisfaction for both the patient and physician. If the deformity resulted from prior hallux valgus surgery, the patient may be angry or frustrated and unenthusiastic about undergoing another surgical procedure.

Classification

Hallux varus deformities can be divided into dynamic and static deformities. Dynamic deformities are usually progressive, resulting from muscular imbalance with disruption of adductor and flexor hallucis brevis function. Static deformities are classified as fixed (uncorrectable) or flexible (passively correctable).

Nonsurgical Treatment

Nonsurgical treatment includes accommodating the hallux varus deformity with a shoe with a wider toe box and taping or splinting the deformity. If motion is limited and arthrosis is present, a stiffer soled, rocker-bottom shoe or a turf toe or carbon graphite orthosis can be used to limit dorsiflexion. If the deformity is secondary to hallux valgus correction, early rather than delayed surgical revision should be considered because the deformity is unlikely to spontaneously resolve.

Surgical Treatment

In patients with hallux varus, the goal of surgical treatment is to restore the function and alignment of the first ray. Treatment options will vary depending on the etiology of the deformity, the flexibility or rigidity of the deformity, prior surgical treatments, and the patient's expectations. Surgical treatment options include soft-tissue release, tendon transfer, tenodesis, metatar-

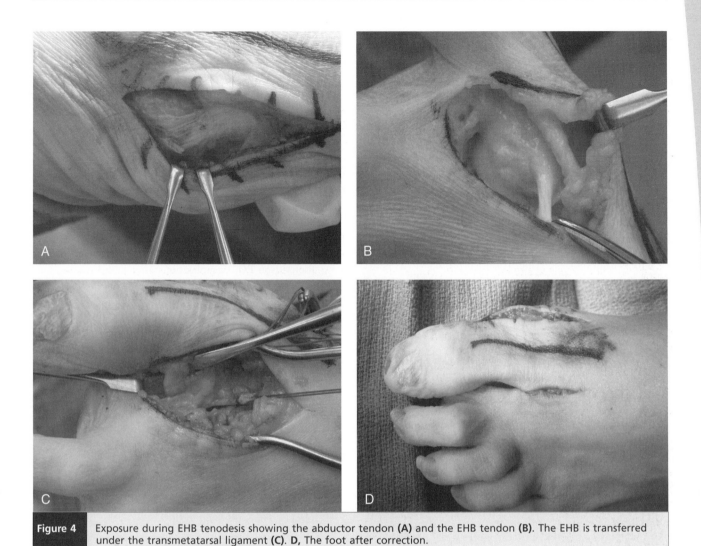

Figure 4 Exposure during EHB tenodesis showing the abductor tendon **(A)** and the EHB tendon **(B)**. The EHB is transferred under the transmetatarsal ligament **(C)**. **D,** The foot after correction.

sal osteotomy, reverse Akin (proximal phalanx) osteotomy, resection arthroplasty, bone grafting to the medial first metatarsal head, and MTP joint arthrodesis.

If the primary cause of the deformity is overcorrection from hallux valgus surgery with overplication of the medial capsule, correction includes soft-tissue release of the medial capsule, extensor hallucis longus (EHL) tenolysis if the EHL is medial to the midline, and lengthening of the abductor hallucis. The goal of soft-tissue correction is to return the sesamoids to their normal position under the facets of the first metatarsal. If this cannot be accomplished, then excision of the medial sesamoid should be considered if the lateral sesamoid is present. Arthrodesis of the first MTP joint is necessary if the lateral sesamoid is absent, especially if the medial sesamoid cannot be reduced.

If the primary cause of the deformity is excessive correction of the intermetatarsal angle by proximal osteotomy or the Lapidus procedure, correction can be accomplished with either a proximal osteotomy or revision of the tarsal-metatarsal fusion. This correction should be combined with distal soft-tissue realignment.

Tendon transfer of the EHL is a reliable method of correcting a flexible, nonarthritic hallux varus deformity. This correction can be accomplished with either a complete EHL transfer to the base of the proximal phalanx with IP joint arthrodesis or with a split-EHL transfer, preserving the medial third of the EHL. Caution is necessary when fusing the IP joint of the hallux if the first MTP joint is arthritic. Fusion of both the IP and MTP joints is usually not well tolerated by patients. Tendon transfers generally pass under the transmetatarsal ligament. Following a distal soft-tissue realignment procedure in hallux valgus surgery, this ligament may be surgically absent, potentially reducing the effectiveness of the tendon transfer.

Extensor hallucis brevis (EHB) tenodesis/transfer also can be performed. This procedure provides a strong force resisting varus displacement (**Figure 4**). The EHB tendon is transected proximally (at the muscle if possible), transferred plantar to the transmetatarsal ligament from distal to proximal, and passed through a drill hole in the first metatarsal head from lateral to medial.[10,11]

A lateral closing wedge proximal phalanx osteotomy (reverse Akin) can be used to treat mild hallux varus deformities that are correctable and have shown no tendency to worsen. Keller resection arthroplasty combined with soft-tissue realignment may be considered for patients with low physical demands. This procedure will significantly reduce the ability of the hallux to transfer weight. It effectively creates an intrinsic minus deformity and loss of medial ray stability at toe-off.

If the primary cause of the hallux varus is excessive excision of the medial first metatarsal head, bone grafting may provide correction of the deformity with maintenance of motion. This surgical procedure is applicable when the varus deformity is related to excessive medial head resection and the deformity is passively correctable to neutral.[2]

The primary salvage operation for hallux varus is first MTP joint arthrodesis. Fusion of the first MTP joint allows reproducible results with good pain reduction, maintenance of toe-off, and restoration of first ray function.[8] The ideal position for first MTP joint arthrodesis is approximately 15° hallux valgus, 15° first MTP extension when measured relative to the plantar surface of the foot, and neutral pronation/supination of the hallux in the axial plane. Multiple options are available to stabilize the first MTP joint. Rigid fixation is desired if possible. Crossed intrafragmentary screws are commonly used. New, low-profile, contoured plating systems have been developed. MTP reamers can be used to create close-fitting surfaces; osteotomies or small burrs also can be used. If the sesamoid articulation has significant arthrosis, first MTP joint arthrodesis is the best treatment for hallux varus. Complications include nonunion, malunion, transfer metatarsalgia, IP arthrosis, infection, neuralgia, and limitations in the choice of shoe wear. In patients with inflammatory arthritis, arthrodesis of the first MTP joint will provide a stable post for the forefoot.

Congenital hallux varus is a rare condition. Z-plasty with dorsal and plantar flaps has been described for hallux varus with preaxial polydactyly of the foot.[4]

Summary

Hallux varus deformities present a challenge for both the patient and treating physician. Avoiding surgical overcorrection of a hallux valgus deformity will prevent the development of hallux varus in many patients. A complete evaluation, careful consideration of treatment options, and an understanding of the patient's expectation will lead to optimal outcomes in treating hallux varus.

Annotated References

1. Donley BG: Acquired hallux varus. *Foot Ankle Int* 1997;18:586-592.

2. Rochwerger A, Curvale G, Groulier P: Application of bone graft to the medial side of the first metatarsal head in the treatment of hallux varus. *J Bone Joint Surg Am* 1999;81:1730-1735.

3. Sammarco GJ, Indusuyi OB: Complications after surgery of the hallux. *Clin Orthop Relat Res* 2001;391:59-71.

4. Toriyama K, Kamei Y, Morishita T, Matsuoka K, Torri S: Z-plasty of dorsal and plantar flaps for hallux varus with preaxial polydactyly of the foot. *Plast Reconstr Surg* 2006;117:112e-115e.

   The authors present a case report on the use of Z-plasty with dorsal and plantar flaps in a 4-year-old child with congenital hallux varus and preaxial polydactyly of the foot.

5. Richardson EG: Complications after hallux valgus surgery. *Instr Course Lect* 1999;48:331-342.

6. Trnka HJ, Zettl R, Hungerford M, Muhlbauer M, Ritschl P: Acquired hallux varus and clinical tolerability. *Foot Ankle Int* 1997;18:593-597.

7. Kopp FJ, Patel MM, Levine DS, Deland JT: The modified Lapidus procedure for hallux valgus: A clinical and radiographic analysis. *Foot Ankle Int* 2005;26:913-917.

   This retrospective study reviewed 32 patients (38 feet) treated with a modified Lapidus procedure for hallux valgus. Hallux varus deformity occurred in three patients, two of whom were symptomatic.

8. Grimes JS, Coughlin MJ: First metatarsophalangeal joint arthrodesis as a treatment for failed hallux valgus surgery. *Foot Ankle Int* 2006;27:887-893.

   The authors present a retrospective review of patients treated by one surgeon using first MTP joint arthrodesis for failed hallux valgus surgery. Symptomatic hallux varus deformity occurred in 24% of patients following initial hallux valgus surgery.

9. Chiodo CP, Schon LC, Myerson MS: Clinical results with the Ludloff osteotomy for correction of adult hallux valgus. *Foot Ankle Int* 2004;25:532-536.

   The authors reviewed 82 cases of hallux valgus treated with the Ludloff osteotomy. Four patients had a hallux varus deformity (range 2° to 10°). One patient was symptomatic and was treated with transfer of the extensor hallucis brevis tendon.

10. Juliano PJ, Myerson MS, Cunningham BW: Biomechanical assessment of a new tenodesis for correction of hallux varus. *Foot Ankle Int* 1996;17:17-20.

11. Myerson MS, Komenda GA: Results of hallux varus correction using an extensor hallucis brevis tenodesis. *Foot Ankle Int* 1996;17:21-27.

    A clinical practice guideline was developed for diagnosing and treating hallux varus based on a consensus of current clinical practice and review of the clinical literature.

Chapter 20
Hallux Rigidus

Paul S. Shurnas, MD

Introduction

The term hallux rigidus describes a painful malady of the great toe metatarsophalangeal (MTP) joint characterized by restricted dorsiflexion and periarticular osteophyte formation. This condition was initially reported in 1887 by Davies-Colley[1] who described a plantar-flexed position of the proximal phalanx relative to the metatarsal head and proposed the term hallux flexus. Cotterill[2] reported on the same condition a few months later and suggested hallux rigidus as the proper nomenclature. The more commonly used terms hallux rigidus and hallux limitus are used interchangeably for this condition. Other than hallux valgus, hallux rigidus is the most common disorder of the first MTP joint and may be more disabling.[3,4] The literature reports an overwhelmingly higher incidence of hallux rigidus in females.[5-10] The authors of a 2003 study found that approximately 80% of patients with bilateral hallux rigidus had a positive family history of great toe disorders and that more than 80% had bilateral disease at long-term follow-up.[7] There is no proven association among hallux rigidus and first ray mobility, metatarsal length, Achilles or gastrocnemius contracture, abnormal foot posture, hallux valgus, metatarsus primus elevatus, adolescent onset of the disorder, or the patient's occupation or type of shoe wear.[7,11]

Etiology and Pathophysiology

The most common cause of hallux rigidus cited in the literature is trauma, which may occur as a single episode, such as an intra-articular fracture and crush injury or as the result of repetitive microtrauma. With an acute injury, forced hyperextension or plantar flexion can create compressive and/or shear forces resulting in chondral or osteochondral injury.[12,13] Arthritis may develop from a sprain or turf toe disorder. Based on long-term follow-up, a clear traumatic episode is most likely the cause of unilateral hallux rigidus.[7] The adolescent patient with hallux rigidus frequently presents with an osteochondral defect that is diagnosed as hallux rigidus based on a high index of suspicion and radiographic and/or MRI evidence.[14-18] The only documented factors associated with hallux rigidus are female gender, a flat or chevron-shaped joint, hallux valgus interphalangeus, metatarsus adductus, bilateral symptoms in those with a positive family history of the disorder, and unilateral symptoms in patients with a traumatic injury.[7,19]

One of the more controversial areas regarding etiology is the condition known as metatarsus primus elevatus, a fixed dorsal elevation of the first metatarsal in relationship to the lesser metatarsals (**Figure 1**). For example, fixed elevation is noted with a dorsiflexion malunion of a first metatarsal osteotomy or fracture, whereas more flexible elevation can occur with poste-

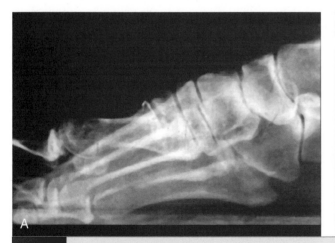
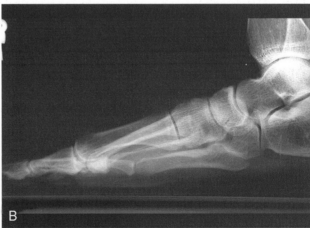

Figure 1   **A,** Lateral radiograph showing metatarsus primus elevatus after a proximal metatarsal osteotomy. **B,** Lateral radiograph showing metatarsus primus elevatus correlated with MTP joint hallux rigidus.

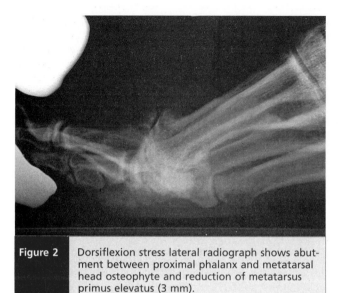

Figure 2 Dorsiflexion stress lateral radiograph shows abutment between proximal phalanx and metatarsal head osteophyte and reduction of metatarsus primus elevatus (3 mm).

rior tibial tendon deficiency, muscle weakness, spasticity, or paralysis. A recent study evaluated metatarsus primus elevatus in patients with hallux rigidus and showed that when elevation was present, it was a secondary condition that correlated with arthritic progression in the first MTP joint.[7,11,19] Metatarsus primus elevatus was nearly eliminated following cheilectomy, interposition arthroplasty, and arthrodesis. No statistical correlation was found between hallux rigidus and first metatarsal elevation (up to 5 mm of elevation was considered normal).[20,21]

Clinical Presentation

In adults with hallux rigidus, the basic pathologic entity is degenerative arthritis.[16] The classic location of cartilage loss occurs on the dorsal one half to two thirds of the metatarsal head.[4,22] As the degenerative process proceeds, osteophytes on the dorsal and dorsolateral metatarsal head develop, creating a prominent bony ridge and abutment with the proximal phalanx (Figure 2).

Physical examination shows a tender, swollen MTP joint with restricted motion; crepitus may be present. MTP joint manipulation may elicit pain during dorsiflexion, plantar flexion, or both. Pain elicited at the midrange of motion with gentle loading indicates extensive cartilage loss in the MTP joint. Bony proliferation around the margin of the affected joint may cause a superficial bursitis, neuritis, or skin ulceration. More information on the clinical presentation of hallux rigidus is available in chapter 16.

Radiographic Examination and Classification

Radiographs often show asymmetric joint-space narrowing or chondrolysis. Increased periarticular ra-

diodensity, subchondral cyst formation, proliferative marginal osteophytes, and intra-articular loose bodies also may be present. Interphalangeal joint hyperextension may develop to compensate for restricted MTP joint dorsiflexion.[23,24] Standing AP and lateral radiographs should be obtained. AP radiographs frequently show asymmetric chondrolysis with widening and flattening of the first metatarsal head. Subchondral cysts and increased radiodensity in the first metatarsal head, widening of the base of the proximal phalanx, and hypertrophy of the sesamoids may develop in more advanced stages of the disorder. The lateral radiograph may show a dorsal metatarsal osteophyte that resembles dripping candle wax, an appearance resulting from the osteophyte as it courses proximally along the dorsal metatarsal metaphyseal-diaphyseal region. A classification system is useful to describe the extent of the arthritic process and for treatment recommendation[19] (Table 1).

Treatment

Nonsurgical
Patients with early stage disease (grades 0 through 2) are treated with nonsteroidal anti-inflammatory drugs and the use of a stiff shoe insole (Morton's extension) to reduce excursion of the MTP joint. Immobilization of the MTP joint with figure-of-8 tape can provide relief when symptoms are related to activity. Orthoses have been shown to provide better and longer-term pain relief than nonsteroidal anti-inflammatory drugs alone.[25] With later disease stages (advanced grade 2 and grades 3 and 4) many orthoses reduce room in the toe box, often increasing pressure on the dorsal prominence.

The authors of one study noted a 6-month benefit using intra-articular steroid injection with joint manipulation for patients with less advanced grades of hallux rigidus.[26] A study of 22 patients (24 feet) treated nonsurgically for hallux rigidus with a mean follow-up of 14 years found that 75% of patients continued to choose nonsurgical treatment.[27] Other investigators have reported successful nonsurgical management in almost 60% of patients treated with shoe wear modifications, orthoses, injections, and taping.[28] More information on the nonsurgical treatment of hallux rigidus is available in chapter 16.

Surgical
The primary indication for surgery is deformity or intractable pain that is not relieved with local or systemic pharmacologic treatment or biomechanical aids such as immobilization or bracing. The selected surgical technique is based on the degree of clinical and radiographic arthritis and correlates well with the grade of hallux rigidus. In the presence of synovial thickening without radiographic changes of degenerative arthritis (grade 0 hallux rigidus), an MTP joint synovectomy

Table 1

Clinical and Radiographic Classification of Hallux Rigidus

Grade	Range of Motion	Radiographic	Clinical
0	Dorsiflexion of 40° to 60° and/or 10% to 20% loss compared with normal side	Normal or minimal findings	No subjective pain, only stiffness Loss of passive motion on examination
1	Dorsiflexion of 30° to 40° and/or 20% to 50% loss compared with normal side	Dorsal spur is main finding Minimal joint narrowing Minimal periarticular sclerosis Minimal flattening of metatarsal head	Mild or occasional subjective pain and stiffness Pain at extremes of dorsiflexion and/or plantar flexion on examination
2	Dorsiflexion of 10° to 30° and/or 50% to 75% loss compared with normal side	Dorsal, lateral, and possibly medial osteophytes give flattened appearance to metatarsal head No more than one fourth dorsal joint-space involvement on lateral radiograph Mild to moderate joint-space narrowing and sclerosis Sesamoids not usually involved but may be irregular in appearance	Moderate to severe subjective pain and stiffness that may be constant Pain just before maximal dorsiflexion and/or plantar flexion on examination
3	Dorsiflexion of 10° or less and/or 75% to 100% loss compared with normal side; notable loss of plantar flexion (often ≤ 10°)	Same as grade 2 but with substantial joint-space narrowing Possibly periarticular cystic changes, more than one fourth of dorsal joint may be involved on lateral side, sesamoids may be enlarged and/or cystic and/or irregular	Nearly constant subjective pain and substantial stiffness Pain throughout range of motion on examination (but not at midrange)
4	Same as grade 3	Same as grade 3	Same as grade 3 but definite pain at midrange of motion

Adapted with permission from Coughlin MJ, Shurnas PS: Hallux rigidus: Grading and long term results of operative treatment. J Bone Joint Surg Am 2003;85:2072-2088.

alone may be used. However, the authors of a 2005 study reported flexor hallucis longus stenosing tenosynovitis as a cause of hallux rigidus in patients without radiographic changes but with restricted passive joint motion.[29] If flexor hallucis longus stenosis is diagnosed in a patient with grade 0 or 1 hallux rigidus, a fibro-osseous tunnel release is performed with or without MTP joint synovectomy, cheilectomy, and/or phalangeal osteotomy depending on the patient.

Removal of osteochondral fragments and microfracture of the osseous base may produce a stable fibrocartilaginous surface and extend the indications for cheilectomy. A 2003 study found no adverse long-term effects in a small number of patients treated with microfracture with cheilectomy; however, any patient with less than 50% of the metatarsal articular surface remaining (grade 3 or 4) had a significantly increased risk of failure of the cheilectomy.[19]

Patients with impingement of the proximal phalanx against a dorsal osteophyte on the metatarsal head (grades 1 through 3) can be treated successfully with cheilectomy. In 1979, the cheilectomy technique of Mann, Coughlin, and DuVries was described and successful results were reported at long-term follow-up.[30]

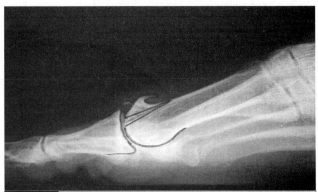

Figure 3 Lateral weight-bearing radiograph shows proper resection of osteophytes and metatarsal head using cheilectomy for hallux rigidus repair.

A 2003 study of 80 patients reported a success rate of 92% at 9.6-year follow-up using cheilectomy.[19] Cheilectomy resects osteophytes and removes bony impingements (25% to 40% of the dorsal metatarsal head) (**Figure 3**). A major reason for failure of cheilectomy is inadequate bone resection, which may explain reported failure rates of more than 30%.[22] Inadequate resection results in suboptimal restoration of MTP joint motion. If impingement persists, the procedure may ultimately fail. Preoperatively, pain that is notable at the midrange of motion with gentle loading indicates that the remaining cartilage surface is inadequate and portends a poor prognosis for the success of treatment with cheilectomy alone.[19] Even if cheilectomy fails, salvage options are available.

For grade 3 hallux rigidus with less than 50% of metatarsal head cartilage remaining at the time of surgery or for grade 4 disease, salvage procedures include arthrodesis, excisional arthroplasty, soft-tissue interposition arthroplasty, or prosthetic replacement. Keller or Mayo-type excisional arthroplasty is not recommended for patients other than nonambulating patients or those who are housebound. Often with excisional arthroplasty, plantar-plate instability of the MTP joint occurs and may lead to transfer metatarsalgia.[6] Generally, poor postoperative results with excisional arthroplasty have been reported with objective improvement in only 9% of patients, no change in 71%, and deterioration in 20%.[31] An association was found between increased phalangeal resection and lateral metatarsalgia.[32] Weight bearing on the hallux was noted in 73% of the feet in which one third or less of the proximal phalanx was resected. Other complications include cock-up deformity of the great toe, stiffness of the interphalangeal joint, marked shortening, impaired control and function, and diminished flexor strength of the great toe. Using a retrospective analysis, the authors of one study reported on the use of the Valenti procedure (a less destructive dorsal resection arthroplasty) and found a high incidence of good and excellent results (33 of 36 procedures) in younger patients at a mean follow-up of 4.2 years.[33]

Limited excision arthroplasty has been combined with capsular interposition, with the tissue serving as a biologic spacer. The relative length of the first and second metatarsals should be equal to avoid a transfer lesion or lateral metatarsalgia. Reported results on 30 patients (34 feet) with severe arthrosis showed increased dorsiflexion with a mean of 40°; 93% of patients were satisfied with the procedure.[34] Similar results were reported using gracilis tendon as a biologic spacer, with conical reaming of the proximal phalanx and metatarsal head to create an effective joint space for graft placement.[11] Seven active, younger patients (mean age, 40 years) reported good to excellent satisfaction with the procedure at a minimum follow-up period of 4 years.

Arthrodesis has been advocated for severe hallux rigidus, preserving the length and stability of the first metatarsal. Other indications for arthrodesis include implant failure or unsuccessful excisional arthroplasty or osteotomy. The success rate for MTP arthrodesis varies significantly depending on the preoperative diagnosis, surgical technique, and method of internal fixation. Reported success rates vary from less than 77% to 100%.[35-38]

A 2003 study of patients with severe hallux rigidus used cup-shaped surfaces achieved after power reaming that were repaired with a low-profile Vitallium plate and oblique derotational screw.[19] Results showed 32 of 34 successful fusions (94%), 100% good or excellent results (including two patients with a fibrous union), and a low complication rate at a mean follow-up period of 6.7 years. Measured first ray mobility was significantly reduced after arthrodesis. First MTP joint arthrodesis has been used with good results for lower grades of hallux rigidus, and a high proportion of good and excellent results have been achieved using screws and/or Steinmann pins alone.[39] In a review of 1,451 cases of hallux rigidus in the literature, a 90% success rate was found for treatment with fusion.[35] With an interfragmentary screw and dorsal plate, a fusion rate of 93% to 100% has been reported.[36]

The main complications of arthrodesis are malalignment, nonunion, and degenerative arthritis of the interphalangeal joint of the hallux. Malunion is poorly tolerated and can occur in any one of three planes: (1) varus/valgus malalignment in the frontal plane (2) dorsiflexion/plantar flexion malalignment in the sagittal plane; and (3) rotational deformity in the transverse plane. Correct varus/valgus alignment also is critical. A threefold increase in the incidence of interphalangeal joint arthrosis was found with an MTP fusion with less than 20° of hallux valgus.[40] However, 10° to 20° of valgus has generally been considered an acceptable position. In contrast, another researcher found that the dorsiflexion angle is the primary determinant of the degree of interphalangeal joint arthritis and reported that 22° of dorsiflexion relative to the metatarsal had the lowest correlation with subsequent interphalangeal joint arthritis.[41]

Joint implant arthroplasty has been advocated for the treatment of hallux rigidus; however, reported complications and severe difficulty with revision surgery have made this procedure less popular.[42-44] Most early MTP joint arthroplasty procedures used the silicone elastomer hemiphalangeal implant introduced by Swanson.[42] Touted as biocompatible and inert, early in vitro and in vivo studies by Swanson and associates[44] led to the widespread use of this implant. Later reports of single-stem implant failure heralded the introduction of the double-stem silicone elastomer implant.[45-47] It is estimated that more than 2 million first MTP joint, hinged, silicone implants were implanted from 1973 through 1993.[48] Later studies with longer follow-up periods have shown high failure rates (57% to 74%) for this implant.[48-50] One study showed a twofold increase in lateral metatarsal weight bearing compared with the contralateral foot after first MTP joint arthroplasty.[50] Initially, it was hoped that joint arthroplasty would facilitate a normal gait pattern; however, normal plantar weight bearing and toe purchase with standing was not restored.[44,50] Pain relief as a primary indication for joint arthroplasty has been reported, but with inconsistent results.[44] One researcher reported moderate and severe first MTP pain in 16 of 51 joints (31%) following MTP arthroplasty.[48] Based on implant survivorship analysis, a 50% failure rate for hinged, silicone implant components was predicted at 4-year follow-up.[50] Because of stress, fatigue, joint overuse, poor fit, abrasion of joint surfaces, and pistoning of the prosthesis, microfragmentation can occur. Migration of these microscopic silicone fragments through the lymphatic system can result in secondary lymphadenopathy caused by foreign body reaction.[49]

One investigator reported that more than 360 metal implants have been used to revise failed silicone implants, but did not report on the subjective or objective results of these revision surgeries.[48] The author of a 2002 study reported five excellent, one good, two fair, and one poor result at 2-year follow-up after total endoprosthetic replacement.[51] Results demonstrated radiographic loosening in one cementless phalangeal component, one prosthetic subluxation, one superficial infection, and one recurrent severe valgus deformity. Another study with longer follow-up found increased shortening from resorption of bone and prosthetic collapse.[50] Only long-term follow-up will provide information on whether cementless first MTP total joint arthroplasties achieve better outcomes than cemented prostheses implanted during the 1970s and 1980s. The paucity of information available with even short-term subjective and objective results makes use of these implants questionable until more published results become available. More information on the surgical treatment of hallux rigidus is available in chapter 16.

Summary

Hallux rigidus is a degenerative arthritic process involving the great toe MTP joint and sesamoid complex. Early in the degenerative process, nonsurgical treatment with shoe wear modifications, judicious use of steroid injections, and figure-of-8 taping can be successful. However, as degeneration progresses, surgery may be necessary. A reliable, well-documented, surgical treatment is hallux rigidus repair or cheilectomy as described by Mann, Coughlin, and DuVries. For more advanced MTP joint deterioration, arthrodesis is the mainstay of surgical treatment; however, interposition arthroplasty should be considered for younger patients who want to maintain some range of motion.

Annotated References

1. Davies-Colley M: Contraction of the metatarsophalangeal joint of the great toe. *BMJ* 1887;1:728.

2. Cotterill J: Stiffness of the great toe in adolescents. *BMJ* 1888;1:1158.

3. DuVries H: Static deformities, in DuVries H (ed): *Sur-*

gery of the Foot. St. Louis, MO, Mosby, 1959, pp 392-398.

4. Moberg E: A simple operation for hallux rigidus. *Clin Orthop Relat Res* 1979;142:55-56.

5. Bonney G, Macnab I: Hallux valgus and hallux rigidus: A critical survey of operative results. *J Bone Joint Surg Br* 1952;34:366-385.

6. Coughlin MJ, Mann RA: Arthrodesis of the first metatarsophalangeal joint as salvage for the failed Keller procedure. *J Bone Joint Surg Am* 1987;69:68-75.

7. Coughlin MJ, Shurnas PS: Hallux rigidus: Demographics, etiology, and radiographic assessment. *Foot Ankle Int* 2003;24:731-743.

   The authors of this retrospective study with a mean follow-up period of 10 years attempted to evaluate the demographics, etiology, and radiographic findings associated with hallux rigidus. The authors concluded that hallux rigidus was associated with hallux valgus interphalangeus and female gender. An association between bilateral involvement in those with a familial history and unilateral involvement in those with a history of trauma was also found. A flat or chevron-shaped metatarsophalangeal joint was more common in patients with hallux rigidus.

8. Drago JJ, Oloff L, Jacobs AM: A comprehensive review of hallux limitus. *J Foot Surg* 1984;23:213-220.

9. Mann RA, Clanton TO: Hallux rigidus: Treatment by cheilectomy. *J Bone Joint Surg Am* 1988;70:400-406.

10. Nilsonne H: Hallux rigidus and its treatment. *Acta Orthop Scand* 1930;1:295-303.

11. Coughlin MJ, Shurnas PS: Soft-tissue arthroplasty for hallux rigidus. *Foot Ankle Int* 2003;24:661-672.

    The authors of this retrospective study evaluated seven patients with severe hallux rigidus who were treated with soft-tissue interposition arthroplasty of the hallux MTP joint. At a mean follow-up of approximately 4 years, all patients reported good or excellent results.

12. Coughlin MJ: Conditions of the forefoot, in DeLee J, Drez D (eds): *Orthopaedic Sports Medicine: Principles and Practice.* Philadelphia, PA, WB Saunders, 1994, pp 221-244.

13. Frey C, Andersen GD, Feder KS: Plantarflexion injury to the metatarsophalangeal joint (sand toe). *Foot Ankle Int* 1996;17:576-581.

14. Goodfellow J: Aetiology of hallux rigidus. *Proc R Soc Med* 1966;59:821-824.

15. Hanft JR, Mason ET, Landsman AS, Kashuk KB: A new radiographic classification for hallux limitus. *J Foot Ankle Surg* 1993;32:397-404.

4: The Forefoot

16. Kessel L, Bonney G: Hallux rigidus in the adolescent. *J Bone Joint Surg Br* 1958;40:669-673.

17. McMaster MJ: The pathogenesis of hallux rigidus. *J Bone Joint Surg Br* 1978;60:82-87.

18. Schweitzer ME, Maheshwari S, Shabshin N: Hallux valgus and hallux rigidus: MRI findings. *Clin Imaging* 1999;23:397-402.

19. Coughlin MJ, Shurnas PS: Hallux rigidus: Grading and long-term results of operative treatment. *J Bone Joint Surg Am* 2003;85:2072-2088.

    The purpose of this retrospective study of 110 patients was to evaluate the long-term outcomes of surgical treatment of hallux rigidus. The authors found that 97% of patients had good or excellent results. Ninety-two percent of those treated with cheilectomy reported pain relief and improved function. Cheilectomy was an effective treatment for patients with grade 1 and 2 hallux rigidus and for selected patients with grade 3 hallux rigidus. The authors recommended arthrodesis for patients with grade 3 disease with less than 50% of metatarsal head cartilage remaining and those with grade 4 hallux rigidus.

20. Meyer JO, Nishon LR, Weiss L, Docks G: Metatarsus primus elevatus and the etiology of hallux rigidus. *J Foot Surg* 1987;26:237-241.

21. Horton GA, Park YW, Myerson MS: Role of metatarsus primus elevatus in the pathogenesis of hallux rigidus. *Foot Ankle Int* 1999;20:777-780.

22. Hattrup SJ, Johnson KA: Subjective results of hallux rigidus following treatment with cheilectomy. *Clin Orthop Relat Res* 1988;226:182-191.

23. Feldman RS, Hutter J, Lapow L, Pour B: Cheilectomy and hallux rigidus. *J Foot Surg* 1983;22:170-174.

24. Gould N: Hallux rigidus: Cheilotomy or implant? *Foot Ankle* 1981;1:315-320.

25. Thompson JA, Jennings MB, Hodge W: Orthotic therapy in the management of osteoarthritis. *J Am Podiatr Med Assoc* 1992;82:136-139.

26. Solan MC, Calder JD, Bendall SP: Manipulation and injection for hallux rigidus: Is it worthwhile? *J Bone Joint Surg Br* 2001;83:706-708.

27. Smith RW, Katchis SD, Ayson LC: Outcomes in hallux rigidus patients treated nonoperatively: A long-term follow-up study. *Foot Ankle Int* 2000;21:906-913.

28. Grady JF, Axe TM, Zager EJ, Sheldon LA: A retrospective analysis of 772 patients with hallux limitus. *J Am Podiatr Med Assoc* 2002;92:102-108.

29. Michelson J, Dunn L: Tenosynovitis of the flexor hallucis longus: A clinical study of the spectrum of presentation and treatment. *Foot Ankle Int* 2005;26:291-303.

    The authors describe the spectrum of clinical presentations that occur in flexor hallucis longus pathology, discuss physical examination findings, and describe an approach to treatment.

30. Mann RA, Coughlin MJ, DuVries HL: Hallux rigidus: A review of the literature and a method of treatment. *Clin Orthop Relat Res* 1979;142:57-63.

31. Rogers W, Joplin R: Hallux valgus, weak foot, and the Keller operations: An end-result study. *Surg Clin North Am* 1947;27:1295-1302.

32. Henry AP, Waugh W, Wood H: The use of footprints in assessing the results of operations for hallux valgus: A comparison of Keller's operation and arthrodesis. *J Bone Joint Surg Br* 1975;57:478-481.

33. Kurtz DH, Harrill JC, Kaczander BI, Solomon MG: The Valenti procedure for hallux limitus: A long-term follow-up and analysis. *J Foot Ankle Surg* 1999;38:123-130.

34. Hamilton WG, O'Malley MJ, Thompson FM, Kovatis PE: Capsular interposition arthroplasty for severe hallux rigidus. *Foot Ankle Int* 1997;18:68-70.

35. Coughlin MJ: Arthrodesis of the first metatarsophalangeal joint with mini-fragment plate fixation. *Orthopedics* 1990;13:1037-1044.

36. Coughlin MJ, Abdo RV: Arthrodesis of the first metatarsophalangeal joint with Vitallium plate fixation. *Foot Ankle Int* 1994;15:18-28.

37. Gimple K, Anspacher J, Kopta J: Metatarsophalangeal joint fusion of the great toe. *Orthopedics* 1978;1:462-467.

38. von Salis-Soglio G, Thomas W: Arthrodesis of the metatarsophalangeal joint of the great toe. *Arch Orthop Trauma Surg* 1979;95:7-12.

39. Lombardi CM, Silhanek AD, Connolly FG, Dennis LN, Keslonsky AJ: First metatarsophalangeal arthrodesis for treatment of hallux rigidus: A retrospective study. *J Foot Ankle Surg* 2001;40:137-143.

40. Fitzgerald JA: A review of long-term results of arthrodesis of the first metatarso-phalangeal joint. *J Bone Joint Surg Br* 1969;51:488-493.

41. Coughlin MJ: Rheumatoid forefoot reconstruction: A long-term follow-up study. *J Bone Joint Surg Am* 2000;82:322-341.

42. Swanson AB: Implant arthroplasty for the great toe. *Clin Orthop Relat Res* 1972;85:75-81.

43. Swanson AB, de Groot Swanson G, Maupin BK, et al:

The use of a grommet bone liner for flexible hinge implant arthroplasty of the great toe. *Foot Ankle* 1991;12: 149-155.

44. Swanson AB, Lumsden RM, Swanson GD: Silicone implant arthroplasty of the great toe: A review of single stem and flexible hinge implants. *Clin Orthop Relat Res* 1979;142:30-43.

45. Lemon RA, Engber WD, McBeath AA: A complication of Silastic hemiarthroplasty in bunion surgery. *Foot Ankle* 1984;4:262-266.

46. Verhaar J, Vermeulen A, Bulstra S, Walenkamp G: Bone reaction to silicone metatarsophalangeal joint-1 hemi-prosthesis. *Clin Orthop Relat Res* 1989;245:228-232.

47. Watermann H: Die arthritis deformans grosszehen-grundgelenkes. *Ztschr Orthop Chir* 1927;48:346-355.

48. Freed JB: The increasing recognition of medullary lysis, cortical osteophytic proliferation, and fragmentation of implanted silicone polymer implants. *J Foot Ankle Surg* 1993;32:171-179.

49. Gordon M, Bullough PG: Synovial and osseous inflammation in failed silicone-rubber prostheses. *J Bone Joint Surg Am* 1982;64:574-580.

50. Granberry WM, Noble PC, Bishop JO, Tullos HS: Use of a hinged silicone prosthesis for replacement arthroplasty of the first metatarsophalangeal joint. *J Bone Joint Surg Am* 1991;73:1453-1459.

51. Ess P, Hamalainen M, Leppilahti J: Non-constrained titanium-polyethylene total endoprosthesis in the treatment of hallux rigidus: A prospective clinical 2-year follow-up study. *Scand J Surg* 2002;91:202-207.

4: The Forefoot

Lesser Toe Deformities, Intractable Plantar Keratosis, Freiberg Infraction, and Bunionette

Jason H. Pleimann, MD   Susan N. Ishikawa, MD   Melanie Sanders, MD

4: The Forefoot

Introduction

Lesser toe (second through fifth toe) deformities and conditions may result from trauma, inflammatory conditions, neurologic disorders, ill-fitting shoe wear, or may have a congenital origin. Such deformities or diseases may be symptomatic and require nonsurgical or surgical treatment to provide pain relief and improved function for the patient.

Mallet Toes, Hammer Toes, and Claw Toes

Pathoanatomy and Etiology

The lesser toes are important for balance and pressure distribution on the plantar surface of the foot. The normal position and function of the toes requires normal balance in both passive and active stabilizers. Imbalances result in various pathologic states. Poorly fitting shoe wear can apply additional deforming forces.[1]

Normal passive stabilizers include extensions of the plantar aponeurosis, joint capsule, plantar plate, and the collateral ligaments. Active stabilizers include the extrinsic muscles (extensor digitorum longus [EDL] and flexor digitorum longus [FDL]) and the intrinsic muscles (flexor digitorum brevis [FDB], extensor digitorum brevis [EDB], interosseous muscles, and the lumbrical muscles). The tibial nerve innervates the extrinsic flexors and the intrinsic muscles. The peroneal nerve innervates the extrinsic extensor muscles.

Dorsally, the EDL and EDB extend the metatarsophalangeal (MTP) joint through their pull on the extensor hood. The EDL continues distally with the central slip inserting into the middle phalanx and the medial and lateral portions merging to insert on the distal phalanx. The EDL and EDB extend the MTP joint, the proximal interphalangeal (PIP) joint, and the distal interphalangeal (DIP) joint. The FDL, which courses deep to the FDB and inserts at the base of the distal phalanx, exerts a strong flexion force at the DIP joint and provides weaker flexion forces at the PIP and

MTP joints. The FDB bifurcates and inserts into the middle phalanx, exerting a strong flexion force at the PIP joint with weaker flexion of the MTP joint. The lumbrical muscles and interossei lie plantar to the axis of motion of the MTP joint, acting as flexors of this articulation (**Figure 1**). Distally, their attachments to the extensor hood lie dorsal to the axis of motion of the PIP and DIP joints, acting as extensors. If the balance between the extrinsic and intrinsic forces is altered, deformities of the lesser toes can result.[2]

Deformities of the lesser toes are typically categorized into three types: mallet toes, hammer toes, and claw toes (**Figure 2**). A mallet toe involves a flexion contracture of the DIP joint with no deformity at the PIP or MTP joints. A hammer toe is characterized by a PIP joint flexion deformity without significant abnormality at the DIP or MTP joints. A claw toe deformity involves hyperextension at the MTP joint and second-

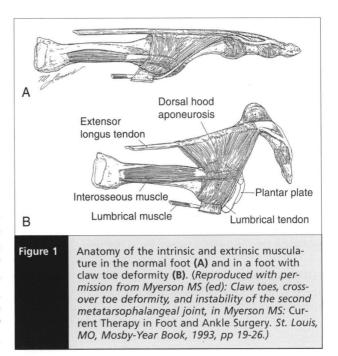

Figure 1   Anatomy of the intrinsic and extrinsic musculature in the normal foot **(A)** and in a foot with claw toe deformity **(B)**. (*Reproduced with permission from Myerson MS (ed): Claw toes, crossover toe deformity, and instability of the second metatarsophalangeal joint, in Myerson MS:* Current Therapy in Foot and Ankle Surgery. *St. Louis, MO, Mosby-Year Book, 1993, pp 19-26.*)

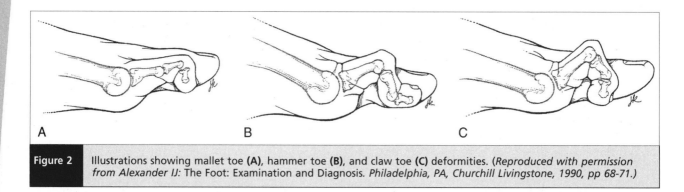

Figure 2 Illustrations showing mallet toe **(A)**, hammer toe **(B)**, and claw toe **(C)** deformities. (*Reproduced with permission from Alexander IJ: The Foot: Examination and Diagnosis. Philadelphia, PA, Churchill Livingstone, 1990, pp 68-71.*)

ary flexion at the PIP joint. These deformities may be subcategorized as flexible or fixed deformities based on an examiner's ability to manually manipulate the toes into a corrected position.

Clinical Presentation and Evaluation

Patients with lesser toe deformities most often describe symptoms associated with wearing closed-toe shoes. Reports include painful calluses or blisters over the dorsal PIP joint or at the tip of the toe, and pain under the metatarsal head related to MTP joint hyperextension. During the physical examination, the position of the toes should be observed with the patient bearing weight because the deformity may be accentuated. It is important to note whether a deformity of the first ray (such as hallux valgus) is present. The degree of flexibility of the lesser toe deformities should be evaluated because the type of surgical correction varies depending on the rigidity of the deformity. Standard radiographs, including standing radiographs of the foot, should be evaluated for degenerative changes or evidence of prior surgery.

Nonsurgical Treatment

Shoes with a deep toe box and proper fit are the foundation for the nonsurgical treatment of lesser toe deformities because pain typically occurs when the toes contact the inner portion of the shoe. Numerous appliances are available to help cushion or protect bony prominences. Various corrective devices such as hammer toe slings, metatarsal pads, and taping techniques may provide relief for deformities with a degree of flexibility. Often, manual stretching exercises are recommended for flexible deformities; however, there is no clear evidence that these exercises provide long-term improvement in toe position or pain. Failure of conservative measures to provide pain relief or a patient's inability to comply with shoe wear restrictions are indications for surgical treatment. Patients often report that corrective devices and cushions are too cumbersome for daily use.

Surgical Treatment

Surgical treatment of lesser toe deformities may combine various soft-tissue and bony procedures to achieve adequate correction. The patient should be appropriately counseled on the potential for complications in-

cluding recurrent deformity, incomplete correction, and vascular compromise of the involved digits.[3] The functional outcome after surgery and the expected postoperative course should be clearly communicated to the patient. Shortened toes, stiff joints, and prolonged swelling are common results of surgical treatment. The patient should be counseled regarding complications and should be made aware that permanent changes in footwear may be necessary to prevent recurrence. Surgical correction of lesser toe abnormalities requires a thoughtful approach based on the etiology of the deformity, with stepwise correction of deforming forces and fixed deformities.

A flexible mallet toe, which most often results in a painful terminal callus, is readily correctable with a percutaneous flexor tenotomy at the level of the distal flexor crease of the toe.[4] This procedure often can be performed in the office setting with the patient under local anesthesia. A rigid mallet toe requires bony correction with resection arthroplasty or DIP arthrodesis, with or without FDL tenotomy. The toe is often held in position with a smooth Kirschner wire (K-wire) that is removed 4 to 6 weeks postoperatively[5] (**Figure 3**).

Flexible hammer toe deformities can be treated with soft-tissue procedures or a combination of soft-tissue and bony procedures. The flexor to extensor tendon transfer involves realignment of the toe with the use of a split FDL transfer to the extensor hood at the proximal phalanx.[6] In this technique, the FDL is exposed at the plantar base of the toe, then percutaneously released from the distal phalanx. The medial and lateral segments of the tendon are then split and passed around the base of the proximal phalanx deep to the neurovascular bundles, but superficial to the extensor hood. Through a separate dorsal incision, the limbs of the FDL are tensioned to correct coronal plane malalignment and sutured to the extensor hood and to one another. The transferred tendon acts as a plantar flexor of the MTP joint and an extensor of the PIP and DIP joints. The procedure typically yields limited motion at interphalangeal joints but maintains functional flexion and extension at the MTP joint. Alternatively, a flexible hammer toe can be repaired through bony removal in the manner described for repair of rigid hammer toe deformity.

The presence of a fixed flexion deformity at the PIP

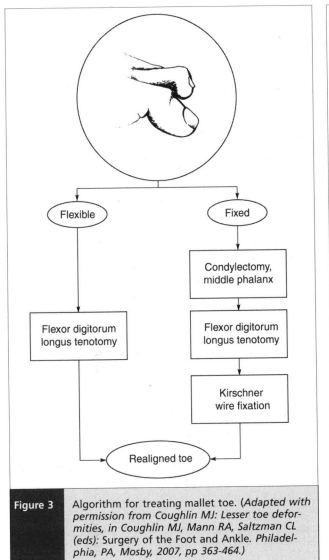

Figure 3 Algorithm for treating mallet toe. (*Adapted with permission from Coughlin MJ: Lesser toe deformities, in Coughlin MJ, Mann RA, Saltzman CL (eds):* Surgery of the Foot and Ankle. *Philadelphia, PA, Mosby, 2007, pp 363-464.*)

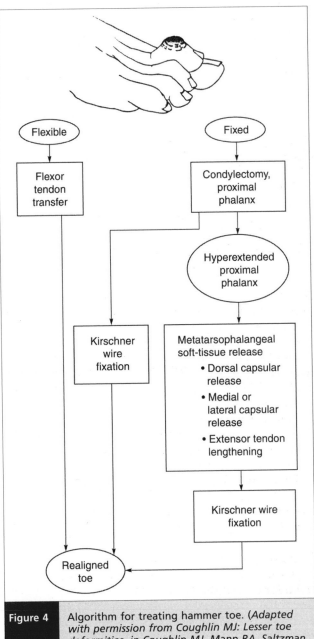

Figure 4 Algorithm for treating hammer toe. (*Adapted with permission from Coughlin MJ: Lesser toe deformities, in Coughlin MJ, Mann RA, Saltzman CL (eds):* Surgery of the Foot and Ankle. *Philadelphia, PA, Mosby, 2007, pp 363-464.*)

joint necessitates bony removal to achieve correction. This can be accomplished with a PIP resection arthroplasty or a formal PIP fusion with or without FDL tenotomy.[7,8] In this procedure, the distal portion of the proximal phalanx is resected just proximal to the condyles and perpendicular to the shaft. Further bony resection may be necessary if there is incomplete passive correction of the toe, or alternatively an FDL tenotomy can be performed either through a separate plantar incision or dorsally through the bony resection site. If PIP fusion is desired, articular cartilage and subchondral bone are removed from the base of the middle phalanx; care should be taken to avoid phalanx overshortening, which can occur with excessive bony resection. If pin fixation is desired to provide stability to the correction, a size 0.045- to 0.062-inch K-wire can be used. If it is anticipated that the pin must cross the MTP joint to correct the deformity, a 0.062-inch K-wire is generally recommended to minimize the risk of pin breakage. The pin is passed in an antegrade fashion through the

base of the middle phalanx and out the tip of the toe. With the toe held in the corrected position, the pin is passed retrograde across the resection site and driven into the proximal phalanx. The K-wire is removed at 4 to 6 weeks postoperatively (**Figure 4**).

When anticipated preoperatively, correction of an MTP contracture should precede correction at the PIP joint to allow better manipulation of the toe during exposure of the MTP joint. Correction of the MTP joint contracture includes dorsal, medial, and lateral capsule release, EDB tenotomy, and EDL Z-lengthening.[9] If frank dislocation exists, a metatarsal shortening osteotomy or DuVries metatarsal head reshaping arthroplasty

4: The Forefoot

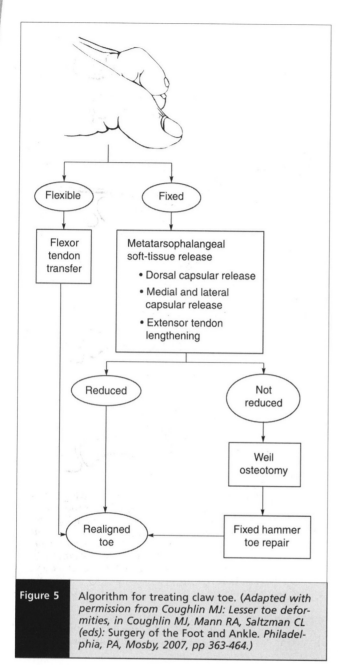

Figure 5 Algorithm for treating claw toe. (*Adapted with permission from Coughlin MJ: Lesser toe deformities, in Coughlin MJ, Mann RA, Saltzman CL (eds): Surgery of the Foot and Ankle. Philadelphia, PA, Mosby, 2007, pp 363-464.*)

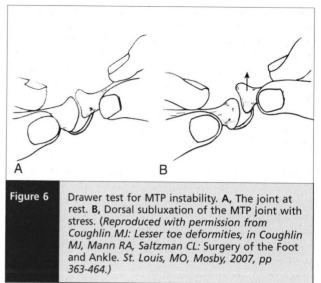

Figure 6 Drawer test for MTP instability. **A,** The joint at rest. **B,** Dorsal subluxation of the MTP joint with stress. (*Reproduced with permission from Coughlin MJ: Lesser toe deformities, in Coughlin MJ, Mann RA, Saltzman CL: Surgery of the Foot and Ankle. St. Louis, MO, Mosby, 2007, pp 363-464.*)

the unique anatomy of the second ray. The second ray is located adjacent to the hallux and is typically longer. The limited motion of the second tarsometatarsal joint subjects the second MTP joint to higher stresses. Repetitive stresses at the second MTP joint result in a reactive synovitis leading to attenuation of the plantar plate, which can lead to instability at the second MTP joint and deformity in the sagittal plane. Continued synovitis can cause frontal and axial plane deformities, which may result in medial deviation (crossover toe) and frank subacute dislocation.

Clinical Presentation and Evaluation

At the time of presentation, patients describe symptoms ranging from a sense of fullness and pain in the area of the second MTP joint to frank deformities that may lead to difficulties with shoe wear and/or intractable keratoses beneath the second metatarsal head.[10] Symptoms may be confused with those of an interdigital neuroma; however, careful palpation typically locates the pain to the joint rather than the second interspace. Provocative tests include eliciting the second MTP drawer sign in which the toe shows painful sagittal plane instability and pain with passive plantar flexion of the second MTP joint[11] (**Figure 6**). The hallux should be assessed for hallux valgus deformity that may encroach on the normal position of the second toe. Imaging should include standing radiographs on which the second MTP joint can be evaluated for widening (indicative of synovitis), narrowing (indicative of subluxation, dislocation, or arthritis), or deviation from the midline (indicative of capsular and collateral ligament attenuation or rupture). The relative length of the second metatarsal compared with the remaining lesser metatarsals and the first metatarsal should be noted.

Nonsurgical Treatment

The goal of nonsurgical treatment in patients with disorders of the second ray should focus on reduction of

should be performed. Correction of the PIP joint deformity should proceed in the same manner as that used for hammer toe deformity (**Figure 5**).

Disorders of the Second Toe

Pathoanatomy and Etiology

A unique set of disorders occurs more frequently in the second toe than in the other lesser toes. These disorders include MTP joint synovitis, which may progress to instability; crossover second toe; and frank dislocation. Although these abnormalities may occasionally originate from an acute traumatic episode, they are more commonly caused by repetitive trauma resulting from inflammation and stress by off-loading the second MTP joint. This goal may be accomplished with metatarsal pads, metatarsal bars, rocker-bottom soles, cast or walker boot immobilization, and short periods with no weight bearing. Highly flexible shoes with narrow toe boxes should be avoided. Taping or strapping the second toe to prevent hyperextension during toe-off may be beneficial. Judicious use of nonsteroidal anti-inflammatory drugs can provide symptomatic relief. Occasionally, a corticosteroid injection may be considered; however, these injections can lead to further attenuation of the plantar plate and capsular ligamentous structures and more rapid instability. Taping or strapping the toe or more aggressive off-loading should be considered for several weeks following the injection.[12] Because these disorders represent a spectrum beginning with synovitis and progressing to dislocation, surgical treatment should be considered if symptoms are not relieved with an adequate trial of conservative care.

Surgical Treatment

When second MTP synovitis persists despite conservative measures, a simple synovectomy may be indicated. Correcting any significant hallux valgus deformity that impinges on the normal resting position of the second toe also should be considered.[13]

When frank instability, deformity, or dislocation of the second MTP joint develops, several surgical options exist. For an unstable second MTP joint without deformity, a flexor-to-extensor transfer may provide sufficient plantar flexion stability to the proximal phalanx. This procedure should be performed in combination with a dorsal capsular release. For a crossover or medially deviated second toe, a progressive soft-tissue release consisting of the dorsal capsule, medial capsule, extensor tendon lengthening, and lumbrical release may restore alignment of the toe. This procedure can be combined with lateral capsular reefing; a collateral ligament reconstruction with an EDB transfer can be added.[14] Pinning of the MTP in a reduced or even overcorrected position with a 0.062-inch K-wire is recommended to maintain joint alignment during soft-tissue healing. The pin is removed at 4 to 6 weeks postoperatively.

In a frankly dislocated second MTP joint, a bony procedure may be necessary. These dislocations often occur in the presence of a relatively long second metatarsal. In the absence of arthritic change of the second MTP joint, a distal oblique (Weil) osteotomy can be used to shorten the second metatarsal, which allows relaxation of the surrounding soft tissues and subsequent relocation of the joint[15] (Figure 7). Associated hammer toe deformity can be corrected with PIP resection arthroplasty, PIP fusion, or flexor-to-extensor tendon transfer. It is important to recognize the possibility of a floating toe deformity that can result from the combination of a hammer toe repair and distal metatarsal osteotomy. When there are arthritic changes at the second MTP joint, a partial resection of the metatarsal head (DuVries arthroplasty) may achieve reduction of the toe. A K-wire is often used to stabilize the joint to allow soft-tissue healing and arthrofibrosis, which pro-

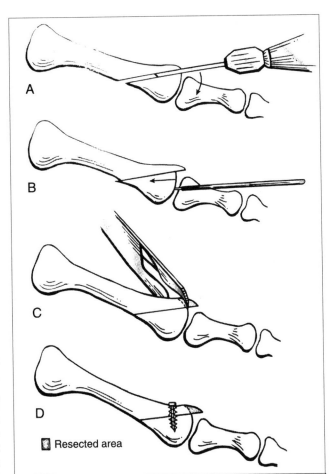

| Figure 7 | Illustration of a Weil osteotomy showing the osteotomy **(A)**, proximal translation of the distal segment **(B)**, resection of the overhanging dorsal bone **(C)**, and fixation **(D)**. *(Reproduced with permission from Coughlin MJ: Lesser toe deformities, in Coughlin MJ, Mann RA, Saltzman CL (eds): Surgery of the Foot and Ankle. St. Louis, MO, 2007, pp 363-464.)* |

◪ Resected area

vides long-term stability to the toe. Overshortening of the second metatarsal can lead to transfer metatarsalgia to the third metatarsal head.

For revision surgery, syndactylization of the second and third toes may achieve sufficient stability. Resection of the second metatarsal head is rarely necessary and can result in development of an intractable plantar keratosis (IPK) under the third metatarsal head and/or subluxation or dislocation of the third MTP joint. In low-demand and elderly patients with severe second toe deformity, a second toe amputation can achieve good results with minimal postoperative morbidity.[16]

Intractable Plantar Keratosis

Pathoanatomy and Etiology

An IPK is a persistent painful callus on the plantar foot, typically beneath a metatarsal head or sesamoid. The epi-

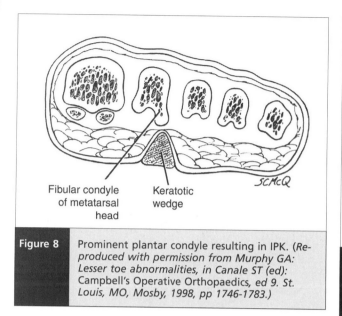

Fibular condyle
of metatarsal
head

Keratotic
wedge

SCMcQ

Figure 8 Prominent plantar condyle resulting in IPK. (*Reproduced with permission from Murphy GA: Lesser toe abnormalities, in Canale ST (ed): Campbell's Operative Orthopaedics, ed 9. St. Louis, MO, Mosby, 1998, pp 1746-1783.*)

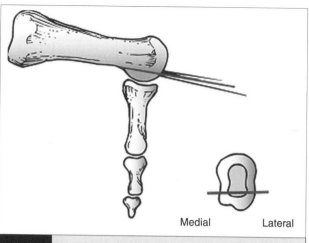

Medial   Lateral

Figure 9 Coughlin's modification of plantar condylectomy. (*Reproduced with permission from Mann RA, Mann JA: Keratotic disorders of the plantar skin, in Coughlin MJ, Mann RA, Saltzman CL (eds): Surgery of the Foot and Ankle. St. Louis, MO, Mosby, 2007, pp 465-490.*)

dermal thickening, which results from pressure, may be discrete or diffuse depending on the underlying etiology. Localized IPKs represent a discrete lesion beneath a single metatarsal head and are characterized by a central keratotic core; they most often result from a prominent lesser metatarsal head fibular condyle (**Figure 8**). Diffuse IPKs, present beneath isolated metatarsal heads, do not demonstrate a central keratotic core and are caused by pressure from the entire metatarsal head. Diffuse IPKs beneath multiple metatarsal heads are typically caused by increased plantar forefoot pressures resulting from biomechanical foot deformities such as contracture of the gastrocnemius or iatrogenic shortening of the first ray after hallux valgus surgery. Plantar fat pad atrophy and systemic disease processes such as inflammatory arthritides may contribute to the condition.[10] Differential diagnoses include plantar warts, epidermal inclusion cysts, and foreign body reaction.

Clinical Presentation and Evaluation

The evaluation of a patient with IPK should include a thorough history for trauma, penetrating injury, systemic inflammatory arthropathy, and prior foot surgery. On physical examination, the exact location of the callus should be identified with palpation to ascertain if it is directly beneath the metatarsal head. Weight-bearing radiographs with a marker placed over the callus can further delineate the exact location relative to the bony anatomy. In-office débridement of the callus with a scalpel is helpful in identifying the presence of a central keratotic core that would confirm a discrete IPK. Standing radiographs should be carefully evaluated for foreign bodies, previous fractures, and for the presence of an excessively long or short metatarsal.

Nonsurgical Treatment

Nonsurgical treatment of IPKs consists of changes in shoe wear including low heels, metatarsal pads or bars,

and rigid or rocker-bottom soles. Use of a pumice stone after bathing or serial débridements with a blade help to debulk the callus and reduce chronic callus buildup that leads to increasing callus formation.[17] Heel cord stretching for a tight Achilles tendon also may provide symptomatic relief.

Surgical Treatment

When conservative treatment fails, surgical treatment may be necessary. Discrete IPKs caused by a prominent metatarsal head fibular condyle are treated with a plantar condylectomy removing 20% to 30% of the plantar metatarsal head (**Figure 9**). Care should be taken to ensure that the cut is made parallel with the sole of the foot and that the metatarsal shaft itself is not violated.[18]

The entire metatarsal head must be considered when surgically treating diffuse IPKs. If the IPK is believed to represent a transfer lesion from decreased weight bearing on an adjacent metatarsal (specifically the first ray), treating the primary abnormality (for example, bunion correction or repair of a metatarsal fracture malunion) may be prudent. For excessively long or plantar-flexed metatarsals, multiple osteotomy options exist.[19,20] A commonly used procedure is the Weil osteotomy that allows elevation and shortening of the metatarsal, reducing the weight-bearing forces.[21] In some instances, such as the presence of arthritic changes, Freiberg infraction, or with osteoporotic bone, an osteotomy is not the best option and DuVries arthroplasty may be used.[18] In this procedure, the distal 2 to 3 mm of the metatarsal head and plantar condyle are removed and the metatarsal head is reshaped to decompress the joint and allow shortening of the metatarsal (**Figure 10**). The joint may be pinned, especially if concurrent hammer toe correction is necessary. DuVries arthroplasty gener-

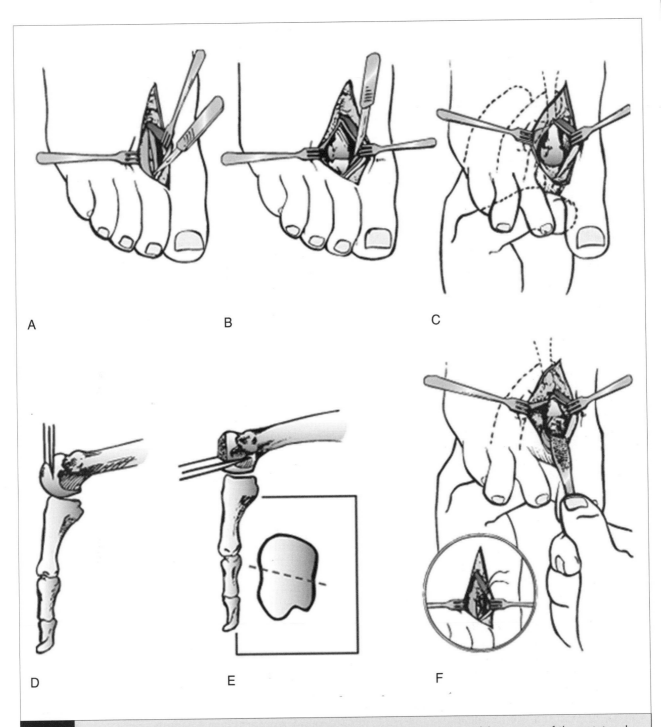

Figure 10   Illustration of DuVries arthroplasty showing the dorsal incision **(A)**, capsulotomy **(B)**, exposure of the metatarsal head through planter flexion of the toe **(C)**, distal metatarsal resection **(D)**, plantar condylectomy **(E)**, and capsular repair **(F)**. *(Reproduced with permission from Mann RA, Mann JA: Keratotic disorders of the plantar skin, in Coughlin MJ, Mann RA, Saltzman CL (eds):* Surgery of the Foot and Ankle. *St. Louis, MO, Mosby, 2007, pp 465-490.)*

ally provides a painless neutral MTP joint with decreased but functional range of motion. With osteotomies or DuVries arthroplasty, care must be taken to avoid overshortening of the metatarsal to prevent the development of a transfer lesion under an adjacent metatarsal.

Freiberg Infraction

Pathoanatomy and Etiology

Osteochondrosis of a lesser metatarsal head typically involves the second metatarsal but may also involve the

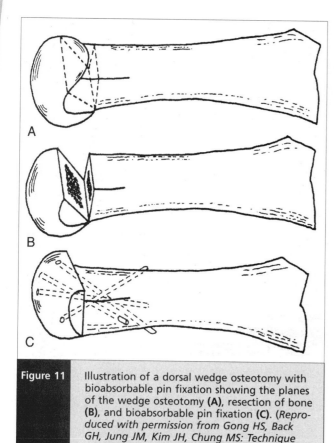

Figure 11 Illustration of a dorsal wedge osteotomy with bioabsorbable pin fixation showing the planes of the wedge osteotomy **(A)**, resection of bone **(B)**, and bioabsorbable pin fixation **(C)**. (*Reproduced with permission from Gong HS, Back GH, Jung JM, Kim JH, Chung MS: Technique tip: Fixation of dorsal wedge osteotomy for Freiberg's disease using bioabsorbable pins. Foot Ankle Int 2003;24:876-877.*)

Nonsurgical Treatment

Early in the disease process, symptoms are treated to provide comfort and minimize the progression of deformity. Protective footwear including metatarsal pads or bars, oral anti-inflammatory medications, toe taping, and occasionally, intra-articular corticosteroid injections, may provide symptomatic improvement. Walking casts with toe extensions, walking boots, or a period of not bearing weight may provide acute relief.[10]

Surgical Treatment

When little or no metatarsal head deformity is present, an MTP joint synovectomy and core decompression of the metatarsal head with 0.045-inch K-wire may be performed; however, there is no evidence in the literature that this treatment provides long-term improvement. In the presence of articular cartilage loss at the dorsal metatarsal head, a dorsiflexion metatarsal neck osteotomy can be performed to rotate the affected portion of the metatarsal head out of the articulation[23,24] (Figure 11). In the end-stage disease process with articular cartilage loss and hypertrophic bone, a joint débridement and exostectomy may provide symptomatic relief. A DuVries-type arthroplasty may be needed if there is complete joint destruction. Maintaining normal metatarsal length is important to prevent the development of transfer lesions.

third or fourth metatarsal heads. This disease most often occurs in adolescent girls or young adult women. Multiple possible etiologies exist including trauma, hypercoagulability, and recent surgery. In this disease, osteonecrosis of the subchondral bone can lead to joint collapse, reactive bony hypertrophy, and degenerative changes.[22]

Clinical Presentation and Evaluation

The patient with Freiberg infraction presents with pain in the forefoot that is exacerbated by activity and weight bearing. Swelling of the MTP joint is often present and may lead to reports of a feeling of fullness under the metatarsal head. Physical examination reveals tenderness and often, fullness at the MTP joint and a limited range of motion, especially late in the disease process. Bony hypertrophy may be palpable and an IPK may be present under the affected metatarsal head. Early in the process, radiographs are normal, making it difficult to discern this disease from other sources of metatarsalgia. When there is clinical suspicion of Freiberg infraction, an MRI or bone scan may help confirm the diagnosis. Later in the process, enlargement and deformity of the metatarsal head may occur with revascularization. Several radiographic classifications exist based on the degree of vascular insult and bone and joint abnormalities.

Congenital Fifth Toe Disorders

Overlapping Fifth Toe

An overlapping fifth toe is a congenital deformity in which the adducted, hyperextended, and externally rotated fifth toe overrides the fourth toe (Figure 12). Although the overall incidence of this deformity is unknown, the condition can be unilateral or bilateral, and equally affects both sexes. Approximately one half of patients with this deformity have symptoms, usually resulting from secondary pressure from shoe wear. Corns can develop over the dorsal aspect of the toe or in the fourth web space. Nonsurgical treatment, consisting of taping, padding, and shoe wear with a wider and deeper toe box, is often unsuccessful. Surgery is often performed to relieve symptoms.

The pathoanatomy of this deformity consists of a contracted dorsomedial capsule, plantar capsular adhesions, a shortened extensor tendon, and a corresponding skin contracture.[25] The extensor tendon may be asymmetric, with a medial band that is thicker than the lateral band.[26]

The choice of surgical treatment depends on the severity of the deformity. For a mild deformity, a soft-tissue release can be performed. The DuVries procedure includes a capsular release and tenotomy of the extensor tendon performed through a longitudinal incision in the web space. The Wilson procedure involves release of the capsule and the extensor tendon, and a V-Y plasty of the skin.[27] The Butler arthroplasty involves re-

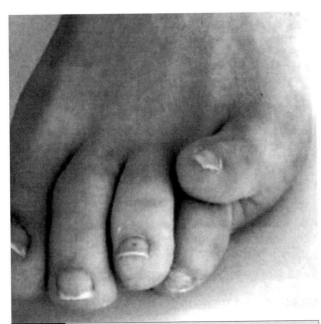

Figure 12   Preoperative appearance of a toe in crossed-over position. (*Reproduced with permission from Thordarson DB: Congenital crossover fifth toe correction with soft tissue release and cutaneous Z-plasty. Foot Ankle Int 2001;22:511-512.*)

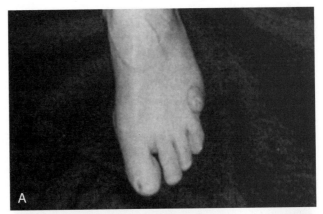

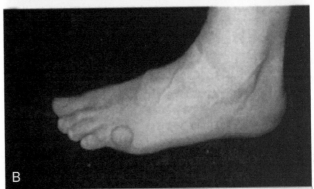

Figure 13   **A,** Dorsal view of the foot of a patient who was dissatisfied with cosmesis after treatment with the Ruiz-Mora procedure. **B,** Lateral view of foot of a patient who was dissatisfied with cosmesis after the Ruiz-Mora procedure. (*Reproduced with permission from Dyal CM, Davis WH, Thompson FM, Bonar SK: Clinical evaluation of the Ruiz-Mora procedure: Long-term follow-up. Foot Ankle Int 1997;18:94-97.*)

lease of the capsule and extensor tendon through a double-racquet incision.[28] The postoperative dressing plays an important role in maintaining the correction in all of these procedures. Although satisfactory results can be achieved, the DuVries and Wilson procedures and Butler arthroplasty are only suitable for patients with mild fifth toe deformities, which are rare.

Several procedures are appropriate to treat more severe deformities. A Lapidus procedure involves proximally transecting the extensor tendon to the fifth toe, then transferring the distal stump under the phalanx of the toe and suturing it to the abductor digiti quinti. A thorough capsular release also is performed.[27] The Ruiz-Mora procedure involves a proximal phalangectomy through a plantar incision. Although this procedure improves function and decreases pain, it can result in a floppy, shortened toe, which many patients find cosmetically unappealing[29] (Figure 13). Syndactylization also can be performed, but is cosmetically unacceptable to most patients.[27] The Ruiz-Mora procedure and syndactylization may be useful when revision surgery is needed. More recently, a soft-tissue release of the capsule with an extensor tendon lengthening and a Z-plasty of the skin have been described. In three patients treated with this procedure, all were satisfied with the surgery and had no recurrence of the deformity[30] (Figure 14).

Biphalangeal Fifth Toe

Another congenital condition is the biphalangeal fifth toe, or the two-boned toe, first described by Leonardo da Vinci in 1492 (Figure 15). Approximately 40% of the

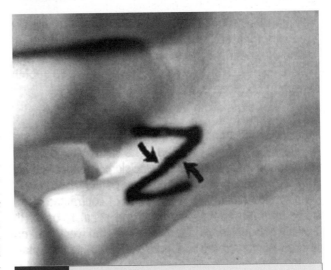

Figure 14   Z-incision with 60° angles drawn. Arrows indicate direction the flaps are transposed to allow lengthening along the longitudinal axis of the Z-plasty. (*Reproduced with permission from Thordarson DB: Congenital crossover fifth toe correction with soft tissue release and cutaneous Z-plasty. Foot Ankle Int 2001;22:511-512.*)

4: The Forefoot

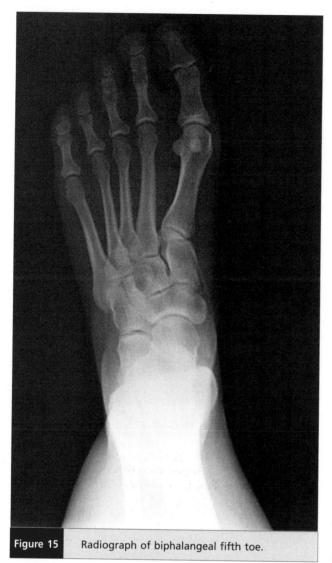

Figure 15   Radiograph of biphalangeal fifth toe.

with compensatory varus deviation of the fifth toe at the MTP joint. With progression of deformity, subluxation of the MTP joint develops in some patients and is associated with laxity of the capsular structures on the lateral side of the joint. When dorsiflexion contractures of the fifth MTP joint occur, stiffness of the joint can contribute to higher pressures under the fifth metatarsal head. Direct pressure from shoes or other structures (such as the floor when sitting with legs crossed) can lead to hypertrophy of the soft tissues overlying the metatarsal head. Less commonly, the clinical appearance of a bunionette is produced by a fifth metatarsal head of unusual size, or outward curving of the distal shaft.

Clinical Presentation and Evaluation

The term bunionette is used to describe the clinical appearance of enlargement of the lateral forefoot directly over the fifth metatarsal head. The apparent enlargement includes the normal metatarsal head, which may be unusually prominent because of lateral deviation of the fifth metatarsal or varus subluxation of the fifth toe, and also thickening of the overlying skin, capsule, and other soft tissues. The association of a bunionette with symptomatic hallux valgus can contribute to the appearance of a splayfoot, with significant widening of the forefoot.

Symptomatic patients often report pain, which is exacerbated by wearing shoes. Patients also may report pain over callosities. Many patients who present with bunionettes are asymptomatic; fewer than one in five require surgical treatment. Bilateral deformity is common with an incidence of more than 45%. The female to male ratio for bunionette deformities is reported to be in the range of 4:1 to 12:1.[33-36] Because the fifth tarsometatarsal joint is the most mobile in the midfoot, patients can more easily tolerate this deformity.

Radiographic Examination

Standard weight-bearing AP and lateral radiographs of the foot are used to evaluate the bunionette. The IMA_{4-5} and the fifth MTP (MTP-5) angle are the most valuable radiographic measurements (**Figure 16**). The average normal IMA_{4-5} is 9.1°.[33] In comparison, patients with a bunionette have an average IMA_{4-5} of 10.7°. Asymptomatic patients with a bunionette often have an average IMA_{4-5} of 9.9°, which is larger than the average normal IMA_{4-5} but is typically smaller than the IMA_{4-5} in patients with symptomatic deformities. The average normal MTP-5 angle is 10.2°, compared with 16.6° in patients with bunionettes. Lateral bowing of the fifth metatarsal and widening of the metatarsal head have not been supported as causes of bunionette deformity when radiographs are carefully evaluated.[33] Similar to the correlations seen in hallux valgus, increasing $IMAs_{4-5}$ are associated with an increase in the MTP-5 angle. Successful surgical procedures reduce the IMA_{4-5} and also reduce the MTP-5 angle. Reduction of the width of the forefoot also is an important goal of surgical correction.

European population has a two-boned toe; in the Japanese population the incidence is approximately 75%. Biphalangeal fifth toe is believed to result from an anatomic variant, with failure of segmentation of the distal interphalangeal joint. It is usually bilateral and is rare in other toes. In two studies, patients undergoing surgery for a symptomatic hammer or claw toe deformity of the fifth toe had a higher prevalence of biphalangealism than that found in a control population. It was hypothesized that the stiffness of a biphalangeal toe may make it less able to adapt to shoe wear.[31,32] There was no significant difference in the prevalence of this condition in patients with bunionette or crossover toe deformities when compared with the control group.[32]

Bunionette Deformities

Pathoanatomy

The anatomic basis for bunionette deformity is widening of the fourth-fifth intermetatarsal angle (IMA_{4-5})

Classification

Bunionettes may be classified into four types.[37] Type I bunionettes have enlargement of the metatarsal head. Type II bunionettes demonstrate lateral bowing with deviation of the metatarsal bone in the distal half of the shaft. Type III is characterized by a widened IMA_{4-5}, and type IV combine two or more characteristics found in type I, II, or III bunionettes. Type III bunionettes are the most common, occurring more often than types I and II combined. Type IV bunionettes are seen in patients with rheumatoid arthritis. The loss of normal mobility of the tarsometatarsal joint can significantly impact nonsurgical treatment and surgical choices.

Nonsurgical Treatment

An ill-fitting shoe is the most common cause of pain with a bunionette deformity. Recommendations for nonsurgical treatment are based on the area of maximal pain and the presence or absence of calluses. Shoes with upper portions fabricated from soft materials and without seams over the area of the deformity are recommended. Selective stretching of the upper portion of the shoe over the prominence can be performed by either the patient or a pedorthist using a ball and ring stretcher. Calluses should be trimmed. If an intractable plantar keratosis is present, a small metatarsal pad can be placed on the insole of the shoe proximal to the plantar keratosis to decrease pressure under the metatarsal head. If a callosity occurs in a direct lateral position in a patient with neuropathy, ulceration may occur. Pads or dressings placed over the metatarsal head can increase the pressure over the bony prominence, worsening the ulcer. To completely relieve pressure over the ulcerated prominence, the upper portion of the shoe leather should be cut or the patient should wear a pressure-relieving sandal until healing occurs.

Surgical Treatment

The goals of surgical treatment include alleviation of pain, maintenance or improvement in activity level, and improved choices in shoe wear. Objective measurement of forefoot width and fifth toe position should improve. The choice of surgical procedure must take into account other deformities or abnormalities in the foot, such as hallux valgus, Morton neuroma, and hammer toes. Bunionette corrections are often performed concurrently with other forefoot procedures; however, aggressive procedures such as metatarsal head resections are not recommended.[38] Long-term follow-up after metatarsal head resections show inconsistent results with failures resulting from transfer metatarsalgia, persistent lateral forefoot prominence, and painful deformity of the fifth toe. Shortening of the fifth toe usually occurs and can be as much as 1 cm.

Simple lateral eminence resection typically will not provide adequate correction for patients with symptoms that require surgery. In the few patients treated with simple resection, care must be taken not to resect too much bone and create an unstable joint. In most patients, the choice of procedure will involve performing an osteotomy at the appropriate level of the fifth metatarsal. Osteotomies at the diaphysis or base of the fifth metatarsal can provide larger corrections than distal osteotomies. Most procedures include repair of the MTP joint capsule, with tightening whenever possible. Release of the medial joint capsule is not necessary. Some procedures spare the lateral eminence from resection, although the lateral eminence resection is usually integral to the procedure to increase the amount of narrowing of the forefoot.

Various distal osteotomies have been described, all achieving reasonable outcomes. Despite the proximity of these osteotomies to the joint, no discernible reduction in joint motion or function has been reported. The chevron osteotomy reduces the IMA_{4-5} by an average of 2.6°, decreases the forefoot width approximately 3.0 mm, and reduces the MTP-5 angle an average of 7.9°.[34,39] Internal fixation with a Kirschner wire is used if the surgeon deems the osteotomy unstable. Other distal osteotomy techniques include a transverse medial slide, an oblique osteotomy without internal fixation, and subcutaneous subcapital partial osteotomy with osteoclasis and translation.[35,40,41]

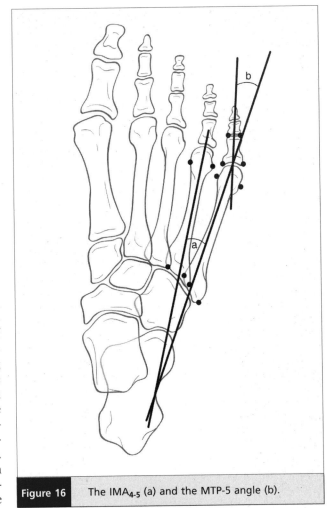

Figure 16   The IMA_{4-5} (a) and the MTP-5 angle (b).

4: The Forefoot

In some patients, an osteotomy within the diaphysis is indicated if the metatarsal head requires dorsomedial translation.[37] The plane of the osteotomy can be altered to change the direction of rotation from directly medial-to-lateral to slightly plantar-to-dorsal. This alteration allows unloading of the metatarsal when an intractable plantar keratosis is present and is indicated in type II or III bunionettes with keratoses. Internal fixation is obtained with a screw.

Proximal osteotomies should be reserved for severe deformities or for failed distal osteotomies.[42] The complication rates (especially nonunion rates) are higher with these procedures and optimal results require internal fixation. The chevron osteotomy has been performed proximally with improvement in all objective measures.[43,44] Another option is a dome-shaped osteotomy technique using a crescentic blade with the cut at the most proximal extent of the diaphysis.[45] Placement of the basilar osteotomy too proximally will increase the rate of nonunion, even with internal fixation.

Nonsurgical management of bunionette deformity is preferred; however, conservative treatment is unsuccessful in approximately 20% of patients. In the symptomatic patient requiring surgical correction, simple lateral eminence resection is usually not adequate and metatarsal head resection is not recommended. The best results are obtained with an osteotomy performed at the appropriate level with stable fixation. The goals of surgical correction are pain relief, improved function, and narrowing of the forefoot. Care should be taken during any procedure to maintain stability of the fifth MTP joint and to provide large and stable bony surfaces to promote high rates of union.

Summary

Lesser toe deformities may be caused by trauma, inflammatory conditions, neurologic disorders, ill-fitting shoe wear, or may have a congenital origin. Lesser toe deformities are usually symptomatic and require nonsurgical management or surgical treatment that may include both bony and soft-tissue procedures. Treatment goals include relieving pain, improving function, and providing patients with the ability to use a wider range of acceptable footwear.

Annotated References

1. Coughlin MJ: Lesser toe abnormalities. *Instr Course Lect* 2003;52:421-444.

   The author provides a review of lesser toe abnormalities including etiology, diagnosis, and treatment.

2. Marks RM: Anatomy and pathophysiology of lesser toe deformities. *Foot Ankle Clin* 1998;3:199-214.

3. Femino JE, Mueller K: Complications of lesser toe surgery. *Clin Orthop Relat Res* 2001;391:72-78.

4. Murphy GA: Mallet toe deformity. *Foot Ankle Clin* 1998;3:279-292.

5. Coughlin MJ: Operative repair of the mallet toe deformity. *Foot Ankle Int* 1995;16:109-116.

6. Padanilam TG: The flexible hammer toe: Flexor-to-extensor transfer. *Foot Ankle Clin* 1998;3:259-268.

7. Coughlin MJ, Dorris J, Polk E: Operative repair of the fixed hammertoe deformity. *Foot Ankle Int* 2000;21:94-104.

8. O'Kane C, Kilmartin T: Review of proximal interphalangeal joint excisional arthroplasty for the correction of second hammer toe deformity in 100 cases. *Foot Ankle Int* 2005;26:320-325.

   PIP resection arthroplasty was used to treat 75 patients with 100 second hammer toe deformities. Results were reviewed at an average follow-up of 44 months. AOFAS scores improved and a high level of patient satisfaction was noted. Floating toe was reported in 18 patients (8 of whom had concurrent metatarsal osteotomies), but none were painful.

9. Dhukaram V, Hossain S, Sampath J, Barrie JL: Correction of hammer toe with an extended release of the metatarsophalangeal joint. *J Bone Joint Surg Br* 2002;84:986-990.

10. Mizel MS, Yodlowski ML: Disorders of the lesser metatarsophalangeal joints. *J Am Acad Orthop Surg* 1995;3:166-173.

11. Kaz AJ, Coughlin MJ: Crossover second toe: Demographics, etiology, and radiographic assessment. *Foot Ankle Int* 2007;28:1223-1237.

    The surgical treatment for crossover second toe was retrospectively reviewed in 169 patients. An increased incidence of both hallux valgus and first MTP joint degenerative arthritis was reported in the cohort. A positive drawer sign was a reliable and consistent examination finding. The most reliable radiographic indicator was medial angular deviation of the second MTP joint.

12. Mizel MS, Michelson JD: Nonsurgical treatment of monarticular nontraumatic synovitis of the second metatarsophalangeal joint. *Foot Ankle Int* 1997;18:424-426.

13. Weinfeld SB: Evaluation and management of crossover second toe deformity. *Foot Ankle Clin* 1998;3:215-228.

14. Haddad SL, Sabbagh RC, Resch S, Myerson B, Myerson MS: Results of flexor-to-extensor and extensor digitorum brevis tendon transfer for correction of the crossover second toe deformity. *Foot Ankle Int* 1999;20:781-788.

15. Myerson MS, Jung HG: The role of toe flexor-to-extensor transfer in correcting metatarsophalangeal joint instability of the second toe. *Foot Ankle Int* 2005;26:675-679.

Fifty-nine patients (64 feet) underwent an FDL transfer as the primary procedure for second MTP joint instability. Secondary procedures were commonly used including Weil osteotomies in 29 feet (45%). Although second toe function improved in most patients, a significant number of patients were dissatisfied with the results because of stiffness.

16. Gallentine JW, DeOrio JK: Removal of the second toe for severe hammertoe deformity in elderly patients. *Foot Ankle Int* 2005;26:353-358.

Twelve patients underwent amputation through the second MTP joint for treatment of severe hammer toe deformity. The authors reported that 10 patients were satisfied with the procedure and 2 were satisfied with reservations. Eleven patients believed that the procedure met their expectations and would recommend it. No significant complications were reported.

17. Mann RA: Intractable plantar keratosis. *Instr Course Lect* 1984;33:287-301.

18. Mann RA, Mann JA: Keratotic disorders of the plantar skin, in Coughlin MJ, Mann RA, Saltzman CL (eds): *Surgery of the Foot and Ankle*, ed 8. Philadelphia, PA, Mosby Elsevier, 2007, pp 465-490.

19. Kitaoka HB, Patzer GL: Chevron osteotomy of the lesser metatarsals for intractable plantar callosities. *J Bone Joint Surg Br* 1998;80:516-518.

20. Idusuyi OB, Kitaoka HB, Patzer GL: Oblique metatarsal osteotomy for intractable plantar keratosis: 10-year follow-up. *Foot Ankle Int* 1998;19:351-355.

21. Vandeputte G, Dereymaeker G, Steenwerckx A, Peeraer L: The Weil osteotomy of the lesser metatarsals: A clinical and pedobarographic follow-up study. *Foot Ankle Int* 2000;21:370-374.

22. Katcherian DA: Treatment of Freiberg's disease. *Orthop Clin North Am* 1994;25:69-81.

23. Chao KH, Lee CH, Lin LC: Surgery for symptomatic Freiberg's disease: Extraarticular dorsal closing-wedge osteotomy in 13 patients followed for 2-4 years. *Acta Orthop Scand* 1999;70:483-486.

24. Lee SK, Chung MS, Baek GH, Oh JH, Lee YH, Gong HS: Treatment of Freiberg disease with intra-articular dorsal wedge osteotomy and absorbable pin fixation. *Foot Ankle Int* 2007;28:43-48.

Twelve patients with symptomatic Freiberg disease were treated with intra-articular dorsal closing wedge osteotomies fixed with polyglycolide pins. All osteotomies healed at an average of 10 weeks. All patients demonstrated decreased pain, increased range of motion, and high satisfaction with the procedure.

25. DeGnore L: The congenital, overlapping fifth toe. *Foot Ankle Clin* 1998;3:313-319.

26. O'Neal ML, Ganey TM, Ogden JA: Asymmetric bifur-cation of the extensor digitorum longus tendon in a case of congenital digitus minimus varus. *Foot Ankle Int* 1994;15:505-507.

27. Coughlin MJ: Lesser toe deformities, in Coughlin MJ, Mann RA, Saltzman CL (eds): *Surgery of the Foot and Ankle*, ed 8. Philadelphia, PA, Mosby Elsevier, 2007, pp 363-464.

The author provides an excellent, comprehensive review of lesser toe deformities.

28. De Boeck H: Butler's operation for congenital overriding of the fifth toe: Retrospective 1- 7-year study of 23 cases. *Acta Orthop Scand* 1993;64:343-344.

29. Dyal CM, Davis WH, Thompson FM, Bonar SK: Clinical evaluation of the Ruiz-Mora procedure: Long-term follow-up. *Foot Ankle Int* 1997;18:94-97.

30. Thordarson DB: Congenital crossover fifth toe correction with soft tissue release and cutaneous Z-plasty. *Foot Ankle Int* 2001;22:511-512.

31. Thompson FM, Chang VK: The two-boned fifth toe: Clinical implications. *Foot Ankle Int* 1995;16:34-36.

32. Dereymaeker G, van der Broek C: Biphalangeal fifth toe. *Foot Ankle Int* 2006;27:948-951.

The authors of this study investigate the prevalence of a biphalangeal fifth toe in patients undergoing surgery for symptomatic hammer or claw fifth toe deformity, bunionette, or crossover deformity compared with a control group.

33. Nestor BJ, Kitaoka HB, Ilstrup DM, Berquist TH, Bergmann AD: Radiologic anatomy of the painful bunionette. *Foot Ankle* 1990;11:6-11.

34. Moran MM, Claridge RJ: Chevron osteotomy for bunionette. *Foot Ankle Int* 1994;15:684-688.

35. Zvijac JE, Janecki CJ, Freeling RM: Distal oblique osteotomy for Tailor's bunion. *Foot Ankle* 1991;12:171-175.

36. Koti M, Maffulli N: Bunionette. *J Bone Joint Surg Am* 2001;83:1076-1082.

37. Coughlin MJ: Treatment of bunionette deformity with longitudinal diaphyseal osteotomy with distal soft tissue repair. *Foot Ankle* 1991;11:195-203.

38. Kitaoka HB, Holiday AD: Metatarsal head resection for bunionette: Long-term follow-up. *Foot Ankle* 1991;11:345-349.

39. Kitaoka HB, Holiday AD, Campbell DC: Distal Chevron metatarsal osteotomy for bunionette. *Foot Ankle* 1991;12:80-84.

40. Weitzel S, Trinka H, Petroutsas J: Transverse medial slide osteotomy for bunionette deformity: Long-term re-

sults. *Foot Ankle Int* 2007;28:794-798.

The authors present the results of 30 patients (44 feet) treated for bunionette deformity using a transverse osteotomy technique buttressed by a longitudinal 1.6-mm Kirschner wire. Follow-up averaged 7 years and 8 months. No shortening was noted, narrowing of the forefoot averaged 5 mm, and the lateral eminence was left intact.

41. Legenstein R, Bonomo J, Huber W, Boesch P: Correction of Tailor's bunion with the Boesch technique: A retrospective study. *Foot Ankle Int* 2007;28:799-803.

   The authors evaluated 77 feet with a tailor bunion treated with a subcutaneous technique using a burr to partially cut the metatarsal neck. Osteoclasis is performed and the metatarsal head is shifted medially and held by a 1.6-mm Kirschner wire driven up the metatarsal shaft. The procedure is done under local anesthesia without a tourniquet.

42. Cohen BE, Nicholson CW: Bunionette deformity. *J Am Acad Orthop Surg* 2007;15:300-307.

   The authors present a literature review, including information on etiology and surgical and nonsurgical management of bunionette deformity.

43. Diebold PF: Basal osteotomy of the fifth metatarsal for the bunionette. *Foot Ankle* 1991;12:74-79.

44. Diebold PF, Bejjani FJ: Basal osteotomy of the fifth metatarsal with the intermetatarsal pinning: A new approach to tailor's bunion. *Foot Ankle* 1987;8:40-45.

45. Okuda R, Kinoshita M: Proximal dome-shaped osteotomy for symptomatic bunionette. *Clin Orthop Relat Res* 2002;396:173-178.

Neuromuscular Disease

SECTION EDITOR:

GREGORY C. BERLET, MD

Chapter 22
The Diabetic Foot

Terrence M. Philbin, DO

Introduction

Diabetes mellitus was first described in Greece in the fifth century BC. In 1922, the discovery of insulin helped to change the course of this chronic disease.[1] The evaluation and treatment of diabetic patients with foot disorders continues to present a substantial challenge to the orthopaedic surgeon.

Diabetes mellitus is a multisystem disease that often progresses in an unpredictable manner. Over the years, the diabetic patient will be at risk for ulcerations, infections, deformities, neuroarthropathy, and amputation. Education is paramount in preventing the sequelae of the disease. Control of comorbid disease is essential and will profoundly impact the success of orthopaedic care. A team approach, including an orthopaedic surgeon, physical therapist, endocrinologist, infectious disease specialist, vascular surgeon, plastic surgeon, orthotist, and pedorthist, is important to increase the rate of successful outcomes. Studies have proven the effectiveness of the team approach in caring for patients with diabetes-related foot disorders.[2-4]

Epidemiology

The American Diabetes Association estimates that 7% of the US population or 20.8 million people have diabetes, and approximately 6.2 million of these people are undiagnosed.[5] Fifteen percent of the population older than 65 years is affected. There were 224,092 deaths attributed to diabetes in 2002. Diabetes has an enormous economic impact on the US health care system; the estimated cost of diabetes annually (direct and indirect) is $132 billion or 1 of every 10 health care dollars.[5]

Foot complications are the most common diagnoses in diabetic patients admitted to hospitals.[6] The severity of the diabetes does not always correlate with the severity of the complications. Most complications occur in patients with type II diabetes, which is the most prevalent disease type. The annual incidence of foot ulcers in patients with diabetes in the United States is 5.6%, with a lifetime incidence of 15% to 25%.[7]

Approximately 82,000 amputations are performed annually in patients with diabetes.[5] The incidence of amputations in diabetic patients is 10 times the incidence in the nondiabetic population. Men with diabetes are 1.4 to 2.7 times more likely to need an amputation than are women with diabetes. The likelihood of a lower extremity amputation is increased 1.8-fold in Mexican Americans, 2.7-fold in African Americans, and threefold for Native Americans compared with whites. Patient education remains one of the most important tools in preventing diabetic amputations.[5]

Pathophysiology of Diabetes Mellitus

Neuropathy is one of the most common comorbidities associated with diabetes mellitus.[8] Diabetic patients with neuropathy have an increased risk of ulceration, amputation, and death.[9] Neuropathic diabetic patients perform worse on functional tests such as walking speed, static and dynamic balance, and coordination. The duration of diabetes strongly affects the occurrence of neuropathy. An 8% prevalence of neuropathy at the time of diabetes diagnosis and the development of neuropathy in 50% of patients within 25 years of diagnosis has been reported in the literature.[10] Patients with diabetic neuropathy can present with symptoms of pain, burning, allodynia, and weakness, which often progress to loss of sensation. Hyperglycemia alone cannot account for the pathogenesis of neuropathy; it likely results from a combination of metabolic and vascular factors[11] (Figure 1). The risk for neuropathy is associated with age, poor control of hyperglycemia, and height.[11]

Sensory neuropathy affects approximately 75% of patients with diabetes. Sensory deficits usually appear first in the distal aspect of the lower extremities and progress proximally in a stockinglike pattern.[12,13] The loss of large sensory fibers leads to decreased awareness of light touch and diminished proprioception, whereas loss of the small fibers decreases pain and temperature perception. Over time, patients may lose deep tendon reflexes and vibratory sense. Patients who have the triad of neuropathy, foot deformity, and repetitive trauma are at high risk for ulcer formation.[14]

Motor neuropathy occurs commonly in combination with sensory and autonomic deficits.[15] The intrinsic muscles of the foot become weak, leading to contracture of the digits, secondary metatarsophalangeal instability, and the development of hammer and claw toes. The development of claw toe deformities creates areas

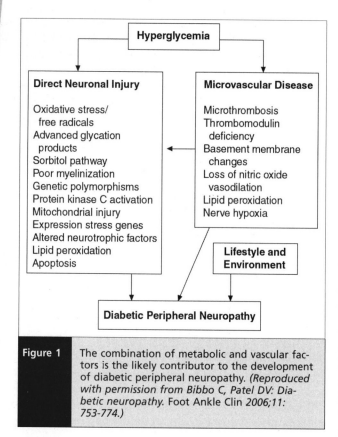

Figure 1 The combination of metabolic and vascular factors is the likely contributor to the development of diabetic peripheral neuropathy. (*Reproduced with permission from Bibbo C, Patel DV: Diabetic neuropathy. Foot Ankle Clin 2006;11: 753-774.*)

of increased pressure at the dorsal aspect of the toe and the plantar aspect of the metatarsal head. Subsequently, this pressure can lead to skin breakdown in as little as 1 hour. Many authors have reported on the effects of motor neuropathy on the Achilles tendon leading to contracture.[16] Increasing evidence suggests that an equinus contracture can lead to increased forefoot pressures and subsequent skin breakdown. Several reports have shown that the treatment of forefoot ulcers with Achilles tendon lengthening reduced the healing time and decreased the rate of recurrent ulceration.[17-19] The authors of one study suggested that equinus of the Achilles tendon plays only a limited role in producing high forefoot pressures and recommended caution in performing tendon-lengthening procedures to decrease peak forefoot plantar pressures in diabetic patients.[20]

Autonomic neuropathy occurs in 20% to 40% of diabetic patients.[12] Deficits of the autonomic system lead to loss of control of the sweat glands in the extremity, blood vessel tone, thermoregulation, and the normal hyperemic response necessary to fight infection. The skin becomes dry and scaly and cracks develop, which enable bacteria to invade and cause infections.

Many diabetic patients have decreased sensation in the lower extremities along with hypersensitivity or painful neuropathy. Painful neuropathy manifests as burning and searing pain that is worse in the evening, commonly bilateral, and symmetric. Treatment can include oral medications such as amitriptyline, carbamazepine, phenytoin, imipramine, nortriptyline, mexile-

tine, and pregabalin.[21-24] In a recent, randomized, double-blind, placebo-controlled study, pregabalin produced significant pain relief within 1 week of administration.[25] Evolving evidence suggests a limited role for nerve decompression in the presence of painful peripheral neuropathy.[26]

Patient Evaluation

Physical Examination
Orthopaedic examination of patients with diabetic foot disorders should include a thorough examination of both lower extremities up to the knee. Gait should be assessed for any deformities, bony prominences, and gross changes in the shape of the foot. A complete examination of the foot includes an evaluation of the skin, hair, vascular status, and protective sensation. Ulcerations should be measured and traced to establish an objective baseline. Shoe wear should be examined for blood or other drainage, abnormal wear, foreign objects, and overall foot protection. Current recommendations advise diabetic patients to have one foot examination annually, with more frequent examinations for high-risk patients.[27] Patients also should examine their feet three to four times daily. Designated risk categories are assigned to patients based on ulceration history, deformity, previous amputation, absence of pulses, and lack of sensation. Risk factors are assigned a value from 0 to 3 based on the possibility of foot complications[28] (Table 1). Patients with a low risk of complications (category 0) should be instructed on basic foot care, have an annual examination, and can use regular footwear. Patients with the highest risk (category 3) require custom, pressure-dissipating, accommodative orthoses; soft leather shoe wear; adjustable-lacing shoes; follow-up evaluations every 2 months; and an evaluation by an orthopaedic foot and ankle specialist.

Sensation from a Semmes-Weinstein 5.07-g monofilament is the accepted threshold for assessing adequate protective sensation to prevent ulcerations. A 4.5-g monofilament indicates protective sensation in diabetic patients.[29] A recent study found performance differences in monofilaments made by four manufacturers.[30] A new 10-g monofilament was tested using a calibrated load cell to determine the maximum buckling force and longevity. Although the Semmes-Weinstein monofilaments are the least expensive and most commonly used technique for assessing sensory neuropathy, the Neuropen monofilament (Owen Mumford; Woodstock, England) and the Bailey Instruments monofilament (Manchester, England) were more accurate, with 100% buckling within ±1.0 g of 10 g. Only 70% of the Semmes-Weinstein monofilaments buckled within that range. The authors of the study recommend the use of Bailey Instruments or Owen Mumford monofilaments, both of which proved superior in terms of longevity of use.[30]

Table 1

Risk Categories for Foot Complications

Category	Risk Factors	Treatment Recommendations
0	No history of ulceration No deformity No previous amputation Pedal pulses present No sensory loss	Instruct in basic foot care Yearly foot examination Regular footwear
1	No history of ulceration No deformity No previous amputation Pedal pulses present Sensory loss	Daily foot self-examination Diabetic foot patient education Depth shoes or running shoes Nonmolded, soft inlays Possible total contact orthoses Foot examination by physician every 6 months
2	No history of ulceration Moderate (prelesion) deformity (for example, hallux rigidus, metatarsal head prominence, claw or hammer toes, callus, plantar bony prominence, hallux valgus, or dorsal exostosis) Pedal pulses present Single lesser ray amputation Sensory loss	Daily foot self-examination Diabetic foot patient education Depth shoes or running shoes Custom-molded foot orthoses Adjuncts: silicon toe sleeves, lamb's wool, foam toe separators, hammer toe crests, or metatarsal pad External shoe modifications: metatarsal bar, rocker sole, extended steel shank, or medial or lateral heel wedges Foot examination by physician every 4 months
3	History of ulceration Presence of deformity (for example, Charcot, hallux rigidus, metatarsal head prominence, claw or hammer toes, callus, plantar bony prominence, hallux valgus, or dorsal exostosis) Previous amputation (multiple ray, first ray, transmetatarsal, or Chopart) Pedal pulses present or absent Sensory loss	Daily foot self-examination Patient-at-risk diabetic foot education Custom fabricated, pressure-dissipating, accommodative foot orthoses Inlay-depth, soft-leather, adjustable-lacing shoes External shoe modifications (rocker soles, extended steel shanks, solid ankle cushion heels, well filled with low-density materials) Off-loading orthoses (patellar tendon bearing brace, ankle-foot orthoses) Foot examination by physician every 2 months Immediate clinical evaluation of any new skin or nail problems Consider evaluation by orthopaedic foot and ankle surgeon

Vascular Evaluation

Vascular disease is approximately 30 times more common in diabetic patients compared with the general population. A comprehensive vascular examination should assess the dorsal pedis and posterior tibial pulses, capillary filling time, and the quality of the skin. Thin, shiny, atrophic, and hairless skin is indicative of diminished vascularity. The main goal of the vascular examination is to determine the ability of the patient to achieve primary healing.[31]

Patients lacking palpable pulses and with nonhealing wounds require additional vascular screening. The most frequently used technique is arterial Doppler ultrasound pressure measurement. The method is reproducible and is not highly operator dependent. Data are collected as both absolute pressures (as detected by an ultrasonic probe) and the ratio of ankle pressure to arm Doppler arterial pressure. A ratio of 0.45 or greater is necessary for favorable healing in diabetic patients.[32,33]

Waveform examination is recommended because calcification of the lower extremity can lead to falsely increased readings. Toe pressures greater than 40 mm Hg indicate adequate inflow to support wound healing. A monophasic waveform indicates the presence of a calcified vessel, whereas a triphasic waveform indicates a more normal vessel. Absolute toe pressures were found to be a more reliable indicator of healing than the ankle-brachial index.[34]

Transcutaneous oxygen readings of more than 30 mm Hg also indicate adequate healing potential. One advantage of this technique compared with Doppler examination is that the measurement does not produce false readings with calcified vessels. To date, no vascular screening tool is 100% accurate at assessing the perfusion of the lower extremity. Patients with significant vascular insufficiency may require arteriography for assessing the severity and level of occlusion. A consultation with a vascular surgeon is necessary to determine possible options for revascularization, including percutaneous transluminal angioplasty or vascular bypass.

Imaging

Radiographic evaluation of the diabetic foot and ankle with three-view, weight-bearing (when possible) radiographs are important in the initial patient evaluation. Often one of the most challenging aspects of treating this patient population is distinguishing between a deep infection and Charcot arthropathy. Labeled white blood cell scans (usually indium 111-labeled leukocytes) have a great specificity for deep infection and osteomyelitis. The combination of technetium Tc 99m and a white blood cell scan is useful in differentiating osteomyelitis from Charcot arthropathy.[35-38] Some of the limitations to a white blood cell scan include higher cost, the time needed to perform the scan, and a possible lack of anatomic resolution. Recently, ^{99m}Tc-ciprofloxacin scanning proved to be a specific and sensitive marker for diagnosing osteomyelitis in diabetic patients; however, care must be taken in situations involving fastidious organisms and ciprofloxacin-resistant bacterial flora.[39]

MRI is most often used for diagnosing diabetic infections, abscesses, and osteomyelitis. MRI scans provide superior anatomic detail and spatial resolution, allowing interpretation of the extent of bone and soft-tissue infection, especially on T1-weighted images (overdiagnosis is possible using T2-weighted images). Ring positron emission tomography (PET) has advantages over MRI because it can be used when patients have metallic implants and is more effective at differentiating bone infection and Charcot arthropathy.[40] Currently, there is no imaging study that is 100% effective in definitively diagnosing diabetic infections and Charcot arthropathy. Occasionally, a bone biopsy may be necessary to rule out osteomyelitis.

Ulceration and Infection

Independent factors related to increasing the risk of a new foot ulcer include a previous history of ulceration, an abnormal Neuropathy Disability Score, prior treatment of the foot, inability to perceive sensation from a 10-g monofilament, diminished pulses, pedal deformities, abnormal reflexes, and advanced patient age.[41] In a 2006 study of the quality of life of adults with unhealed and healed diabetic ulcers, the author found that patient anxiety and frustration about unhealed ulcers resulted in a negative impact on well-being scores.[42]

The classic diabetic foot infection usually begins with a loss of skin integrity and the development of diabetic foot ulceration. Causes of diabetic foot ulcerations are multifactorial and are associated with neuropathy, insulin usage, foot deformity, increased body weight, decreased vascularity, and poor vision. Other factors include impaired leukocyte function, poor glu-

cose regulation, malnutrition, and the use of immunosuppressive drugs and/or tobacco. Compared with the nondiabetic population, diabetic patients have an 80% increased risk for cellulitis, a fourfold increased risk of osteomyelitis, and a twofold increased risk of both sepsis and death resulting from infection.[43] The depth of the ulcer, vascularity, and the presence of severe infection must be determined to achieve a successful outcome in patients with diabetic ulcerations. The three most common reasons that a diabetic ulcer does not heal are decreased vascular supply, deep infection, and failure to unload the affected area.

Wound and Vascular Classification

The initial step in treating a diabetic foot ulceration is to classify the wound[44] (**Figures 2 and 3**) and (**Table 2**). The evaluation begins with a visual inspection of the ulcer to document the size, location, margins, and depth (if the bone can be probed, there is a high probability of osteomyelitis and a grade 3 lesion). The physician should examine the foot for any exposed tendon, drainage, and any signs of deep infection. Most grade 0 and grade 1 lesions can be treated on an outpatient basis, whereas lesions graded 2 and above require inpatient care. The vascular supply to the lower extremity is then assessed. Based on the results of vascular studies performed on ischemic patients, the physician can determine the likelihood of wound healing and successful infection treatment, and if amputation will be needed. Consultation with a vascular surgeon may be necessary to determine if revascularization is an option.

Laboratory Evaluation

Laboratory studies should include a white blood cell count with differential, albumin, and prealbumin. Leukocytosis can occur in fewer than 50% of diabetic patients with infections.[45,46] Erythrocyte sedimentation rate and C-reactive protein levels should be obtained; elevated levels indicate a sensitivity for bone infection, but the specificity is debatable.

Débridement

Most diabetic ulcers without deep infection require serial débridement for successful healing. Removing all of the necrotic tissue and callus formation is paramount in converting a chronic wound to an acute wound or a grade 1 lesion. Currently, there is no wound-healing agent or topical dressing system that can replace proper débridement. Healing can be increased by converting circular wounds into elliptical wounds. After the initial débridement, further débridement should occur weekly or biweekly until healing is complete.

Pressure Off-Loading

Total contact casting remains the gold standard and most commonly used form of off-loading pressure from a diabetic plantar ulceration. In a 2006 study, the mechanism of plantar off-loading in a total contact cast resulted primarily from the transfer of the load to the leg

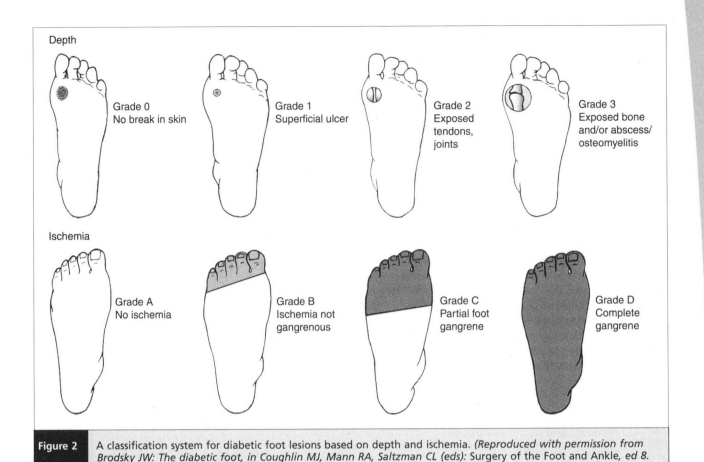

Figure 2 A classification system for diabetic foot lesions based on depth and ischemia. *(Reproduced with permission from Brodsky JW: The diabetic foot, in Coughlin MJ, Mann RA, Saltzman CL (eds): Surgery of the Foot and Ankle, ed 8. Philadelphia, PA, Mosby, 2007, vol 2, pp 1281-1368.)*

portion of the cast rather than from molding of the plantar surface.[47] Another study reported that moderate, early weight bearing in a total contact cast slows healing minimally and that allowing immediate ambulation in a total contact cast may make treatment more acceptable to patients.[48] A prospective, randomized study comparing a total contact cast, a half-shoe, and a removable cast walker for the treatment of 63 diabetic foot ulcers reported an 89.5%, 65%, and 58.3% healing rate, respectively.[49] The time to healing of the ulcers was statistically shorter in patients using a total contact cast.

However, the use of a total contact cast can result in complications. The authors of one study reported a 17% rate of complications, including skin irritation and a cast that was too tight.[50] It was concluded that serious complications can be minimized with good casting technique, close follow-up, and patient education. In a 2003 study, total contact casting was found to be a successful tool in healing diabetic foot ulcers; however, there was a high ulcer recurrence rate.[51] Routine, outpatient follow-up and custom-made footwear to decrease recurrence rates was recommended. Another study reported that an initial total contact cast had an 85% healing rate in patients with diabetic ulcers, but a recurrence rate of 57%.[52] In that study, patients treated with surgical corrections after primary healing became ulcer free.

Removable cast walkers have proven to be as effective as total contact casts in reducing pressure to the plantar aspect of the foot. Off-the-shelf diabetic walker boots performed as well as fiberglass total contact casts in decreasing pressures on the plantar aspect of the foot.[53] Similar results were reported when comparing an off-the-shelf instant contact casting device to a fiberglass cast.[54] In a prospective, randomized, controlled trial, an irremovable cast walker boot (wrapped in fiberglass) was compared with a standard total contact cast in the treatment of diabetic plantar ulcers.[55] The irremovable cast walker boot achieved equal ulcer healing, was faster to don, and was less costly than the total contact cast.

Microbiology

Diabetic foot infections are often polymicrobial. In a review of 825 infected diabetic foot ulcers, 75% of the wounds had multiple bacteria, with an average of 2.4 organisms per wound.[56] Gram-positive aerobic bacteria were the most prevalent (68%), followed by gram-negative aerobes (24%); anaerobes (6%) and fungal species (3%) were less common. In another study, evaluation of superficial wound cultures identified the deep tissue organism in 75% of patients and the osseous organisms in only 30%.[57] The most dependable method of obtaining cultures and biopsy material is

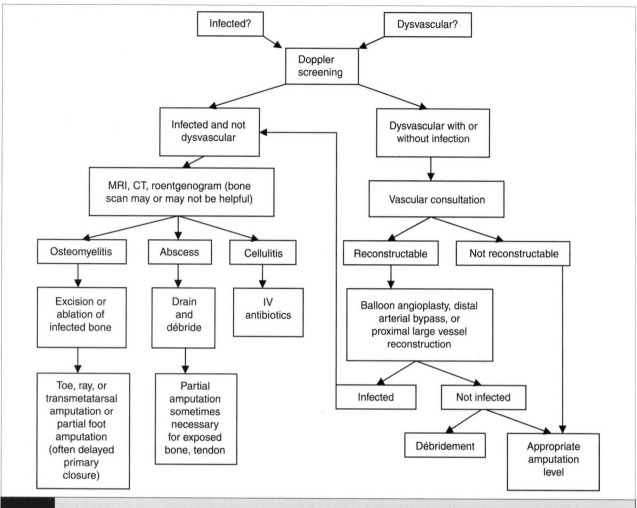

Figure 3 Algorithm showing the principles of care for the diabetic foot. (*Reproduced with permission from Brodsky JW: The diabetic foot, in Coughlin MJ, Mann RA, Saltzman CL (eds): Surgery of the Foot and Ankle, ed 8. Philadelphia, PA, Mosby, 2007, vol 2, pp 1281-1368.*)

from deep in the wound and from the bone if osteomyelitis is suspected.

Non–limb-threatening infections can be treated with oral antibiotics. Infections that do not respond to oral antibiotics and that are limb threatening or life threatening should be treated with intravenous antibiotic therapy. A recent study found that 75 of 93 episodes of diabetic osteomyelitis (80.5%) went into remission with oral antimicrobial therapy.[58] This therapy is recommended, especially in areas of the country with limited access to infectious disease physicians and foot and ankle specialists.

Multidrug-resistant bacteria, most commonly methicillin-resistant *Staphylococcus aureus* (MRSA), are becoming more common in diabetic foot infections. Three recent studies found no difference in the clinical outcome of wounds infected with MRSA compared with other organisms if proper treatment is administered.[59-61] An infectious disease specialist is an important member of the team for managing diabetic foot infections.

Surgical Treatment

Surgical treatment of diabetic foot infections is appropriate if traditional nonsurgical care is unsuccessful, if an abscess is present that requires drainage, and if the primary goal is salvaging optimal foot function. Although antibiotic therapy can result in remission of deep infections, surgical débridement is often necessary to fully eradicate many deep diabetes-related infections and osteomyelitis. Often, bony prominences must be resected to properly internally unload an ulcer. Vacuum-assisted closure (VAC) is a successful adjunct in healing ulcers in patients with diabetes or peripheral vascular disease. Multiple studies have shown this modality to be a good option for salvaging difficult wounds.[62] Local muscle flaps and microvascular free flaps also are viable treatment options in patients with diabetic foot infections requiring soft-tissue coverage for foot salvage.[63] The use of hyperbaric oxygen also has been advocated in the management of diabetic wounds and infection.[64]

Table 2

The Depth-Ischemia Classification System of Diabetic Foot Lesions

Grade	Definition	Treatment
0	The at-risk foot: previous ulcer or neuropathy with deformity that can cause ulcerations	Patient education, regular examination, appropriate footwear and insoles
1	Superficial ulceration, not infected	External pressure relief: total contact cast, walking brace, special footwear
2	Deep ulceration exposing a tendon or joint (with or without superficial infection)	Surgical débridement, wound care, pressure relief if the lesion closes and converts to grade 1 (appropriate antibiotics as needed)
3	Extensive ulceration with exposed bone and/or deep infection (osteomyelitis) or abscess	Surgical débridement, ray or partial foot amputation, antibiotics, pressure relief if wound converts to grade 1
Depth	Ischemia Classification	Treatment
A	Not ischemic	None
B	Ischemia without gangrene	Vascular evaluation (such as Doppler, transcutaneous oxygen pressure, arteriogram), vascular reconstruction as needed
C	Partial (forefoot) gangrene of the foot	Vascular evaluation, vascular reconstruction (such as proximal and/or distal bypass or angioplasty), partial foot amputation
D	Complete foot gangrene	Vascular evaluation, major extremity amputation (below or above knee), possible proximal vascular reconstruction

(Adapted from Brodsky JW: The diabetic foot, in Coughlin MJ, Mann RA, Saltzman CL (eds): Surgery of the Foot and Ankle, ed 8. Philadelphia, PA, Mosby, 2007, vol 2, pp 1281-1368.)

Amputations

More than 60% of all lower extremity amputations are performed in patients with diabetes; the rate of amputation in diabetic patients is 10 times higher than in the nondiabetic population.[5] There is a strong correlation between morbid obesity and diabetes-associated morbidity.[65] Minor environmental trauma also is a factor in amputation rates in diabetic patients.[66] Poverty is a contributing factor affecting lower extremity amputation rates in minority patients age 50 years and older.[67]

The energy consumption required for ambulation in a patient with an amputated limb is inversely proportional to the length of the residual limb and the number of functional joints preserved.[68] Following an amputation, 30% of amputees will undergo amputation of their contralateral limb within 3 years, and approximately two thirds of patients will die within 5 years.[69] Previously, amputation had been viewed as a sign of failed treatment and the beginning of a lifelong bout with disability and disfigurement. Currently, because of advancements in diagnosis, surgical techniques, rehabilitation, and orthotic and prosthetic hardware, positive outcomes for diabetic amputees have increased.

One of the paramount decisions necessary for a successful outcome following a diabetes-related amputation is determining the level at which an amputation will heal and permit optimum residual limb function. The preoperative assessment should include evaluating the quality of the tissue; the extent of infection; the amount of vas-

cularity; and the patient's nutritional, immune, and ambulatory status. A serum albumin level of 3.0 g/dL is the currently accepted nutritional parameter for wound healing; however, a 2003 study reported an 88% healing rate in 83 diabetic patients treated with a Syme amputation who had a serum albumin threshold of 2.5 g/dL.[70] A total lymphocyte count of more than 1,500 correlates with immunocompetence for wound healing. The different levels of amputation include partial-digital, digital, ray resection, transmetatarsal, Chopart (midtarsal), Syme, below knee, and above knee.

The energy expended following an amputation is inversely proportional to the length of the residual limb. Amputations of the midfoot and more proximally may require tendon transfers to balance the foot and Achilles tendon lengthening to prevent uneven load to the residua. Successful healing was reported in 82 of 97 diabetic patients (84.5%) treated with one-stage Syme amputation.[71] Postamputation care requires close follow-up; the proper choice of orthotics, prosthetics, and footwear; and rehabilitation. A multidisciplinary diabetic foot team can help decrease the rate of major amputations.[4]

Charcot Arthropathy

Charcot joint was first described in 1868. In 1936, the first case of Charcot joint in a patient with diabetic neuropathy was reported.[72] Charcot arthropathy, also

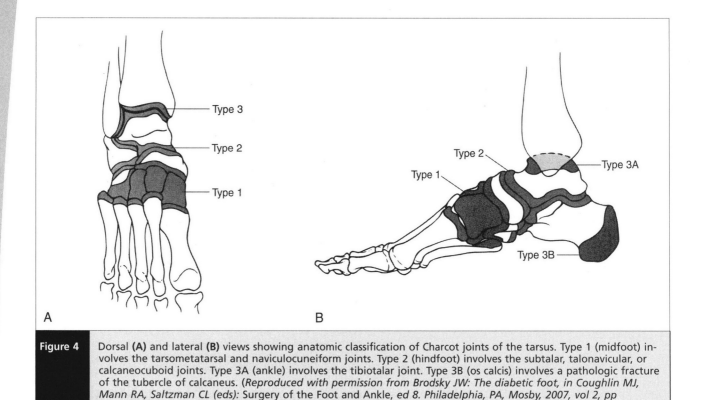

Figure 4 Dorsal **(A)** and lateral **(B)** views showing anatomic classification of Charcot joints of the tarsus. Type 1 (midfoot) involves the tarsometatarsal and naviculocuneiform joints. Type 2 (hindfoot) involves the subtalar, talonavicular, or calcaneocuboid joints. Type 3A (ankle) involves the tibiotalar joint. Type 3B (os calcis) involves a pathologic fracture of the tubercle of calcaneus. *(Reproduced with permission from Brodsky JW: The diabetic foot, in Coughlin MJ, Mann RA, Saltzman CL (eds):* Surgery of the Foot and Ankle, *ed 8. Philadelphia, PA, Mosby, 2007, vol 2, pp 1281-1368.)*

known as neuropathic arthropathy, is a progressive destruction of joints that most commonly occurs in the feet and ankles of diabetic patients. The incidence of Charcot arthropathy in the diabetic population ranges from 1% to 37%, with a rate of approximately 30% for bilateral involvement.[73,74] Charcot arthropathy occurs at a similar rate in men and women with diabetes.

The incidence of neuroarthropathy is increasing and is often unrecognized and misdiagnosed. Two basic theories exist regarding the cause of neuroarthropathy. The first theory, neurotraumatic destruction, postulates that joint deterioration occurs as a consequence of cumulative trauma unrecognized by an insensate foot. The second theory, neurovascular destruction, hypothesizes that joint destruction occurs from bone resorption and ligament loosening related to a neurally controlled vascular reflex. Currently, it is believed that a combination of both mechanisms is responsible for the changes associated with Charcot arthropathy. Researchers have investigated osteopenia as a potential contributor to the development of Charcot arthropathy.[75,76] The authors of a 2006 study reported excessive osteoclastic activity in the environment of cytokine mediators in bone resorption of Charcot reactive bone.[77] This finding indicated that pharmacologic agents could be used to decrease cytokine activation and osteoclastic resorption, helping to prevent destruction and collapse. Other authors reported an increased expression of a nuclear transcription factor that results in increased osteoclastogenesis and helps to confirm the role of proin-flammatory cytokines.[78] Patients often have localized osteopenia, making them more prone to fracture.[79] Charcot dislocations were associated with normal bone density, whereas fractures were associated with decreased bone density. Clinically, the severity of the diabetic neuropathy is not necessarily related to the development of Charcot arthropathy. Some patients who are most severely affected by Charcot arthropathy have mild type 2 diabetes that is being treated with oral hypoglycemic medications or changes in diet.

Staging

In 1966, Eichenholtz first described the three classic stages of Charcot arthropathy.[80] Stage one is known as the acute Charcot phase. Patients present with hyperemia, edema, increased warmth, and erythema around the affected joint. Radiographs usually show fracture, joint subluxation, and fragmentation (another name for stage one). Stage two, the subacute or coalescence phase, is characterized by a decrease in the acute inflammatory changes occurring in stage one, resorption of bone debris, and radiographically confirmed new bone formation. Stage three, the chronic Charcot or consolidation phase, is characterized by the resolution of the inflammatory response and radiographic consolidation with frequent deformity.[80]

Classification

The anatomic classification of Charcot joints of the foot and ankle helps the treating physician break down

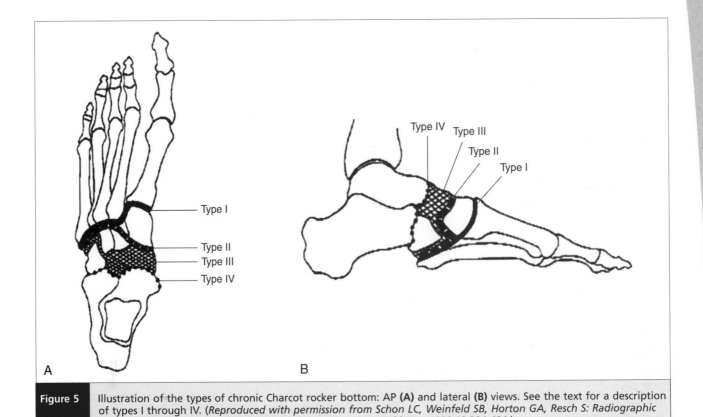

Figure 5 | Illustration of the types of chronic Charcot rocker bottom: AP **(A)** and lateral **(B)** views. See the text for a description of types I through IV. (*Reproduced with permission from Schon LC, Weinfeld SB, Horton GA, Resch S: Radiographic and clinical classification of acquired midfoot tarsus.* Foot Ankle Int *1998:19:394-404.*)

this serious disorder into four anatomic areas that are most commonly affected[44] (**Figure 4**). Type 1 Charcot joints affect the midfoot, tarsometatarsal, and naviculo-cuneiform joints and account for 60% of Charcot arthropathy of the foot. In type 1, the plantar medial bony exostosis resulting from sagittal plane collapse can increase the risk of ulceration. Type 2 Charcot arthropathy involves the hindfoot, occurring in 30% to 35% of patients with Charcot joints. Hindfoot instability can be a difficult problem for patients because it is associated with foot subluxation and ulcer formation. Type 3A affects approximately 5% of patients with Charcot joints in the foot and is the most unstable pattern. Type 3B is characterized by a fracture of the calcaneal tuberosity, which can be caused by trauma or, usually, a missed or delayed diagnosis. Type 3B Charcot joints result in weak push-off, pes planus, and bony prominence leading to ulceration. More proximal Charcot joints in the foot and ankle correlate with a higher risk of joint instability.

The anatomic classification of Charcot foot by Schon and associates[81] is based on the type and stage of the Charcot joint (**Figure 5**). Type I affects the metatarsocuneiform joints and usually results in a medial plantar prominence and an abduction deformity. Type II affects the naviculocuneiform joint and is characterized by a plantar lateral prominence under the fourth and fifth metatarsocuboid joints (**Figure 6**). Type III affects the navicular, with a collapse of the medial column, resulting in an adducted-supinated deformity and a plan-

tar lateral prominence under the cuboid. Type IV affects the transverse tarsal joints with an associated prominence under the calcaneocuboid or talonavicular joint. The staging portion of the classification is based on the severity of the deformity. **Figure 7** shows stages A through C.[81]

Treatment

The main goals in treating Charcot arthropathy of the foot are to achieve a stable, plantigrade foot that is either amenable to bracing or an accommodative orthotic and is free of infection or ulceration. Many feet affected with Charcot arthropathy can be treated nonsurgically, with the goal of converting Eichenholtz stage one arthropathy to stage three with bone healing and stability. The time frame of this treatment period can be unpredictable and can lead to patient frustration and noncompliance. Educating patients about the treatment time span and goals is paramount to a successful outcome.

Nonsurgical treatment of a stage one Charcot foot includes rest, elevation, and the use of a total contact cast with protected weight bearing. The initial cast changes occur at weekly intervals as redness and swelling fluctuate; cast change intervals are increased gradually from 1 week to several weeks as the process becomes less acute. Total contact casting continues until the onset of stage two (coalescence, decreased edema and warmth). Prefabricated walking boots can diminish forefoot and midfoot pressures in a manner similar to

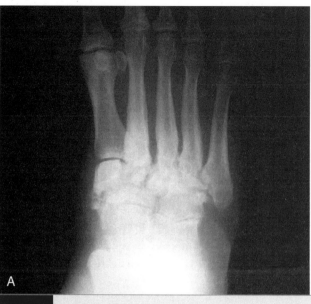
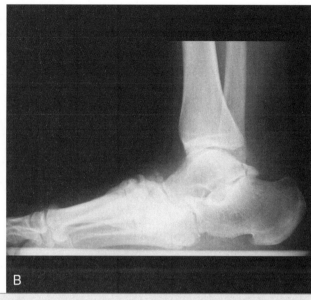

Figure 6 Dorsal **(A)** and lateral **(B)** radiographic views of a Charcot deformity. *(Courtesy of Terrence M. Philbin, DO, Columbus, OH.)*

Figure 7 Illustration showing the classification of staging of chronic Charcot rocker bottom deformity. *(Reproduced with permission from Schon LC, Weinfeld SB, Horton GA, Resch S: Radiographic and clinical classification of acquired midfoot tarsus. Foot Ankle Int 1998;19:394-404.)*

Stage A

Stage B

Stage C

that of a total contact cast. The prefabricated boots allow wound dressing changes and more frequent wound surveillance. However, the prefabricated boots are not customized and cannot accommodate some severe deformities. At stage two, patients can ambulate in an ankle-foot orthosis. Once the bony healing of stage three is achieved, the patient can transfer from an ankle-foot orthosis to a custom-molded accommodative orthotic.

Although conservative treatment can be successful, disappointing findings were reported in a retrospective study of 115 patients (127 limbs) with Charcot arthropathy treated under a protocol incorporating structured, intensive, nonsurgical treatment.[82] A 2.7% annual rate of amputation and a 49% risk of recurrent ulcers were reported.

The main indications for surgical treatment of Charcot joints are infection, osteomyelitis, recurrent or impending ulceration, and an unbraceable or unstable deformity. A 17% yearly rate of ulceration in 115 diabetic patients with Charcot joints was reported in one study.[83] Exostectomy is indicated when there is a failure to heal or unload ulcers related to bony prominences. It is important to understand the balance between removing enough bone to decrease the pressure on the soft tissues while preserving adequate bone to prevent instability.

Surgical reconstruction has historically been reserved for stage three deformities because of the high risk of complications seen in earlier stages of Charcot, such as nonunion, infection, and wound complications. However, with some significant Charcot deformities occurring in stage one and two, standard conservative care is likely to fail. Some acute dislocations will have imminent skin compromise. The more proximal the defor-

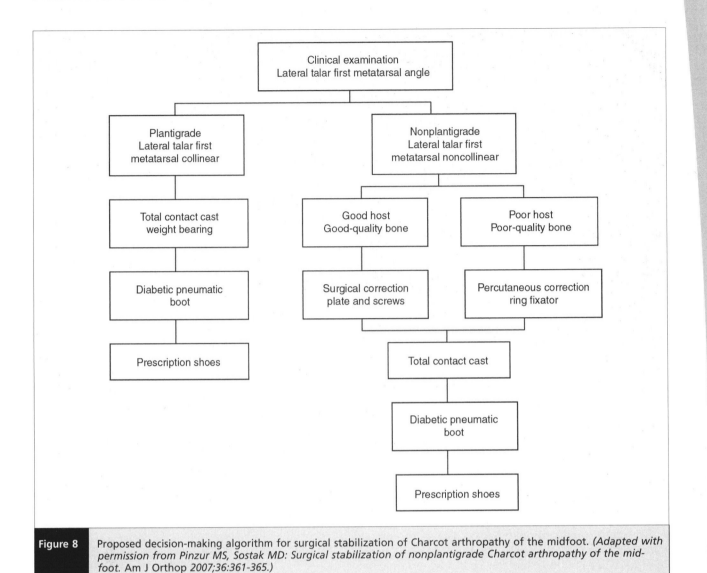

Figure 8 Proposed decision-making algorithm for surgical stabilization of Charcot arthropathy of the midfoot. *(Adapted with permission from Pinzur MS, Sostak MD: Surgical stabilization of nonplantigrade Charcot arthropathy of the midfoot. Am J Orthop 2007;36:361-365.)*

mity, the more challenging it is to achieve stability with a total contact cast and brace. Early reconstruction of Charcot joints using external fixation and limited skin incisions can minimize complications. In one study, single-stage correction using surgical débridement, osteotomy, external fixation, and antibiotic therapy was used to treat 11 patients with midfoot Charcot joints, collapse, and ulceration who were at risk for amputation.[84] Ten of the 11 patients had sufficient improvement to allow the use of therapeutic footwear at an average of 24 months postoperatively. Fine wire fixators have been advocated for the salvage of Charcot joints with wound infections.[85] In another study, good results were reported using early arthrodesis in 14 patients with midfoot Charcot arthropathy.[86]

Outcomes
Quality of life is a key factor in assessing treatment outcomes in patients with Charcot arthropathy. In a 2004 study, the author reported the results of 198 patients treated for diabetes-associated Charcot foot arthropathy.[87] The deformity in patients with nonplantigrade feet was treated with surgery, whereas those with plantigrade feet were treated with accommodative orthotic methods. Results showed that in 87 of 147 feet with midfoot disease (59.2%), the patients achieved the desired end point (long-term management with appropriate inserts) without surgical correction. The authors of a 2007 study proposed a treatment algorithm for the surgical stabilization of nonplantigrade midfoot Charcot arthropathy[88] (**Figure 8**). In another study, the algorithm was used to treat 26 diabetic patients who had multiple comorbidities and nonplantigrade midfoot Charcot deformity.[89] The patients were treated using a neutrally applied three-level ring external fixator along with appropriate antibiotic administration and surgeries, including Achilles tendon lengthening, excision of infected bone, and correction of deformities. At 1 year postoperatively, 24 patients were free of infection and were able to ambulate with accommodative footwear.

In another 2007 study, 18 patients with Charcot

5: Neuromuscular Disease

neuroarthropathy and unstable ankles were treated with retrograde transcalcaneal nailing for ankle arthrodesis in a limb-salvage effort.[90] With a mean follow-up of 14 ± 10 months, 100% successful limb salvage was achieved with no major complications.

Another study evaluated the reliability of the American Orthopaedic Foot and Ankle Society diabetic foot questionnaire with regard to quality of life for patients with Charcot arthropathy.[91] Results showed that the quality of life for patients with Charcot arthropathy is poor with respect to physical functioning.

Prophylactic Care and Patient Education

The prevention of diabetic foot disorders begins with the proper screening of patients and providing education concerning complication risk factors. Patients most at risk for complications are those with foot deformities, a history of ulceration or infection, loss of protective sensation, and peripheral vascular disease. Diabetic patients, their families, and care providers must all be involved in the treatment and prevention of these disorders. To prevent ulcers and infection in the diabetic foot, multiple screening methods are recommended, including assessing peripheral vascular disease, reviewing proper footwear, and checking for increased plantar pressure.[7] Effective interventions include patient education, optimizing glycemic control, smoking cessation, and appropriate skin and nail care. Current American Orthopaedic Foot and Ankle Society guidelines for foot care in diabetic patients are based on the level of risk.[27,28]

Diabetic patients should be instructed to inspect their feet daily for skin breakdown or signs of infection, to avoid bathing their feet in hot water, to avoid trimming their own calluses, and to apply lotion to their feet to help maintain skin moisture (but not interdigitally). Improperly fitting shoes can be a substantial cause of diabetic foot disorders. Patients at high risk for complications may benefit from specialized footwear, including extra-depth or custom-molded shoes. Shoe wear should accommodate the size and shape of the foot, including the toes. Insoles also play a key role in preventing ulcerations by reducing shear and pressure on the plantar aspect of the foot.

Summary

Diabetes mellitus is a multisystem disease that is insidious in nature. Its incidence is increasing dramatically in the United States. Foot complications are the most common reason for hospital admission for diabetic patients, and the treatment of foot disorders can be challenging. Up to 25% of diabetic patients may be affected by foot disorders at some point during their lifetime. Patient education is important in preventing diabetic foot complications and in achieving successful outcomes after nonsurgical and surgical treatment. The likelihood of successful outcomes can be greatly enhanced by using a multidisciplinary team approach to patient education and treatment.

Annotated References

1. Medvei V: *History of Endocrinology.* Lancaster, UK, MTP Press, 1982.

2. Apelqvist J, Ragnarson-Tennvall G, Persson U, Larsson J: Diabetic foot ulcers in a multidisciplinary setting: An economic analysis of primary healing and healing with amputation. *J Intern Med* 1994;235:463-471.

3. Edmonds ME, Blundell MP, Morris ME, Thomas EM, Cotton LT, Watkins PJ: Improved survival of the diabetic foot: The role of a specialized foot clinic. *Q J Med* 1986;60:763-771.

4. Aksoy DY, Gürlek A, Çetinkaya Y, et al: Change in the amputation profile in diabetic foot in a tertiary reference center: Efficacy of team working. *Exp Clin Endocrinol Diabetes* 2004;112:526-530.

   The authors of this study compared lower extremity amputation rates at the Hacettepe University Hospital before and after establishment of a multidisciplinary foot care team. Although amputation was still performed frequently, interventions by the foot care team resulted in a relatively decreased rate of major amputations.

5. American Diabetes Association. Diabetes statistics. http://www.diabetes.org/diabetes-statistics.jsp. Accessed August 14, 2007.

   This Website provides statistics concerning the prevalence of diabetes, the complications associated with diabetes, diabetes-associated deaths, and the economic impact of this disease.

6. Centers for Disease Control and Prevention Website: National Diabetes Fact Sheet, United States, 2005. http://www.cdc.gov/diabetes/pubs/pdf/ndfs_2005.pdf. Accessed July 2, 2008.

   This Website provides general information about diabetes, including an explanation of the types, treatments, and prevalence of the disease. It also includes estimated data concerning diabetes according to age and ethnicity, complications, and economic consequences.

7. Singh N, Armstrong DG, Lipsky BA: Preventing foot ulcers in patients with diabetes. *JAMA* 2005;293:217-228.

   The efficacy of methods for preventing diabetic foot ulcers in the primary care setting is presented based on a review of the literature published between 1980 and 2004. Evidence supports screening all diabetic patients for foot disorders. Patient education about proper foot care and the importance of regular foot examinations is paramount; screening also involves prescription footwear, podiatric care, and assessing the need for surgical treatment.

8. Adler A: Risk factors for diabetic neuropathy and foot ulceration. *Curr Diab Rep* 2001;1:202-207.

9. Simmons Z, Feldman E: Update on diabetic neuropathy. *Curr Opin Neurol* 2002;15:595-603.

10. Pirat J: Diabetes mellitus and its degenerative complications: A prospective study of 4,400 patients observed between 1947 and 1973. *Diabetes Cases* 1987;1:252-258.

11. Bibbo C, Patel DV: Diabetic neuropathy. *Foot Ankle Clin* 2006;11:753-774.

The anatomic and molecular pathogenesis of diabetic neuropathy is described. The authors present classifications of diabetic neuropathy and the subset of painful neuropathies along with pharmacologic treatments and the current status of research.

12. Ross MA: Neuropathies associated with diabetes. *Med Clin North Am* 1993;77:111-124.

13. Cameron NE, Eaton SE, Cotter MA, Tesfaye S: Vascular factors and metabolic interactions in the pathogenesis of diabetic neuropathy. *Diabetologia* 2001;44:1973-1988.

14. Reiber GE, Smith DG, Wallace C, et al: Effect of therapeutic footwear on foot reulceration in patients with diabetes: A randomized controlled trial. *JAMA* 2002;287:2552-2558.

15. Ishii DN: Implications of insulin-like growth factors in the pathogenesis of diabetic neuropathy. *Brain Res Rev* 1995;20:47-67.

16. Lin SS, Lee TH, Wapner KL: Plantar forefoot ulceration with equinus deformity of the ankle in diabetic patients: The effect of tendo-Achilles lengthening and total contact casting. *Orthopedics* 1996;19:465-475.

17. Mueller MJ, Sinacore DR, Hastings MK, Strube MJ, Johnson JE: Effect of Achilles tendon lengthening on neuropathic plantar ulcers: A randomized clinical trial. *J Bone Joint Surg Am* 2003;85-A:1436-1445.

The authors hypothesized that Achilles tendon lengthening would result in a lower rate of recurrent foot ulcers. Thirty-three patients were treated with a total contact cast only, and 31 were treated with the cast and Achilles tendon lengthening. Casting alone resulted in an 88% rate of ulcer healing. All of those treated with casting and surgery had healed ulcers. The authors concluded that Achilles tendon lengthening should be considered to reduce recurrent ulceration in diabetic patients with dorsiflexion of 5° or less.

18. Mueller MJ, Strube MJ: Therapeutic footwear: Enhanced function in people with diabetes and transmetatarsal amputation. *Arch Phys Med Rehabil* 1997;78:952-956.

19. Hastings MK, Mueller MJ, Sinacore DR, Salsich GB, Engsberg JR, Johnson JE: Effects of a tendo-Achilles lengthening procedure on muscle function and gait char-

acteristics in a patient with diabetes mellitus. *J Orthop Sports Phys Ther* 2000;30:85-90.

20. Orendurff MS, Rohr ES, Sangeorzan BJ, Weaver K, Czerniecki JM: An equinus deformity of the ankle accounts for only a small amount of the increased forefoot plantar pressure in patients with diabetes. *J Bone Joint Surg Br* 2006;88:65-68.

Flexion contractures (equinus) can result in increased forefoot pressure when ambulating. Forefoot pressures during walking were measured in 27 patients. Statistical analysis of the results suggested that equinus plays a limited role in increased forefoot pressures. More research is needed to establish high forefoot pressure as an indication for tendon lengthening.

21. Dejgard A, Petersen P, Kastrup J: Mexiletine for treatment of chronic painful diabetic neuropathy. *Lancet* 1988;1:9-11.

22. Oskarsson P, Ljunggren GJ, Lins PE: Efficacy and safety of mexiletine in the treatment of painful diabetic neuropathy: The Mexiletine Study Group. *Diabetes Care* 1997;20:1594-1597.

23. Stracke H, Meyer UE, Schumacher HE, Federlin J: Mexiletine in the treatment of diabetic neuropathy. *Diabetes Care* 1992;15:1550-1555.

24. Wright JM, Oki JC, Graves L III: Mexiletine in the symptomatic treatment of diabetic peripheral neuropathy. *Ann Pharmacother* 1997;31:29-34.

25. Rosenstock J, Tuchman M, LaMoreaux L, Sharma U: Pregabalin for the treatment of painful diabetic peripheral neuropathy: A double-blind, placebo-controlled trial. *Pain* 2004;110:628-638.

In an 8-week, randomized, double-blind, placebo-controlled, parallel-group, multicenter study, the researchers evaluated pregabalin in relieving pain caused by diabetic peripheral neuropathy. Seventy-six patients were randomized to receive 300 mg/day pregabalin and 70 patients received a placebo. The pregabalin group show statistically significant improvements compared with the placebo group for mean pain scores. Pregabalin also improved the mood, rate of sleep disturbance, and quality of life of patients.

26. Biddinger KR, Amend KJ: The role of surgical decompression for diabetic neuropathy. *Foot Ankle Clin* 2004;9:239-254.

Metabolic changes in diabetes cause external compression of peripheral nerves in particular, resulting in peripheral neuropathy. Pain can be reduced and sensation improved by the surgical release of multiple nerves. The authors present a review of their study and previous studies and discuss surgical techniques for releasing the common peroneal nerve, deep peroneal nerve, and tarsal tunnel. Indications for proper patient selection also are presented.

27. Pinzur MS, Slovenkai MP, Trepman E, Shields NN: Guidelines for diabetic foot care: Recommendations en-

dorsed by the Diabetes Committee of the American Orthopaedic Foot and Ankle Society. *Foot Ankle Int* 2005; 26:113-119.

Physician and patient self-screening for foot disorders and treatment guidelines are presented. Treatment should be based on the presence of peripheral neuropathy, deformity, and ulcer history. Ongoing treatments involve patient education and skin and nail care; a multidisciplinary team approach may be required.

28. Berlet GC, Shields NN: The diabetic foot, in Richardson EG (ed): *Orthopaedic Knowledge Update: Foot and Ankle 3*. Rosemont, IL, American Academy of Orthopaedic Surgeons, 2003, pp 123-134.

The authors provide a thorough overview of all issues concerning the diabetic foot. Prevention or early treatment of ulcers and infection is the most important factor in decreasing the likelihood of subsequent amputation.

29. Saltzman CL, Rashid R, Hayes A, et al: 4.5-gram monofilament sensation beneath both first metatarsal heads indicates protective foot sensation in diabetic patients. *J Bone Joint Surg Am* 2004;86-A:717-723.

The authors tested 47 diabetic patients with a history of foot ulcers and 45 with no history of foot ulcers to determine if testing at fewer than 10 test sites would produce results as accurate as those obtained from testing at 10 sites. Sensitivity to 4.5-g monofilament under both first metatarsal heads showed 100% sensitivity in predicting the risk of ulceration (specificity, 67%). A patient who cannot sense the 4.5-g monofilament at either of those sites is at risk for injury and/or ulceration.

30. Booth J, Young MJ: Differences in the performance of commercially available 10-g monofilaments. *Diabetes Care* 2000;23:984-988.

31. Shapiro SA, Stansberry KB, Hill MA, et al: Normal blood flow response and vasomotion in the diabetic Charcot foot. *J Diabetes Complications* 1998;12:147-153.

32. Wagner F: A classification and treatment program for diabetic, neuropathic and dysvascular foot problems. *Instr Course Lect* 1979;28:143-165.

33. Wagner FW: Amputation of the foot and ankle: Current status. *Clin Orthop Relat Res* 1977;122:62-69.

34. Apelqvist J, Castenfors J, Larsson J, Stenström A, Agardh CD: Prognostic value of systolic ankle and toe blood pressure levels in outcome of diabetic foot ulcer. *Diabetes Care* 1989;12:373-378.

35. Crerand S, Dolan M, Laing P, Bird M, Smith ML, Klenerman L: Diagnosis of osteotomy in neuropathic foot ulcers. *J Bone Joint Surg Br* 1996;78:51-55.

36. Johnson JE, Kennedy EJ, Shereff MJ, Patel NC, Collier BD: Prospective study of bone, indium-111-labeled white blood cell, and gallium-67 scanning for the evaluation of osteomyelitis in the diabetic foot. *Foot Ankle Int* 1996;17:10-16.

37. Maurer AH, Millmond SH, Knight LC, et al: Infection in diabetic osteoarthropathy: Use of indium-labeled leukocytes for diagnosis. *Radiology* 1986;161:221-225.

38. Splittgerber GF, Spiegelhoff DR, Buggy BP: Combined leukocyte and bone imaging used to evaluate diabetic osteoarthropathy and osteomyelitis. *Clin Nucl Med* 1989;14:156-160.

39. Dutta P, Bhansali A, Mittal BR, Singh B, Masoodi SR: Instant 99mTc-ciprofloxacin scintigraphy for the diagnosis of osteomyelitis in the diabetic foot. *Foot Ankle Int* 2006;27:716-722.

The authors tested 25 patients with type 3 diabetes and foot ulcers with ^{99m}TC-ciprofloxacin scintigraphy to determine its effectiveness in diagnosing osteomyelitis. The scan was true-positive in 12 patients, true-negative in 6, false-positive in 1, and false-negative in 6. They concluded that the test is sensitive and specific in diagnosing bone infection in diabetic patients but caution that inaccurate results may occur when fastidious organisms and ciprofloxacin-resistant bacteria are present.

40. Hopfner S, Krolak C, Kessler S, et al: Preoperative imaging of Charcot neuroarthropathy in diabetic patients: Comparison of ring PET, hybrid PET, and magnetic resonance imaging. *Foot Ankle Int* 2004;25:890-895.

This prospective study assessed the value of two types of PET imaging in the preoperative evaluation of Charcot deformities. Ring and hybrid PET imaging were compared with MRI in 16 patients. Surgery subsequently identified 39 Charcot lesions; 37 were detected by ring PET, 30 by hybrid PET, and 31 by MRI. PET is more effective than MRI because it can be used if a patient has a metal implant and can distinguish inflammatory versus infectious soft-tissue lesions, along with osteomyelitis versus Charcot neuroarthropathy. Ring PET is preferred over hybrid PET.

41. Abbott CA, Carrington AL, Ashe H, et al: The northwest diabetes foot care study: Incidence of and risk factors for new diabetic foot ulceration in a community-based patient cohort. *Diabet Med* 2002;19:377-384.

42. Goodridge D, Trepman E, Sloan J, et al : Quality of life of adults with unhealed and healed diabetic foot ulcers. *Foot Ankle Int* 2006;27:274-280.

The authors evaluated 57 patients with unhealed foot ulcers and 47 with healed ulcers using the Medical Outcomes Study 12-Item Short Form questionnaire and a wound impact scale to assess quality of life. The unhealed group had significantly lower physical component scores on the questionnaire. The scores of both groups were significantly lower than published scores for the general, diabetic, and hypertensive populations. It was concluded that unhealed and healed ulcers negatively impact the quality of life; unhealed ulcers have a greater negative impact.

43. Shah BR, Hux JE: Quantifying the risk of infectious diseases for people with diabetes. *Diabetes Care* 2003;26: 510-513.

Using an administrative data cohort that included all

people with diabetes in Ontario, Canada, on April 1, 1999, researchers retrospectively determined the risk ratios of having an infectious disease and death from an infectious disease by comparison to a cohort of people without diabetes (n = 513,749 in each group). The same analysis was performed in a second set of cohorts from 1996 to confirm estimated risks. People with diabetes had a risk ratio for hospitalization of 1.21 and a risk ratio for death resulting from infection of 1.92 compared with nondiabetic individuals.

44. Brodsky JW: The diabetic foot, in Coughlin MJ, Mann RA, Saltzman CL (eds): *Surgery of the Foot and Ankle,* ed 8. Philadelphia, PA, Mosby, 2007, pp 1281-1368.

A thorough discussion of all aspects of the diabetic foot, including the pathophysiology, diagnosis, classification systems, clinical problems and their treatment methods, wound closure, Charcot joints, neuropathic fractures and their complications, skin and nail disorders, footwear, and the importance of a true team approach to treatment are presented.

45. Eneroth M, Apelqvist J, Stenström A: Clinical characteristics and outcome in 223 diabetic patients with deep foot infections. *Foot Ankle Int* 1997;18:716-722.

46. Armstrong DG, Lavery LA, Sariaya M, Ashry H: Leukocytosis is a poor indicator of acute osteomyelitis of the foot in diabetes mellitus. *J Foot Ankle Surg* 1996; 35:280-283.

47. Leibner ED, Brodsky JW, Pollo FE, Baum BS, Edmonds BW: Unloading mechanism in the total contact cast. *Foot Ankle Int* 2006;27:281-285.

The authors measured plantar pressures and forces during standing and ambulation in 12 healthy individuals wearing total contact casts and again after removing the shank of the cast. Although the effectiveness of the total contact cast is believed to result from reduced plantar pressure, the results of this study indicated that the effectiveness is probably a result of reduced ankle motion provided by the shank of the cast.

48. Saltzman CL, Zimmerman MB, Holdsworth RL, Beck S, Hartsell HD, Frantz RA: Effect of initial weight-bearing in a total contact cast on healing of diabetic foot ulcers. *J Bone Joint Surg Am* 2004;86:2714-2719.

This study evaluated the effects of early weight bearing in a total contact cast on ulcer healing. Forty patients with noninfected foot ulcers were treated with total contact casting until healing or for 13 weeks. A step counting device was embedded in the cast, and the patient was instructed not to bear weight for 48 hours. Although most patients walked during the immediate period after cast application, healing was only minimally affected by moderate early weight bearing. Level of evidence: II.

49. Armstrong DG, Nguyen HC, Lavery LA, van Schie CH, Boulton AJ, Harkless LB: Off-loading the diabetic foot wound: A randomized clinical trial. *Diabetes Care* 2001;24:1019-1022.

50. Wukich DK, Motko J: Safety of total contact casting in high-risk patients with neuropathic foot ulcers. *Foot Ankle Int* 2004;25:556-560.

This prospective study treated 13 patients (18 neuropathic ulcers) with total contact casting to evaluate the frequency of complications. The first cast was changed in 3 to 4 days and subsequently each week. There were 14 complications (13 skin irritations, 1 cast too tight); 15 of the 18 ulcers healed. The authors concluded that total contact casting is safe for high-risk patients.

51. Matricali GA, Deroo K, Dereymaeker G: Outcome and recurrence rate of diabetic foot ulcers treated by a total contact cast: Short-term follow-up. *Foot Ankle Int* 2003;24:680-684.

Healing and outcome of total contact casting in 15 patients with diabetic foot ulcers (17 ulcers) was assessed. Three patients were lost to follow-up. At a mean follow-up period of 91 weeks, all ulcers healed. On longer follow-up after casting was discontinued, only 4 of the 12 patients had no new ulcers.

52. Frigg A, Pagenstert G, Schäfer D, Valderrabano V, Hintermann B: Recurrence and prevention of diabetic foot ulcers after total contact casting. *Foot Ankle Int* 2007; 28:64-69.

The authors treated 28 patients (34 ulcers) with total contact casting for a mean period of 4 months. Complete healing was achieved in 85% of ulcers, but 57% of patients had 26 recurrences, and 18 new ulcers occurred in other areas of the foot. Sixteen recurrent ulcers were successfully treated with casting. The rate of new recurrences was 50%. In the eight recurrent ulcers treated by surgically correcting deformities, patients remained ulcer free. The authors concluded that surgical correction of deformities should be performed after primary healing.

53. Pollo FE, Brodsky JW, Crenshaw SJ, Kirksey C: Plantar pressures in fiberglass total contact casts vs. a new diabetic walking boot. *Foot Ankle Int* 2003;24:45-49.

The authors evaluated plantar pressures in 18 healthy individuals who wore the Bledsoe Conformer Diabetic Boot (Bledsoe Medical Technology; Grand Prairie, TX). Results showed that this orthotic device performs as well as (and in some cases better than) a total contact cast in reducing plantar forces and pressures.

54. Piaggesi A, Macchiarini S, Rizzo L, et al: An off-the-shelf instant contact casting device for the treatment of diabetic foot ulcers: A randomized prospective trial versus traditional fiberglass cast. *Diabetes Care* 2007;30: 586-590.

The authors compared the Optima Diab Walker (Molliter; Civitanova Marche, Italy) to total contact casting in 40 diabetic outpatients over a 12-week period. They found no difference in healing rates, time to healing, and number of adverse events. The Optima Diab Walker was 78% less expensive than casting, required 77% less time to apply and 58% less time to remove, and achieved higher rates of patient satisfaction.

5: Neuromuscular Disease

55. Katz IA, Harlan A, Miranda-Palma B, et al: A randomized trial of two irremovable off-loading devices in the management of plantar neuropathic diabetic foot ulcers. *Diabetes Care* 2005;28:555-559.

They authors compared a removable cast walker wrapped with fiberglass casting material (to make it irremovable) to a total contact cast in 41 patients. In patients who completed the 12-week trial, healing and complication rates were equal. The cost of the irremovable device was lower, and less time was required to place and ultimately remove the device compared with the total contact cast.

56. Ge Y, MacDonald H, Lipsky B, Zasloff M, Holroyd K: Microbiological profile of infected diabetic foot ulcers. *Diabet Med* 2002;19:1032-1034.

57. Senneville E, Melliez H, Beltrand E, et al: Culture of percutaneous bone biopsy specimens for diagnosis of diabetic foot osteomyelitis: Concordance with ulcer swab cultures. *Clin Infect Dis* 2006;42:57-62.

The authors compared the results of percutaneous bone biopsy and ulcer swab cultures in 69 patients with osteomyelitis. Results were identical for 12 patients (17.4%), indicating that superficial swab cultures are inadequate in reliably detecting bone bacteria.

58. Embil JM, Rose G, Trepman E, et al: Oral antimicrobial therapy for diabetic foot osteomyelitis. *Foot Ankle Int* 2006;27:771-779.

The authors reviewed the records of 79 patients (93 episodes of osteomyelitis) treated with oral antibiotics (with or without an initial short course of intravenous antibiotics). The mean duration of oral antibiotic therapy was 40 ± 30 weeks, and relapse-free follow-up was 50 ± 50 weeks. Of the 93 episodes of osteomyelitis, 75 (80.5%) went into remission. The authors concluded that osteomyelitis can be treated effectively with oral antibiotics.

59. Dang CN, Prasad YD, Boulton AJ, Jude EB: Methicillin-resistant Staphylococcus aureus in the diabetic foot clinic: A worsening problem. *Diabet Med* 2003;20:159-161.

The authors reviewed the records of 63 patients with positive wound swabs to determine if there had been a change in the prevalence of pathogens in foot ulcers occurring from 1998 to 2001. The rate of *Staphylococcus aureus* was higher in 2001, and the incidence of MRSA was almost double the 1998 rate. The authors cite the need for a multicenter study to determine methods of reducing MRSA in diabetic foot ulcers.

60. Game FL, Boswell T, Soar C, et al: Outcome in diabetic foot ulcers with and without methicillin resistant Staphylococcus aureus (MRSA). *Diabet Med* 2003; 20(suppl 2):30.

The authors analyzed 147 ulcers (96 patients) to compare outcomes of those with MRSA versus those without MRSA. The outcomes for patients with MRSA and diabetic foot ulcers were no worse than outcomes for patients without MRSA.

61. Hartemann-Heurtier A, Robert J, Jacqueminet S, et al: Diabetic foot ulcer and multidrug-resistant organisms: Risk factors and impact. *Diabet Med* 2004;21:710-715.

Records of 180 patients admitted to a specialized diabetic foot unit who had microbiologic specimens taken on admission were reviewed. Multidrug-resistant organisms were present in 18% of specimens. Previous hospitalization for the same wound and osteomyelitis showed a statistically significant association with the presence of multidrug-resistant organisms; however, the presence of multidrug-resistant organisms was not associated with a longer time to healing.

62. Mendonca DA, Cosker T, Makwana NK: Vacuum-assisted closure to aid wound healing in foot and ankle surgery. *Foot Ankle Int* 2005;26:761-766.

Fifteen patients (18 wounds/ulcers) underwent surgical débridement and VAC. Satisfactory wound healing occurred in 13 of the 18 wounds/ulcers at an average follow-up of 2.5 months. VAC therapy was unsuccessful in five patients (five class III ulcers) and three subsequently required below-knee amputations. The authors concluded that VAC therapy is useful in patients with diabetes or peripheral vascular disease, result in more rapid healing, and often prevent the need for additional surgery.

63. Verhelle NA, Lemaire V, Nelissen X, Vandamme H, Heymans O: Combined reconstruction of the diabetic foot including revascularization and free-tissue transfer. *J Reconstr Microsurg* 2004;20:511-517.

Over a 4-year period, the authors treated 19 diabetic patients with large soft-tissue defects of the foot with revascularization and free-tissue transfer. They report 100% flap survival, 3 (16.6%) early local wound problems, and a recurrence rate of approximately 18.7%; no other flap procedures were needed. With a mean follow-up of 38 months (range, 23 to 55 months), the limb salvage rate was 94.4%. There was one amputation and one patient had difficulty with ambulation. Sixteen patients (84.2%) were fully rehabilitated and could function independently.

64. Strauss MB: Hyperbaric oxygen as an intervention for managing wound hypoxia: Its role and usefulness in diabetic foot wounds. *Foot Ankle Int* 2005;26:15-18.

The authors reviewed 12 reports of the use of hyperbaric oxygen in treating diabetic wounds and reported that the healing of problematic diabetic foot wounds improved from 48% to 76% and amputation rates decreased from 45% to 19% in patients treated with hyperbaric oxygen treatments. Hyperbaric oxygen treatment is an effective adjunct to traditional treatments when wound hypoxia may interfere with healing.

65. Pinzur M, Freeland R, Juknelis D: The association between body mass index and foot disorders in diabetic patients. *Foot Ankle Int* 2005;26:375-377.

The authors reviewed the records of 133 patients admitted to a tertiary care facility over a 66-month period. Data allowed calculation of body mass index for 82 of the patients. Forty-six of the 82 patients (56%) were obese, a significantly higher percentage than the percentage of adults nationwide (20.9%, $P < 0.001$). The authors reported a strong correlation between morbid obesity and diabetes foot morbidity.

66. Smith DG, Assai M, Reiber GE, Vath LE, Master J, Wallace C: Minor environmental trauma and lower extremity amputation in high-risk patients with diabetes: Incidence, pivotal events, etiology, and amputation level in a prospectively followed cohort. *Foot Ankle Int* 2003;24:690-695.

In this study, 400 diabetic patients in a footwear trial were followed for a period of 2 years. Eleven patients required lower limb amputation (one amputation was related to footwear). Other causes were minor environmental trauma (six patients), vascular disease (two patients), injury during toenail cutting (one patient), and decubitus ulcer (one patient). The authors concluded that patient education should emphasize the avoidance of environmental trauma, particularly for patients with neuropathy and vascular disease.

67. Wachtel MS: Family poverty accounts for differences in lower-extremity amputation rates of minorities 50 years old or more with diabetes. *J Natl Med Assoc* 2005;97:334-338.

The author reviewed the records of 107 diabetic patients (age 50 years and older) from the same zip code who underwent their first amputations at the same hospital. Statistical analysis of demographic characteristics revealed no differences in age, atherosclerosis severity, sex, or type of amputation. However, the amputees included a significantly higher percentage of African Americans, Hispanic Americans, and other ethnicities. The author concluded that family poverty accounts for higher diabetic amputation rates in those ethnic groups.

68. Smith DG, Ehde DM, Legro MW, Reiber GE, del Aguila M, Boone DA: Phantom limb, residual limb, and back pain after lower extremity amputations. *Clin Orthop Relat Res* 1999;361:29-38.

69. Philbin TM, Leyes M, Sferra JJ, Donley BG: Orthotic and prosthetic devices in partial foot amputations. *Foot Ankle Clin* 2001;6:215-228.

70. Pinzur MS, Stuck RM, Sage R, Hunt N, Rabinovich Z: Syme ankle disarticulation in patients with diabetes. *J Bone Joint Surg Am* 2003;85-A:1667-1672.

The authors retrospectively reviewed 97 Syme amputations performed over an 11-year period. Wounds healed in 82 patients (84.5%). With an ultrasound Doppler ischemic index of 0.5 or transcutaneous partial pressure of oxygen between 20 to 30 mm Hg and serum albumin of 2.5 g/dL, the overall success rate was 88%. Patients who smoke had three times the infection rate of nonsmokers, but smoking did not affect wound healing. Syme amputations allow better ambulation than more proximal amputations.

71. Pinzur MS, Smith D, Osterman H: Syme ankle disarticulation in peripheral vascular disease and diabetic foot infection: The one-stage versus two-stage procedure. *Foot Ankle Int* 1995;16:124-127.

72. Jordan W: Neuritic manifestations in diabetes mellitus. *Arch Intern Med* 1936;57:307.

73. Cavanagh PR, Young MJ, Adams JE, Vickers KL, Boulton AJ: Radiographic abnormalities in the feet of patients with diabetic neuropathy. *Diabetes Care* 1994;17:201-209.

74. Brodsky JW, Kwong PK, Wagner FW, Chambers RB: Patterns of breakdown in the Charcot tarsus of diabetes and relation to treatment. *Orthop Trans* 1987;2:484.

75. Childs M, Armstrong DG, Edelson GW: Is Charcot arthropathy a late sequela of osteoporosis in patients with diabetes mellitus? *J Foot Ankle Surg* 1998;37:437-439.

76. Jirkovská A, Kasalicky P, Boucek P, Hosová J, Skiborá J: Calcaneal ultrasonometry in patients with Charcot osteoarthropathy and its relationship with densitometry in the lumber spine and femoral neck and with markers of bone turnover. *Diabet Med* 2001;18:495-500.

77. Baumhauer JF, O'Keefe RJ, Schon LC, Pinzur MS: Cytokine-induced osteoclastic bone resorption in Charcot arthropathy: An immunohistochemical study. *Foot Ankle Int* 2006;27:797-800.

Tissue samples with Charcot arthropathy were examined to determine cell type and immunoreactivity of known cytokine mediators of bone resorption. Twenty specimens were stained with hematoxylin and eosin, nine with interleukin-1 (IL-1) antibody, nine with tumor necrosis factor alpha antibody, and nine with IL-6 antibody. The author reported increased osteoclastic activity in the environment of cytokine mediators of bone resorption (IL-1, IL-6, and tumor necrosis factor alpha), which may indicate enhanced bone resorption. Pharmacologic agents may alter bone loss and lead to healing.

78. Jeffcoate WJ, Game F, Cavanagh PR: The role of proinflammatory cytokines in the cause of neuropathic osteoarthropathy (acute Charcot foot) in diabetes. *Lancet* 2005;366:2058-2061.

The authors hypothesized that an excessive inflammatory response to trauma leads to the development of acute Charcot foot and a subsequent process results in increases in osteoclasts. The osteoclasts cause bone lysis, resulting in fracture. Proinflammatory cytokines may lead to new markers of Charcot activity and new treatments.

79. Herbst SA, Jones KB, Saltzman CL: Pattern of diabetic neuropathic arthropathy associated with the peripheral bone mineral density. *J Bone Joint Surg Br* 2004;86:378-383.

The authors prospectively studied 55 diabetic patients with Charcot arthropathy with dual-energy x-ray absorptiometry in the affected and unaffected extremities. There were 23 fracture patterns, 23 dislocation patterns, and 9 combined fracture-dislocation patterns. There was an odds ratio of 9.5 for the development of a Charcot joint with a fracture pattern versus dislocation pattern in osteopenic bone. Fracture pattern is associated with deficient bone mineral density, whereas the dislocation pattern is associated with normal bone mineral density.

80. Eichenholtz S: *Charcot Joints*. Springfield, IL, Charles C. Thomas, 1966.

81. Schon LC, Weinfeld SB, Horton GA, Resch S: Radiographic and clinical classification of acquired midfoot tarsus. *Foot Ankle Int* 1998;19:394-404.

82. Saltzman CL, Hagy ML, Zimmerman B, Estin M, Cooper R: How effective is intensive nonoperative initial treatment of patients with diabetes and Charcot arthropathy of the feet? *Clin Orthop Relat Res* 2005;435: 185-190.

    The authors retrospectively reviewed the records of 115 patients (127 limbs) to determine clinical outcome after nonsurgical treatment using an intensive, disease-specific protocol. They reported a 49% risk of recurrent ulceration, a 2.7% annual rate of amputation, and a 23% risk of bracing required for more than 18 months. Level of evidence: IV.

83. Larsen K, Fabrin J, Holstein PE: Incidence and management of ulcers in diabetic Charcot feet. *J Wound Care* 2001;10:323-328.

84. Farber DC, Juliano PJ, Cavanagh PR, Ulbrecht J, Caputo G: Single stage correction with external fixation of the ulcerated foot in individuals with Charcot neuroarthropathy. *Foot Ankle Int* 2002;23:130-134.

85. Cooper PS: Application of external fixators for management of Charcot deformities of the foot and ankle. *Foot Ankle Clin* 2002;7:207-254.

86. Simon SR, Tejwani SG, Wilson DL, Santner TJ, Denniston NL: Arthrodesis as an early alternative to nonoperative management of Charcot arthropathy of the diabetic foot. *J Bone Joint Surg Am* 2000;82:939-950.

87. Pinzur M: Surgical versus accommodative treatment for Charcot arthropathy of the midfoot. *Foot Ankle Int* 2004;25:545-549.

    Patients with Charcot arthropathy were treated with surgery (nonplantigrade feet) and accommodative orthotic methods (plantigrade feet) with the goal of long-term management with standard accommodative shoes and custom orthoses. Over a 6-year period, 198 patients (201 feet) were treated. With a minimum 1-year follow-up, more than 50% of the patients with midfoot Charcot arthropathy achieved the goal without surgery.

88. Pinzur MS, Sostak MD: Surgical stabilization of nonplantigrade Charcot arthropathy of the midfoot. *Am J Orthop* 2007;36:361-365.

    Fifty-one patients with Charcot arthropathy between the talonavicular and tarsometatarsal joints were treated with surgical stabilization. The treatment goal was to allow patients to walk wearing commercially available accommodative footwear while remaining free of ulcers and infections. At a mean follow-up of 33.2 months, 44 patients achieved the goal. The authors present a decision-making algorithm to help orthopaedic surgeons avoid surgical procedures in patients without deformity.

89. Pinzur MS: Neutral ring fixation for high-risk nonplantigrade Charcot midfoot deformity. *Foot Ankle Int* 2007;28:961-966.

    The Charcot treatment algorithm of Pinzur and associates was used to treat 26 diabetic patients with multiple comorbidities and nonplantigrade midfoot deformities. Using a neutrally applied, three-level ring external fixator along with surgical correction of deformities, 24 patients achieved ambulatory status with accommodative footwear at 1-year follow-up.

90. Dalla Paola L, Volpe A, Varotto D, et al: Use of a retrograde nail for ankle arthrodesis in Charcot neuroarthropathy: A limb salvage procedure. *Foot Ankle Int* 2007; 28:967-970.

    The authors achieved limb salvage in 18 patients with Charcot neuroarthropathy and unstable ankles who were treated with retrograde transcalcaneal nailing.

91. Dhawan V, Spratt KF, Pinzur MS, Baumhauer J, Rudicel S, Saltzman CL: Reliability of AOFAS diabetic foot questionnaire in Charcot arthropathy: Stability, internal consistency, and measurable difference. *Foot Ankle Int* 2005;26:717-731.

    Patients with Charcot arthropathy completed a questionnaire that assessed health-related quality of life, and the researchers completed an observational survey. Fifty-seven patients completed the initial questionnaire and returned at 3-month follow-up to complete a second questionnaire. Patients with Charcot arthropathy scored much lower on the physical component areas than the reported scores for other diseases, including diabetes. It is important to consider quality of life when assessing the effectiveness of Charcot treatments. Further studies to create an effective assessment questionnaire are needed.

Chapter 23

Charcot-Marie-Tooth Disease and the Cavovarus Foot

Wolfram Wenz, MD   Thomas Dreher, MD

Introduction

Charcot-Marie-Tooth disease is also known as hereditary motor and sensory neuropathy (HMSN) or peroneal muscular atrophy. This disease was first described in 1886 by Jean-Martin Charcot, a celebrated professor of neurology, and his student, Pierre Marie, a famous French neurologist.[1] In the same year, Howard Henry Tooth, an English physician, published an independent description of peroneal muscular atrophy.[2] In 1889, a German neurologist, Johann Hoffmann, confirmed that this disease was a disorder of the peripheral nervous system.[3]

Neurologic Characteristics and Genetic Basis

Charcot-Marie-Tooth disease is a heterogeneous inherited neuropathy that is characterized by the loss of muscle tissue and touch sensation, predominantly in the feet and legs but also occurring in the hands and arms. It is one of the most common inherited neurologic disorders, affecting approximately 36 in 100,000 people, and is the most common inherited disorder of the peripheral nerves.[4-6] Charcot-Marie-Tooth disease is caused by the absence or malfunction of essential molecules (caused by mutations in the genes coding these molecules) that are necessary for physiologic function of the nerves. The dysfunction can be located either in

the axon or the myelin sheath of the nerve cell. Charcot-Marie-Tooth disease is the most common cause of cavovarus feet.[7]

Charcot-Marie-Tooth disease belongs to the group of HMSNs and includes both types 1 and 2.[8] HMSN type 1 is the most common, affecting approximately 80% of patients with Charcot-Marie-Tooth disease.[6,7] Type 1 HMSN is transmitted as an autosomal dominant disorder (Figure 1) and causes demyelination, which diffusely and homogeneously lowers the nerve conduction velocity below 38 m/s.[9] The measurement of nerve conduction velocities is the most important primary tool for diagnosing this disorder.

Classification

Charcot-Marie-Tooth disease can be classified into primary demyelinating neuropathies and axonal neuropathies; however, recent studies elucidate the frequent intermingling of the pathologies of these two classes because of the dependence and close cellular interaction of Schwann cells and neurons in regulating myelin formation.[10,11] The interaction between demyelinating Schwann cells and fibroblasts causes the expression of abnormal axonal structure and function. It appears that the weakness and sensory loss in patients with Charcot-Marie-Tooth disease is a result of axonal degradation. Axonal dysfunction also can be induced by

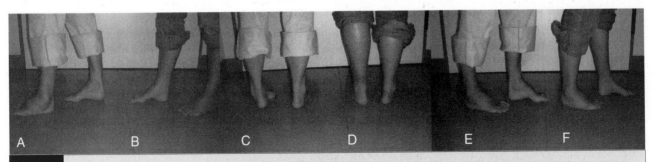

Figure 1 HMSN type I affects approximately 80% of patients with Charcot-Marie-Tooth disease. Its autosomal dominant transmission is illustrated in clinical photographs of the feet of a 63-year-old woman (**A, C,** and **E**) and her 36-year-old daughter (**B, D,** and **F**). The mother's foot deformity is more severe and has progressed further compared with the daughter's foot deformity.

American Academy of Orthopaedic Surgeons

5: Neuromuscular Disease

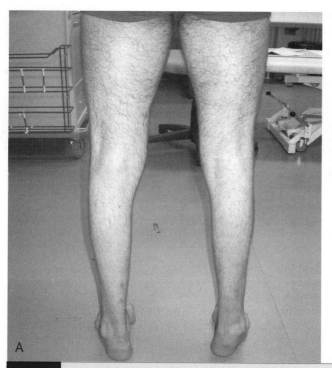
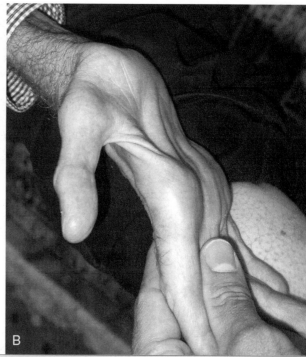

Figure 2 **A,** There is typically a discrepancy between the relatively strong thigh muscles and early degenerated shank muscles in a patient with Charcot-Marie-Tooth disease. **B,** The atrophy of the upper limb muscle leads to the typical "monkey hand."

demyelinating Schwann cells.[12] Penetrance of the genes in involved families is 30% in the first decade and essentially complete by the middle of the third decade.[13] Patients with Charcot-Marie-Tooth disease show substantial variations in clinical penetrance within the same family.[14] The gene defect leads to malfunction of the peripheral nerves, resulting in atrophy of the corresponding supplied muscles. The peroneal nerve is one of the first nerves to be affected. In an examination of the distribution patterns of muscular atrophy using CT analyses, two patterns of affliction were found: earlier involvement of the peroneal muscle and primary involvement of the tibial nerves and corresponding muscles.[15]

Clinical Presentation, Signs, and Symptoms

Patients with Charcot-Marie-Tooth disease most commonly present for treatment because of ankle and foot deformities and weakness, painful callosities, difficulty with shoe wear, and ankle instability.[16,17] The signs of distal wasting and a proximal sparing pattern of muscular atrophy are typical characteristics of the disease and result in an "inverted champagne bottle" appearance in the lower limbs (**Figure 2, A**). Typically, symmetric bilateral involvement occurs, first in the intrinsic foot muscles, followed by the peroneal muscle group, the extensor group (anterior tibial muscle and long toe extensors), and lastly by the calf muscles and the posterior tibial muscle. Usually, early drop foot occurs be-

cause of weakness of the anterior tibialis muscle, which may be compensated for or substituted by the long toe flexors in patients with remaining function. During ambulation, this extensor substitution pattern is seen mainly in the swing phase of the gait cycle. Another common problem encountered during ambulation is caused by the varus component of the hindfoot, which affects stance phase stability by increasing the tendency for ankle twisting. Dorsiflexion also may be limited by bony impingement of the talus and the anterior aspect of the tibia or by a hindfoot equinus component (often caused by short calf muscles).

Symptoms of Charcot-Marie-Tooth disease usually begin in late childhood or early adulthood, but symptom onset and progression of the disease can vary among patients. As the disease progresses, muscular atrophy with weakness in the hands and forearms affects many patients, usually near the end of the adolescent period. Atrophy of the intrinsic hand muscles leads to the intrinsic-minus of the fingers and to the loss of thumb opposition (Figure 2, B). Involvement of the upper extremity impairs the patient's ability to use supportive walking aids; therefore, providing optimal treatment of the foot deformities is essential.

In patients with severe Charcot-Marie-Tooth disease, distal accented involvement of the lower extremity often occurs in early childhood. Dysplasia of the hip(s) and/or scoliosis should be considered when planning further examinations and treatment. Clinical and radiographic examinations of the pelvis and spine are suggested for patients with severe forms of the disease.

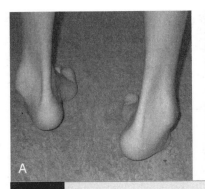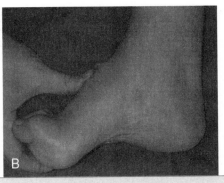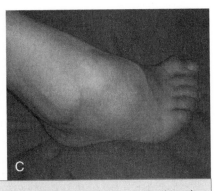

Figure 3 The typical anatomic characteristics of the cavovarus foot in Charcot-Marie-Tooth disease are shown. **A,** Equinus deformity of the ankle, hindfoot varus, external rotation of the talus, retraction of the lateral malleolus, medial dislocation of the Chopart joint, and cavus deformity. **B,** Plantar flexed position of the first column. **C,** Pronation and adduction of the forefoot and claw toes.

In a study of 66 patients with Charcot-Marie-Tooth disease, 31 patients had involvement of the hands and 36 patients had kyphoscoliosis.[18] The deformities in patients with Charcot-Marie-Tooth disease tend to worsen during periods of growth, as is the situation in patients with other neurologic disorders such as cerebral palsy or myelomeningocele.

In addition to muscular atrophy, the sensory and autonomic nervous systems also are involved, leading to common disorders such as ataxia; tremor; loss of vibratory sensation, two-point discrimination, and proprioception; hand and upper limb weakness; and scoliosis. The loss of sensation in the feet with the concomitant foot deformity often results in chronic ulceration. Early loss of Achilles tendon reflex is common, whereas the patellar tendon reflex survives for a longer period.

The Cavovarus Foot

The most common foot deformity seen in patients with Charcot-Marie-Tooth disease is a cavovarus foot with concomitant claw toes. Charcot-Marie-Tooth disease is the most common cause of cavovarus foot deformity. A 2006 study reported that 116 of 148 children (78%) (mean age, 10 years; range, 3 to 18 years) with bilateral cavovarus deformity had Charcot-Marie-Tooth disease.[7]

Anatomy

The foot deformity in Charcot-Marie-Tooth disease is characterized by a combination of hindfoot varus (subtalar), forefoot equinus (cavus), and plantar flexion of the first metatarsal, which can result in forefoot valgus.[16,19] The cavus component is characterized by increased plantar flexion of the forefoot and midfoot in relationship to the hindfoot. In most patients, there is concomitant limited dorsiflexion of the ankle joint (hindfoot equinus, dorsal impingement), and forefoot/midfoot adductus and/or pronatus occurs.

Pathomechanics

The foot deformity develops slowly because of the muscular imbalance and the influence of the ground reaction force (**Figure 3**). In early childhood, a slight valgus foot with shortened calf muscles may be the only clinical finding; remodeling into a cavovarus foot occurs during the following years. There is a typical pattern of muscular involvement. The pathogenesis of cavovarus deformities in Charcot-Marie-Tooth disease can be attributed to the imbalance between the strong peroneus longus and weak anterior tibialis muscle couple, and strong tibialis posterior and weak peroneus brevis couple.[19] MRI has shown that the ratio of the cross-sectional area of the lateral to anterior compartments in patients with Charcot-Marie-Tooth disease with a cavovarus foot is twice that of healthy individuals. This finding indicates a relative imbalance between the bulk of the peroneus longus compared with the tibialis anterior.[20] This discrepancy is present in most patients with Charcot-Marie-Tooth disease and cavovarus foot deformity (**Figure 4**).

Although the calf muscles, the posterior tibialis muscle, and the long toe flexors are spared in the early stages of the disease, the dorsiflexors (anterior tibialis muscle, long toe extensors, and the peroneus tertius muscle) and the everters (long and short peroneal muscles) of the foot show early involvement. The muscular imbalance between the peroneus brevis and the posterior tibialis muscles leads to a medial shift of the talonavicular and the calcaneocuboid complex and locks the subtalar joint in supination. At the same time, the weakness of the anterior tibialis muscle and the concomitant relative overactivity of the peroneus longus muscle force the forefoot into increased pronation. The increased plantar flexion of the first metatarsal bone (resulting from forefoot pronation) augments hindfoot inversion during standing or the stance phase of walking. Severe hindfoot varus stresses the ankle joint and causes lateral opening in situations of prostrated compensation. The loss of activity in the short foot muscles leads to claw toes, which are augmented by extensor substitution (**Figure 5**).

Because of a weak anterior tibial tendon that leads to drop foot, the long toe extensors are activated to compensate for this deficiency (extensor substitution). The toes are hyperextended in the metatarsophalangeal joints. At the same time, the long toe flexors pull the end phalangeal bone into plantar flexion, leading to claw toes. The higher the muscular imbalance, the broader is the resulting foot deformity. All components of the cavovarus foot in Charcot-Marie-Tooth disease are flexible in the early stage of the disease and become rigid after a period of years.

Diagnosis

The diagnosis of Charcot-Marie-Tooth disease is based on the results of a physical examination, neurologic assessment, family history, and diagnostic tests, which include electromyography, nerve conduction velocity studies, and/or DNA analysis.[9,21] Genetic markers have been identified for some but not all forms of the disease. The diagnosis is established by an electromyographic examination showing decreased velocity of nerve impulse conduction and increased charging time of the nerve. Biopsy of the sural nerve represents the ultimate diagnostic test for many patients with Charcot-Marie-Tooth disease. The presence of several well-formed "onion bulbs" consisting of Schwann-cell extensions on nerve biopsy is a typical finding in type 1 HMSN (**Figure 6**). The differential diagnoses for cavovarus foot are shown in **Table 1**.

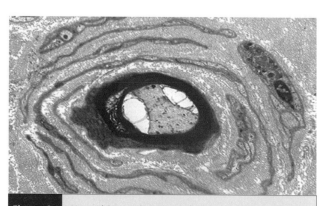

Figure 4 MRI scan shows typical degeneration of the anterior compartments involving the tibialis anterior, the hallux extensors, and part of the peroneal tendons. The ratio of the cross-sectional area of the lateral to anterior compartments in a patient with Charcot-Marie-Tooth disease is twice that found in healthy individuals. (*Reproduced with permission from Döderlein L, Wenz W, Schneider U: Pathogenere der hohlfußes, in Döderlein L, Wenz W: Der Hohlfuß. Berlin, Germany, Springer-Verlag, 2007, vol 3, pp 25-28.*)

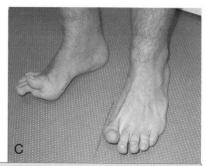

Figure 6 Nerve biopsy showing Schwann cell extensions that are a typical characteristic in type 1 HMSN. (*Courtesy of Dimitri Agamanolis, Akron, OH. http://www.neuropathologyweb.org.*)

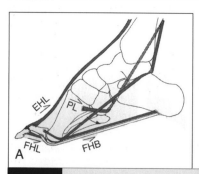
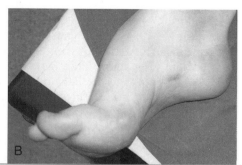

Figure 5 Illustration (**A**) and clinical photograph (**B**) showing the pathomechanics of a cavovarus foot. The muscular imbalance between the peroneus brevis and the tibialis posterior muscles leads to a medial shift of the Chopart joint. The subtalar joint is locked in supination. The weakness of the tibialis anterior muscle and the relative overactivity of the peroneus longus (PL) muscle pronate the forefoot and lead to increased plantar flexion of the first metatarsal bone. This augments hindfoot inversion while standing or during the stance phase of ambulation. The loss of activity in the short foot muscles causes claw toes, which are augmented by extensor substitution, shown in (**C**). EHL = extensor hallucis longus, FHL = flexor hallucis longus, FHB = flexor hallucis brevis. (*Reproduced with permission from Döderlein L, Wenz W, Schneider U: Pathogenere der hohlfußes, in Döderlein L, Wenz W: Der Hohlfuß. Berlin, Germany, Springer-Verlag, 2007, vol 3, pp 25-28.*)

Clinical Examination

The clinical examination of the foot includes inspection in all three planes and functional, muscular, and special tests, including the Coleman block test, the first metatarsal redression test, and the Silfverskiöld test (**Figures 7** through **9**). The skin also should be examined for ulcerations. The clinical examination findings of cavovarus foot are shown in **Figure 10**.

Assessing the actions of individual muscles is ineffective and inappropriate because muscle action is primarily synergistic.[22] The most important muscle groups should be tested (dorsiflexors, plantar flexors, everters, inverters, toe flexors, and extensors) to obtain information about muscular imbalance, which is essential in planning tendon transfers. Another important aspect of the clinical examination is the dynamic observation of gait, which should include the identification of abnormalities during the stance and swing phases of the gait (**Table 2**).

Imaging Studies

The views and findings of the radiographic evaluation for diagnosis and preoperative planning are shown in **Table 3** and **Figure 11**. CT scans and three-dimensional reconstruction images may be helpful in evaluating patients with severe forms of the disease (**Figure 12**). Dynamic pedobarography is a useful objective method to measure the dynamic pressure distribution pattern of the foot during ambulation (**Figure 13**). It is used to identify the main pressure points of the foot and the abnormal distribution caused by deformity.[23] In addition to dynamic pedobarography, three-dimensional foot analysis in instrumented gait analysis (for example, the Heidelberg Foot Model) is an important tool for surgical planning (**Figures 14** and **15**).

Nonsurgical Treatment

Nonsurgical treatment of the cavovarus foot in Charcot-Marie-Tooth disease is usually unsuccessful because it does not prevent disease progression and further deformity.[24,25] Nonsurgical treatment merely compensates for the functional problems occurring in pes cavovarus and does not prevent its progression. The most common nonsurgical treatment options are the use of orthopaedic arch supports (reducing the head of the first metatarsal bone and providing a smooth bedding) and custom-made orthopaedic shoes.

Surgical Treatment

The goals of surgical treatment are to restore normal function of the foot and create a plantigrade foot. Because the disease progresses rapidly in many patients, early surgical correction of the deformity in the second decade of life should be considered. Tendon transfers are used for soft-tissue balancing. If active function cannot be achieved, tenodesis is needed to stabilize the foot. Single-event surgical treatment of both feet is possible and should be discussed with the patient along with information on the difficulties of postoperative re-

Table 1

Differential Diagnoses of Cavovarus Foot

Central Nervous System
Cerebral palsy
Traumatic brain injuries
Stroke
Multiple sclerosis
Friedreich ataxia (central symptoms, ataxia)
Roussy-Levy syndrome (tremor of the hands)
Malignant or benign tumors (angioma, lipoma)
Refsum-syndrome (heredopathia atactica polyneuritiformis)

Spinal Cord and Peripheral Nervous System
Myelomeningocele (spina bifida)
Syringomyelia
Diastematomyelia
Poliomyelitis (not progressive and no sensory deficiency)
Spinal dysraphism
Malignant or benign spinal cord tumor
Tethered cord syndrome
Spinal muscular atrophy
Polyneuropathy
Dejerine-Sottas interstitial hypertrophic neuritis (HMSN type 3)

Other
Muscular dystrophy
Arthrogryposis multiplex congenita
Compartment syndrome
Burn injuries
Rheumatic diseases
Diabetic foot syndrome

Idiopathic
Diagnosis of exclusion

covery in bilateral non–weight-bearing casts. To achieve optimal treatment results, extensive and thorough preoperative planning consisting of clinical and radiologic examinations and functional and dynamic testing is essential.

Soft-tissue procedures are performed before bony procedures. In patients with mildly deformed feet, soft-tissue procedures may correct foot deformities without the need for bony procedures. In more severely deformed feet, this approach will diminish the amount of bony correction necessary. For optimal soft-tissue balancing, tendon transfers are generally sutured after the bony procedures. Performing bony procedures without soft-tissue balancing will cause recurrence of the deformity.

Surgical procedures used in the treatment of cavovarus foot include the Steindler, split posterior tibial tendon transfer, modified Jones, Cole, Lambrinudi, and Hibbs procedures; Achilles tendon lengthening; and Chopart fusion.

The first step in treating cavovarus feet is the Steindler procedure (dissection of the planter aponeurosis, which corrects the soft-tissue component of the cavus, especially in patients with mild deformity.[26] In patients with more severe deformity, the Steindler procedure is

5: Neuromuscular Disease

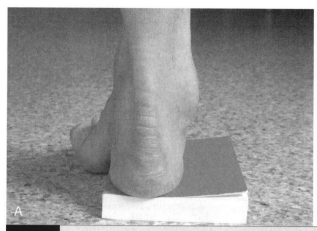
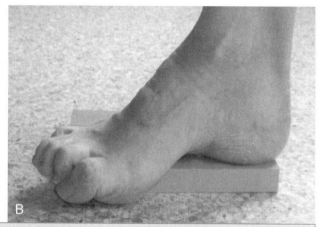

Figure 7   Clinical photographs showing the Coleman block test to determine the compensation of the hindfoot in fixed fore-foot pronation and compensation of the plantar flexion of the first metatarsal bone. **A,** The patient's foot is placed on a block 2.5 to 6 cm thick, with the heel and lateral border of the foot bearing weight on the block. **B,** The first, second, and third metatarsals are allowed to hang freely into plantar flexion and pronation.

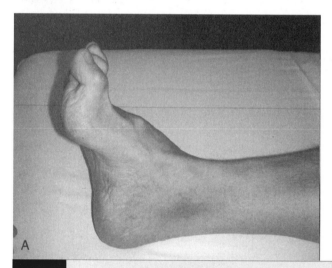
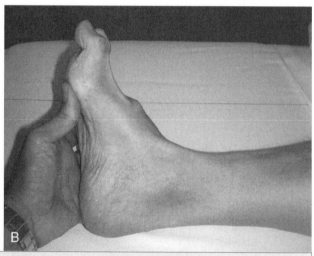

Figure 8   **A** and **B,** First metatarsal redression testing is shown. The flexibility of the plantar-flexed first metatarsal bone is tested by manual extension and pressure on the first metatarsophalangeal joint.

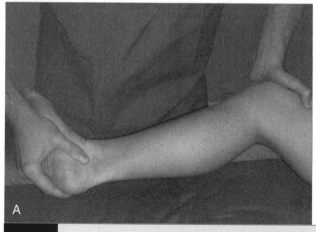
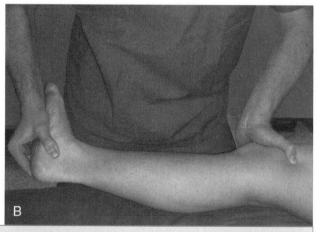

Figure 9   The Silfverskiöld test should be performed preoperatively and intraoperatively to evaluate knee flexion **(A)** and extension **(B)** to detect equinus deformity and for the differentiation between gastrocnemius and soleus muscle involvement.

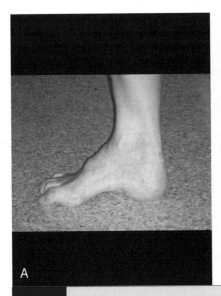
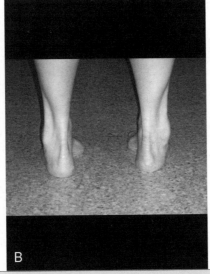
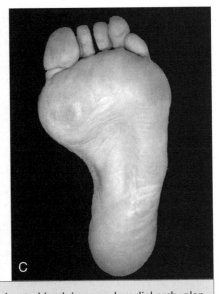

Figure 10 Clinical examination findings of a cavovarus foot. **A,** Medial view shows elevated heel, increased medial arch, plantar flexion of the first metatarsal bone, and claw toe deformity of the first column. **B,** Posterior view shows varus deformity of the heel, prominent lateral malleolus, pronation of the forefoot, elevation of the heel, and "hello big toe" sign. **C,** Plantar view shows convex lateral border of the foot, prominent basis of the fifth metatarsal bone, increased weight bearing of the heads of the first and fifth metatarsal bones, increased skin weal, and hindfoot equinus (missing weight bearing of the heel).

Table 2

Gait Analysis

Gait Phase	Abnormality Observed
Stance	The ankle position at initial contact (hindfoot equinus, limited dorsiflexion)
	Hyperextension of the knee (genu recurvatum)
	An overload of the lateral border of the foot (varus deformity)
	Instability during loading response of the gait cycle
	Limited second rocker movement caused by reduced dorsiflexion in midstance
	Internal rotation moment caused by second rocker movement over the lateral border of the foot
Swing	Drop foot (weak anterior tibial muscle) with foot clearance problems
	Compensation for drop foot (increased knee flexion and/or hip flexion, circumduction)
	Equinus foot at the end of the swing phase (leads to forefoot initial contact)
	Extensor substitution (compensation of decreased dorsiflexion, leads to claw toes)

Table 3

Radiologic Findings in Cavovarus Foot

View	Findings
Sagittal	Posterior shift of the lateral malleolus
	Longitudinal talus axis parallel to axis of the calcaneus
	Seemingly shortened calcaneus cause by the varus position
	Decreased distance between the navicular bone and the medial malleolus
	Visible calcaneocuboid joint, normally overlaid by the talonavicular joint
	Plantar-flexed and prominent first metatarsal bone
	Claw toes
	Posterior subtalar joint projected horizontally
	Opened sinus tarsi (sinus tarsi window)
	Talus-first metatarsal angle
	Calcaneus-first metatarsal angle
	Calcaneal pitch
AP	Longitudinal axis of the talus parallel to the calcaneus bone axis
	Medial shift of the talonavicular joint and, in some instances, shift of the calcaneocuboid joint
	Seemingly shortened appearance of the first metatarsal bone caused by its plantar-flexed position
	Overlapping of the metatarsal bones
AP ankle	Varus deformity of the hindfoot, gaping in the ankle in severe varus
	Osteophytes
	Osteoarthritis

5: Neuromuscular Disease

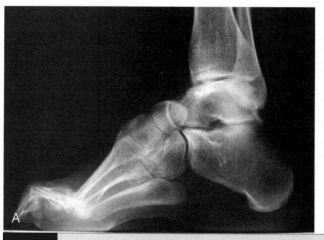
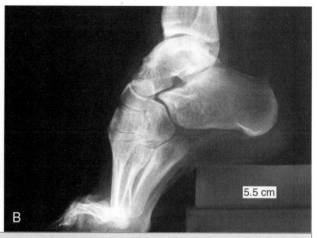

5.5 cm

Figure 11   Radiographic views of a cavovarus foot. Sagittal view **(A)** and sagittal view with the foot on a block **(B)**.

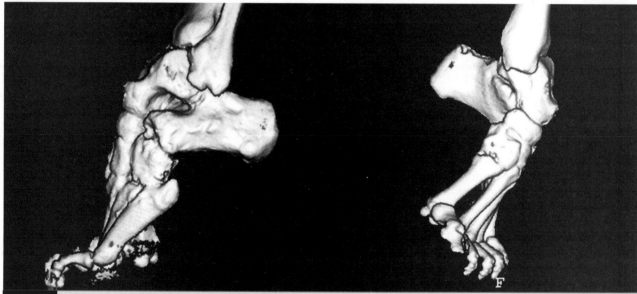

Figure 12   Three-dimensional reconstruction CT scans can be helpful in preoperative planning in patients with severe Charcot-Marie-Tooth deformities. These CT scans are of a 25-year-old patient with a severe equinocavovarus foot deformity.

often inadequate for total correction. Additional bony procedures, such as a Cole osteotomy or a Chopart/ triple fusion, are needed.[27,28] Next, the tendon transfers are advanced. The purpose of the split posterior tibial tendon transfer procedure is to eliminate the overactive posterior tibial muscle, which is responsible for hindfoot varus, and to augment the usually weak dorsiflexor muscles.[29] After advancement of the tendon transfers, correction of the first column should be accomplished with a modified Jones procedure, which eliminates the overactive extensor hallucis longus muscle and corrects the claw toe deformity of the first toe.[30,31] Before suturing the backward transfer of the extensor hallucis longus tendon, the correction is tested. If full correction of first metatarsal flexion is not possible with the modified Jones procedure, an addi-

tional extension osteotomy of the first metatarsal bone should be performed at the conclusion of the surgical procedure.[32] Bony correction of the midfoot and hindfoot are then performed with attention to the dominating deformities of the varus and the cavus components. Sparing and resecting procedures may be used. Persistent cavus after the Steindler procedure can be corrected by a Cole[27] procedure or Chopart fusion.[27,28] The sparing Cole procedure is indicated in patients with a stable Chopart joint, isolated cavus without hindfoot varus, and/or more distally located apex of the cavus. If the cavus affects only the first column, an extension osteotomy of the first metatarsal bone will achieve adequate correction.[32] In patients with severe involvement and/or instability, Chopart fusion with a dorsally based wedge resection is required. In patients with moderate

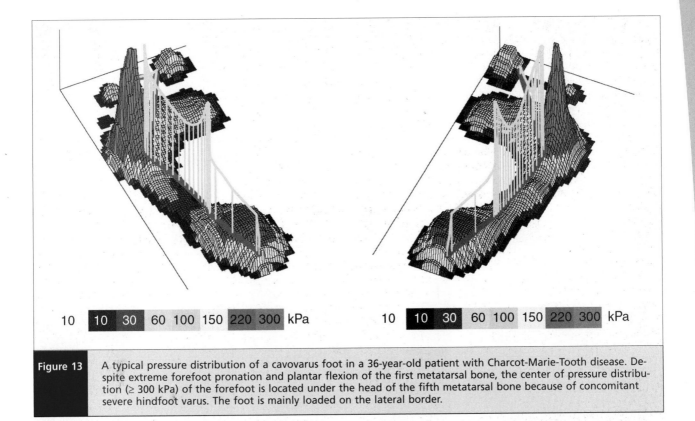

10 | 10 | 30 | 60 | 100 | 150 | 220 | 300 | kPa   10 | 10 | 30 | 60 | 100 | 150 | 220 | 300 | kPa

Figure 13 A typical pressure distribution of a cavovarus foot in a 36-year-old patient with Charcot-Marie-Tooth disease. Despite extreme forefoot pronation and plantar flexion of the first metatarsal bone, the center of pressure distribution (≥ 300 kPa) of the forefoot is located under the head of the fifth metatarsal bone because of concomitant severe hindfoot varus. The foot is mainly loaded on the lateral border.

hindfoot varus and a stable subtalar joint, this component can be corrected by a Dwyer osteotomy if the hindfoot cannot be totally redressed and correction of hindfoot varus cannot be achieved by tendon transfer.[33] In more severe deformities, triple arthrodesis is the only procedure that can possibly achieve acceptable correction.[28] This procedure is key for successful management of very severe pes cavus resulting from Charcot-Marie-Tooth disease. In patients with ventral impingement of the talus on the tibia and limited dorsiflexion or extreme hindfoot equinus, a modified Lambrinudi procedure is appropriate.[34] After bony correction of the midfoot and hindfoot, an intraoperative Silfverskiöld test should be performed to identify residual hindfoot equinus. An additional Achilles tendon lengthening can be performed if both calf muscles are shortened and equinus is severe and fixed. In patients with flexible and mild equinus, an intramuscular recession (Baumann technique) is indicated.[35]

After correcting deformities of the hindfoot and midfoot, deformities of the forefoot should be treated. If there are shortened long toe flexors (once hidden because of equinus deformity), intramuscular lengthening of the long digitorum and hallucis flexor tendons can be performed through the incision used for Achilles tendon lengthening. If the second through fifth toes are clawed because of overactivity of the extrinsic (long extensor and flexor digitorum) muscles in comparison with the intrinsic muscle groups, the Hibbs procedure should be used.[36] An extension osteotomy of the first metatarsal bone, which corrects the flexion deformity

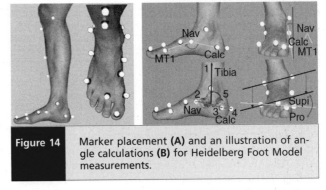

Figure 14 Marker placement **(A)** and an illustration of angle calculations **(B)** for Heidelberg Foot Model measurements.

of the first column, is then performed. Before wound closure, all tendon transfers are sutured with the foot held in the corrected position.

Steindler Procedure
In the Steindler procedure, a slightly dorsally convex, 3- to 4-cm long incision is made at the medial border of the foot.[26] After retraction of the subcutaneous tissue, the origin of the plantar aponeurosis at the calcaneus and the short flexor digitorum muscle are exposed as proximally as possible and released sharply with a strong scissors. A redression grasp is needed to obtain the lengthening effect.

Modified Split Posterior Tibial Tendon Transfer Procedure
In a modified split posterior tibial tendon transfer procedure (**Figure 16**), a 3- to 4-cm long incision is made

5: Neuromuscular Disease

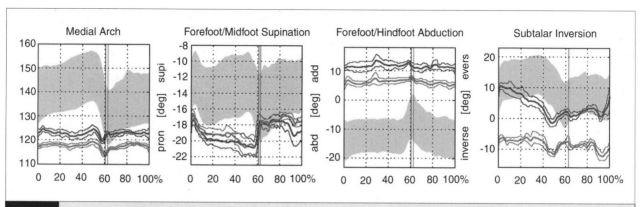

Figure 15 Graphs showing typical motion curves for different foot segments in three planes. This tool is important for objective recording of dynamic data for outcome evaluation and is helpful in determining the need for surgery.

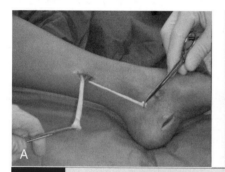
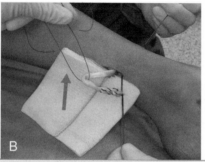
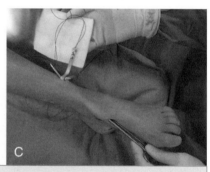

Figure 16 The split posterior tibial tendon transfer procedure. **A,** Distal release, proximal exposition of the posterior tibial tendon, and bisection. **B,** Slim corn forceps are driven through the interosseous membrane behind the tibia, and both tendon halves are transferred to the extensor compartment. Security thread for the backward transfer is shown (*arrow*). **C,** One half of the tibialis posterior tendon is transferred to the medial border of the foot through the tendon sheath of the anterior tibial muscle with a slim corn forceps.

over the distal insertion of the posterior tibial tendon at the navicular bone.[29] The tendon is loaded on an Overholt clamp and released at its insertion point, with the scalpel positioned as distally as possible. Another 3-cm skin incision is made at the distal medial shank, three to four fingers proximal to the ankle, directly behind the posterior edge of the tibial bone. After incising the fascia, the tendon of the long toe flexor muscle is identified and retracted. The posterior tibial muscle is exposed, retracted, and bisected; both halves are tagged with No. 1 polyglycolic acid sutures.

A third skin incision 3 cm in length is made on the lateral side of the shank at the same height directly ventral to the fibula. The fascia is incised and retracted. Subsequently, a slim corn forceps is driven through the interosseous membrane, from the medial wound to the lateral wound. A single thread is grabbed with the forceps and pulled through the medial wound. Next, the tag sutures of the two halves of the posterior tibial tendon can be contrived to the loop, and the tendons are transferred to the lateral wound by pulling the end of the single thread. The anterior tibial tendon is then exposed with a 2- to 3-cm skin incision. When planning this incision, the need for talonavicular fusion should be considered. If fusion is needed, the incision should

run into the proximal incision, where the posterior tibial tendon was previously exposed. The slim corn forceps is driven through the sheath of the anterior tibial tendon toward the extensor compartment, and the tagging suture strings of one half of the posterior tibial tendon are grabbed and transferred distally. An additional skin incision is made on the back of the foot, exposing the long toe extensor tendons. The other half of the posterior tibial tendon is transferred using the same technique. The peroneal tendons are exposed, and the peroneus brevis tendon is tagged with a vessel loop. Any other needed concomitant procedures should be performed at this point, before suturing the tendon transfers. At the end of the procedure, the medial half of the posterior tibial tendon is sutured to the anterior tibial tendon, and the lateral half is sutured to the peroneus brevis tendon. It is important that the foot is held in the correct position. Tension on the transfer should not be too great to avoid overcorrection; however, tension should be adequate to achieve the desired effect.

The Modified Jones Procedure

In the modified Jones procedure (**Figure 17**), a crosswise S-shaped skin incision is made over the first meta-

5: Neuromuscular Disease

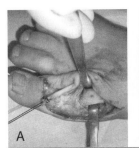
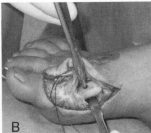
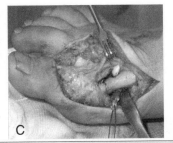
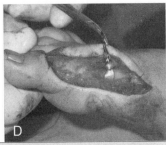

Figure 17 The modified Jones procedure. **A,** Exposition of the extensor hallucis longus tendon, tagging, distal release, and exposure of the first metatarsal bone. **B,** A hole is drilled through the first metatarsal bone. **C,** The extensor hallucis longus tendon is transferred through the hole with a strong needle. **D,** With the first column in a dorsiflexed position, the transferred tendon is sutured with itself.

tarsophalangeal joint, extending to the first interphalangeal joint distally and to the base of the first metatarsal bone.[30,31] The extensor hallucis tendon is exposed, tagged distally with No. 0 polyglycolic acid sutures, and released as distally as possible. The first interphalangeal joint is opened by an incision of the capsule, and the articular cartilage is removed from both joint surfaces. The fusion is fixed in neutral extension and rotation by the retrograde drilling of two crossing Kirschner wires (K-wires) (1.4 mm for children; 1.8 mm for adults). The first metatarsal bone is then exposed subperiosteally with two fibula Hohmann levers. A 3.2-mm hole is drilled centrally in the first metatarsal bone. The tagged tendon of the long extensor hallucis muscle is transferred through the hole with a large needle. After all bony procedures are completed, the tendon is sutured with itself using No. 1 polyglycolic thread; the distal end can be readapted to the periosteum of the distal phalanx as a tenodesis to avoid postoperative flexion position of the hallux. If plantar flexion of the first metatarsal bone cannot be satisfactorily corrected, an extension osteotomy of the metatarsal bone is needed.

Fusion of the Chopart Joint/Triple-Fusion/Lambrinudi Procedures

The lateral approach is made by a crosswise S-shaped skin incision, beginning 2 cm distal and dorsal to the lateral malleolus, which arches to the navicular bone, distal to the palpable head of the talus. The sural nerve bundle is exposed and retracted. The origin of the short extensor digitorum muscle at the anterior process of the calcaneus is released with an L-shaped incision and detached with a concave chisel. The Chopart joint is then exposed by inserting two retractors. The fusion can be a conservative resection of the cartilage or a correcting wedge resection. If cavus cannot be corrected by the Steindler procedure, a dorsally based wedge resection is needed. If there is extreme forefoot/midfoot adduction, the wedge is more laterally based. The conservative resection of the cartilage is done with a concave chisel by sparing the joint contour. For wedge resection, an oscillating power bone saw is used. After complete release of the Chopart joint, the cavus foot can be cor-

rected manually, and the navicular bone can be centered to the head of the talus. The transfixation can be done using four K-wires (two through the talonavicular joint and two through the calcaneocuboid joint); alternatively, fixation can be achieved with screws. If complete correction is not possible with Chopart fusion, especially in patients with severe hindfoot varus, triple fusion is necessary. In the case of ventral impingement with limited dorsiflexion or extreme hindfoot equinus, an additional modified Lambrinudi procedure should be performed.

For both procedures, the sinus tarsi is freed from all soft-tissue structures (interosseous ligaments and fat), including the talocalcaneal interosseous ligament. An arthrodesis spreader is inserted, and the subtalar joint is exposed. Cartilage is removed with a concave chisel or oscillating bone saw if wedge resection is needed. Severe hindfoot varus is corrected by removing a laterally based wedge from the subtalar joint (**Figure 18**). If a Lambrinudi fusion is needed, a ventrally based wedge is removed from the subtalar joint (**Figure 19**). The first osteotomy runs parallel to the ankle joint line through the head of the talus bone, ending in the posterior edge of the subtalar joint, and should not include more than 50% of the talus head. The next osteotomy runs parallel to the subtalar joint line through the calcaneal bone and unites with the first cut, forming a ventrally based wedge with its apex in the posterior aspect of the subtalar joint. The subtalar and the Chopart joint fragments are then repositioned. The cavus, the hindfoot varus, and the equinus components should be correctable. Osteosynthesis can be performed with six K-wires (two for the talonavicular joint, two for the calcaneocuboid joint, and two for the subtalar joint). Alternatively, fixation can be achieved with screws or an angle locking plate.

Cole Osteotomy

The surgical approach for a Cole osteotomy is a lazy-S incision at the lateral border of the foot.[27] The sural nerve is exposed and retracted. An incision between the sheath of the peroneal tendons and the short extensor digitorum muscle belly is made and the cuboid bone is exposed. The osteotomies are accomplished with an os-

5: Neuromuscular Disease

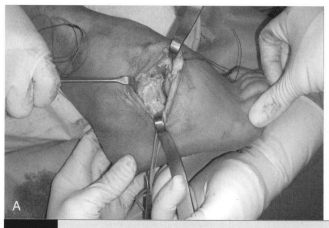

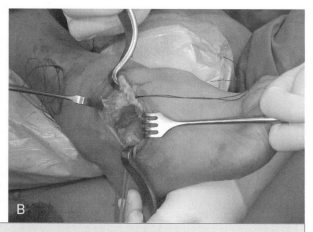

Figure 18 Triple arthrodesis. **A,** The calcaneocuboid and talonavicular joint viewed from a lateral approach. The anterior process of the calcaneus is released and retracted. **B,** The talus and calcaneus after resection of a laterally based and dorsally based bony wedge for hindfoot varus and cavus correction.

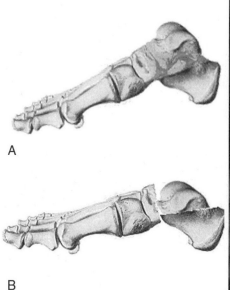

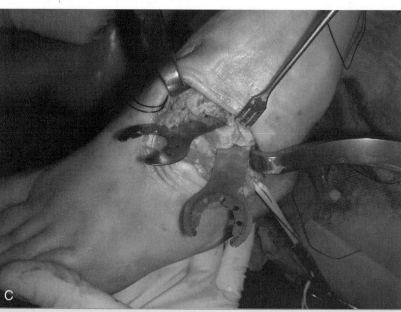

Figure 19 Lambrinudi procedure. A ventrally based wedge is removed from the subtalar joint to correct ventral impingement of the talus or extreme hindfoot equinus. Illustrations showing the foot before **(A)** and after **(B)** the ventrally based wedge resection from the subtalar joint. **C,** Intraoperative view of the ventrally based wedge.

teotome or an oscillating bone saw (Figure 20). The distal osteotomy should be driven exactly through the cuneiform bones and the cuboid bone; the proximal osteotomy runs through the cuboid and the navicular bone, where there should be at least 0.5 cm of distance between the proximal osteotomy and the talonavicular joint. A dorsally based bony wedge is removed, and the osteotomy is closed and fixed analogous to the Chopart fusion.

Dwyer Osteotomy

In a Dwyer osteotomy (**Figure 21**), a skin incision (approximately 5 cm) is made at the lateral border of the hindfoot above the peroneal tendons, vertical to the longitudinal axis of the calcaneus bone.[33] After retracting the sural nerve, the neck of the calcaneus bone is revealed subperiosteally, and a laterally based bony wedge is resected from the calcaneal neck with the oscillating bone saw. The osteotomy is opened with a flat chisel. The hindfoot is redressed under valgus stress while the osteotomy closes. Two K-wires are drilled in posteriorly.

Calf Muscle Lengthening (Baumann Procedure/ Achilles Tendon Lengthening)

When using the Baumann procedure, a 4- to 5-cm skin incision is made at the medial aspect of the first one third of the shank.[35] The calf fascia is incised, the inter-

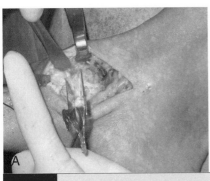
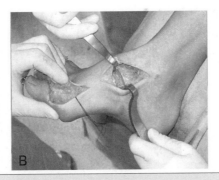
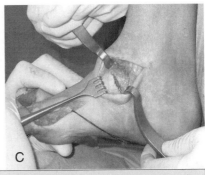

Figure 20   Cole osteotomy. **A** and **B**, A dorsal-based wedge is removed by two osteotomies. The distal osteotomy runs through the cuneiform bones and the cuboid bone. The proximal osteotomy runs through the cuboid and navicular bone. **C**, After resection, the cavus can be corrected.

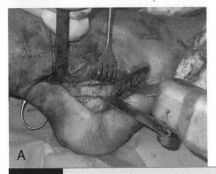
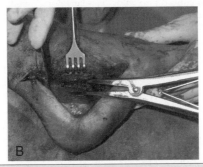
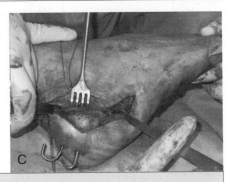

Figure 21   Dwyer osteotomy. **A**, A laterally based bony wedge is resected from the calcaneal neck with an oscillating bone saw. **B**, The osteotomy is opened with a spreader. **C**, The hindfoot is redressed and fixed with two K-wires.

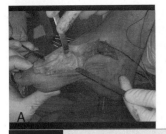
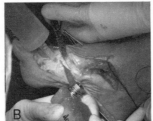
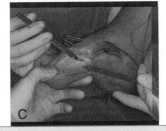
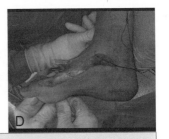

Figure 22   Extension osteotomy of the first metatarsal bone to correct a flexion deformity of the first column. **A**, The first metatarsal bone is subperiosteally exposed by inserting two Hohmann levers. **B** and **C**, A dorsally based wedge is resected with an oscillating bone saw. **D**, The osteotomy is closed by applying plantar pressure.

val between the gastrocnemius and the soleus muscles is opened, and two broad Langenbeck levers are inserted. The intramuscular recession of the aponeurosis of the gastrocnemius and/or soleus is performed using the scissors. After recession, the ankle should be correctable into neutral position.

The approach for an open Achilles tendon lengthening is made with a 6- to 10-cm skin incision at the medial aspect of the distal shank, approximately 3 to 4 cm above the ankle (the length of the incision varies depending on the amount of Achilles tendon lengthening needed). The fascia is incised and divided proximally and distally, and the Achilles tendon is identified and elevated with two Langenbeck hooks that are inserted under the tendon proximally and distally. Z-lengthening is then done with a small scalpel, and

both halves are tagged with No. 1 polyglycolic acid sutures. The ankle joint can then be redressed in 10° to 20° of dorsiflexion. With the ankle joint in neutral position, both tendon halves are sutured together under tension.

Basis Extension Osteotomy

The approach to the basis extension osteotomy of the first metatarsal bone is made by lengthening the incision for the Jones procedure proximally to the basis of the first metatarsal bone[32] (**Figure 22**). After incising the periosteum of the first metatarsal bone and exposing it with fibula Hohmann levers, the first osteotomy is performed with an oscillating power bone saw, vertically to the first metatarsal bone, approximately 0.5 cm distal to the cuneiform-metatarsal joint in adults and

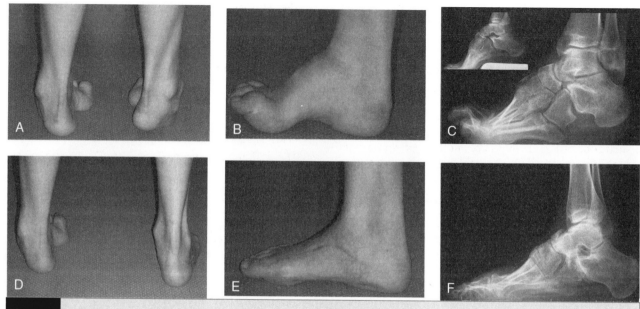

Figure 23 Clinical photographs (**A** and **B**) and radiograph (**C**) of a 16-year-old female patient with Charcot-Marie-Tooth disease and bilateral cavovarus foot with preoperative hindfoot varus and equinus, cavus deformity, plantar flexion of the first metatarsal bone, and claw toes. Preoperatively, the patient had pain under the first and the fifth metatarsophalangeal joint, especially after walking long distances. The patient was treated with a Steindler procedure, a Jones procedure, a posterior tibial tendon transfer, Chopart-fusion, and an extending metatarsal bone osteotomy, beginning with the right side. Postoperative clinical photographs (**D** and **E**) and radiograph (**F**) showing good clinical and radiologic results on the treated right foot compared with the untreated left foot.

the growth plate in children. It is important to spare the plantar cortex to avoid a rotational error. The second osteotomy is accomplished by converging to the first osteotomy with a dorsal basis. The width of the basis is chosen according to the angle of planned correction. In most situations, 2 to 3 mm is sufficient for correction. At this point, the osteotomy can be closed and fixed with two crossing K-wires or with an angle locking plate with four screws.

Hibbs Procedure

The approach in the Hibbs procedure is made above the fourth metatarsal bone.[36] The extensor digitorum longus tendons II through V are exposed and tagged together proximally and distally with atraumatic No. 1 polyglycolic acid sutures. The tendons are cut between the two sutures. The short digitorum extensor muscle then is dissected carefully, and the bone is exposed. In children, the proximal ends of the tendons can be sutured to the periosteum. In adults, a hole must be driven into the bone (using a drill or awl), and the tendons are fixed with a bone anchor. The distal part of the tagged tendons also should be sutured to the periosteum or the anchor to achieve a distal tenodesis.

Postoperative Treatment

The foot is immobilized in a non–weight-bearing shank plaster cast in neutral ankle position with the heel held slightly in eversion. On the first postoperative day, a radiograph is obtained and the plaster cast is changed. If bony procedures were performed, the affected limb(s) must not bear weight for 6 weeks in adults or 4 weeks in children. After this time, if a second radiographic evaluation shows satisfactory healing, the K-wires are removed and a weight-bearing plaster cast is applied for an additional 6 weeks in adults or 4 weeks in children. If bony procedures were not performed, the weight-bearing plaster cast is applied directly after surgery. After the final plaster cast is removed, a shank orthosis is used for approximately 6 months. **Figure 23** shows clinical photographs and radiographs before and after treatment of a typical patient with Charcot-Marie-Tooth disease with a cavovarus foot.

Complications

Possible complications include infection, vessel/nerve-bundle injury, nonunion, overcorrection (flatfoot, valgus foot, or calcaneal foot), undercorrection, recurrence, ulceration caused by the plaster cast, and K-wire infection. All of these possible complications should be discussed with the patient prior to surgery.

Outcome Studies

Studies reporting the long-term outcomes after complex foot reconstruction surgery in pes cavovarus are rare. A 2007 study reported significant improvements in the cavovarus deformity after radiographic assessment (talus-first metatarsal angle, calcaneus-first metatarsal angle, calcaneal pitch) and pedobarography.[37] Postoperative improvements in pressure patterns were unsatisfactory and abnormal, showing increased heel pressures. Study limitations included a small number of patients (nine) and the absence of a three-dimensional foot analysis model. In a 2005 study, 25 patients with Charcot-Marie-Tooth disease were evaluated.[38] The authors reported substantial improvement in radiographic parameters after surgical correction and emphasized the importance of graded treatment, with soft-tissue procedures more appropriate for young children and bony correction more appropriate for older patients. Because pain and arthritic signs were reported after triple arthrodesis, the authors concluded that this procedure should be avoided if possible. Another study also reported poor results after triple arthrodesis in 50% of patients with Charcot-Marie-Tooth disease.[39] The authors recommended that triple arthrodesis be used only for patients who have progressive peripheral neuropathy and a severe, rigid deformity. Sparing procedures are preferred for treating cavovarus foot in patients with Charcot-Marie-Tooth disease. Prospective, controlled studies based on clinical, radiographic, and functional data comparing different treatment strategies are needed.

Summary

Charcot-Marie-Tooth disease is an inherited peripheral neuropathy and the most common cause of pes cavovarus. The disease can be diagnosed based on clinical observation of the classic foot deformities (cavovarus and claw toes) and by measuring nerve conduction velocities. Symptoms of Charcot-Marie-Tooth disease typically begin in late childhood or early adulthood. Nonsurgical treatment is ineffective and does not prevent disease progression. Preoperative planning should include clinical examination, radiography, CT and dynamic examinations (such as pedobarography and three-dimensional foot analysis). The goals of surgical treatment include stopping disease progression and creating a functional, plantigrade foot. Tendon transfers are mandatory to correct a cavovarus foot (soft-tissue balancing). Bony procedures also may be needed to achieve a total correction in patients with more severe conditions, but lead to recurrence when performed without soft-tissue balancing. Triple arthrodesis has achieved mixed results and should be reserved for patients with more severe deformities.

Annotated References

1. Charcot JM, Marie P: Sur une forme particulière d'atrophie musculaire progressive, souvent familiale débutant par les pieds et les jambes et atteignant plus tard les mains. *Rev Med (Paris)* 1886;6:97-138.

2. Tooth HH: Dissertation: The peroneal type of progressive muscular atrophy. London, England, HK Lewis, 1886.

3. Hoffmann J: Über progressive neurotische Muskelatrophie. *Arch Psychiatr Nervenkr* 1889;20:660.

4. Skre H: Genetic and clinical aspects of Charcot-Marie-Tooth's disease. *Clin Genet* 1974;6:98-118.

5. Lupski JR, de Oca-Luna RM, Slaugenhaupt S, et al: DNA duplication associated with Charcot-Marie-Tooth disease type 1A. *Cell* 1991;66:219-232.

6. Wines AP, Chen D, Lynch B, Stephens MM: Foot deformities in children with hereditary motor and sensory neuropathy. *J Pediatr Orthop* 2005;25:241-244.

   The authors reviewed the feet of 52 children with HMSN and found the cavovarus deformity to be the most common in HMSN types I, III, IV, and V and in X-linked HMSN.

7. Nagai MK, Chan G, Guille JT, Kumar SJ, Scavina M, Mackenzie WG: Prevalence of Charcot-Marie-Tooth disease in patients who have bilateral cavovarus feet. *J Pediatr Orthop* 2006;26:438-443.

   Using a chart review, the authors determined the prevalence of Charcot-Marie-Tooth disease in 116 children with bilateral cavovarus feet. They found that, regardless of family history, there was a 78% probability of a patient with bilateral cavovarus feet having Charcot-Marie-Tooth disease.

8. Buchthal F, Behse F: Peroneal muscular atrophy (PMA) and related disorders: I. Clinical manifestations as related to biopsy findings, nerve conduction and electromyography. *Brain* 1977;100:41-66.

9. Pareyson D: Diagnosis of hereditary neuropathies in adult patients. *J Neurol* 2003;250:148-160.

   The author reviews the clinical diagnostic approach to hereditary neuropathies in adults. Heredity, different modalities of presentation, laboratory and instrumental diagnostic tests, symptoms, and the involvement of other organs are discussed.

10. Berger P, Niemann A, Suter U: Schwann cells and the pathogenesis of inherited motor and sensory neuropathies (Charcot-Marie-Tooth disease). *Glia* 2006;54:243-257.

    The authors investigated the molecular pathomechanisms of HMSN. Different proteins showed mutations in different subtypes of HMSN.

11. Berger P, Young P, Suter U: Molecular cell biology of Charcot-Marie-Tooth disease. *Neurogenetics* 2002;4:1-15.

12. Krajewski KM, Lewis RA, Fuerst DR, et al: Neurological dysfunction and axonal degeneration in Charcot-Marie-Tooth disease type 1A. *Brain* 2000;123:1516-1527.

13. Bird TD, Kraft GH: Charcot-Marie-Tooth disease: Data for genetic counselling relating age to risk. *Clin Genet* 1978;14:43-49.

14. Dehne R: Congenital and acquired neurological disorders, in Couglin MJ, Mann RA (eds): *Surgery of the*

5: Neuromuscular Disease

Foot and Ankle. St. Louis, MO, Mosby, 1999, pp 525-557.

15. Price AE, Maisel R, Drennan JC: Computed tomographic analysis of pes cavus. *J Pediatr Orthop* 1993; 13:646-653.

16. Holmes JR, Hansen ST: Foot and ankle manifestations of Charcot-Marie-Tooth disease. *Foot Ankle* 1993;14: 476-486.

17. Alexander IJ, Johnson KA: Assessment and management of pes cavus in Charcot-Marie-Tooth disease. *Clin Orthop Relat Res* 1989;246:273-281.

18. Ghanem I, Zeller R, Seringe R: The foot in hereditary motor and sensory neuropathies in children. *Rev Chir Orthop Reparatrice Appar Mot* 1996;82:152-160.

19. Mann RA, Missirian J: Pathophysiology of Charcot-Marie-Tooth disease. *Clin Orthop Relat Res* 1988;234: 221-228.

20. Tynan MC, Klenerman L, Helliwell TR, Edwards RH, Hayward M: Investigation of muscle imbalance in the leg in symptomatic forefoot pes cavus: A multidisciplinary study. *Foot Ankle* 1992;13:489-501.

21. Houlden H, King R, Blake J, et al: Clinical, pathological and genetic characterization of hereditary sensory and autonomic neuropathy type 1 (HSAN I). *Brain* 2006; 129:411-425.

    The authors analyzed the *SPTLC1* gene for mutations in families with hereditary sensory and autonomic neuropathy types I and II and Charcot-Marie-Tooth disease types I and II. They found mutations of the *SPTLC1* gene in six of eight families with hereditary sensory and autonomic neuropathy type I and in none of the other types. The approach for diagnosing hereditary neuropathies also is described.

22. Dwyer FC: The present status of the problem of pes cavus. *Clin Orthop Relat Res* 1975;106:254-275.

23. Metaxiotis D, Accles W, Pappas A, Doederlein L: Dynamic pedobarography (DPB) in operative management of cavovarus foot deformity. *Foot Ankle Int* 2000;21: 935-947.

24. Samilson RL, Dillon W: Cavus, cavovarus and calcaneocavus: An update. *Clin Orthop Relat Res* 1983;177: 125-132.

25. Thometz JG, Gould JS: Cavus deformity, in Drennan JC (ed): *The Child's Foot and Ankle.* New York, NY, Raven Press, 1992, pp 343-353.

26. Steindler A: The treatment of pes cavus (hollow claw foot). *Arch Surg* 1921;2:325-337.

27. Cole WH: The treatment of claw foot. *J Bone Joint Surg* 1940;22:895-908.

28. Hoke M: An operation for stabilizing paralytic feet. *J Orthop Surg (Hong Kong)* 1921;3:494.

29. Hsu JD, Hoffer MM: Posterior tibial tendon transfer anteriorly through the interosseus membrane. *Clin Orthop Relat Res* 1978;131:202-204.

30. Jones R: An Operation for paralytic calcaneo-cavus. *Am J Orthop Surg* 1908;190:371-376.

31. DePalma L, Colonna E, Travasi M: The modified Jones procedure for pes cavovarus with claw hallux. *J Foot Ankle Surg* 1997;36:279-283.

32. Tubby AH: *Deformities Including Diseases of Bones and Joints,* ed 2. London, England, MacMillan, 1912.

33. Dwyer FC: Osteotomy of the calcaneum for pes cavus. *J Bone Joint Surg Br* 1959;41:80-86.

34. Lambrinudi C: New operation for drop foot. *Br J Surg* 1927;15:193.

35. Baumann JU, Koch HG: Ventrale aponeurotische Verlängerung des Musculus gastrocnemius. *Oper Orthop Traumatol* 1989;4:254-258.

36. Hibbs RA: An operation for claw foot. *J Am Med Assoc* 1919;73:1583-1585.

37. Chan G, Sampath J, Miller F, Riddle EC, Nagai MK, Kumar SJ: The role of the dynamic pedobarography in assessing treatment of cavovarus feet in children with Charcot-Marie-Tooth disease. *J Pediatr Orthop* 2007; 27:510-516.

    The authors evaluated 9 children (14 feet) in whom Charcot-Marie-Tooth disease was diagnosed and who had been surgically treated with a combination of osteotomies and muscle transfers. Heel pressures displayed an inverse relationship to ankle power generation. The amount of correction measured radiographically showed no correlation with pedobarography.

38. Azmaipairashvili Z, Riddle EC, Scavina M, Kumar SJ: Correction of cavovarus foot deformity in Charcot-Marie-Tooth disease. *J Pediatr Orthop* 2005;25: 360-365.

    Twenty-five patients (41 feet) with Charcot-Marie-Tooth disease and cavovarus foot deformity were evaluated before and after surgery. The authors studied a new radiographic technique in some of these patients to determine the usefulness of this imaging modality. The new imaging method was useful in determining the optimal surgical choice for correcting this complex deformity.

39. Wetmore RS, Drennan JC: Long-term results of triple arthrodesis in Charcot-Marie-Tooth disease. *J Bone Joint Surg Am* 1989;71:417-422.

Chapter 24
Peripheral Nerve Disorders

Keith J. Hill, MD

Interdigital Plantar Neuralgia

Forefoot pain in the distal metatarsal interspace has been attributed to an abnormality within the digital nerves. In 1845, a neuralgic pain in the plantar nerve between the third and fourth metatarsal bones was described.[1] In 1876, Morton hypothesized that the pain was caused by a neuroma or hypertrophy of the digital branches of the lateral plantar nerve. The condition has since been referred to as a Morton neuroma. The cause of pain between the distal metatarsals has been ascribed to many causes, including congestion and thickening of the digital nerves, neuritis, nerve entrapment, and neuroma. However, the interdigital neuroma is not necessarily a neuroma but rather a painful clinical entity that involves the common digital nerve. The suffixes -oma and -itis imply that a neoplastic or inflammatory state is involved; however, because the condition can occur as an entrapment without inflammation, inflammatory mediators, or a neoplasm, the suffix -algia, is more accurate. The term interdigital neuralgia is, therefore, recognized as a more appropriate name. Recently proposed nomenclature suggests that the term nerve compression be used. This term can be further distinguished by naming the involved nerve, such as compression of the interdigital nerve to the third web space.[1]

Anatomic Factors

A common presumption has been that the transverse metatarsal ligament is a major causative factor in the development of interdigital neuralgia. Histologic changes have been shown to occur distal to the transverse metatarsal ligament, whereas the nerve proximal to the ligament appears normal. Although it is not clear if the transverse metatarsal ligament is the cause, entrapment of the nerve at some point is suspected. A decrease in the number of thick myelinated fibers, decreased diameter in the individual nerve fibers, and increased nerve width have been reported.[2,3] A recent study demonstrated that, histopathologically, the distal nerve shows intraneural fibrosis and sclerohyalinosis with an increase of the elastic fibers in the stroma.[4] These findings suggest that changes are probably caused by an entrapment neuropathy resulting in deposition of an eosinophilic substance within the nerve followed by a slow degeneration of the nerve fibers. How-

ever, the precise etiology of the interdigital neuralgia remains obscure, and compression from the transverse metatarsal ligament has not been demonstrable.

Another recent study evaluated the anatomic location of interdigital neuralgia.[5] This report showed that interdigital neuralgias remained distal to the deep transverse metatarsal ligament (DTML) in both the midstance and the heel-off stage during walking. The authors reported that the main lesion was located between the metatarsal head and the metatarsophalangeal (MTP) joint and more distal than the DTML. It was questioned whether the DTML could be a major cause in the development of interdigital neuralgia because the nerve did not appear to be compressed by this structure.

Risk factors for the development of interdigital neuralgia are equally as enigmatic. There has been no demonstrable increase in the incidence of neuralgia symptoms in runners, workers who stand for a prolonged duration, recreational or professional athletes, dancers, or those with fat pad atrophy. It has been postulated that the nerve in the third interspace is thicker because it has communicating branches from both the medial and lateral plantar nerves;[6] however, this has not been demonstrated clinically. It has been noted that the second and third interspaces are significantly narrower than the first and fourth interspaces, suggesting a possible area of entrapment.[7] Communicating branches between the third and fourth common plantar digital nerves have been reported in 28% of feet;[8] an injury to these communicating branches may be a cause of symptoms but also may be a reason for recurrent pain after excision of the common digital nerve.

Increased mobility between the third and fourth rays has been suggested as a reason for the increased incidence of neuromas in the third web space. The medial three rays are more firmly fixed in position at the metatarsocuneiform joints; the fourth and fifth metatarsocuboid articulation is more mobile. The relative increased motion in the third web space may potentially result in trauma to the distal nerve, resulting in neuralgic symptoms. This model of nerve trauma is less likely because a significant number of neuromas occur in the second interspace, which has far less motion in this area. A more likely scenario is that the nerve is tethered under the metatarsal heads as the toes are dorsiflexed during normal gait. This scenario is supported by the fact that the incidence of neuromas in women is much more common than in men. It is likely that fashionable footwear forces plantar flexion of the metatarsal heads and hyperdorsiflexion of the MTP joints, causing recurrent trauma to the nerves, which results in an entrapment neuropathy.[9]

History and Physical Examination

Symptoms of interdigital neuralgia occur far more frequently in women (4 to 15 times) than in men, with a reported average age at occurrence of 55 years. Neuralgia usually is unilateral but has been reported bilaterally in 15% of patients. The presence of two neuromas simultaneously in one foot is believed to occur infrequently, with a reported incidence of 3%.[10] Most authors agree that symptoms occur more frequently in the third interspace; however, there is little agreement as to how often symptoms occur in the second interspace. It is generally accepted that a neuralgia in the first and fourth interspaces is rare.

The most common symptom of interdigital neuralgia is pain localized to the plantar aspect of the foot between the metatarsal heads. The pain usually radiates to the toes of the involved interspace. The pain can be variable but is generally described as burning, stabbing, tingling, or electrical in nature. Symptoms are aggravated by weight-bearing activities and are particularly exacerbated by wearing a tight-fitting, high-heeled shoe. This pain is often relieved by removing the shoe and rubbing the forefoot. Often, the patient finds that pain during gait can be limited by voluntarily curling the toes or by avoiding rolling through to a normal toe-off position. The patient often reports no symptoms when walking barefoot on a soft surface.

The physical examination begins with a careful observation of the foot, noting deviation, subluxation, or clawing of the toes or evidence of fullness in the involved web space. Palpation of the MTP joints and plantar fat pad should be performed carefully to elicit tenderness associated with synovitis and pain from degeneration of the fat pad. Special attention should be directed to the second MTP joint because synovitis is more common in this area; the joint is also adjacent to a commonly occurring location of interdigital neuralgia; therefore, it can be a confounding factor in the diagnosis. A drawer test of the MTP joints should help determine if joint instability is the cause of the pain.

A sensory examination rarely shows any deficit in a patient with interdigital neuralgia. Interdigital neuralgia does not typically cause tenderness over the dorsal or plantar metatarsal heads; instead, tenderness is localized within the web space. If palpation of the web space reproduces the character and quality of symptoms, interdigital neuralgia should be suspected. Simultaneous medial and lateral compression of the metatarsal heads while gently palpating the plantar web space may create a palpable "click" (Mulder sign) that reproduces the patient's symptoms; this finding is considered diagnostic of interdigital neuralgia. A click without the presence of pain can be a normal finding.

Diagnostic Studies

Weight-bearing radiographs of the foot should be obtained to evaluate osseous abnormalities, such as subluxation, dislocation, or arthritis of the MTP joint, which may contribute to the patient's symptoms. The use of MRI in diagnosing interdigital neuralgia is controversial. The positive diagnosis of interdigital neuralgia by MRI does not necessarily translate to positive symptoms. Because MRI has resulted in 33% positive findings of neuroma in patients with no clinical evidence of this condition, the diagnosis cannot be made on the basis of MRI alone.[11]

Ultrasound also is controversial for diagnosing interdigital neuralgia. Its use is operator dependent, making it difficult to reproduce results. Ultrasound correctly identified interdigital neuralgia in 92% of patients when preoperative ultrasound reports were compared with postoperative histopathologic reports.[12] However, other studies have shown that ultrasound is especially inaccurate for detecting small lesions. Diagnostic accuracy improves when there is a strong clinical suspicion of interdigital neuralgia.[13]

Other reports have questioned the use of MRI in combination with ultrasound for diagnosing interdigital neuralgia.[14] Studies have shown that the accuracy of ultrasound and MRI are similar and both are dependent on the size of the lesion that is being evaluated.[13,14] A 2003 study showed that imaging with both modalities failed to meet the predictive values attained by clinical assessment.[14] Clinical assessment was reported to be the most sensitive and specific diagnostic modality, leading the authors to conclude that ultrasound or MRI is not needed to make a diagnosis in patients who are believed to have interdigital neuralgia. These findings supported an earlier study that evaluated the histomorphology of resected intermetatarsal neuromas compared with normal autopsy specimens.[15] The authors reported that, qualitatively, the nerves from autopsy specimens showed the same findings as those of the surgically excised specimens. Measurements of swelling in the nerves were 80% specific and 78% sensitive. Because there was no significant difference in size between clinically symptomatic neuromas and normal specimens, it was concluded that neither MRI nor ultrasound was necessary for making a diagnosis or treatment decision. MRI continues to play a primary role in the differential diagnosis of other diseases that cause similar symptoms, such as stress fractures, bursitis, ganglion cysts, or tumors of the tendon sheaths.

Electrodiagnostic testing to confirm interdigital neuralgia has generally been accepted as unreliable. Recently, a near-nerve needle sensory conduction test was reported to be a highly sensitive diagnostic test for interdigital neuralgia.[16] An abnormal dip phenomenon (a selective decrease of 50% or more in the sensory compound nerve action potential amplitude of the affected nerve compared with that of the preceding interdigital nerve) is the most characteristic electrophysiologic marker for diagnosing interdigital neuralgia. Although electrodiagnostic tests may not play a large role in diagnosing interdigital neuralgia, they can be useful in identifying a proximal entrapment, radiculopathy, or neuropathy when these conditions are suspected. Selective injections of the interspace with a local anesthetic may be a useful diagnostic tool.

Nonsurgical Treatment

Initial treatment of interdigital neuralgia should always be nonsurgical. Because this condition is considered to be caused by mechanical pressure, compression should be relieved. This relief can often be achieved by wearing a shoe with a wide toe box that allows splaying of the metatarsal heads. A pad placed proximal to the metatarsal heads also may off-load the pressure on the forefoot, thereby relieving painful symptoms. Oral anti-inflammatory medications may provide some relief. Other medications used off label, such as tricyclic antidepressants, selective serotonin reuptake inhibitors, and antiseizure medications, are useful in diminishing nerve excitation and lessening the severity of nerve-related symptoms.

Corticosteroid injection into the area of the interdigital neuralgia can occasionally be helpful. There are contradictory reports regarding the long-term results of this treatment. Although pain relief has been reported in 60% to 80% of patients, other investigators have reported that only 30% of patients obtain pain relief that lasts more than 2 years.[17] A recent study evaluated ultrasound-guided injection of local anesthetic and corticosteroid into the area of interdigital neuralgias.[18] Follow-up at 11.4 months showed that 63% of patients had no limitation in activity and did not require shoe wear modifications; however, corticosteroid injections have the potential for adverse side effects.

Neuroma alcohol-sclerosing therapy has been reported as a safe and effective method of treating interdigital neuralgia.[19-21] One study evaluated a sclerosing solution composed of anesthetic (mepivacaine hydrochloride–adrenaline 70%) and ethylic alcohol (30%), which was injected inside the interdigital neuroma using ultrasound guidance.[20] The procedure was repeated every 15 days until resolution of the symptoms was achieved. Total or partial symptomatic relief was obtained in 90% of patients. A 20% to 30% reduction in mass volume was reported at 10-month follow-up. Another study of ultrasound-guided injection with an alcohol-sclerosing agent reported a 61% improvement or resolution of symptoms.[19] Feet that received five or more injections were more likely to improve (74%) than those that received fewer than five injections (39%). A large prospective study (101 patients) of sonographically guided alcohol injections into an interdigital neuroma reported partial or total symptom improvement in 94% of patients; 84% were totally free of pain.[21] An average of 4.1 treatments per patient was administered. Although neuroma alcohol-sclerosing therapy has been shown to have good results, these studies all used ultrasound guidance and required multiple treatments to provide symptom relief.

Surgical Treatment

If nonsurgical treatment fails to provide long-term relief, surgery may be warranted. Surgical treatment is eventually elected by 60% to 70% of patients with interdigital neuralgia.[9] Excision of the interdigital nerve is the most frequently performed surgery. Some physicians have advocated release of the transverse metatarsal ligament as an isolated procedure or in combination with neurolysis as an effective way to relieve symptoms. Endoscopic decompression of the interdigital nerve has excellent results with minimal complications.[22] A procedure that uses an instrument designed to release the transverse carpal ligament has been described. In 14 patients with a mean follow-up of 26 months, pain relief was reported in 79% of patients.[23]

Dorsal and plantar incisions both provide adequate exposure to the interdigital nerve. The main advantage of the dorsal approach is that it prevents scar formation on the plantar aspect of the foot. The plantar approach provides some advantage in revision surgery because it allows more proximal exposure to the nerve and is usually not encumbered by scarring from a previous dorsal incision (**Figure 1**). For a very proximal focal tender trigger point, a plantar transverse approach proximal to the metatarsal plantar fat pad is recommended. This approach permits more direct exposure of the nerve, allows the nerve resection to be performed off the weight-bearing surface at a more proximal level, allows identification of anomalous nerve branches, and improves the surgeon's ability to avoid the artery and vein. Development of a painful plantar scar is a potential disadvantage. Because of the minimal histomorphologic differences reported between surgically resected symptomatic interdigital nerves and asymptomatic autopsy specimens, one study questioned the value of postoperative histologic examinations of surgical specimens.[15] The authors concluded that postoperative microscopic examination provided little additional information other than merely proving that the nerve was resected.

Clinical Outcomes

Generally, 80% of patients treated with interdigital neuralgia excision become asymptomatic or have significant improvement; 20% of patients report minimal improvement or no pain relief.[24] In a 5-year follow-up study, good to excellent results were reported in 85% of patients.[25] Seventy percent of the patients required some modification in footwear to remain pain free; however, most patients had no limitation in their activity level. Subjective numbness occurred in 50% of the operated feet, although the pattern of numbness was variable. Similar results were reported in a study of 60 patients who were treated with excision of the interdigital neuroma.[4] The authors noted excellent or good results in 78%, fair results in 19%, and poor results in

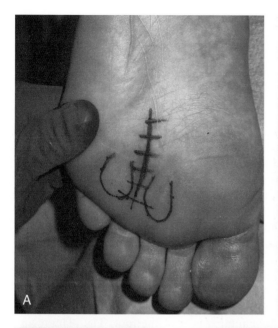
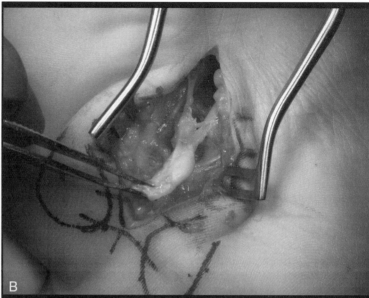
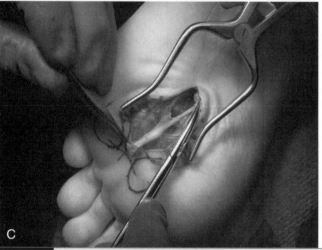
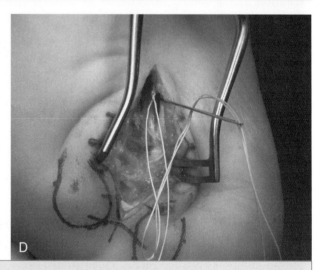

Figure 1 Photographs of the foot of a patient with a recurrent interdigital neuroma. **A,** The plantar approach for a revision procedure is shown. **B,** The recurrent neuroma is identified and dissected from surrounding tissues. Visibility is excellent using this approach. **C,** The nerve is transected proximally. **D,** The free end of the nerve is secured with suture. A Keith needle is passed through the midfoot, exiting dorsally. The cut end of the nerve is subsequently buried in soft tissues of the midfoot where neuroma formation is less likely to be symptomatic.

3% of patients. Notably, 62% of patients had normal sensation and no paresthesias postoperatively despite excision of the digital nerve, 38% had numbness, 57% had no difficulty with footwear, and 40% had some limitation.

Outcomes following surgery for recurrence of an interdigital neuralgia are much less satisfying than the results reported for primary nerve excision. In one study, 60 interspaces were reexplored for recurring or persistent symptoms after a previous excision of an interdigital neuroma.[26] Ten patients had simultaneous excision of an adjacent primary neuroma, and 19 underwent additional forefoot surgery. At an average follow-up of 39.7 months, 31% of patients were completely satis-

fied, 27% were satisfied with minor reservations, 20% were satisfied with major reservations, and 22% were dissatisfied with the outcome. No pain or mild pain was reported in 57% of patients; 59% had moderate or severe restrictions in the choice of footwear. In another study, the authors described a technique that combined resecting the interdigital neuroma through a plantar approach and implantation of the proximal end of the nerve into an intrinsic muscle in the arch of the foot.[27] Eighty percent of patients had excellent relief of symptoms, returned to their regular jobs, and wore usual footwear. Twenty percent of the patients had good relief of symptoms, changed jobs, and had to change their choice of footwear.

Complications

Complications in the treatment of interdigital neuralgia can occur with nonsurgical and surgical management. Corticosteroid injections into the forefoot can lead to atrophy of the fat pad, discoloration of the skin, and disruption of the joint capsule, which can lead to deviation of the toe. Follow-up studies of surgical treatment of interdigital neuralgia report that 2% to 20% of patients have residual pain.[26] Initial symptoms or those that recur shortly after surgical excision of the interdigital nerve may be caused by a variety of factors. An inaccurate initial diagnosis may play a role in unsuccessful surgical treatment. Many other disorders can mimic the symptoms of interdigital neuralgia (Table 1). A preoperative and postoperative history and physical examination are necessary to guide the accurate treatment of the patient. A diagnosis other than interdigital neuralgia should be considered if pain persists in the immediate postoperative period before a recurrent neuroma can develop.

The bulb neuroma that inevitably forms at the end of the cut nerve probably does not grow to sufficient size to become symptomatic until 12 months after surgery. This accounts for some late surgical failures. Patients with recurrent symptoms of neuralgia have a focal area of tenderness, usually either beneath the metatarsal head or adjacent to it. Palpation of this area usually elicits an electriclike pain that reproduces the patient's symptoms. Nonsurgical management of a recurrent neuralgia is similar to the treatment given at the initial presentation. Patients who have well-localized findings with a Tinel sign usually respond better to repeat surgery than patients with poorly defined symptoms. Causes for recurrence noted on reexploration of the metatarsal interspace include a second primary symptomatic interdigital nerve in an adjacent interspace; intact or distally transected nerves (under the deep transverse metatarsal ligament); stump neuromas; formation of a neuroma attached to an area of movement, friction, pressure, or tension; and synovial cysts.[26] Accessory nerves traveling obliquely under the metatarsal heads may retract directly under the weight-bearing surface of the metatarsal head and cause a painful neuroma stump after excision of the primary nerve.

A retrospective analysis of 674 consecutive primary interdigital neurectomies showed that 38.9% of specimens included the digital artery.[28] No difference was observed between dorsal and plantar surgical approaches used for excision. No complications related to vascular perfusion to the digits were reported, most likely because extensive collateralization of the digital vessels maintains vascular perfusion of the toes. In patients with decreased vascularity to the toes and in those with adjacent interdigital neuromas, care should be taken to avoid possible vascular compromise.

Several surgical techniques have been suggested to improve the success of reexploration of the interdigital neuroma. A plantar approach may provide a better view of the digital nerve at its most proximal level in

Table 1
Differential Diagnosis of Interdigital Neuralgia Symptoms
Lipoma
Ganglion
Synovial cyst
Hypertrophy of transverse tarsal ligament
MTP joint synovitis
Instability of the MTP joint
Interdigital bursitis
Fracture malunion
Deviated toe
Inflamed intermetatarsal bursa
Osteonecrosis of the metatarsal head
Arthrosis of the metatarsal head
Stress fracture of the metatarsal

the interspace. Adequate transection of the small cutaneous nerves arising from the interdigital nerve may result in better retraction of the transected nerve from the weight-bearing area. Release of the transverse metatarsal ligament alone or in combination with neurolysis can improve outcomes.[26] Intramuscular transposition of the transected nerve can eliminate its predilection to grow toward the distal side of the cut surface.

Regardless of the chosen technique, revision surgery is better avoided than fixed. It is critical that the patient be informed preoperatively of the relatively high rates of failure and the increased likelihood of residual pain after revision surgery. Patients should have realistic expectations concerning the possible need for a decreased activity level and restrictions in footwear choices.

Tarsal Tunnel Syndrome

Tarsal tunnel syndrome is an entrapment neuropathy involving the posterior tibial nerve within the tarsal canal, or entrapment of one of its terminal branches after the nerve leaves the tarsal canal. First described in 1960, this condition has received considerable attention and is sometimes compared with carpal tunnel syndrome in the wrist.[29] This comparison is misleading because tarsal tunnel syndrome differs from carpal tunnel syndrome in its frequency, presentation, clinical symptoms, diagnostic study results, causes, and response to treatment.

Anatomy

The tarsal tunnel is a fibro-osseous canal located posterior to the medial malleolus. Its borders are created by the tibia (anteriorly) and the posterior process of the talus and calcaneus (laterally). The tunnel is created as

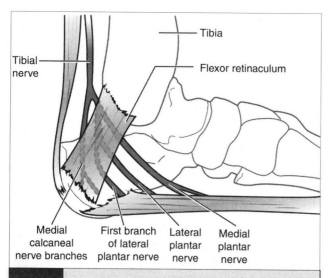

Tibia

Tibial nerve

Flexor retinaculum

Medial calcaneal nerve branches   First branch of lateral plantar nerve   Lateral plantar nerve   Medial plantar nerve

Figure 2   The contents of the tarsal tunnel. The flexor retinaculum passes posteriorly over the tarsal tunnel. The medial calcaneal nerve may originate from the tibial nerve proximal to the tarsal tunnel and may have multiple branches. The first branch of the LPN may originate within the tarsal tunnel. The MPN frequently provides one or more calcaneal branches.

Table 2
Causes of Local Tibial Nerve Entrapment Resulting in Tarsal Tunnel Syndrome
Ganglion or synovial cyst
Lipoma within the tarsal canal
Exostosis or fracture fragment
Medial talocalcaneal bar
Enlarged venous complex
Neurilemoma of the tibial nerve
Hindfoot valgus causing tension of the tibial nerve
Hindfoot varus causing compression of the tibial nerve
Accessory muscle within the tarsal canal

the flexor retinaculum passes posteriorly from its attachment on the tibia, creating an enclosed space over the tibial nerve and the flexor tendons of the medial ankle.

The tibial nerve enters the canal proximally and then branches within the tunnel into its three terminal branches: the medial plantar nerve (MPN), the lateral plantar nerve (LPN), and medial calcaneal nerve, which shows significant variability in its branches and course (Figure 2). The medial calcaneal nerve originates from the tibial nerve approximately 75% of the time and from the LPN about 25% of the time.[9] Cadaver studies have shown that 60% of specimens have multiple calcaneal nerve branches, and 20% of specimens have aberrant innervation of the abductor hallucis muscle.[30] Another study of the calcaneal nerve showed that 37% of specimens had a single branch, 41% had two branches, 19% had three branches, and 3% had four branches.[31] In addition, the MPN gave origin to a calcaneal nerve in 46% of feet.

The topographic anatomy of the tibial nerve has been mapped to show the position of the various nerves before ramification. The calcaneal nerve descends from medial to posteromedial, is never located anterolaterally, and is only rarely located laterally. The LPN rotates externally from lateral and posterolateral to lateral and posteromedial as it descends. The LPN is not found medially or anteromedially. The MPN internally rotates from anteromedial (proximal) to anterior (distally); it is never found posteriorly.[32]

History and Physical Examination

Patients with tarsal tunnel syndrome can present with a wide variety of symptoms. Patients usually report dif-

fuse pain on the plantar aspect of the foot and medial ankle. The pain is often diffuse and poorly localized and is characterized as a spectrum of burning, shooting, searing, electric, shocking, stabbing, tingling, or numbing pain. The pain is usually aggravated by standing or walking and is relieved by rest. Some patients report that the pain is worse when lying in bed and that relief is obtained by arising and walking. About one third of patients with tarsal tunnel syndrome have pain that radiates proximally, extending to the medial middle calf region.[9]

Patients should be evaluated for systemic disorders such as diabetes, obesity, thyroid disease, rheumatologic disorders, and Lyme disease. Medication usage, alcohol abuse, or back pain with radiculopathy should be documented to rule out other nonfocal causes of tibial neuralgia. Although systemic causes are less common, an identifiable cause of tarsal tunnel syndrome has been reported in 80% of symptomatic patients.[33] More commonly, causes include trauma, such as a severe ankle sprain; crush injury; calcaneal fractures; varicosities, ganglions, or other space-occupying lesions; heel varus or valgus; and fibrosis (Table 2). An accessory muscle within the tarsal tunnel, such as an accessory soleus or accessory flexor digitorum longus, also can compress the nerve.[34]

A thorough physical examination should identify activities and specific movements or positions that exacerbate the pain of tarsal tunnel syndrome. Athletes who place a heavy load on the ankle, such as sprinters, jumpers, and those using certain martial arts kicking techniques, have increased symptoms. A flatfoot deformity, talocalcaneal coalition, or accessory muscles or bony fragments around the tarsal tunnel predispose both athletes and nonathletes to symptoms of tarsal tunnel syndrome.[35] The physical examination should critically evaluate the overall posture of the foot, especially any significant varus or valgus deformity of the hindfoot. The position of the foot in relation to the ankle can increase pressure within the tarsal canal, and symptoms can be further exacerbated with both passive inversion and eversion of the hindfoot.[36] MRI studies of the tarsal canal have shown that the volume of the tarsal tunnel is decreased with both inversion and eversion, thereby increasing the pressure on a nerve that may already have little available space.[37] With additional hindfoot instability, eversion, dorsiflexion-eversion, and cyclical loading will increase tibial nerve tension in an unstable hindfoot.[38,39] Dynamic hindfoot instability has been implicated as a cause of the "heel pain triad" (plantar fasciitis, posterior tibial tendon dysfunction, and tarsal tunnel syndrome). Instability caused by failure of the static (plantar fascia) and dynamic (posterior tibial tendon) supports of the longitudinal arch of the foot results in traction on the tibial nerve, causing tarsal tunnel syndrome.[40] Abnormalities in electrodiagnostic test results in patients with pes planus support these findings, which suggest that dynamic instability plays a role in exacerbating tarsal tunnel syndrome, and that this instability should be considered in the treatment plan.[41]

Provocative maneuvers, such as passive hindfoot inversion or eversion, can generate dysesthesias in the tibial nerve distribution. Another more specific test for tarsal tunnel syndrome combines passive dorsiflexion of the ankle, heel eversion, and dorsiflexion of all the toes. This dorsiflexion-eversion test can induce symptoms after a few seconds.[42] The windlass test (dorsiflexion and MTP joint extension) that is used to evaluate plantar fasciitis increases tension on the tibial nerve and can reproduce the symptoms of tarsal tunnel syndrome.

The entire course of the tibial nerve should be carefully palpated beginning proximal to the tarsal tunnel and continuing distally along the terminal branches. Swelling may indicate a space-occupying lesion such as a ganglion (**Figure 3**). Rarely, a bony ridge may be noted along the course of the tibial nerve. Percussion over an area of nerve entrapment or irritability can cause radiating pain along the distribution of the MPN or LPN. Sensory examination of the foot usually does not reveal a focal defect of the nerve. Although patients often report dysesthesias and numbness, it is difficult to demonstrate actual areas of numbness on the bottom of the foot. If there is specific involvement of the MPN or LPN, it is occasionally possible to detect a localized sensory loss in the foot. Semmes-Weinstein monofilament or two-point discrimination testing of distal sensory branches can show tibial nerve deficits.[9] Motor weakness is also difficult to clinically demonstrate. Atrophy of the abductor hallucis muscle or abductor digiti quinti muscle may be present.

Diagnostic Studies

Radiographic studies of the foot and ankle should be obtained to evaluate fractures or degenerative changes. MRI is needed if a space-occupying lesion is suspected. In one study, MRI showed pathologic conditions in 88% of patients with suspected tarsal tunnel syndrome; these MRI findings were confirmed in 90% of patients at the time of surgery.[43]

Ultrasound is useful in evaluating tarsal tunnel syndrome. A recent study reported that ultrasound was used to accurately diagnose ganglia, talocalcaneal coalitions, and varicose veins in patients with tarsal tunnel syndrome.[44] These findings were confirmed intraoperatively. Although ultrasound is a useful adjunct in confirming suspected causes of tarsal tunnel syndrome, ultrasound is a more technician-dependent study than MRI, which provides more soft-tissue and bony detail. High-resolution techniques for both MRI and ultrasound are recommended, and knowledge of the anatomy of the fibro-osseous tunnels is important to establish the correct diagnosis.

Electrodiagnostic Studies

It is generally recommended that electrodiagnostic testing be performed to confirm the diagnosis of tarsal tunnel syndrome. The sensory nerve conduction velocity (NCV) study is probably the most accurate study for evaluating tarsal tunnel syndrome and has a reported sensitivity of 90%.[45] However, questions concerning the reliability of electrodiagnostic testing have been raised. A recent analysis of 317 published articles evaluated the use of NCV studies and needle electromyography (EMG) in diagnosing tibial neuropathy at the ankle.[46] This extensive review determined that NCV studies were abnormal in only some patients. Sensory NCV studies were more likely to be abnormal than motor NCV studies, but the actual sensitivity and specificity of these studies could not be determined from the data available. The sensitivity of needle EMG studies could not be determined. The authors concluded that although NCV studies may be useful, there are no good prospective reports available that evaluate the reliability and reproducibility of electrodiagnostic techniques in tarsal tunnel syndrome.[46] The diagnosis of tarsal tunnel syndrome cannot be determined based only on electrodiagnostic results; it must be made in conjunction with the patient's history and physical examination findings.

The diagnosis of tarsal tunnel syndrome can be supported by NCV studies if the history and physical examination findings are consistent with this diagnosis. The diagnosis can often be determined by applying three criteria: (1) a strong history of neuritic symptoms in the tibial nerve or branches, (2) objective Tinel sign along the course of the nerve, and (3) supportive NCV studies. If none of the criteria are met, the diagnosis of tarsal tunnel syndrome should be excluded. If only one criterion is met, a different diagnosis should be considered. If two of the three criteria are met, and if the findings are reproducible, the diagnosis of tarsal tunnel syndrome can be considered.

Nonsurgical Treatment

If a mass is present and causing symptoms of tarsal tunnel syndrome, surgical excision should be considered. If no lesion is present, nonsurgical management is indicated. Initial nonsurgical management can include non-

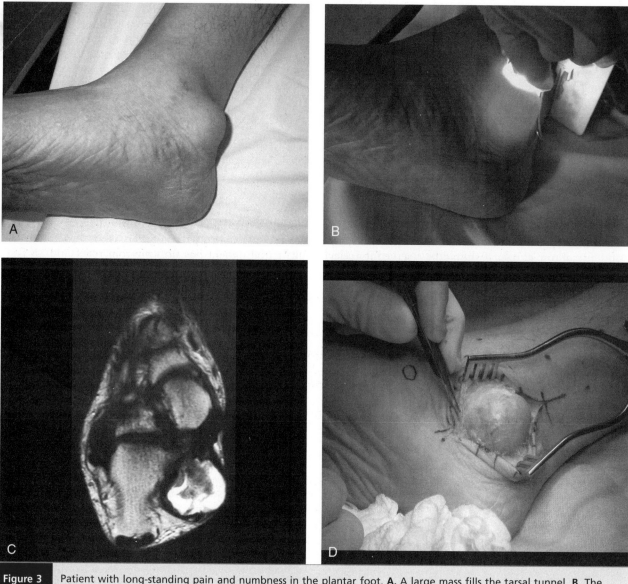

Figure 3 Patient with long-standing pain and numbness in the plantar foot. **A,** A large mass fills the tarsal tunnel. **B,** The mass easily transilluminates, suggesting a ganglion cyst. **C,** MRI shows high intensity signal of mass within the tarsal tunnel. **D,** Intraoperative dissection shows attenuation of flexor retinaculum with mass bulging through the roof of the tarsal tunnel.

steroidal anti-inflammatory drugs, oral vitamin B$_6$, and tricyclic antidepressants. Selective serotonin reuptake inhibitors or antiseizure medications (such as gabapentin) may be beneficial. Injection of a corticosteroid into the tarsal tunnel, alone or in combination with immobilization in a walking boot or cast, may provide relief. Hindfoot instability that exacerbates symptoms can be stabilized with an orthotic device that holds the foot in a neutral position.

Surgical Treatment

If the patient has neuritic pain, positive physical examination findings, confirmatory studies of tarsal tunnel syndrome, and has been unsuccessfully treated with

nonsurgical modalities, surgery can be considered. An obvious space-occupying lesion should be removed (such as a ganglion or lipoma), varicosities ligated, and nerve constrictions released. Other pathologic findings, such as hindfoot instability, must be treated at the time of surgery to obtain a successful outcome. Release of the tibial nerve may not provide complete symptom relief if there is a secondary structural cause of symptoms that is unrecognized.[40]

Tarsal tunnel release for the treatment of diabetic neuropathy has been proposed for patients who have not been successfully treated with nonsurgical modalities. Indications for surgery in diabetic patients include decreased plantar sensation, a positive Tinel sign, and pain in the tibial nerve distribution. This procedure is contraindicated in patients with vascular disease.[47-50] Endoscopic tarsal tunnel release has provided good to excellent short-term results, although there have been only a small number of patients treated with this procedure.[51]

Complications

Complications following tarsal tunnel release are similar to those of any nerve decompression surgery. Complications include increased pain, numbness, paresthesias, dysesthesias, painful incision or scar, failure to relieve symptoms, vascular injury, infection, delayed wound healing, difficulty with footwear, or type 2 complex regional pain syndrome (CRPS). Occasionally, the resulting symptoms are worse than the original symptoms. Tarsal tunnel release should be reserved for select patients who have been unsuccessfully managed with less invasive treatments.

Clinical Outcomes

When a discrete localized lesion is removed during surgical treatment, such as a ganglion or lipoma, relief of symptoms is generally successful. However, even if no specific cause of nerve compression is identified, approximately 75% of patients obtain some pain relief after surgery.[9] A small number of patients have increased symptoms following surgery, whereas others have initially satisfactory relief of symptoms after surgery only to have symptoms recur. Some patients have reported recurrence as late as 5 years after their surgical procedure.

One review of the literature reported that 69% of patients had good results, 22% were improved, 7% had poor results, and 2% had a recurrence of symptoms.[33] Another study reported that early satisfactory results deteriorated with long-term follow-up, eventually leading to a 38% dissatisfaction rate and no long-term relief of the pain.[52] Patients with a traumatic cause of tarsal tunnel syndrome have poorer results, presumably because the hemorrhage and crushing of the nerve leads to adhesions and intraneural disease.[53] In contrast, a recent study reported that a history of trauma had no negative effect on outcomes for patients treated with tarsal tunnel release.[54] The authors reported that the most common surgical findings included arterial vascular leashes indenting the nerve and scarring about the nerve. The absence of a discrete space-occupying lesion and long-standing preoperative symptoms were not associated with a poor outcome.

Ultimately, the success of the surgical release of the tarsal tunnel is predicated on the patient's perception of the outcome and may not necessarily match the objective findings. One study of 60 patients who underwent tarsal tunnel release for a positive Tinel sign and an abnormal motor NCV study reported decreased subjective success.[55] Despite objectively measured complete relief of symptoms in 85% of patients, only 51% reported symptom relief on a questionnaire. Improvements in work quality in 51% of patients, job productivity in 47%, and interpersonal relationships in 46% were reported. Even with a successful surgical outcome, patients may not perceive significant improvement, making follow-up care frustrating for both the patient and the surgeon.

Recurrence

Surgical failures for tarsal tunnel syndrome are better prevented than treated. Outcomes for revision surgeries are significantly worse than for the primary procedure. A patient with a failed surgery should initially be treated conservatively. Repeat surgical procedures should only be considered for patients with refractory symptoms. An adequate release must be ensured, and all other associated pathologies must be treated. Generally, if the patient has no symptom relief and an adequate surgical incision was performed, repeat surgery for tibial nerve release and neurolysis produces poor results. However, if the initial surgical incision was inadequate, repeat tarsal tunnel release achieves better results. If tibial nerve scarring is present, a poor prognosis should be expected despite the adequacy of the previous release.

CRPS type 2 should be considered in patients with recurrent or persistent symptoms. Sympathetically mediated symptoms of edema, allodynia, and hyperalgesia, along with changes in extremity temperature, skin color, or hair quality, suggest CRPS. These symptoms should be treated before any repeat surgical procedure is considered.

Complex Regional Pain Syndrome

CRPS, most recently referred to as reflex sympathetic dystrophy, is known by many names, including sympathetic dystrophy, posttraumatic dystrophy, algoneurodystrophy, Sudeck atrophy, acute bone atrophy, sympathetic trophoneurosis, peripheral trophoneurosis, painful osteoporosis, minor causalgia, and sympathalgia. These numerous terms reflect the confusion surrounding this condition. The term reflex sympathetic dystrophy, established in 1946, has been the most commonly used term for referring to this complex and challenging condition. However, the International Association for the Study of Pain proposed the term complex regional pain syndrome, which deliberately avoids suggesting the etiology of the condition. CRPS used to be considered a rare, sympathetically mediated, devastating complication of injury, which mainly affected psychologically abnormal patients. Current research has provided a new perspective on this enigmatic disease.

CRPS is an exaggerated response to the injury of a limb, manifested by intense prolonged pain, vasomotor disturbances, delayed functional recovery, and trophic changes. Acute pain is the normal protective response to injury. Physical trauma begins as a cascade of chemical releases, mediated by prostaglandins that lead to

5: Neuromuscular Disease

peripheral sensitization and hyperalgesia (increased sensitivity to a noxious stimulus) at the site of the damage. In patients with CRPS, repeated, unrelieved, peripheral nerve firings cause central sensitization, hyperalgesia, and allodynia distant to the damaged site. If central sensitization continues, neuronal pathways undergo plastic modification, and acute pain is converted to chronic neuropathic pain.

Etiology

An injury produces an initial barrage of afferent pain signals and generates a secondary inflammatory response. If these stimuli continue unchecked, prolonged changes in both the peripheral and the central nervous system may amplify and prolong the pain response. Peripheral sensitization can then decrease the threshold necessary to generate a painful sensation. Central sensitization can occur as a result of the continuous input from the peripheral afferent nerves. Together, these two processes contribute to the postinjury hypersensitivity state (spinal windup). In this way, pain may be prolonged beyond the duration normally expected following an acute insult. Prolonged central sensitization can lead to permanent alterations in the central nervous system, including the death of inhibitory neurons, replacement with new afferent excitatory neurons, and establishment of aberrant excitatory synaptic connections. These alterations lead to a prolonged state of sensitization, resulting in intractable pain that is unresponsive to many analgesics.[56] Although responses vary in different patients, if left untreated, irreversible anatomic and physiologic changes can occur, and symptoms can continue for years. CRPS that develops in this hyperexcited state exists in two forms: CRPS type 1 and CRPS type 2. CRPS type 1 is an inappropriate, nonspecific pain syndrome following trauma. CRPS type 2 develops after an injury to a specific nerve (causalgia) and causes pain in that nerve's distribution.

History and Physical Examination

CRPS type 1 develops after a precipitating traumatic event or noxious stimulus. The injury can be very minor, and the pain response may seem out of proportion to the inciting event. Patients may be viewed with initial skepticism concerning the reported pain. CRPS is characterized by acute onset, usually within 1 month after a noxious event, but symptoms may occur almost immediately after the initial trauma. A delay of 6 to 12 months in the development of symptoms in the lower limb is not unusual. Conditions that may lead to CRPS include fractures, sprains, tendinitis, surgical procedures, peripheral nerve injury, immobilization, infection, deep venous thrombosis, malignancy, vasculitis, herpes zoster, or polymyalgia rheumatica.

CRPS Type 1

CRPS type 1 is characterized by changes in sensory, autonomic, and motor responses, which occur in a generalized distribution in the extremity. The symptoms are independent of the location of the preceding trauma and are not limited to the distribution of a single peripheral nerve. Pain is present in more than 90% of patients and is routinely disproportionate to the inciting event. Pain is unremitting, although sleep is often unaffected. The pain is deep, spontaneous, burning, and diffuse and is frequently triggered by a breeze, light touch, or temperature change.[57]

Following an inciting event, several different physical changes can occur depending on how CRPS is expressed. Commonly, the associated changes in sensation, hypoesthesia, hyperesthesia, allodynia, and anesthesia dolorosa suggest the diagnosis of CRPS. Changes that occur in the autonomically controlled nervous system can lead to extremity swelling, vasodilation, skin warming, and changes in sweating patterns. In the classic presentation, the limb is initially dry, hot, and pink. As vasoconstriction occurs later in the disease, the limb becomes blue, cold, and sweaty. Motor changes cause decreased active range of motion, decreased strength, increased tremor, and difficulty in initiating motion. Dramatic changes in appearance (trophic changes) frequently occur late in the condition and include muscle atrophy, joint contractures, osteoporosis, nail changes, and shiny skin. In a fully developed case of CRPS, the foot and ankle can display any combination of these symptoms.

CRPS Type 2

CRPS type 2 is a pain syndrome that develops after an injury to a specific peripheral nerve, resulting in CRPS type 2 pathophysiologic phenomena. Sensory, autonomic, and motor deficits occur but develop in the specific distribution of the peripheral nerve, not throughout the limb. Spontaneous pain, allodynia, sensory deficits, and skin blood flow and sweating abnormalities are usually limited to the territory of the nerve. Motor function deficits are usually the result of a direct injury to motor axons. Swelling and trophic changes are discrete.

Incidence

The true incidence of CRPS is unknown, presumably because this condition is frequently misdiagnosed. In adults, CRPS occurs three times more frequently in women than in men; CRPS occurs much less frequently in children. CRPS occurs in 1% to 2% of patients with fractures and in 2% to 5% of those with peripheral nerve injuries.[57] Prospective studies show that mild CRPS occurs after 30% to 40% of fractures and surgical trauma.[58] Occurrence is strongly associated with cigarette smoking.

Physical Examination

CRPS is confirmed by a diagnosis of exclusion. The differential diagnosis includes direct effects of trauma, fracture, cellulitis, arthritis, and malignancy. Causes of referred pain must be considered and investigated, including nerve compression caused by spinal pathology or peripheral entrapment. Many patients present with only one or two of the classic symptoms of CRPS. Good evidence indicates that true CRPS types 1 or 2 are not psychogenic; no personality disorder is specific to patients with CRPS. A thorough physical examination is critical to determine if there is any underlying pathology that would rule out the diagnosis of CRPS.

Sensory examination is vital in evaluating the distribution of symptoms because changes in sensation are commonly associated with CRPS. A diffuse area of involvement versus a single dermatome distribution can help distinguish between CRPS types 1 and 2. Hypoesthesia (diminished pain in response to normally painful stimulus), hyperesthesia (abnormally increased sensitivity to stimulation), allodynia (pain from a stimulus that does not normally evoke pain), and anesthesia dolorosa (sensitivity to touch is absent, whereas severe pain is present in an anesthetized area) are some of the common symptoms that should cause the physician to consider a diagnosis of CRPS.

Further changes that occur in the autonomically controlled nerves can lead to edema, vasodilation, skin warming, and changes in sweating patterns. These differences can be assessed by palpation and by comparing the affected extremity with the unaffected side. Thermography with or without cold challenge is useful. In patients with CRPS, considerable asymmetry of skin temperature is created during controlled thermoregulation. This characteristic can be used as a supplementary bedside test to assist in the diagnosis, with a high sensitivity and specificity (76% and 93%, respectively).[56] A limb surface temperature differential of 1°F or more is believed to be significant.[59] Discoloration of the skin is a commonly reported finding. Vasoconstriction occurs later in the disease process and can manifest as nail changes, shiny skin, and a cool, pale extremity. Motor evaluation should assess the foot and ankle for decreased active range of motion, decreased strength, increased tremor, and difficulty in initiating motion. Significant muscle atrophy and joint contractures are common late findings.

Diagnostic Evaluation

CRPS is a clinical diagnosis. Diagnostic tests can be misleading and misinterpreted. The patient is generally systemically well, and no abnormal biochemical markers or indices of infection are present. To exclude systemic causes of pain, a complete blood count, erythrocyte sedimentation rate, and measurements of fasting blood glucose and serum calcium levels should be obtained along with a thyroid function test; these tests are normal in patients with CRPS.

A three-phase technetium Tc 99m bone scan is the prime imaging technique used to confirm CRPS. Bone scanning in early CRPS shows increased isotope uptake in the delayed phase (phase 3), demonstrating increased

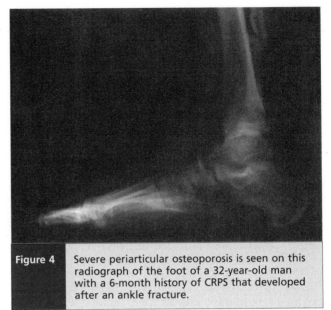

Figure 4 Severe periarticular osteoporosis is seen on this radiograph of the foot of a 32-year-old man with a 6-month history of CRPS that developed after an ankle fracture.

bone metabolism. The accuracy of bone scans is variable, ranging from 44% to 96% sensitivity and 75% to 98% specificity.[60] Later in the disease, the bone scan returns to normal levels, making this technique less reliable.

Radiographs show rapid bone loss, including visible demineralization with patchy subchondral or subperiosteal osteoporosis, metaphyseal banding, and profound bone loss (**Figure 4**). Despite the osteoporosis, fractures are uncommon. CRPS does not cause arthritis, and the joint space is preserved. A normal bone scan without radiographic evidence of osteoporosis virtually excludes adult CRPS.[58] MRI shows early bone and soft-tissue edema earlier than the bone scan but is not diagnostic. Clinical assessment is the most important diagnostic tool.

Sympathetic blockade may be helpful in determining the extent of sympathetic involvement in CRPS.[61] Sympatholysis can be achieved by alpha-blocking agents (phentolamine), intravenous regional blockade with guanethidine or bretylium, epidural blockade, and local anesthetic blockade. A paravertebral lumbar sympathetic chain block is the most effective technique because it does not block the sensory and motor nerves. A documented increase in the skin temperature of 1°C to 3°C confirms the success of the sympathetic nerve block. Differential spinal blockade is considered unreliable. The usefulness of regional blockade has been questioned. Response to the block indicates that sympathetically maintained pain is involved; pain conditions that do not respond to a sympathetic block are defined as sympathetically independent pain states.

EMG and NCV testing can assist in evaluating an underlying discrete nerve lesion. This testing is especially beneficial in the diagnosis of CRPS type 2 when a specific nerve is involved. Because EMG and NCV tests measure large-fiber disease, these tests are less helpful in CRPS type 1, where much of the neuropathic pain is small-fiber mediated. Skin biopsies performed at selected laboratories show damage to the neural elements in affected patients, but their clinical role is unclear.[57]

Treatment

A wide variety of treatments for CRPS have been proposed, but few are founded on well-constructed scientific studies. The goal of treatment in CRPS is to diminish the exaggerated pain symptoms and improve the function of the extremity. Early recognition and aggressive treatment are critical. Fifty percent of the patients who are untreated in the first year have significant long-term effects. Treatment of CRPS no longer concentrates on manipulation of the sympathetic nervous system but now focuses on functional rehabilitation of the limb to break the vicious cycle of disuse.[58] A multimodal approach of physical therapy, sympathetic blocks, pharmacologic agents, and reassessment of the patient's symptoms is critical for a successful outcome.

Physical therapy should be the first line of treatment, concentrating on controlling edema, preventing joint contractures, desensitization, and reestablishing voluntary motor control. Gentle motion and strengthening exercises should progress slowly to avoid the pain caused from forced passive motion, which can cause a mechanoreceptor barrage and subsequent increase in perceived pain. Cryotherapy and immobilization should be avoided because these treatments may exacerbate the patient's symptoms.

Mirror visual feedback has been used in the early stages of CRPS type 1. This technique is based on the finding that visual input from a moving, unaffected limb reestablishes the pain-free relationship between sensory feedback and motor execution in the affected limb. In a study of eight patients with CRPS type 1, five patients with early and intermediate disease had good results from mirror visual feedback after other treatments had failed.[62] Three patients with chronic disease did not benefit from mirror visual feedback.

Transcutaneous electrical nerve stimulation has shown some usefulness in a small study in the pediatric literature, but there is little evidence to support its use in adults.[60,63] Transcutaneous electrical nerve stimulation releases endorphins and can overload nerves with benign impulses, preventing their use for pain transfer. Ultrasound treatments have shown some usefulness in the treatment of CRPS of the foot. Relaxation therapy, biofeedback, cognitive-behavioral modification, acupuncture, and electroacupuncture have been suggested as concurrent treatment options in a multimodal approach to treating CRPS.

Pharmacologic agents are used to modify sympathetic and nonsympathetic symptoms. Numerous systemic medications have been studied for pain relief in patients with CRPS, but no clear evidence advocates the use of any of these drug therapies. The clinical management of CRPS usually involves the intravenous regional administration of sympatholytic agents and the use of nonsteroidal anti-inflammatory drugs and corticosteroids. Other published studies support the use of gabapentin (an anticonvulsant), prazosin (an alpha-adrenergic blocking agent), propranolol (an oral beta blocker), nifedipine (a calcium channel blocker), and mexiletine (an antiarrhythmic).[57-59,61,64] Results with bisphosphonates have been encouraging. Desensitization of peripheral nerve receptors with capsaicin, which depletes substance P, also has been advocated.

Pain control is essential for successful treatment and a combination of drugs, such as a tricyclic antidepressant, gabapentin, and a strong opiate may be needed to achieve this control. Opiate medications should be used throughout the period that a patient has pain rather than on an as-needed basis. Fixed doses of long-acting medications (such as a transdermal fentanyl patch or time-released oxycodone) with supplemental short-acting medicine for breakthrough pain (oxycodone, hydromorphone, or hydrocodone) is recommended.[56,64]

Surgical treatment should be directed at any continuing pain generators (such as tarsal tunnel syndrome or fractures). Surgery generally creates a painful stimulus that can exacerbate CRPS or precipitate a new attack; however, a few surgical procedures are indicated to treat CRPS. Implantable spinal electrodes for dorsal column stimulation to control intractable pain should be considered in patients with refractory pain.[65] Chemical or surgical lumbar sympathectomy has shown benefits in patients with CRPS in the foot and ankle. Amputation of a limb affected by severe CRPS should be considered with great caution. Relief of pain is rare and unpredictable. CRPS often recurs in the stump, especially if the amputation level was symptomatic at the time of surgery. This procedure is not predictable and is generally not recommended.

MPN Entrapment

The pain reported in MPN entrapment (jogger's foot) is usually the result of a neuroma formed in the nerve from a transection or severe crush injury of the MPN. Transient neuralgia is more common than a transection injury.

Anatomy

On the medial side of the foot, the MPN and LPN branch from the tibial nerve in the tarsal tunnel. The MPN travels deep to the abductor hallucis muscle, coursing along the plantar surface of the flexor digitorum longus tendon as it passes through the knot of Henry. The MPN then travels along the medial border of the foot, branching around the medial and lateral aspects of the flexor hallucis longus tendon.

Etiology

MPN entrapment often affects joggers. Recurrent trauma to the nerve from repetitive impact received during running is the likely cause. MPN entrapment occurs in the region of the knot of Henry. Most patients with this condition have excessive heel valgus or hyperpronation of the foot. Orthotics with large arch supports can exacerbate symptoms by compressing the MPN.

Incidence

This condition has no gender predilection, although it is more frequently reported in men. No specific age distribution has been reported.

Clinical Symptoms

Patients with MPN entrapment describe aching or shooting pain in the medial aspect of the arch. The pain often radiates distally into the medial three toes and also can cause the radiation of proximal pain into the ankle. The pain is usually worse with running on level ground but may be caused by workouts on stairs. Occasionally, patients report new onset of symptoms after switching to a new orthosis or shoe.

Diagnosis

The presence of hindfoot valgus should be determined because it is often a predisposing position for MPN entrapment. The patient's running shoes and orthotics should be examined for areas that may lead to compression. Palpation along the MPN usually reproduces symptoms consisting of medial arch tenderness with radiation, dysesthesia, or paresthesia to the medial three toes. Symptoms may worsen when the patient performs a single limb heel rise that tightens the abductor hallucis muscle and compresses the MPN. Because of the close proximity of the MPN and the medial tendons, it can be difficult to distinguish between neuralgia and tendinitis. Directing the patient to run for a prolonged period immediately before the examination may reproduce pain and numbness in the MPN distribution.

Treatment

Activity and shoe modifications usually relieve compression on the nerve and provide pain relief. If pain is not relieved, surgical decompression of the MPN is performed by releasing the superficial fascia over the abductor muscle and the deep fascia around the knot of Henry. Neuroma formation can be resected, and the proximal nerve can be buried into the deep muscle layer.

LPN Entrapment

Entrapment of the first branch of the LPN can cause heel pain similar to pain reported in plantar fasciitis, calcaneal stress fractures, or subcalcaneal bursitis. This obscure condition can be the source of intractable heel pain. Accurate diagnosis is difficult because symptoms overlap with other more common conditions.

Anatomy

The tibial nerve divides into three branches posterior to the medial malleolus in or around the tarsal tunnel. After separating from the tibial nerve, the LPN branches still further. The first branch of the LPN ramifies into three major branches, with one innervating the periosteum of the medial process of the calcaneal tuberosity, one innervating the flexor digitorum brevis as it passes dorsally over the muscle, and one branch terminating in the abductor digiti minimi muscle.

Etiology

Entrapment of the first branch of the LPN occurs between the deep fascia of the abductor hallucis muscle and the medial caudal margin of the quadratus plantae muscle. Chronic stretching of the nerve may occur in patients with hypermobile pronated feet. Hypertrophy of the abductor hallucis muscle or the quadratus plantae muscle may also place pressure on the nerve. Accessory muscles, abnormal bursae, and phlebitis in the calcaneal venous plexus can cause symptoms.

Incidence

Approximately 5% to 15% of patients with chronic, unresolved heel pain have entrapment of the first branch of the LPN.[9] As is the situation in those with MPN entrapment, most patients with LPN entrapment are runners and joggers, but nonathletes can also be affected. This condition occurs in men 88% of the time. Patients usually are 26 to 38 years of age.

Clinical Symptoms

Patients with entrapment of the first branch of the LPN report chronic heel pain exacerbated by walking or running. Patients describe a pain that radiates proximally from the medial plantar aspect of the heel into the medial ankle region. The pain can radiate laterally across the plantar aspect of the foot. As in plantar fasciitis, entrapment of the first branch of the LPN produces pain that is frequently worse in the morning; numbness in the heel or the foot is usually not present. Most patients present with persistent pain despite the use of extensive stretching programs, heel cups, anti-inflammatory medications, and corticosteroid injections.

Diagnosis

The pathognomonic finding for entrapment of the first branch of the LPN is tenderness over the nerve deep to the abductor hallucis muscle. Pressure on this point reproduces symptoms and radiates pain proximally and distally. More proximal and distal nerve entrapments must be excluded by palpation along the entire course of the posterior tibial nerve and its branches. Symptoms are exacerbated by hyperpronation.

Treatment

Nonsurgical treatment of subcalcaneal pain syndrome is recommended for 12 to 18 months before considering surgery. In one study, surgical release of the first branch of the LPN and the medial plantar fascia achieved good to excellent results in 88% of patients.[66] Some level of satisfaction was obtained in 93% of patients. Recovery from the procedure can be lengthy despite the patient's ability to return to work; 52% of patients require more than 6 months for maximal improvement. This lengthy recovery period does not appear to be associated with the preoperative duration of symptoms. Complete resolution of pain following nerve release occurred in 83% of patients.[67]

Superficial Peroneal Nerve Entrapment

The common peroneal nerve divides into the deep peroneal nerve and the superficial peroneal nerve (SPN) in the proximal leg. It passes through the lateral leg compartment, providing motor innervation to the peroneus brevis and peroneus longus muscles. The nerve then continues as a sensory branch to the lateral leg and the dorsal foot. To pass from the lateral compartment to the dorsal foot, the nerve must transition from subfascial to subcutaneous areas, passing between the anterior intermuscular septum and the fascia of the lateral compartment. The nerve pierces the deep fascia approximately 8 to 12 cm proximal to the tip of the lateral malleolus as it exits the lateral compartment. At this point, the SPN takes a subcutaneous path around the lateral fibula as it continues distally. Approximately 6 cm proximal to the lateral malleolus, the nerve divides into the intermediate and the medial dorsal cutaneous nerves. These two nerves then split to fan out over the dorsum of the foot. The intermediate dorsal cutaneous nerve provides sensory innervation to the dorsolateral aspect of the ankle, the fourth toe, and portions of the third and fifth toes. The medial dorsal cutaneous nerve provides sensation to the dorsomedial aspect of the ankle, the medial aspect of the hallux, and the second and third toes.

Etiology

The most common site of entrapment of the SPN occurs at its exit point from the deep fascia in the lateral leg. The sharp fascial edge impinges the nerve as it pierces through the lateral fascia. This opening for the nerve passage also is a point of weakness in the fascia. This weakness can lead to attenuation of the fascia, ultimately creating a large fascial defect. During exercise, increased pressure in the muscle can cause it to herniate through the opening and pinch the nerve. Entrapment of the SPN in this fascial defect may be part of a chronic exertional compartment syndrome.

Other anatomic abnormalities, such as a fibrotic tunnel passing between the anterior intermuscular septum and the fascia of the lateral compartment, also can contribute to entrapment of the SPN.[68] In one anatomic study of patients with entrapment of the SPN, the position of the nerve was located in the lateral compartment in 57% of patients, in the lateral and anterior compartments in 26%, and in the anterior compartment in 17%.[69] In 43% of patients, at least one branch, if not the entire SPN, was located in the anterior compartment. Although this anatomic variability may not predispose the nerve to entrapment, it does reinforce the recommendation that surgical release of the SPN should be evaluated in all of these areas.

Approximately 25% of patients with SPN symptoms have a history of prior trauma to the extremity, most commonly an ankle sprain.[70] Chronic ankle sprains cause recurrent stretching of the nerve, leading to persistent pain. A previous anterior compartment fasciotomy can shift the fascia, with resultant stretching and impingement of the nerve. Superficial peroneal nerve entrapment also can be caused by direct pressure from a ganglion, a fibular fracture, syndesmotic sprains, and lower extremity edema. Chemotherapy induced neuropathy, especially with the use of cisplatin, carboplatin, paclitaxel, and vincristine, can cause a painful sensory neuropathy.[71]

Incidence

Entrapment of the SPN was reported in 17 of 480 patients (3.5%) with chronic leg pain.[72] Entrapment of the SPN occurs equally in men and women, with patients usually age 28 to 36 years. Symptoms occur most frequently in runners, but this condition also has been reported in soccer, hockey, tennis, and racquetball players.[9]

Clinical Symptoms

Patients report radiating pain on the dorsolateral foot and the lateral calf, especially in the middle and distal thirds of the leg, with approximately one third of patients reporting numbness and paresthesias. Occasionally, swelling in the foot or leg is reported, but nocturnal pain is uncommon. The pain is typically worse with physical activities, such as walking, running, or squatting. Relief from pain occurs with cessation of the exacerbating activity.

Diagnosis

Symptoms can be related to a complication along the course of the peroneal component of the sciatic nerve or to an L5-S1 nerve root disorder. It should be determined if there is a history of back, hip, knee, or leg surgery; direct trauma to the leg; or numbness or pain radiating from the back into the foot. Common peroneal nerve entrapment should be evaluated by palpating around the head of the fibula. Point tenderness is usually elicited where the nerve pierces the deep fascia on the lateral leg. Paresthesias and numbness are frequently noted in this area. A fascial defect can be palpated in approximately 60% of patients.

Three provocative tests for SPN entrapment have

been described: (1) The patient actively dorsiflexes and everts the foot against resistance while the site of nerve impingement is palpated. (2) The patient's foot is passively plantar flexed and inverted without pressure over the nerve. (3) The patient's foot is passively plantar flexed and inverted with percussion along the course of the nerve.[68]

Electrodiagnostic testing can be beneficial, although findings may be normal. Neurosensory testing with a Pressure-Specified Sensory Device (Sensory Management Services, LLC; Baltimore, MD) has demonstrated nerve compression even when other electrodiagnostic tests are normal.[73] This testing measures the cutaneous pressure threshold for one-point static and one-point moving touch and for two-point static and two-point moving touch.

Nonsurgical Treatment

Nonsurgical treatment of SPN injuries includes improving ankle proprioception and strength to decrease recurrent sprains. A supportive ankle brace and a lateral heel and sole wedge in the shoe may help prevent inversion of the ankle. Neuropathic drugs, such as gabapentin and selective serotonin reuptake inhibitors, may be useful. Complete relief of a true entrapment with nonsurgical treatment is uncommon.

Surgical Treatment

Surgical treatment of SPN entrapment involves fasciotomy and nerve decompression through an incision made in the area of maximal symptoms. Improvement of symptoms after surgical release of the SPN has been reported in 75% to 100% of patients.[68,70-72] Because the SPN or a branch of the SPN is present in the anterior compartment in 43% of patients, release of the fascia in both the anterior and lateral leg compartments is recommended to decompress the SPN entrapment.[69] Recurrent SPN pain following fasciotomy for exertional compartment syndrome can be satisfactorily treated with reexploration.[70] If symptoms persist after release, the nerve can be reexplored, transected, and buried into the deep muscle to minimize possible symptoms from the inevitable stump neuroma that will form.

Sural Nerve Entrapment

Anatomy

A recent anatomic study reported that in 60% of specimens, the sural nerve was formed by the union of the medial cutaneous nerve (tibial branch) and the lateral cutaneous nerve (peroneal branch) in the upper two thirds of the leg.[74] The study also reported that the lateral cutaneous nerve was absent in 16.7% of specimens, the medial cutaneous nerve was absent in 6.7%, and nerves had a separate course in 6.7% of specimens. In general, the sural nerve travels along the midline of the calf bordering the Achilles tendon. Approximately

10 cm from the calcaneus, the sural nerve passes over the lateral edge of the Achilles tendon and passes subcutaneously posterior and then inferior to the lateral malleolus.

Branches of the sural nerve supply sensation to the lateral aspect of the heel and often have anastomoses with the lateral branch of the superficial peroneal nerve. As it reaches the tuberosity of the fifth metatarsal, the nerve ramifies. The most common distribution of the sural nerve in the foot is to the lateral side of the fifth toe in 60% of feet and to the lateral two and one half toes in 26.7% of feet.[74] Along its course, the sural nerve supplies sensation to the posterior lateral lower leg and ankle, the lateral foot and heel, and the lateral two or three toes.

Etiology

Despite its largely superficial course, sural nerve entrapment generally occurs near the lateral ankle and foot. Injuries to surrounding structures can lead to nerve compression. As in other peripheral nerve injuries, recurrent ankle instability can lead to traction injuries and fibrous tissue entrapment of the nerve. Proximal fifth metatarsal fractures have been reported as a cause of sural nerve entrapment.[75] Other reported causes of entrapment include ganglions of the peroneal sheath or calcaneocuboid joint and recurrent ankle sprains. Symptoms of superficial peroneal nerve compression may present as sural nerve pain.

The sural nerve is vulnerable to direct injury during surgical procedures, such as a Strayer-type Achilles tendon lengthening procedure, Achilles tendon reconstructions, open reduction of a calcaneal fracture, calcaneal osteotomy (Dwyer procedure), lateral ankle ligament reconstruction, peroneal tendon repairs, and subtalar fusion. Injury can occur from transection or traction or from scarring that entraps the nerve. In a recent report evaluating percutaneous placement of posterolateral screws for ankle fusion, the authors recommended placing a guide pin close to the fibula to avoid injury to the sural nerve.[76] No direct injury to the sural nerve was noted in any specimen.

Clinical Symptoms

Patients with sural nerve entrapment report radiating pain along the lateral ankle and foot. Most patients report a previous ankle sprain and may report persistent pain and paresthesias associated with instability. Pain is frequently exacerbated by running or walking on uneven terrain. Although the pain pattern may be poorly localized, a focal area of tenderness is occasionally noted along the course of the nerve.[9]

Diagnosis

A history of surgery performed on the posterior calf, lateral heel, ankle, or foot should raise suspicion that a sural nerve injury may be involved. The surgical scar area should be palpated to determine if the symptoms are reproducible. The entire course of the sural nerve should be palpated to evaluate for local tenderness and a positive Tinel sign. These findings are characteristic of entrapment and may be magnified by having the patient run or walk on a treadmill. Occasionally, numbness is present. Concomitant conditions, such as ankle instability and Achilles or peroneal tendinosis should be evaluated.

Plain radiographs should be obtained for evaluating subtalar arthritis, lateral wall compression from a previous calcaneal fracture, and fifth metatarsal nonunion, which may cause symptoms. MRI and EMG studies may be helpful. Typically, electrodiagnostic tests are most useful in diagnosing more proximal nerve compression. Selective lidocaine injections into the tendon sheath, the joints, or the area around the nerve can assist in isolating the symptomatic area.

Nonsurgical Treatment

Much like the other superficial nerve compression syndromes, nonsurgical management of sural nerve entrapment should treat the specific area of entrapment or the exacerbating cause. Because ankle instability frequently is associated with sural nerve symptoms, improving ankle proprioception and strength to decrease recurrent sprains is recommended. A supportive ankle brace and a lateral heel and sole wedge in the shoe may help prevent ankle inversion; however, because the nerve is superficial, external compression from a brace can exacerbate pain. Rarely, symptoms are severe and diffuse enough to require administration of a tricyclic antidepressant medication to decrease nerve irritability. Capsaicin, lidocaine patches, or other topical agents may take advantage of the superficial position of the nerve to provide symptomatic relief.

Surgical Treatment

In patients who have not responded to conservative treatment and have well-localized neurologic findings, surgery may be indicated. Surgical decompression of the sural nerve should be directed to the area of maximal symptoms. An adequate nerve decompression should provide relief of tension and focal constriction on the nerve without disturbing the surrounding veins, arteries, and fat. The nerve itself should be minimally manipulated. Release of constricting tissue or decompression from a mass typically results in satisfactory symptom relief.[77,78] Concomitant procedures (such as peroneal tendon repair, lateral calcaneal wall decompression, and lateral ankle stabilization) should be performed as indicated. Lateral ankle ligament stabilization may provide relief of sural neuralgia without directly exploring the nerve. When the symptoms are the result of previous surgery, decompression of the nerve is not as predictable.[9]

Summary

CRPS should be considered in patients presenting with reports of pain that seem out of proportion to expected symptoms. This condition is probably underdiagnosed.

Aggressive treatment should be instituted as early as possible and includes physical therapy with early motion exercises.

Interdigital plantar neuralgia can be initially treated with footwear modifications. Injections of a corticosteroid or a sclerosing agent into the nerve may provide relief. If nonsurgical treatment is unsuccessful, excision of the digital nerve can provide good results.

Tarsal tunnel syndrome should be confirmed clinically. Hindfoot instability should be considered as a contributing factor to tarsal tunnel syndrome symptoms. Peripheral nerve disorders in the lower extremity can cause a wide variety of painful symptoms, ranging from a local interdigital compression to a diffuse dystrophic limb. In general, peripheral nerve disorders are better avoided than treated. Careful surgical technique may avoid injuries to specific peripheral nerves that may lead to painful nerve entrapment syndromes. Nonsurgical treatment for nerve compression should be considered initially. Outcomes following decompression are generally better when a mass effect, such as a ganglion, is the source of painful stimulation.

Annotated References

1. Larson EE, Barrett SL, Battiston B, Maloney CT Jr, Dellon AL: Accurate nomenclature for forefoot nerve entrapment: A historical perspective. *J Am Podiatr Med Assoc* 2005;95:298-306.

   The authors review the historic impetus for the terminology being used for Morton neuroma and propose terminology based on the current understanding of the pathogenesis of the condition. The authors prefer the term nerve compression rather than neuroma. The condition is further distinguished by naming the involved nerve. Level of evidence: IV.

2. Graham CE, Graham DM: Morton's neuroma: A microscopic evaluation. *Foot Ankle* 1984;5:150-153.

3. Lassmann G: Morton's toe: Clinical, light, and electron microscopic investigations in 133 cases. *Clin Orthop Relat Res* 1979;142:73-84.

4. Giannini S, Bacchini P, Ceccarelli F, Vannini F: Interdigital neuroma: Clinical examination and histopathologic results in 63 cases treated with excision. *Foot Ankle Int* 2004;25:79-84.

   Results of 60 consecutive patients (63 neuromas) treated with excision of interdigital neuroma are reported. The clinical results were excellent or good in 49 feet (78%), fair in 12 (19%), and poor in 2 (3%) based on a specifically developed clinical rating system. The authors also reported histopathology findings, including intraneural fibrosis, sclerohyalinosis in the interstitium, and an increase of elastic fibers in the stroma. Level of evidence: III.

5. Kim JY, Choi JH, Park J, Wang J, Lee I: An anatomical study of Morton's interdigital neuroma: The relation-

ship between the occurring site and the deep transverse metatarsal ligament. *Foot Ankle Int* 2007;28:1007-1010.

This cadaver study examined the anatomic relationship between interdigital neuromas and the DTML, which is considered a major causative factor in neuroma formation. The location of the interdigital neuroma and the DTML were evaluated at two phases of the gait cycle (60° of MTP dorsiflexion and 15° of ankle dorsiflexion). Interdigital neuromas were located between the metatarsal head and the MTP joint and more distal than the DTML. This finding questioned previous studies suggesting that the DTML is the major causative factor in the development of Morton interdigital neuroma. Level of evidence: IV.

6. Jones JR, Klenerman L: A study of the communicating branch between the medial and lateral plantar nerves. *Foot Ankle* 1984;4:313-315.

7. Levitsky KA, Alman BA, Jesevar DS, Morehead J: Digital nerves of the foot: Anatomic variations and implications regarding the pathogenesis of the interdigital neuroma. *Foot Ankle* 1993;14:208-214.

8. Govsa F, Bilge O, Ozer MA: Anatomical study of the communicating branches between the medial and lateral plantar nerves. *Surg Radiol Anat* 2005;27:377-381.

    The authors of this cadaver study noted a communicating branch between the third and fourth common plantar digital nerves in 28% of feet. Communications were most frequent from the lateral to the medial plantar nerve. Communicating branches may be more susceptible to surgical injury and may explain recurrence or persistence of symptoms. Level of evidence: IV.

9. Schon L, Mann RA: Diseases of the nerves, in Coughlin M, Mann R, Saltzman C (eds): *Surgery of the Foot and Ankle*, ed 8. Philadelphia, PA, Mosby, 2007, pp 613-686.

    This book is an updated version of the quintessential classic text on the foot and ankle. This chapter discusses all issues relevant to the evaluation and management of nerve disorders in the lower extremity. Thorough and well written, this chapter is an excellent analysis and overview of the literature on foot and ankle nerve disorders. Level of evidence: IV.

10. Thompson FM, Deland JT: Occurrence of two interdigital neuromas in one foot. *Foot Ankle* 1993;14:15-17.

11. Bencardino J, Rosenberg ZS, Beltran J, Liu X, Marty-Delfaut E: Morton's neuroma: Is it always symptomatic? *AJR Am J Roentgenol* 2000;175:649-653.

12. Kankanala G, Jain AS: The operational characteristics of ultrasonography for the diagnosis of plantar intermetatarsal neuroma. *J Foot Ankle Surg* 2007;46:213-217.

    The usefulness of ultrasound in diagnosing Morton interdigital neuroma was evaluated in this retrospective study. Preoperative ultrasound findings were compared with postoperative histopathologic findings in resected interdigital neuromas. Statistical analysis reported a sensitivity of 91.48%, a specificity of 100%, and 100% positive and 20% negative predictive values. The authors report that the probability that ultrasound will confirm the presence of plantar intermetatarsal neuroma is 91.67%. Level of evidence: IV.

13. Quinn TJ, Jacobson JA, Craig JG, van Holsbeeck MT: Sonography of Morton's neuromas. *AJR Am J Roentgenol* 2000;174:1723-1728.

14. Sharp RJ, Wade CM, Hennessy MS, Saxby TS: The role of MRI and ultrasound imaging in Morton's neuroma and the effect of size of lesion on symptoms. *J Bone Joint Surg Br* 2003;85:999-1005.

    In this study, clinical assessment, ultrasound, and MRI were compared for accuracy in diagnosing interdigital neuromas. The accuracy of ultrasound and MRI was similar and dependent on lesion size; ultrasound was especially inaccurate for small lesions. Clinical assessment was the most sensitive and specific modality measured in this study. The authors concluded that there is no requirement for ultrasound or MRI to diagnose a Morton neuroma. Level of evidence: III.

15. Morscher E, Ulrich J, Dick W: Morton's intermetatarsal neuroma: Morphology and histological substrate. *Foot Ankle Int* 2000;21:558-562.

16. Almeida DF, Kurokawa K, Hatanaka Y, Hemmi S, Claussen GC, Oh SJ: Abnormal dip phenomenon: A characteristic electrophysiological marker in interdigital neuropathy of the foot. *Arq Neuropsiquiatr* 2007;65:771-778.

    This study reported the usefulness of electrodiagnostic tests in diagnosing interdigital neuralgia. Near-nerve needle nerve conduction showed abnormality in the affected interdigital nerves in all patients with a definite diagnosis of interdigital neuralgia. The authors reported that an abnormal dip phenomenon is the most characteristic electrophysiologic marker for diagnosing interdigital neuralgia. Level of evidence: IV.

17. Greenfield J, Rea J Jr, Ilfeld FW: Morton's interdigital neuroma: Indications for treatment by local injections versus surgery. *Clin Orthop Relat Res* 1984;185:142-144.

18. Hassouna H, Singh D, Taylor H, Johnson S: Ultrasound guided steroid injection in the treatment of interdigital neuralgia. *Acta Orthop Belg* 2007;73:224-229.

    This study reports the clinical effectiveness of ultrasound-guided injection of local anesthetic and steroid in the management of interdigital neuralgia. At a mean follow-up of 11.4 months, 67% of patients were satisfied with the results of treatment, and 63% of patients had no activity limitations and did not need modifications in shoe wear. Level of evidence: IV.

19. Mozena JD, Clifford JT: Efficacy of chemical neurolysis for the treatment of interdigital nerve compression of the foot: A retrospective study. *J Am Podiatr Med Assoc* 2007;97:203-206.

5: Neuromuscular Disease

This historic cohort study evaluated the safety and efficacy of dilute alcohol injections into the foot for the treatment of interdigital neuralgia. Three of 49 patients (6%) reported mild complications, all of which resolved spontaneously within 2 days of the injection. The authors concluded that dilute alcohol injections are a safe and effective treatment option for patients, but the procedure may be more successful if the patient receives at least five injections. Level of evidence: IV.

20. Fanucci E, Masala S, Fabiano S, et al: Treatment of intermetatarsal Morton's neuroma with alcohol injection under US guide: 10-month follow-up. *Eur Radiol* 2004; 14:514-518.

This study evaluated the efficacy of neuroma alcohol-sclerosing therapy injected inside interdigital neuromas using ultrasound guidance. Total or partial symptom relief was achieved in 90% of patients. At 10-month follow-up, there was a 20% to 30% reduction in mass volume. Transitory plantar pain caused by a reaction induced by the sclerosing solution occurred in 15% of patients. Level of evidence: IV.

21. Hughes RJ, Ali K, Jones H, Kendall S, Connell DA: Treatment of Morton's neuroma with alcohol injection under sonographic guidance: Follow-up of 101 cases. *AJR Am J Roentgenol* 2007;188:1535-1539.

This prospective study of 101 patients evaluated the use of ultrasound-guided alcohol injections into interdigital neuromas. Partial or total symptom improvement was achieved in 94% of the patients; 84% reported complete pain relief. An average of 4.1 treatments per person was administered. No major complications were reported. Level of evidence: III.

22. Shapiro SL: Endoscopic decompression of the intermetatarsal nerve for Morton's neuroma. *Foot Ankle Clin* 2004;9:297-304.

Endoscopic decompression of interdigital neuroma has shown promising results in early reports. Indications, advantages, and preliminary results in the first 40 patients are discussed. No hematomas or infections were reported. Level of evidence: IV.

23. Zelent ME, Kane RM, Neese DJ, Lockner WB: Minimally invasive Morton's intermetatarsal neuroma decompression. *Foot Ankle Int* 2007;28:263-265.

A technique for decompression of interdigital neuromas using an instrument designed to release the transverse carpal ligament for carpal tunnel syndrome is described. After this minimally invasive procedure, 11 of the 14 patients (79%) reported an absence of neuroma symptoms. Level of evidence: IV.

24. Mann RA, Reynolds JD: Interdigital neuroma: A critical clinical analysis. *Foot Ankle* 1983;3:238.

25. Coughlin MJ, Pinsonneault T: Operative treatment of interdigital neuroma: A long-term follow-up study. *J Bone Joint Surg Am* 2001;83:1321-1328.

26. Stamatis ED, Myerson MS: Treatment of recurrence of symptoms after excision of an interdigital neuroma: A retrospective review. *J Bone Joint Surg Br* 2004;86: 48-53.

The results of treating recurring or persistent symptoms after a previous excision of an interdigital neuroma are reported. Sixty interspaces were reexplored, and other concomitant procedures were performed. The authors report that 31% of patients were completely satisfied, 27% were satisfied with minor reservations, 20% were satisfied with major reservations, and 22% were dissatisfied with the outcome. No pain or mild pain was reported in 57% of patients, and 59% had moderate or severe restrictions in the choice of footwear; 16% had moderate restriction of activity. The authors noted that revision surgery for relieving the symptoms of interdigital neuroma is less successful than primary procedures. Level of evidence: IV.

27. Wolfort SF, Dellon AL: Treatment of recurrent neuroma of the interdigital nerve by implantation of the proximal nerve into muscle in the arch of the foot. *J Foot Ankle Surg* 2001;40:404-410.

28. Su E, Di Carlo E, O'Malley M, Bohne WH, Deland JT, Kennedy JG: The frequency of digital artery resection in Morton interdigital neurectomy. *Foot Ankle Int* 2006; 27:801-803.

A review of 674 consecutive pathologic specimens obtained after resection of an interdigital neuroma showed that the digital artery was simultaneously resected in 39% of specimens. Although no adverse effect was recorded following these arterial resections, the authors cautioned that care was needed to decrease the risk of vascular compromise. Level of evidence: IV.

29. Kopell HP, Thompson WA: Peripheral entrapment neuropathies of the lower extremity. *N Engl J Med* 1960; 262:56-60.

30. Davis TJ, Schon LC: Branches of the tibial nerve: Anatomic variations. *Foot Ankle Int* 1995;16:21-29.

31. Dellon AL, Kim J, Spaulding CM: Variations in the origin of the medial calcaneal nerve. *J Am Podiatr Med Assoc* 2002;92:97-101.

32. Lumsden DB, Schon LC, Easley ME, et al: Topography of the distal tibial nerve and its branches. *Foot Ankle Int* 2003;24:696-700.

The topographic anatomy of the distal tibial nerve and its branches is reported in this anatomic study. Knowledge of this anatomy is helpful in understanding the position of the various branches before ramification. Damaged nerve fascicles may be localized within the trunk of the nerve. Level of evidence: IV.

33. Cimino WR: Tarsal tunnel syndrome: Review of the literature. *Foot Ankle* 1990;11:47-52.

34. Kinoshita M, Okuda R, Morikawa J, Abe M: Tarsal tunnel syndrome associated with an accessory muscle. *Foot Ankle Int* 2003;24:132-136.

The authors report on patients with tarsal tunnel syndrome resulting from an accessory muscle within the tarsal canal. An accessory flexor digitorum longus muscle was present in six patients, and an accessory soleus muscle was present in one patient (both feet). No functional deficit was observed after tarsal tunnel release and accessory muscle excision. Level of evidence: IV.

35. Kinoshita M, Okuda R, Yasuda T, Abe M: Tarsal tunnel syndrome in athletes. *Am J Sports Med* 2006;34:1307-1312.

   This review of the medical charts of athletes with tarsal tunnel syndrome found predisposing underlying physical factors, such as flatfoot deformity, talocalcaneal coalition, accessory muscles, and bony fragments around the tarsal tunnel that exacerbated symptoms. Tarsal tunnel syndrome was triggered by activities that applied a heavy burden on the ankle joint, such as sprinting, jumping, and performing ashibarai in judo. Level of evidence: IV.

36. Trepman E, Kadel NJ, Chisholm K, Razzano L: Effect of foot and ankle position on tarsal tunnel compartment pressure. *Foot Ankle Int* 1999;20:721-726.

37. Bracilovic A, Nihal A, Houston VL, Beattie AC, Rosenberg ZS, Trepman E: Effect of foot and ankle position on tarsal tunnel compartment volume. *Foot Ankle Int* 2006;27:431-437.

   This MRI study showed that positional change of the foot and ankle from neutral to eversion or inversion causes decreased tarsal tunnel compartment volume. Decreased compartment volume of the tarsal tunnel with inversion and eversion of the foot can contribute to symptoms of tibial nerve entrapment in tarsal tunnel syndrome. Level of evidence: IV.

38. Daniels TR, Lau JT, Hearn TC: The effects of foot position and load on tibial nerve tension. *Foot Ankle Int* 1998;19:73-78.

39. Lau JT, Daniels TR: Effects of tarsal tunnel release and stabilization procedures on tibial nerve tension in a surgically created pes planus foot. *Foot Ankle Int* 1998;19:770-777.

40. Labib SA, Gould JS, Rodriguez-del-Rio FA, Lyman S: Heel pain triad (HPT): The combination of plantar fasciitis, posterior tibial tendon dysfunction and tarsal tunnel syndrome. *Foot Ankle Int* 2002;23:212-220.

41. Budak F, Bamac B, Ozbek A, Kutluay P, Komsuoglu S: Nerve conduction studies of lower extremities in pes planus subjects. *Electromyogr Clin Neurophysiol* 2001; 41:443-446.

42. Kinoshita M, Okuda R, Morikawa J, Jotoku T, Abe M: The dorsiflexion-eversion test for diagnosis of tarsal tunnel syndrome. *J Bone Joint Surg Am* 2001;83:1835-1839.

43. Frey C, Kerr R: Magnetic resonance imaging and the evaluation of tarsal tunnel syndrome. *Foot Ankle* 1993; 14:159-164.

44. Nagaoka M, Matsuzaki H: Ultrasonography in tarsal tunnel syndrome. *J Ultrasound Med* 2005;24:1035-1040.

   To clarify the diagnostic value of ultrasound in tarsal tunnel syndrome, preoperative ultrasound findings were confirmed by intraoperative findings. Ganglia, talocalcaneal coalition, talocalcaneal coalition associated with ganglia, and varicose veins were confirmed by surgery as causes of tarsal tunnel syndrome. The authors concluded that as a diagnostic imaging technique for tarsal tunnel syndrome, ultrasonography is extremely useful for identifying space-occupying lesions. Level of evidence: IV.

45. Oh SJ, Savaria PK, Kuba T, Elmore RS: Tarsal tunnel syndrome: Electrophysiologic study. *Ann Neurol* 1979; 5:327-330.

46. Patel AT, Gaines K, Malamut R, et al: Usefulness of electrodiagnostic techniques in the evaluation of suspected tarsal tunnel syndrome: An evidence-based review. *Muscle Nerve* 2005;32:236-240.

   This evidence-based review was performed to evaluate the use of NCV studies and needle EMG in diagnosing tarsal tunnel syndrome. The authors reviewed 317 articles on tarsal tunnel syndrome. Four articles met class III level of evidence and were included in the study. These articles examined the use of electrodiagnostic techniques for evaluating patients with clinically suspected tarsal tunnel syndrome. It was noted that sensory NCV studies were more likely to be abnormal than motor NCV studies; however, the actual sensitivity and specificity could not be determined. The sensitivity of needle EMG abnormalities could not be determined. Level of evidence: III.

47. Aszmann O, Tassler PL, Dellon AL: Changing the natural history of diabetic neuropathy: Incidence of ulcer/amputation in the contralateral limb of patients with a unilateral nerve decompression procedure. *Ann Plast Surg* 2004;53:517-522.

   This retrospective analysis evaluates a patient population treated with peripheral nerve decompression for symptomatic diabetic neuropathy. No ulcerations developed and no amputations were performed on the foot treated with peripheral nerve decompression. Indications for surgical treatment of diabetic neuropathy are discussed. The authors conclude that surgical nerve decompression holds the promise of effectively preventing ulceration and amputation caused from the naturally occurring neuropathy of diabetes. Level of evidence: IV.

48. Biddinger KR, Amend KJ: The role of surgical decompression for diabetic neuropathy. *Foot Ankle Clin* 2004; 9:239-254.

   The authors review previous studies of surgical decompression of peripheral nerves for the treatment of diabetic peripheral neuropathy. The controversies surrounding this topic are discussed. Level of evidence: IV.

49. Dellon AL: Diabetic neuropathy: Review of a surgical approach to restore sensation, relieve pain, and prevent ulceration and amputation. *Foot Ankle Int* 2004;25: 749-755.

5: Neuromuscular Disease

This article presents a review of the basic scientific and clinical research that supports the concepts that metabolic neuropathy renders the peripheral nerve susceptible to compression in patients with diabetes and that decompression of lower extremity peripheral nerves in these patients can relieve pain, restore sensation, and prevent ulceration and amputation. Level of evidence: IV.

50. Lee CH, Dellon AL: Prognostic ability of Tinel sign in determining outcome for decompression surgery in diabetic and nondiabetic neuropathy. *Ann Plast Surg* 2004; 53:523-527.

Outcomes of patients with and without a Tinel sign who were treated with surgical decompression of the tibial nerve and its branches in the tarsal tunnel are presented. The presence of a positive Tinel sign demonstrates that 92% of the patients can expect a good to excellent outcome. If the preoperative Tinel sign is negative, 33% of the patients can expect a good to excellent outcome. This finding was true for patients with diabetic and idiopathic tibial neuropathy. Level of evidence:IV.

51. Krishnan KG, Pinzer T, Schackert G: A novel endoscopic technique in treating single nerve entrapment syndromes with special attention to ulnar nerve transposition and tarsal tunnel release: Clinical application. *Neurosurgery* 2006;59(suppl 1):ONS89-100.

Endoscopic tarsal tunnel release techniques and outcomes are described in this article. Results showed scores of excellent in 62.5% and good in 37.5% of patients treated with this procedure for tarsal tunnel syndrome. Level of evidence: IV.

52. Pfeiffer WH, Cracchiolo A III: Clinical results after tarsal tunnel decompression. *J Bone Joint Surg Am* 1994; 76:1222-1230.

53. Takakura Y, Kitada C, Sugimoto K, Tanaka Y, Tamai S: Tarsal tunnel syndrome: Causes and results of operative treatment. *J Bone Joint Surg Br* 1991;73:125-128.

54. Sammarco GJ, Chang L: Outcome of surgical treatment of tarsal tunnel syndrome. *Foot Ankle Int* 2003;24: 125-131.

Long-term outcome data based on clinical findings and positive electrodiagnostic studies after tarsal tunnel release are reported. The most common surgical findings included arterial vascular leashes indenting the nerve and scarring about the nerve. Level of evidence: IV.

55. Gondring WH, Shields B, Wenger S: An outcomes analysis of surgical treatment of tarsal tunnel syndrome. *Foot Ankle Int* 2003;24:545-550.

Outcomes following tarsal tunnel release are reported. A clinical dichotomy was noted by the authors. Although 85% of patients had objectively measured complete symptom relief, only 51% of the patients reported subjective symptom relief. Level of evidence: IV.

56. Reuben SS, Buvanendran A: Preventing the development of chronic pain after orthopaedic surgery with preventive multimodal analgesic techniques. *J Bone Joint Surg Am* 2007;89:1343-1358.

This article presents an in-depth strategy for controlling postoperative pain and focuses on a multimodal approach. Level of evidence: IV.

57. Pedowitz W, Pedowitz D: Soft tissue disorders of the foot, in Coughlin M, Mann R, Saltzman C (eds): *Surgery of the Foot and Ankle,* ed 8. Philadelphia, PA, Mosby, 2007, pp 1826-1841.

This chapter discusses all issues relevant to the evaluation and management of CRPS in the lower extremity. It is a thorough and indispensable reference for treating patients with CRPS. Level of evidence: IV.

58. Atkins RM: Complex regional pain syndrome. *J Bone Joint Surg Br* 2003;85:1100-1106.

The author summarizes the current understanding and approach to treating the enigmatic problems of CRPS from an orthopaedic perspective. Level of evidence: IV.

59. Stanton-Hicks M: Complex regional pain syndrome. *Anesthesiol Clin North America* 2003;21:733-744.

A review of the advances in clinical management and research of CRPS is presented. Attention is given to a treatment algorithm that focuses on a rehabilitation model. The authors report that sympatholysis itself is not a diagnostic test for CRPS. Level of evidence: IV.

60. Hogan CJ, Hurwitz SR: Treatment of complex regional pain syndrome of the lower extremity. *J Am Acad Orthop Surg* 2002;10:281-289.

61. Dowd GS, Hussein R, Khanduja V, Ordman AJ: Complex regional pain syndrome with special emphasis on the knee. *J Bone Joint Surg Br* 2007;89;285-290.

The pathophysiology, diagnosis, and current treatment options for CRPS are discussed in this article. Level of evidence: IV.

62. McCabe CS, Haigh RC, Ring EF, Halligan PW, Wall PD, Blake DR: A controlled pilot study of the utility of mirror visual feedback in the treatment of complex regional pain syndrome. *Rheumatology (Oxford)* 2003;42:97-101.

Congruent visual feedback of the moving unaffected limb via a mirror significantly reduces the perception of pain in early CRPS type 1 and stiffness in the intermediate stages of the disease. The extent of the analgesic effect was unexpected by both patients and investigators in this study. Level of evidence: III.

63. Wilder RT, Berde CB, Wolohan M, Vieyra MA, Masek BJ, Micheli LJ: Reflex sympathetic dystrophy in children: Clinical characteristics and follow-up of seventy patients. *J Bone Joint Surg Am* 1992;74:910-919.

64. Phillips WJ, Currier BL: Analgesic pharmacology: II. Specific analgesics. *J Am Acad Orthop Surg* 2004;12: 221-233.

This extensive review article discusses current medications and their indications and uses in treating pain. Level of evidence: IV.

65. Grabow TS, Tella PK, Raja SN: Spinal cord stimulation for complex regional pain syndrome: An evidence-based medicine review of the literature. *Clin J Pain* 2003;19: 371-383.

This critical review of the published literature discusses the efficacy of spinal cord stimulation in the treatment of CRPS and scrutinizes the rationale behind the widespread use of spinal cord stimulation as a therapeutic modality in the management of CRPS. Level of evidence: III.

66. Watson TS, Anderson RB, Davis WH, Kiebzak GM: Distal tarsal tunnel release with partial plantar fasciotomy for chronic heel pain: An outcome analysis. *Foot Ankle Int* 2002;23:530-537.

67. Baxter DE, Pfeffer GB: Treatment of chronic heel pain by surgical release of the first branch of the lateral plantar nerve. *Clin Orthop Relat Res* 1992;279:229-236.

68. Styf J: Entrapment of the superficial peroneal nerve: Diagnosis and results of decompression. *J Bone Joint Surg Br* 1989;71:131-135.

69. Rosson GD, Dellon AL: Superficial peroneal nerve anatomic variability changes surgical technique. *Clin Orthop Relat Res* 2005;438:248-252.

Anatomic variability in the location of the SPN is evaluated in this study. The SPN was found in the lateral compartment in 57% of patients, the lateral and anterior compartments in 26%, and in the anterior compartment in 17%. The authors note the importance of releasing the anterior compartment during surgical decompression of the nerve. Level of evidence: IV.

70. Schepsis AA, Fitzgerald M, Nicoletta R: Revision surgery for exertional anterior compartment syndrome of the lower leg: Technique, findings, and results. *Am J Sports Med* 2005;33:1040-1047.

Patients with a recurrence of symptoms following fasciotomy for exertional compartment syndrome were reported to have symptoms, signs, and surgical findings of SPN entrapment in 44% of patients. Level of evidence:IV.

71. Dellon AL, Swier P, Maloney CT Jr, Livengood M, Werter S: Chemotherapy-induced neuropathy: Treatment by decompression of peripheral nerves. *Plast Reconstr Surg* 2004;114:478-483.

The authors review the various causes for neuropathy and their treatment by surgical nerve decompression.

Patients with a positive Tinel sign over the site of entrapment have better outcomes. Level of evidence: IV.

72. Styf J, Morberg P: The superficial peroneal tunnel syndrome: Results of treatment by decompression. *J Bone Joint Surg Br* 1997;79:801-803.

73. Coert JH, Meek MF, Gibeault D, Dellon AL: Documentation of posttraumatic nerve compression in patients with normal electrodiagnostic studies. *J Trauma* 2004; 56:339-344.

This study discusses the use of neurosensory testing with a Pressure-Specified Sensory Device. The authors report that this testing documents the presence of neuropathy and can demonstrate axonal loss by measuring increasing distances in two-point discrimination. Level of evidence: IV.

74. Aktan Ikiz ZA, Ucerler H, Bilge O: The anatomic features of the sural nerve with an emphasis on its clinical importance. *Foot Ankle Int* 2005;26:560-567.

This anatomic study discusses the variability of the sural nerve in the lower extremity. Level of evidence: IV.

75. Gould N, Trevino S: Sural nerve entrapment by avulsion fracture of the base of the fifth metatarsal bone. *Foot Ankle* 1981;2:153-155.

76. Keeling JJ, Schon LC: Risk to neurovascular structures using posterolateral percutaneous ankle screw placement: A cadaver study. *Foot Ankle Int* 2007;28: 614-616.

This cadaver study identifies the risks to local neurovascular structures using standard surgical approaches for percutaneous guide pin placement during ankle arthrodesis. The authors recommend starting the posterolateral guide pin more lateral or closer to the fibula to avoid injury to the sural nerve. The tibial nerve is potentially at risk for injury if the percutaneous pin insertion crosses medial to the coronal midline plane. Level of evidence: IV.

77. Fabre T, Montero C, Gaujard E, Gervais-Dellion F, Durandeau A: Chronic calf pain in athletes due to sural nerve entrapment: A report of 18 cases. *Am J Sports Med* 2000;28:679-682.

78. Schon LC: Nerve entrapment, neuropathy, and nerve dysfunction in athletes. *Orthop Clin North Am* 1994; 25:47-59.

5: Neuromuscular Disease

Section 6

Special Problems
of the Foot and Ankle

SECTION EDITOR:

STUART D. MILLER, MD

Chapter 25

Nondiabetic Foot Infections

Daniel C. Farber, MD   Sharon Henry, MD

Introduction

Infection, the pathologic condition resulting from invasion of a host organism by a foreign species, is both a common cause of disorders of the foot and ankle and a potential complication of treatment. Infections result from an imbalance between the host immunity and the virility of the invading organisms. Understanding the methods of prevention, detection, diagnosis, and treatment of infection is a crucial part of any foot and ankle practice. A thorough history and physical examination play an important role in identifying factors that increase a patient's susceptibility to infection and can help direct treatment. Based on the medical condition of a specific patient population, preventive measures may be available to minimize the incidence of infection. Diagnostic modalities help to determine affected areas and causative organisms. This information is used in planning treatment, which may include surgical and nonsurgical modalities. This chapter will review strategies for preventing infection and evaluating and treating infections in the foot and ankle.

History and Physical Examination

A thorough history and physical examination are crucial elements in evaluating a patient with a suspected infection of the foot and ankle. The duration of symptoms will help differentiate acute, subacute, and more chronic disorders. An acute disorder may evolve into a rapidly progressive condition, such as an abscess or necrotizing fasciitis, which requires urgent evaluation and treatment. A lengthy prodromal period may indicate chronic osteomyelitis or a slowly progressing fungal infection. Evidence of systemic involvement (such as fever, chills, fatigue, and nausea) should prompt more rapid evaluation and treatment. Numerous underlying medical conditions, especially those that compromise the patient's ability to effectively combat pathogens, increase the risks of infection. Conditions such as acquired immunodeficiency syndrome, diabetes, chronic kidney disease, peripheral vascular disease, and autoimmune dermatologic conditions such as psoriasis (which predispose the patient to bacterial entry by compromising the skin) are known to increase the risks of infection. Certain medications, particularly those affecting the host immune system, including antirejection transplant medications, chemotherapeutic agents, and disease-modifying antirheumatologic medications, are established risk factors for certain types of opportunistic infections. Previous trauma (acute or remote) increases the risk of infection by providing an opportunity for tissue contamination or the formation of a hematoma, which may be susceptible to hematogenous seeding. Recent antibiotic use can affect diagnostic tests and mask underlying infection or lead to the growth of resistant bacteria. Insect or animal exposure or bites, recent travel, exposure to ill individuals, previous institutionalization, work in the health care environment, and previous infections may expose patients to specific, unique infectious diseases. Prior surgery in the affected area also is important in evaluating the potential chronicity and extent of tissue involvement. For patients undergoing surgery, tobacco use is associated with an increased risk of complications, including infection, and also is a barrier to healing of an active infection.[1] Nutritional status, which can have a significant effect on both susceptibility to infection and the ability to overcome it, should also be assessed through either direct questioning or laboratory evaluation.[2] Screening devices, such as the Nutritional Risk Index or the Maastricht Index, are effective in determining nutritional status.[3] A history of vascular insufficiency or bypass surgery should be determined. The characteristics of local symptoms, including location, pain, warmth, and swelling, are important factors. If an open wound is present, a history of the type and quality of drainage from the area and any recent changes in the quality or location of discomfort should be elicited from the patient.

The physical examination may reveal obvious signs in fulminant infections, but findings may be less apparent in patients with chronic infection. Evidence of systemic involvement includes pyrexia (not always seen in elderly patients), hypotension, tachycardia, and a change in mental status. More focal examination should include evaluation for areas of skin compromise, erythema, edema, drainage, local tenderness, fluctuant tissue, and the presence of old scars that may indicate prior trauma or surgical procedures. Wounds should be inspected and assessed for size, color, exudate, and odor. Sinus tracts should be probed. A positive probe-to-bone test (such that the probe encounters the bone) is highly suggestive of osteomyelitis.[4] Local

6: Special Problems of the Foot and Ankle

spread of disease may be evidenced by streaking erythema or subcutaneous air. Cellulitis may extend to distant areas. Lymphadenopathy of the corresponding lymph nodes should be assessed. Joint range of motion and the quality and level of pain caused by motion should be noted to differentiate soft-tissue involvement from joint involvement. A vascular examination should be performed by evaluating pulses, capillary refill, hair distribution, and, if appropriate, ankle-brachial indices. Marking the extent of erythema or other skin changes assists in evaluating the efficacy of treatment and the progression of the disease process.

Diagnostic Studies

Laboratory Studies

Laboratory testing can play an important role in evaluating a patient with suspected infection and is useful for monitoring treatment efficacy. A complete blood count with differential will provide information about the systemic response to infection. In a normal host, acute infection will be characterized by an elevated white blood cell count with acute bacterial infections yielding an increase in neutrophils (a left shift). Elderly patients or immunocompromised patients may not produce leukocytosis. An increased lymphocyte count may reflect viral or chronic bacterial infection. Abundant eosinophils suggest a potential parasitic or allergic condition.

Inflammatory markers, such as erythrocyte sedimentation rate (ESR) and quantitative C-reactive protein (CRP), provide important but nonspecific information. A positive result may confirm the clinical suspicion of infection and can help identify the efficacy of therapy. In general, the ESR is slower to respond to the systemic infectious process and slower to return to normal after effective treatment compared with CRP. CRP correlates more acutely with the body's inflammatory response and will decline rapidly with the initiation of effective treatment. A recent study suggests that ESR may decrease as early as the second day of treatment and should continue to trend downward with successful healing.[5] ESR, however, may remain elevated above normal levels, whereas CRP should normalize with successful treatment. Some elevation of ESR and CRP occurs with surgery, even in the absence of infection.[6] Patients with other comorbidities, especially autoimmune disease, may have chronically elevated levels of these markers. Interpretation of absolute values may be difficult without knowing the patient's baseline levels, including nutritional markers such as albumin, prealbumin, and transferrin.

Results of bacterial cultures are often important in the treatment of infection. Isolation of the infectious organism and its antibiotic susceptibility profile can be crucial to successful treatment. Cultures should be obtained in as clean a fashion as possible. Cultures obtained from chronic wounds will often yield polymicrobial growth that will not be beneficial in guiding treatment. Deep cultures obtained via aspiration or through surgical débridement yield the best results. Ideally, these cultures should be obtained before the initiation of antibiotic therapy to avoid false-negative results. Cultures should be evaluated for aerobic and anaerobic bacteria, fungi, and mycobacteria as indicated by the clinical situation.

Autoimmune disorders, including gout, can present with inflammatory symptoms that mimic infection. Appropriate laboratory testing, including analysis of serum and joint aspirate, can help differentiate the etiology of the inflammatory process.

Imaging Studies

Radiography plays an important role in the diagnosis of foot and ankle infections. Plain radiographs may show gas in the local tissues, soft-tissue shadows representing edema or abscess, or bony changes. Localized osteopenia, bony erosion, or periosteal reaction are helpful radiographic signs, but their absence does not preclude the diagnosis of infection because these findings are generally absent in the acute phases of osteomyelitis. Bony findings may lag 2 to 4 weeks behind the disease process. The presence of a prior fracture or retained implants also is important in formulating an appropriate treatment plan.

CT is more sensitive than a plain radiograph for showing bony changes, including the identification of sequestrum, nonunion, and periosteal reactions. CT also may help detect gas in soft-tissue planes and soft-tissue swelling and can localize abscesses for aspiration or surgical planning. Although few studies are available to support the effectiveness of CT for evaluating osteomyelitis, sensitivity is estimated at approximately 70% and specificity from 50% to 70%.[7,8] CT can be affected by metal implants that create local interference affecting the usefulness of this modality.

MRI is effective at evaluating edema within the bone and soft tissues. Abscesses and bony involvement are readily detectable; however, the changes seen are often nonspecific and may result from fractures, tumors, reactive changes, or local soft-tissue injury. The most valuable findings are destruction of a bony cortex, especially when contiguous with a soft-tissue mass (usually representative of abscess formation). Sensitivity of 77% to 100% and specificity of 40% to 100% in diagnosing osteomyelitis has been reported.[9,10] Metal implants also can distort the images obtained with MRI, although titanium implants may produce only local signal dropout.

Ultrasound may be useful for detecting abscesses for image-guided aspiration. The probe, however, may not be tolerated by some patients because of the sensitivity of the skin and soft tissues. Ultrasound is unreliable for detecting subtle changes in bone integrity.

Nuclear Medicine

Nuclear medicine studies can provide valuable information about infection. Three-phase technetium bone scans are often the first investigative tool and will show subtle bony destruction before changes can be identified with plain radiographs; however, these studies are nonspecific because uptake can be caused by fracture, stress, or injury. The sensitivity of a triple-phase bone scan is approximately 82%, with a 25% specificity in chronic osteomyelitis.[7] Technetium, exametazime, or indium-labeled white blood cell scans are more specific for infection, with values ranging from 77% to 84% for chronic osteomyelitis.[7,11] The combination of a triple-phase bone scan, followed by an indium (leucocyte-labeled) study can help differentiate bone edema (as seen in patients with Charcot foot) from active bone infection. Sulfur colloid studies may help to determine the amount of background marrow reaction if questions remain concerning the etiology of increased uptake with other modalities. Quiescent marrow on sulfur colloid scanning suggests that the uptake is caused by the labeled white blood cells, whereas active marrow suggests a false-positive white blood cell scan. Nuclear medicine studies often are helpful in localizing pathology and in assessing the nature of the disease process. These studies also can guide more focused evaluation with MRI, CT, or ultrasound. The use of single photon emission CT and positron emission tomography scanning (sensitivity and specificity values in chronic osteomyelitis of 96% and 91%, respectively), often combined with CT imaging, has received recent attention; however, these modalities are not yet widely available.[7]

It is important to realize that no single imaging or nuclear medicine test is routinely accurate for evaluating infection. These studies must always be correlated with the clinical situation to avoid inappropriate treatment.

Common Infections

Minor infections about the foot and ankle are common. Some of the most prevalent include ingrown toenails, felons, fungal infections of the skin and nails, puncture wounds, secondarily infected abrasions, and bites from animals or insects.

Ingrown Toenails

Ingrown toenail infections result from impaction of the nail into the surrounding tissue caused by improper nail trimming or the inherent shape of the nail. The traumatized tissue is colonized by local bacteria, which can lead to a painful infection (paronychia). Early infection of ingrown toenails may respond to soaking in warm water and oral antibiotics; however, surgical drainage and removal of the nail edge is necessary when there is fluctuant tissue or gross purulence. Incision and drainage often can be accomplished in the office setting using digital block anesthesia. Recurrent complications can be managed with partial nail removal and ablation of the appropriate area of the nail matrix.

Felons

A felon is an infection occurring within the septated tissue of the pulp space of the distal phalanx of the toe. *Staphylococcus aureus* is the most common infecting organism. Patients present with severe pain around a tense and erythematous distal toe. Surgical treatment is necessary, and the wound is usually left open to drain during administration of antibiotics. The incision should be transverse, releasing the multiple septae involved with this condition. Failure to recognize and treat this infection can result in subsequent osteomyelitis of the distal phalanx.

Fungal Infections

Fungal infections of the skin and nails can be difficult to treat. Slow growing fungal species such as *Trichophyton rubrum* and other dermatophytes can become entrenched in nail tissue and skin. Topical treatment with antifungal agents such as amorolfine, ciclopirox, terbinafine, or imidazoles requires prolonged and regular treatment, with skin infections responding better than nail infections. Systemic treatment with terbinafine is superior to itraconazole and griseofulvin, but the risk of liver toxicity necessitates careful monitoring of liver function during treatment. Duration of treatment ranges from 3 to 9 months, and adverse side effects, such as taste disturbance and gastrointestinal upset, are common. These factors may further complicate treatment by affecting the patient's willingness to undergo treatment and complete the course of treatment.

Puncture Wound Infections

Puncture wounds of the foot are common and frequently occur in barefoot individuals. Hard objects such as metal nails, wood splinters, or other debris can penetrate the shoe before breaking the skin, thus bringing additional contaminants to the wound. Animal bites also can cause puncture wounds. Therapeutic attention should be directed toward contamination from the penetrating object, contamination from the shoe material (commonly *Pseudomonas aeruginosa*), and displaced skin flora. The patient's tetanus immunization status should be determined, and a booster shot should be considered. The offending object should be removed if still in place, and the wound copiously irrigated. It is critical to ensure that no foreign body is retained; this can be challenging when radiolucent material is involved. Retained foreign bodies can cause chronic nonhealing wounds. Surgical exploration is unnecessary if there is no residual foreign material or injury to tendons, nerves, or blood vessels. A short course of cephalosporin or another antibiotic, depending on the level of contamination, is recommended.

Secondary infection of minor cuts or abrasions of the foot or ankle will usually respond to local wound débridement and oral antibiotics. Cultures may be helpful in directing antibiotic therapy. Rapidly progressive infection may represent necrotizing fasciitis.

Animal bites may be treated similarly to other traumatic injuries to the soft tissues. Débridement of the wound should be performed as needed. The animal should be identified and tested for rabies; if any suspicion of rabies exists, prophylactic vaccination should be initiated. Early treatment will usually avoid late complications. Patients presenting in a delayed fashion may require further wound débridement, immobilization, and parenteral antibiotics. The most common infecting organism following a cat or dog bite is *Pasteurella multocida*. Antibiotic treatment with amoxicillin/clavulanic acid should cover most potential gram-negative and gram-positive organisms. Patients sustaining a cat bite are at risk of infection with *Bartonella henselae*, the organism that causes cat-scratch fever, and should be counseled about the signs and symptoms of this infection, which include a sore at the bite area and local lymphadenopathy.

The initial reaction to insect bites is an envenomation or allergic response. Infection occurs from secondary contamination. The bite of the brown recluse spider causes subcutaneous tissue necrosis that can mimic necrotizing fasciitis. The transmission of disease processes such as Lyme disease, Rocky Mountain spotted fever, filariasis, and dengue fever should also be considered in patients with insect bites.[12]

Cellulitis

Cellulitis involves infection of the skin and subcutaneous tissues and can arise from major or minor trauma to the skin or from hematogeneous or lymphatic sources. The risk of cellulitis increases with age, with a 43% increase per 10-year increment.[13] Toe-web intertrigo has been identified as a risk factor for cellulitis, and, in some instances, the same organisms have been identified at the site of cellulitis.[14,15] Pain, swelling, erythema, and induration are common characteristics of this infection, and signs and symptoms are usually well localized and nonsystemic. Fevers or other sites of involvement require a septic workup to determine the source of a disseminating infection.

A leg with cellulitis shows localized erythema with possible lymphangitic spread and lymphadenopathy. Care should be taken to observe any areas of fluctuant tissue to rule out an abscess as the source of the cellulitis. It is often helpful to mark the extent of erythema on the skin so that improvement or worsening of the condition following treatment can be observed and documented. Cellulitis spanning a joint may decrease range of motion, but pain is usually more superficial and less focal than in septic arthritis. Aspiration of the joint through unaffected skin should be considered only if there is high suspicion of joint infection. Aspiration through cellulitic tissue should be avoided because of potential contamination of the joint that could precipitate septic arthritis.

Cellulitis can be determined by clinical diagnosis and may not require radiographic evaluation. Radiographs may be helpful to detect foreign bodies or air in the soft tissues. CT or MRI provides less information at this stage of the infection but may be useful if abscess or fascial involvement is suspected.

S aureus and *Streptococcus* are the most common organisms responsible for localized cellulitis. Most patients will respond to oral antibiotic treatment in combination with local care, including immobilization and elevation of the affected limb. Clinical response may take 2 to 3 days for resolution of the erythema. Empirically, first-generation cephalosporins are appropriate therapy, but clindamycin and ciprofloxacin may be substituted in patients who are allergic to penicillin. Ciprofloxacin should be used when *Pseudomonas* is suspected. Methicillin-resistant *S aureus* (MRSA) is becoming an increasingly common cause of cellulitis, and appropriate antibiotics should be given to patients with risk factors. If the disease process is advanced or severe, parenteral antibiotics may be warranted, with broad-spectrum coverage using antibiotics such as ampicillin-sulbactam or piperacillin-tazobactam. Rapid progression of cellulitis may represent a more severe infection, such as necrotizing fasciitis, and must be vigorously treated.

Necrotizing Fasciitis

Necrotizing fasciitis is an extremely aggressive infection that can be classified into two groups. Type I is a polymicrobial infection in which *Escherichia coli*, *Pseudomonas, Klebsiella, S aureus*, streptococci, and anaerobic organisms may be the causative agents; type II is caused by group A, β-hemolytic *Streptococcus pyogenes* alone or in combination with *S aureus*.[16] Early recognition is critical because this infection progresses rapidly by traveling along fascial planes. Initial symptoms include pain that may be out of proportion to the clinical appearance of the leg. Patients are often misdiagnosed with muscle strains and later present with severe involvement and shock. Typically, the affected limb will become swollen and erythematous, and dark fluid-filled blisters may arise. Necrosis of the subcutaneous tissues and fascia can progress at up to 1 inch per hour with visible skin changes lagging considerably behind the deeper tissues. The infecting organisms may secrete toxins that damage endothelial linings and activate the complementary cascade, resulting in systemic involvement. This can lead to septic shock, multisystem organ failure, and a high mortality rate. Immunocompromised patients, such as those with diabetes, human immunodeficiency virus, malignancy, malnutrition, chronic kidney disease, and patients receiving chemotherapy or corticosteroids are at high risk for necrotizing fasciitis. Patients with multiple trauma and those in the peripartum period also are at greater risk for necrotizing fasciitis.

Although necrotizing fasciitis is a clinical diagnosis, radiographic imaging may be helpful in defining the extent of necrosis or fluid collections. Aggressive care should not be delayed while waiting for the results of diagnostic studies. Antibiotic treatment alone is inadequate; rapid surgical débridement combined with appropriate antibiotic therapy and intensive medical care is required. There is evidence to support the use of adjunctive hyperbaric oxygen therapy following adequate surgery. Repeated débridements are often necessary to fully control this infection, and amputation may be needed to treat rapidly progressive infections. Extensive soft-tissue reconstruction is often necessary after the infection is eradicated.

Recruitment of other specialists, including a general surgeon, an infectious disease consultant, and a critical care specialist, is appropriate. Referral to a tertiary care center may be necessary for reconstruction; however, because of the rapid progression of the disease, the treating physician should begin aggressive care; delaying surgical débridement is associated with increased mortality.[16]

Osteomyelitis

Osteomyelitis is an infection of bone by pyogenic organisms that may be either acute or chronic and may arise from local inoculation or hematogenous spread. Local inoculation can occur as a complication from surgery, trauma, skin ulceration, or other lesions. Hematogenous spread may result from intravenous drug use, systemic infection, or seeding from a distant infected site. Diabetes, acquired immunodeficiency syndrome, sickle cell disease, peripheral vascular disease, intravenous drug abuse, alcoholism, chronic steroid use, or any immune-compromising condition can predispose patients to osteomyelitis. Retained hardware also poses a risk factor for osteomyelitis because glycocalyx formation can prevent antibiotic effectiveness on colonized metal.

Acute hematogenous osteomyelitis occurs primarily in children, affecting the highly vascularized metaphyseal area of bone. When promptly diagnosed, osteomyelitis in children can often be treated with intravenous antibiotics alone. However, the presence of intramedullary abscess, bone necrosis, or sequestrum may necessitate surgical débridement. Hematogenous osteomyelitis is rare in adults, although it occasionally occurs in the spine. Hematogenous spread in adults is more likely to progress to chronic osteomyelitis.

Acute osteomyelitis is characterized by a relatively rapid onset (1 to 4 weeks) of pain and is usually preceded by local trauma or surgery. Patients may have tenderness over the involved bone and local signs of inflammation. Restricted range of motion and an antalgic gait may be observed. Prompt recognition, before the onset of purulence or necrosis, may allow treatment with antibiotics alone.

Chronic osteomyelitis often follows a more indolent course that can progress over months to years. Patients may present with a draining sinus tract, bony instability, gait abnormalities, or chronic soft-tissue changes in the affected area. In some instances, the clinical examination may be quite benign, and only an appropriate history yields clues to the diagnosis. In patients with both acute and chronic osteomyelitis, a radiographic workup is important to assess the extent of bone involvement, the presence of purulence or sequestrum, and the presence of surgical implants or other foreign material. Diagnostic imaging may include plain radiographs, nuclear medicine imaging, CT, or MRI. In many patients with osteomyelitis, débridement is required in addition to parenteral or highly bioavailable oral antibiotics. Surgical treatment of osteomyelitis has several goals. The removal of all purulent and nonviable tissue and any implants or other contaminants is crucial. Obtaining a specimen for cultures allows directed treatment with the most effective and appropriate antibiotic. Care should be taken to treat any potential instability or fracture; this may require casting or external fixation. Dead spaces should be drained or filled with antibiotic-impregnated bone cement, calcium sulfate, or other resorbable material. These materials usually are combined with vancomycin, gentamicin, and/or tobramycin to provide high concentrations of antibiotics at the site of infection. Recent studies have evaluated the use of daptomycin, which may be helpful in infections from methicillin- or vancomycin-resistant organisms.[17,18] Elution rates are highest in the first 24 hours and taper off significantly after that period.[19] Methylmethacrylate beads must be removed before definitive treatment, whereas calcium sulfate beads will be reabsorbed over time. It is important to note that using calcium sulfate beads to deliver antibiotics is an off-label use because it has not been approved by the US Food and Drug Administration. Anecdotally, calcium sulfate resorbable delivery mechanisms are known to drain from the wound with a creamy white discharge, which is suggestive of purulence. This discharge can be disconcerting to the patient and surgeon but should not require additional surgery if clinical signs do not warrant such action. Consideration of external fixation is appropriate when hardware removal will result in an unstable construct (**Figure 1**). Current research is investigating the use of resorbable microspheres, collagen scaffolds, and gels for antibiotic delivery as both prophylaxis and treatment.

In some instances, the extent of disease combined with the poor health, comorbidities, and vascularity of the host may indicate that amputation is the more prudent treatment. The level of amputation should ensure adequate removal of the affected tissue, appropriate soft-tissue coverage, and an adequate blood supply for healing.

In similar settings, chronic suppression of infection with oral antibiotics should be considered when the host cannot tolerate or does not desire extensive reconstruction. In such instances, adequate surveillance must be instituted to guard against progression to fulminant

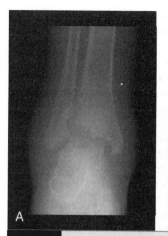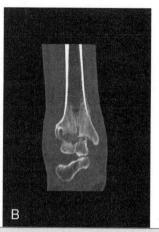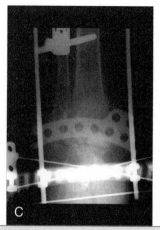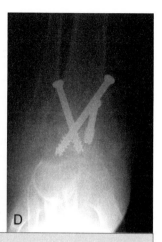

Figure 1 Osteomyelitis of the talus developed in a 58-year-old woman following septic arthritis. **A,** Radiograph shows destructive changes in the talus. **B,** A CT scan confirms and better defines the area of involvement. **C,** The patient was treated with débridement, placement of antibiotic methylmethacrylate beads, and application of an external fixator. **D,** After eradication of the infection, successful ankle arthrodesis was achieved.

infection and the patient should also be monitored for antibiotic toxicities.

Septic Arthritis

Acute joint infection may arise from either local inoculation or hematogenous spread. The fact that the tibiotalar and first metatarsophalangeal joints are the more commonly involved sites of infection may be attributable to their more capacious joint capsules compared with most other joints in the foot. Patients typically present with an acutely swollen, erythematous, and painful joint with significant limitation of motion and difficulty in weight bearing. The differential diagnosis includes gout and other crystalline arthropathies, toxic synovitis, or rheumatic disease. Joint aspiration is the most effective tool for diagnosis. Aspirations should be performed in a sterile manner, and the fluid should be analyzed for cell count, Gram stain, culture, and crystals. The quality of the fluid aspirated is often a good indicator of infection. A white blood cell count of more than 100,000 is generally diagnostic of septic arthritis, but lower counts with a shift toward 75% neutrophils should be viewed with suspicion. An aspirate with less than 50,000 white blood cells in an immunocompetent patient is more likely to indicate an inflammatory as opposed to an infectious pathology. The results of the Gram stain and culture are also helpful in differentiating the type of infection and may be used to aid in antibiotic selection. Radiographs may show effusion in the affected joint, but other changes are unlikely in the acute setting. MRI is not helpful in differentiating inflammatory from infectious causes except in the presence of bony involvement, such as erosions or bone edema.

Once a diagnosis of septic arthritis is confirmed, surgical drainage should be accomplished as soon as medically feasible. Delays in treatment risk destruction of the articular cartilage because it is exposed to a harsh purulent environment. If a significant delay is anticipated, serial aspirations should be considered. Drainage can be performed via open or arthroscopic techniques, depending on the joint involved and the surgeon's familiarity with arthroscopy. The joint should be closed over a drain when feasible to prevent the creation of an environment that is ripe for repeat infection. Duration of postoperative antibiotic treatment is variable and depends on the offending organism and host factors.

Surgical Infections

The best treatment for surgical infections is prevention. Interventions to eliminate the patient's use of tobacco products will reduce the risk of infection and wound healing complications. Surgeons should recognize that patients may deny smoking yet will be actively using nicotine replacement or other forms of tobacco. Counseling patients about the negative effects of nicotine and tobacco products is essential. The use of supplemental oxygen in the perioperative period may reduce the incidence of wound infection and other complications.

A second aspect of prevention involves appropriate preoperative antibiotic prophylaxis. Current guidelines from the Centers for Disease Control and Prevention and Centers for Medicare and Medicaid Services recommend cefazolin or cefuroxime administered within 1 hour prior to surgery.[20] Clindamycin or vancomycin may be used in patients with a β-lactam allergy or in patients with preexisting resistant pathogens. The literature does not support administering postoperative antibiotics after clean surgical procedures.

The use of chlorhexidine followed by isopropyl alcohol has been shown to be an effective method for disinfecting the surgical site.[21] However, some other preparations appear to provide adequate disinfection for surgical procedures of the foot and ankle.[22] Some controversy exists concerning the need to cover the toes when operating on the foot and ankle. Recent evidence suggests this is unnecessary, although some recolonization can occur during the procedure.[23,24]

Care must be taken by the surgical staff to avoid breaks in sterile technique. A culture of open communication is important to ensure that the surgeon is aware of any contamination problems so that effective recovery mechanisms can be promptly instituted.

Prompt recognition of postoperative infections is crucial. Patient education about the signs and symptoms of infections will help patients seek appropriate care quickly. If recognized early, most superficial infections or early cellulitis can be treated to completion with antibiotics and local wound care. Unrecognized infections can progress to deep infections involving muscle and/or bone and may require drainage and débridement. Postoperative infections are most commonly caused by *S aureus*, *Staphylococcus epidermidis*, coagulase-negative *Staphylococcus*, *Streptococcus*, and *P aeruginosa*. These infections can arise from the patient's own skin flora, by contamination from operating room personnel, or by postoperative contamination of the wound caused by poor patient self-care, pet contamination, or unclean environments. Deep infections usually require the removal of any implanted hardware because the metal implant serves as a nidus for bacterial growth and compromises antibiotic action. These infections likely involve infected or necrotic bone and should be treated in a manner similar to osteomyelitis, as was previously discussed. Alternatively, attempts can be made to suppress the infection until the bone is adequately healed; hardware removal can be delayed if infection control can be maintained.

Methicillin-Resistant *S Aureus*

Although health care–associated MRSA has become a common pathogen, the prevalence of community-associated strains is increasing and drawing public attention. Recent epidemiologic data suggest that up to 85% of MRSA infections are health care–associated MRSA and 14% are community-associated MRSA.[25] Strains of community-associated MRSA often affect younger and healthier individuals than do the nosocomial varieties. This pathogen is commonly associated with a cytotoxin that can increase the incidence of tissue necrosis. Groups at risk for community-associated MRSA include people in day care facilities, military personnel, those in prison, athletes who participate in contact sports, and several minority groups.[26] Risk factors of MRSA associated with health care include hospitalization or institutionalization, an indwelling catheter or percutaneous device, contact with an infected patient, or recent antimicrobial treatment. Unlike health care–associated MRSA, which appears to spread by contamination from colonized individuals and envi-

ronmental factors, community-associated MRSA is associated with skin-to-skin contact, especially in the setting of abrasion, other trauma, skin breaks, or from spread via fomites (whirlpool baths, towels, benches).[27] People in close contact with one another are at risk. Preventive measures, such as preoperative showers with 4% hexachlorophene and decolonization of the nares of MRSA carriers may be effective for health care–associated MRSA; however, such measures are more difficult to execute in the community setting. With the increasing prevalence of community-associated MRSA, it may be necessary to reevaluate empiric antibiotic treatment, especially in at-risk groups. β-lactam penicillins and cephalosporins are not effective against MRSA, may delay effective treatment, and allow infections to progress. Other established antibiotics, such as trimethoprim sulfamethoxazole, clindamycin, tetracycline, doxycycline, tigecycline, and rifampin, have shown effectiveness against community-associated MRSA in both intravenous and oral forms. Vancomycin is the standard treatment for MRSA but must be administered intravenously. Newer agents, such as daptomycin and linezolid, also have been used to successfully treat both health care–associated and community-associated MRSA.[26] Linezolid has excellent oral bioavailability and has been effective in implant-related osteomyelitis.[28] Daptomycin is effective for both MRSA and vancomycin-resistant septic arthritis in foot and ankle osteomyelitis.[17] MRSA in all its forms is an important and prevalent pathogen. High suspicion of MRSA infection in susceptible groups and early initiation of appropriate treatment, often with the assistance of an infectious disease consultant, will help to achieve a successful outcome.

Acinetobacter

Acinetobacter has received special attention recently because many military personnel have returned with wounds infected by these gram-negative bacteria. Found in soil and water, *Acinetobacter baumannii* is the most common species associated with human infections. *A baumannii* is an opportunistic pathogen that can be found on the skin and generally does not cause infection in immunocompetent hosts. Serious infections can develop in immunocompromised patients and are associated with a 75% mortality rate in those with bacteremia.[29]

Acinetobacter has played an increasing role in nosocomial infections over the past 40 years. *A baumannii* was reported to be the most common gram-negative bacillus recovered from traumatic injuries to extremities during the Vietnam War.[30] Often colonizing open wounds and spread by person-to-person contact, *Acinetobacter* can survive for prolonged periods of time on environmental surfaces (such as keyboards and telephones) and has contributed to protracted outbreaks in hospitals and intensive care facilities. This organism has the capacity to adhere to epithelial cells and kill them by apoptosis while producing toxins that damage host tissues. It remains unclear what role these activities play in virulence, but *Acinetobacter* has shown an increasing resistance to many antibiotics.[31] *Acinetobacter* is generally sensitive to meropenem, polymyxin B and E, amikacin, rifampin, minocycline, and tigecycline. Resistant strains may require therapy with multiple drugs, combining polymyxin B with a second drug; however, polymyxin can potentially cause renal and neurologic toxicities.

Summary

Nondiabetic infections of the foot and ankle are a common source of morbidity. In the surgical setting, prevention is paramount. In other settings, prompt recognition of the infectious process combined with appropriate clinical, radiographic, and laboratory evaluations will lead to an accurate diagnosis. Treatment can range from antibiotic administration alone to extensive surgical débridement with external fixator stabilization and the use of antibiotic-impregnated implants. In some instances, amputation may be necessary. A multidisciplinary approach incorporating an infectious disease specialist and other appropriate consultants will help to achieve an optimal outcome.

Annotated References

1. Møller AM, Villebro N, Pedersen T, Tønnesen H: Effect of preoperative smoking intervention on postoperative complications: A randomised clinical trial. *Lancet* 2002; 359:114-117.

2. Lawson RM, Doshi MK, Barton JR, Cobden I: The effect of unselected post-operative nutritional supplementation on nutritional status and clinical outcome of orthopaedic patients. *Clin Nutr* 2003;22:39-46.

   The authors of this prospective controlled study evaluated the effectiveness of nutritional supplements in orthopaedic patients. There was a reduction in major complications and decreased cost of care in patients receiving supplements. Level of evidence: II.

3. Kuzu MA, Terzioglu H, Genc V, et al: Preoperative nutritional risk assessment in predicting postoperative outcome in patients undergoing major surgery. *World J Surg* 2006;30:378-390.

   Prospectively administered nutritional screening tests for patients undergoing elective surgery were helpful in predicting morbidity in malnourished patients. Level of evidence: I.

4. Grayson ML, Gibbons GW, Balogh K, Levin E, Karchmer AW: Probing to bone in infected pedal ulcers: A clinical sign of underlying osteomyelitis in diabetic patients. *JAMA* 1995;273:721-723.

5. Rabjohn L, Roberts K, Troiano M, Schoenhaus H: Diagnostic and prognostic value of erythrocyte sedimentation rate in contiguous osteomyelitis of the foot and ankle. *J Foot Ankle Surg* 2007;46:230-237.

   The authors of this prospective study tracked ESR in patients with osteomyelitis and documented decreases in ESR in a small subset of patients who showed resolution of infection. No decline in ESR was seen in patients with persistent infection. Level of evidence: II.

6. Larsson S, Thelander U, Friberg S: C-reactive protein (CRP) levels after elective orthopedic surgery. *Clin Orthop Relat Res* 1992;275:237-242.

7. Termaat MF, Raijmakers PG, Scholten HJ, Bakker FC, Patka P, Haarman HJ: The accuracy of diagnostic imaging for the assessment of chronic osteomyelitis: A systematic review and meta-analysis. *J Bone Joint Surg Am* 2005;87:2464-2471.

   In this study, meta-analysis was used to assess the accuracy of multiple imaging modalities in patients with chronic osteomyelitis. The authors provide a helpful review of diagnostic options. Level of evidence: III.

8. El-Maghraby TA, Moustafa HM, Pauwels EK: Nuclear medicine methods for evaluation of skeletal infection among other diagnostic modalities. *Q J Nucl Med Mol Imaging* 2006;50:167-192.

   A review of nuclear medicine tests for musculoskeletal infections that may be helpful in choosing the appropriate scanning technique is presented.

9. Liu PT, Dorsey ML: MRI of the foot for suspected osteomyelitis: Improving radiology reports for orthopaedic surgeons. *Semin Musculoskelet Radiol* 2007;11: 28-35.

   This thorough review of MRI evaluation for osteomyelitis focuses on how radiologists can provide useful feedback to orthopaedic surgeons.

10. Kapoor A, Page S, Lavalley M, Gale DR, Felson DT: Magnetic resonance imaging for diagnosing foot osteomyelitis: A meta-analysis. *Arch Intern Med* 2007;167: 125-132.

    This meta-analysis showed good results with MRI in diagnosing osteomyelitis. MRI was clearly superior to radiographs and nuclear medicine imaging. Level of evidence: II.

11. Pakos EE, Koumoulis HD, Fotopoulos AD, Ionnidis J: Osteomyelitis: Antigranulocyte scintigraphy with 99mTc radiolabeled monoclonal antibodies for diagnosis. Meta-analysis. *Radiology* 2007;245:732-734.

    A meta-analysis evaluating 19 studies showed an 81% sensitivity and 77% specificity of white cell scans for osteomyelitis. Level of evidence: II.

12. Dreyer G, Addiss D, Gadelha P, Lapa E, Williamson J, Dreyer A: Interdigital skin lesions of the lower limbs among patients with lymphoedema in an area endemic for bancroftian filariasis. *Trop Med Int Health* 2006;11: 1475-1481.

The authors of this observational study examined interdigital lesions as a risk factor for filariasis in an endemic area of Brazil. Level of evidence: III.

13. McNamara DR, Tleyjeh IM, Berbari EF, et al: Incidence of lower-extremity cellulitis: A population-based study in Olmsted county, Minnesota. *Mayo Clin Proc* 2007; 82:817-821.

This retrospective population-based study examined risk factors that contributed to the development of cellulitis. Increasing age was noted as the most significant risk factor. Level of evidence: III.

14. Hilmarsdóttir I, Valsdóttir F: Molecular typing of Beta-hemolytic streptococci from two patients with lower-limb cellulitis: Identical isolates from toe web and blood specimens. *J Clin Microbiol* 2007;45:3131-3132.

Bacteria found in the toe web space were compared with the causative organism in two patients with cellulitis. The web space was documented as the portal of entry for more proximal leg cellulitis. Level of evidence: IV.

15. Björnsdóttir S, Gottfredsson M, Thórisdóttir AS, et al: Risk factors for acute cellulitis of the lower limb: A prospective case-control study. *Clin Infect Dis* 2005;41: 1416-1422.

This prospective case-controlled study showed web-space intertrigo as a risk factor for cellulitis. Level of evidence: IV.

16. Wong CH, Chang HC, Pasupathy S, Khin LW, Tan JL, Low CO: Necrotizing fasciitis: Clinical presentation, microbiology, and determinants of mortality. *J Bone Joint Surg Am* 2003;85-A:1454-1460.

Early surgical débridement is shown to be the most important factor to decrease mortality in patients with necrotizing fasciitis. Level of evidence: II.

17. Holtom PD, Zalavras CG, Lamp KC, Park N, Friedrich LV: Clinical experience with daptomycin treatment of foot or ankle osteomyelitis: A preliminary study. *Clin Orthop Relat Res* 2007;461:35-39.

This preliminary study showed the effectiveness of daptomycin in foot and ankle osteomyelitis caused by gram-positive bacteria. Level of evidence: IV.

18. Richelsoph KC, Webb ND, Haggard WO: Elution behavior of daptomycin-loaded calcium sulfate pellets: A preliminary study. *Clin Orthop Relat Res* 2007;461: 68-73.

The authors of this in vitro study examined an effective method of mixing daptomycin within resorbable calcium sulfate pellets for the treatment of osteomyelitis and compared the elution of this drug with tobramycin.

19. Joseph TN, Chen AL, Di Cesare PE: Use of antibiotic-impregnated cement in total joint arthroplasty. *J Am Acad Orthop Surg* 2003;11:38-47.

This review article focuses on the use of methyl-methacrylate cement in total joint arthroplasty. A good overview of the effect of adding antibiotics to cement and the elution characteristics of several antibiotics also are presented.

20. Bratzler DW, Hunt DR: The surgical infection prevention and surgical care improvement projects: National initiatives to improve outcomes for patients having surgery. *Clin Infect Dis* 2006;43:322-330.

The authors present a report on the surgical infection prevention program including the Centers for Disease Control and Prevention guidelines for prophylaxis in surgical patients.

21. Bibbo C, Patel DV, Gehrmann RM, Lin SS: Chlorhexidine provides superior skin decontamination in foot and ankle surgery: A prospective randomized study. *Clin Orthop Relat Res* 2005;438:204-208.

For decontamination of the foot and ankle before surgery, chlorhexidine was shown to be superior to povidone-iodine with approximately one half the incidences of positive cultures from the foot after prepping and draping the patient. Level of evidence: I.

22. Ostrander RV, Botte MJ, Brage ME: Efficacy of surgical preparation solutions in foot and ankle surgery. *J Bone Joint Surg Am* 2005;87:980-985.

In foot and ankle surgery, chlorhexidine was shown to be superior to an iodine and isopropyl alcohol solution for eliminating bacterial pathogens, with approximately one half the incidences of positive cultures from the foot. Level of evidence: I.

23. Goucher NR, Coughlin MJ: Covering of the toes during hindfoot and ankle surgery: A randomized, controlled, clinical study. *Foot Ankle Int* 2007;28:413-415.

This prospective randomized study showed no benefit to covering the toes for foot and ankle surgery. The authors examined recolonization of the second toe web space and conducted patient follow-ups for evidence of postoperative infection. Level of evidence: I.

24. Hort KR, DeOrio JK: Residual bacterial contamination after surgical preparation of the foot or ankle with or without alcohol. *Foot Ankle Int* 2002;23:946-948.

25. Klevens RM, Morrison MA, Nadle J, et al: Invasive methicillin-resistant Staphylococcus aureus infections in the United States. *JAMA* 2007;298:1763-1771.

The authors present the results of population-based surveillance of nine communities to determine the incidence of health care–associated and community-associated MRSA in the United States.

26. Marcotte AL, Trzeciak MA: Community-acquired methicillin-resistant Staphylococcus aureus: An emerging pathogen in orthopaedics. *J Am Acad Orthop Surg* 2008;16:98-106.

An excellent review of community-associated MRSA with clinical and microbiological details is presented.

27. Miller LG, Diep BA: Clinical practice: Colonization, fomites, and virulence. Rethinking the pathogenesis of community-associated methicillin-resistant Staphylococ-

6: Special Problems of the Foot and Ankle

cus aureus infection. *Clin Infect Dis* 2008;46:752-760.

The authors review the differences in etiology of health care–associated MRSA versus community-associated MRSA and comment on different prevention and treatment strategies.

28. Vercillo M, Patzakis MJ, Holtom P, Zalavras CG: Linezolid in the treatment of implant-related chronic osteomyelitis. *Clin Orthop Relat Res* 2007;461:40-43.

In this retrospective study of 22 patients treated with linezolid for implant-related infections, successful control of the infection was achieved in 14 patients; 8 patients were lost to follow-up. Level of evidence: IV.

29. Cisneros JM, Reyes MJ, Pachón J, et al: Bacteremia due to Acinetobacter baumannii: Epidemiology, clinical findings, and prognostic features. *Clin Infect Dis* 1996; 22:1026-1032.

30. Centers for Disease Control and Prevention (CDC): Acinetobacter baumannii infections among patients at military medical facilities treating injured U.S. service members, 2002-2004. *MMWR Morb Mortal Wkly Rep* 2004;53:1063-1066.

This publication presents data on specific infectious diseases as reported by state and territorial health departments. This report provides demographic data on 102 patients with *A baumannii* bacteremia at military medical facilities treating service personnel injured in Afghanistan, Iraq, and Kuwait.

31. Gerischer U (ed): *Acinetobacter Molecular Biology.* Norwich, United Kingdom, Caister Academic Press, 2008.

Aspects of the molecular biology of *Acinetobacter* are presented, along with an extensive list of the available literature regarding this organism.

Chapter 26

Plantar Heel Pain

Alan C. League, MD

Introduction

Plantar heel pain is a common condition that is believed to affect 2 million Americans each year and 10% of the general population during their lifetime. Plantar fasciitis is the most recognized cause of plantar heel pain; it is estimated that 11% to 15% of all reports of foot ailments requiring medical attention can be attributed to this condition.[1,2] Plantar fasciitis is considered a self-limiting condition because symptoms resolve in 80% to 90% of patients within 10 months of onset.[3-6] However, this long time interval for symptom resolution causes frustration for patients and physicians. Many other etiologies also can cause plantar heel pain (Table 1). A thorough patient history and physical examination usually results in an accurate diagnosis. Treatment can then be initiated.

Anatomy

Understanding the complex anatomy of the plantar heel is necessary for accurately diagnosing and treating a patient with plantar heel pain (Figure 1). The heel fat pad is a highly specialized structure. The elastic adipose tissue is organized as spiral fibrous septa, which are anchored to the calcaneus, the skin, and to each other. The septa are reinforced with elastic fibers that connect the walls and create separate fat compartments. The thickness of the fat pad begins to deteriorate in people older than 40 years, resulting in a diminished ability to absorb impact.

The plantar fascia is a strong, fibrous aponeurosis that originates from the plantar tuberosity of the calcaneus and fans out into three bands that insert into the bases of the proximal phalanges. The central band anatomically and structurally dominates the medial and lateral bands, and the thick plantar fat pad protects and cushions the origin. The midsubstance can be palpated subcutaneously when the plantar fascia is tensioned. Dorsiflexion of the toes (especially the hallux) activates the windlass mechanism, which passively tensions the plantar fascia and elevates the medial longitudinal arch.

An understanding of the neuroanatomy of the heel also is imperative when diagnosing plantar heel pain (Figure 2). The posterior tibial nerve within the tarsal tunnel is divided into three branches: medial calcaneal, medial plantar, and lateral plantar nerves. The medial calcaneal branch is the most posterior of the three and provides sensation to the medial and plantar heel. The medial plantar nerve is the anterior branch of the posterior tibial nerve; it passes deep to the abductor hallucis muscle and distally where it divides. The lateral plantar nerve is located posterior and lateral to the medial plantar branch. The first branch of the lateral plantar nerve (FBLPN), the nerve to the abductor digiti quinti, has been implicated in plantar heel pain.[7] Entrapment of this nerve can occur as it passes between the deep fascia of the abductor hallucis muscle and the medial caudal margin of the quadratus plantae muscle.

Histopathology

Plantar fasciitis is defined as a localized inflammation and degeneration of the proximal plantar aponeurosis. The most common site of involvement is near the origin

---

Table 1

Differential Diagnosis for Plantar Heel Pain

Plantar fascia
  Plantar fasciitis
  Rupture of plantar fascia
  Enthesopathy
    Rheumatoid arthritis
    Seronegative spondyloarthropathy
    Systemic lupus erythematosus
    Crystalline arthropathies
    Psoriatic arthritis

Bone
  Calcaneus stress fracture
  Calcaneus contusion
  Osteomyelitis
  Neoplasm

Soft tissue
  Fat pad atrophy

Circulation
  Ischemia

Nerve
  Entrapment of the first branch of the lateral plantar nerve
  Tarsal tunnel syndrome
  Neuropathy (metabolic)
  Radiculopathy

6: Special Problems of the Foot and Ankle

at the medial tuberosity of the calcaneus. Similar to chronic tendon disorders, pathologic findings have included degenerative changes in the plantar fascia with fibroblastic proliferation and limited inflammatory tissue.[8-10] There is general agreement in the literature that a process of mechanical overload and excessive strain produces microtears within the fascia, which eventually incites an inflammatory response.[11,12] Repeated heel strikes can hinder or prevent normal healing,[13] resulting in chronic inflammation followed by degeneration.[14-16] Pathologic changes also have been reported in patients with FBLPN entrapment; evidence of perineural fibrosis and hypertrophy has been observed.[17]

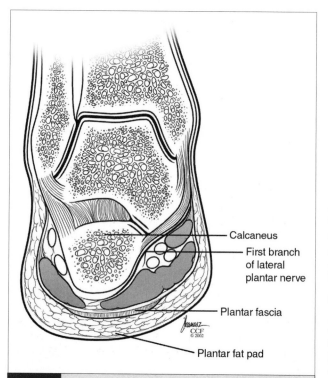

Figure 1 Coronal cross section of the hindfoot shows the relationships among the plantar fascia, plantar heel pad, and the FBLPN. (Reproduced with permission from the Cleveland Clinic Foundation, Cleveland, OH.)

Patient Evaluation

History

Although the differential diagnosis of plantar heel pain is broad, a thorough history and physical examination can usually provide the clinician with the correct diagnosis. Most differential diagnoses can be included or excluded based on the patient's history; however, it is important to consider unusual causes. The presence of constitutional symptoms such as fevers, chills, or weight loss can be indicative of a neoplasm or infection. A recent increase in activity or training may predispose patients to stress fractures, which are often present with medial and lateral calcaneal wall pain. A warm and swollen heel should be evaluated to exclude stress fracture or infection from the diagnosis.

Plantar fasciitis is the most common cause of plantar heel pain and typically presents with the insidious onset of "start-up" pain. This sharp, stabbing pain is localized to the plantar medial aspect of the heel and occurs when arising from bed in the morning or from a chair after sitting for an extended period. Start-up pain dissipates after a short period of weight bearing. Patients frequently describe an achy pain at the end of the day, especially following prolonged weight-bearing activities. If untreated, the pain may worsen over time, re-

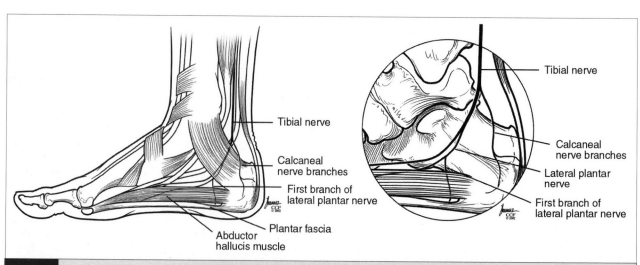

Figure 2 The medial view of the foot and ankle with detailed close-up of the tibial nerve and its branches. Note the relationship between the FBLPN and the abductor hallucis muscle. (Reproduced with permission from the Cleveland Clinic Foundation, Cleveland, OH.)

sulting in an antalgic gait. Subsequent compensatory gait changes can produce painful symptoms in the ipsilateral or contralateral lower extremity or the low back.

Central heel pain syndrome may develop in elderly patients because of heel pad atrophy. Heel pad atrophy is present to some degree in most elderly patients, but can be accelerated in patients with connective tissue disorders or those treated with corticosteroid injections in that area. The clinical presentation typically involves central plantar heel pain associated with barefoot walking or the use of hard-soled shoes. Unlike patients with plantar fasciitis, the pain does not improve after the first few steps, but is usually relieved by rest or with the use of well-padded shoes.

Entrapment of the FBLPN also causes inferior heel pain.[7] The nerve becomes entrapped between the stout deep fascia of the abductor hallucis muscle and the medial head of the quadratus plantae muscle. Athletes who spend a significant amount of time on their toes (sprinters, dancers, gymnasts, and skaters) are more prone to this type of nerve entrapment because they have a well-developed abductor hallucis muscle. Unlike plantar fasciitis, this condition may result in paresthesias, although the occurrence of abnormal sensations is variable. With isolated entrapment of the FBLPN, start-up pain is unusual; however, if simultaneous involvement of the fasciae occur, the clinical scenario can mimic plantar fasciitis.

Physical Examination

The key to the examination of the painful plantar heel is determining the location of maximal tenderness (Figure 3). Each diagnosis has a specific location of maximal tenderness. Percussion and compression should be performed over the medial and lateral calcaneal tuberosities, proximal and distal plantar fascia, proximal abductor hallucis muscle, plantar heel fat pad, tarsal tunnel, and any surgical scar near the heel. The precise location of maximal tenderness will often provide the diagnosis. Plantar fasciitis is usually indicated by pain with deep palpation at the origin of the plantar fascia on the plantar medial calcaneus tuberosity. Pain appreciated more medially and cranially to this point, over the origin of the abductor hallucis muscle, may indicate entrapment of the FBLPN. Pain with palpation in the central plantar heel is often associated with a thinning of the fat pad and is consistent with fat pad atrophy.

The windlass mechanism should be tensioned through dorsiflexion of the metatarsophalangeal joints. This maneuver can detect defects or masses in the plantar fascia midsubstance. Achilles tendon contracture is commonly associated with plantar fasciitis and should be evaluated by measuring ankle dorsiflexion with the knee in flexion and extension. A positive Tinel sign along an incision is consistent with a surgically injured nerve.

Weight-bearing alignment of the entire lower extremity should be observed during gait and while the

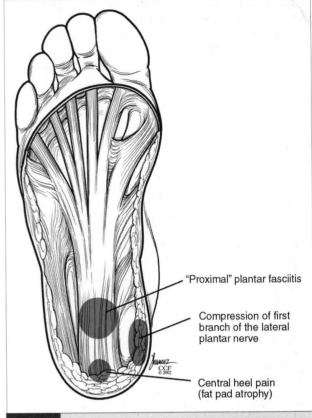

"Proximal" plantar fasciitis

Compression of first branch of the lateral plantar nerve

Central heel pain (fat pad atrophy)

Figure 3 Common locations of tenderness in patients with plantar heel pain. (*Reproduced with permission from the Cleveland Clinic Foundation, Cleveland, OH.*)

patient is standing. A thorough neurologic and vascular examination should be performed. Range of motion of the ankle and subtalar joint should be measured to evaluate intra-articular pathology. Unilateral heel symptoms are most common; bilateral involvement may indicate a systemic rheumatologic condition.

Imaging

A thorough history and physical examination is usually sufficient to properly identify the etiology of plantar heel pain; however, imaging can be helpful in ruling out or confirming a diagnosis. Weight-bearing radiographs are typically normal in patients with plantar heel pain syndromes but may show arthritis, neoplasm, trauma, infection, or prior surgery. The lateral image will occasionally show a plantar heel spur, although its clinical relevance is unknown.

Technetium bone scans have a 60% to 98% sensitivity and up to an 86% specificity in diagnosing plantar fasciitis, and may be helpful in detecting a calcaneus stress fracture or neoplasm.[18] A heel with plantar fasciitis shows increased uptake at the origin of the fascia, whereas a stress fracture shows increased uptake throughout a much larger portion of the calcaneus. MRI may show thickening of the plantar fascia. The

6: Special Problems of the Foot and Ankle

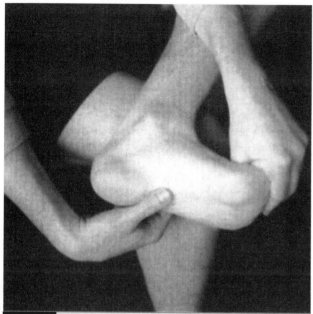

Figure 4 Achilles stretching exercise. (Reproduced with permission from DiGiovanni BF, Nawoczenski DA, Lintal ME, et al: Tissue-specific plantar fascia-stretching exercise enhances outcomes in patients with chronic heel pain: A prospective, randomized study. J Bone Joint Surg Am 2003;85:1270-1277.)

fascia in patients with plantar fasciitis has been measured at 6 to 8 mm, whereas the fascia measures less than 4 mm in asymptomatic individuals.[19] MRI also is useful in detecting a stress fracture of the calcaneus. Ultrasonography has received increased attention for its diagnostic capabilities and its role in guiding the location of extracorporeal shock wave therapy (ESWT). With ultrasound, the fascia can easily be differentiated from the superficial fat pad and the underlying calcaneus. The normal thickness of the plantar fascia is 2 to 4 mm, whereas a thickness from 5 to 7 mm is found in patients with plantar fasciitis.[18,20]

Who Is at Risk for Plantar Fasciitis?

Although mechanical overload is frequently implicated as a primary factor, the etiology of plantar fasciitis is believed to be multifactorial. Intrinsic factors such as older age, abnormal foot posture, an elevated body mass index, and a tight Achilles tendon, as well as extrinsic factors such as the use of improper footwear, the type and intensity of daily activity, and incidence of isolated or repetitive trauma have been proposed as risk factors for plantar fasciitis. No single risk factor has been reliably identified across multiple studies. Static and dynamic cadaver studies have linked Achilles tendon tension and plantar fascia loading to plantar fasciitis; the clinical significance of this relationship continues to draw investigative interest.[21,22] A recent,

retrospective, case-controlled study of 50 patients in whom unilateral plantar fasciitis was clinically diagnosed, evaluated three factors commonly believed to predispose an individual to the disorder.[23] Two control subjects were matched to each patient on the basis of age and gender. The study showed that individuals who stand during most of their workday had a significantly increased risk of plantar fasciitis compared with those who do not stand for long periods. The risk of plantar fasciitis also increases as the amount of ankle dorsiflexion decreases or as the body mass index increases. Each of these three variables was determined to be an independent risk factor for plantar fasciitis, with reduced ankle dorsiflexion being the most important.

Nonsurgical Treatment

Plantar fasciitis is believed to be a self-limiting condition in most patients. Nonsurgical treatment is successful in 90% of patients; however, complete resolution of pain often takes several months and sometimes more than 1 year. Initiation of treatment within the first 6 weeks after symptoms appear may speed recovery, although this has yet to be proven.[24,25] An important element of successful management is patient education, which includes establishing realistic patient expectations. Patients who expect rapid resolution of pain will usually be disappointed and frustrated; these expectations can have a negative impact on compliance with treatment and on the relationship with the physician. Many previous clinical studies evaluating the efficacy of nonsurgical treatment lacked high-level evidence; however, the quality of recent research has improved. Data from several high-quality, randomized, controlled studies are available to assess the efficacy of specific treatment options.

Stretching Exercises

Stretching exercises are a simple and inexpensive component of many treatment protocols for plantar fasciitis. Favorable results have been reported with Achilles tendon and plantar fascia stretching, but an optimal regimen has not been established. Recent randomized clinical trials compared the results of Achilles stretching (**Figure 4**) with plantar fascia-specific stretching (**Figure 5**) in patients with chronic plantar fasciitis.[26,27] All patients in the study used prefabricated insoles, underwent 3 weeks of nonsteroidal anti-inflammatory drug (NSAID) therapy, and viewed an educational video on plantar fasciitis. By 8 weeks, the plantar fascia-specific group showed significant improvement compared with the Achilles tendon stretching group. At 8 weeks, the Achilles tendon group also was instructed in plantar fascia stretching. By 2 years, both groups showed significant improvement and no significant differences were noted between the groups. Because these studies did not use a control group, the benefit of stretching versus not stretching was not evaluated.

Another recent study evaluating the effectiveness of

stretching in the treatment of plantar fasciitis included a sham control group.[28] Participants were blinded as to whether they were in the treatment group or the sham group. The treatment group performed calf stretching and received sham ultrasound treatment, whereas the control group received sham ultrasound treatment alone. After 2 weeks, no difference was found between the two groups. Although stretching remains a safe and relatively easy treatment option, its efficacy in the treatment of plantar fasciitis is undetermined.

Night Dorsiflexion Splints

A tight Achilles tendon is implicated as one possible etiology of plantar fasciitis. A night splint can be used to hold the ankle in maximum dorsiflexion in an attempt to prevent contracture of the plantar fascia and gastrocnemius-soleus complex. The reduction of start-up pain is considered a direct benefit of nocturnal splinting. A prospective crossover study showed significant improvement when using a night splint as compared with no treatment.[29] After the crossover, both groups showed significant improvement, which was maintained after 6 months. A randomized, controlled study compared the use of NSAIDs, Achilles tendon stretching, and footwear modification with and without the use of night splints.[30] No differences were found between the two groups. The evidence supporting the use of night splints in treating plantar fasciitis is mixed.

Orthoses

Heel cups, prefabricated insoles, and custom orthotics are used to treat plantar fasciitis. The goal of these devices is to elevate and cushion the heel, provide medial arch support, or both. A multicenter study found prefabricated orthotic devices to be superior to custom-made orthotic devices in treating plantar fasciitis in patients who stand more than 8 hours per day.[2] However, outside this subgroup, no difference was detected. A more recent randomized study compared the use of a custom-made orthosis to a night dorsiflexion splint. The authors found no difference in pain or function between the groups; however, a much higher rate of compliance was reported for patients using the orthosis compared with those treated with the night splint. Neither study used a sham control group.

A recent randomized controlled study compared a sham orthosis (thin, soft foam), a prefabricated orthosis (thick, firm foam), and a customized semirigid orthosis in a population of patients who did not receive any other treatment (such as NSAIDs and stretching exercises).[31] At 3- and 12-month follow-up, all three groups had improvement in pain and function. At 3 months, the groups using the prefabricated and customized orthoses had significant improvement in function compared with the sham group, but no difference in pain level. By 12 months, no difference in function or pain was reported among the groups. The short-term use of custom or prefabricated orthoses is sup-

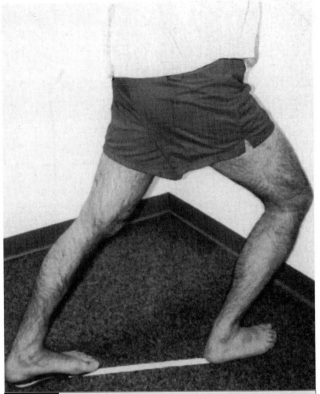

Figure 5 | Plantar fascia-specific stretching exercise. *(Reproduced with permission from DiGiovanni BF, Nawoczenski DA, Lintal ME, et al: Tissue-specific plantar fascia-stretching exercise enhances outcomes in patients with chronic heel pain: A prospective, randomized study. J Bone Joint Surg Am 2003;85:1270-1277.)*

ported by high-quality clinical evidence, but the long-term benefits of these devices have not been established.

Anti-inflammatory Agents and Other Modalities

Anti-inflammatory agents are often used in clinical practice, but limited data are available to evaluate their efficacy in treating plantar fasciitis. A recent double blind, prospective, placebo-controlled study evaluated a nonsurgical protocol (heel cord stretching, heel cups, night splinting) with or without the administration of oral celecoxib.[32] Over time, pain and disability scores improved significantly in both groups. Although the NSAID group showed a trend for improved function and pain scores, there was no statistical significance between the placebo and NSAID groups at 1-, 2- or 6-month follow-up.

Corticosteroid injection, usually mixed with local anesthetic, is another common treatment for plantar fasciitis. To avoid injection into the plantar fat pad and subsequent atrophy, a medial approach is advocated. The needle tip should be placed at the medial origin of the plantar fascia. One study found significantly improved pain at 1 month, but no difference at 3- and 6-month follow-up when compared with the use of a local anesthetic alone.[33] This apparent short-term benefit must be weighed against the potential complications of plantar fat pad atrophy and plantar fascia rupture.[34,35]

Topically applied steroid, propelled into the tissues with a small electric charge (iontophoresis), may provide a safer alternative. The authors of one study found significant improvement in pain control and function at the time of treatment compared with a placebo group.[36] At 1-month follow-up, no significant difference was reported between the two groups. Although it may not alter the natural history of the disease, iontophoresis may be helpful in allowing athletes to return to play more quickly.

Patients with central heel pain secondary to fat atrophy can be treated nonsurgically. Interventions mainly involve alteration in footwear, with options including gel heel cups, prefabricated shock-absorbing shoe inserts, and custom-made orthotic devices. Combined with activity modification, these devices can reduce the impact and pain associated with this condition.

Nonsurgical management of entrapment of the FBLPN typically involves activity modification, the use of heel cups, NSAIDs, and corticosteroid injections; however, the clinical response to these treatments is unclear.

When patients do not adequately respond to nonsurgical treatments, additional medical studies may be performed to rule out less common etiologies of heel pain. Rheumatoid arthritis and other inflammatory conditions are associated with heel pain. These conditions can be diagnosed with laboratory studies, including a complete blood cell count with differential white blood cell count, and evaluation of erythrocyte sedimentation rate, rheumatoid factor, antinuclear antibodies, and human leukocyte antigen B27 and uric acid levels. If the findings are positive, consultation with a rheumatology specialist is recommended.

Extracorporeal Shock Wave Therapy

Proponents of ESWT, also referred to as orthotripsy, claim it offers an effective means of treatment of chronic plantar fasciitis in patients who have been unresponsive to other nonsurgical treatments. The mechanism of action of orthotripsy is similar to lithotripsy for treating kidney stones. Acoustic waves dissipate mechanical energy at the interface of two substances of differing acoustic impedance. An electrohydraulic, electromagnetic, or piezoelectric generator can be used to produce the shock waves. Currently, all three wave production techniques are available for clinical use. ESWT is classified as either high- or low-energy therapy based on the magnitude of the shock wave generated by the device. High-energy ESWT requires local or general anesthesia and is administered in a single session, whereas low-energy treatment does not require anesthesia and is usually administered in three weekly sessions.

ESWT has been actively investigated in recent years; however, the results of several randomized, controlled trials have produced conflicting results.[37-39] A recent meta-analysis examined the efficacy of ESWT for plantar fasciitis.[40] This systemic review of all randomized, controlled trials published from 1966 to 2004 evaluated 15 published studies. Six studies (897 patients) had sufficient statistical analysis to allow pooling of the data and met the inclusion criteria. Outcomes showed a significant effect with respect to morning pain; however, despite this statistical significance ($P = 0.04$), the clinical benefit was small. At 12 weeks, the observed difference was less than 0.50 cm on a 10-cm visual analog scale.

ESWT remains a viable option for treating chronic plantar fasciitis when other nonsurgical measures have failed; however, consistent reports of good outcomes from high-quality studies are needed to make this therapy a more attractive treatment option.

Surgical Treatment

In most patients, plantar fasciitis resolves with nonsurgical treatment. For patients who do not achieve pain relief after at least 6 to 12 months of conservative management, surgical treatment may be considered. Surgical treatment options for recalcitrant plantar fasciitis include isolated partial or complete release of the plantar fascia, a fascial release combined with resection of a calcaneal spur, excision of abnormal tissue, or nerve decompression. These procedures can be performed either open or using an endoscopic approach. Most studies on the surgical treatment of plantar fasciitis have been case series evaluating a single surgical technique or retrospective comparisons of two different techniques.[7,17,41-43] These types of studies produce low-level evidence (level III and IV evidence). To date, no randomized, controlled studies on the surgical management of plantar fasciitis have been published.

Open release of the plantar fascia is performed through a medial incision that allows direct visualization of the fascia. Preservation of the lateral 50% of the plantar fascia fibers may prevent collapse of the longitudinal arch. One technique that releases the entire plantar fascia requires no weight bearing for 6 months, followed by the use of arch support for 1 year.[43] Removal of the plantar calcaneal spur introduces additional surgical trauma and delays recovery without improving outcomes.[44] In patients with isolated plantar fasciitis, endoscopic release may offer a shorter recovery time; however, the ability to view surrounding structures is impaired, and the lateral plantar nerve may be at risk for injury. Patients with symptoms of nerve compression and plantar fasciitis are not appropriate candidates for endoscopic release.

Success rates for surgical treatment of plantar fasciitis are variable, and the use of different outcome measures prevents direct comparisons between studies. A recent case study of endoscopic plantar fascia releases found improvement in the American Orthopaedic Foot and Ankle Society ankle-hindfoot score (66 to 88).[41] Complications in this group included one patient with complex regional pain syndrome who required consultation with a pain specialist. Other potential complications from open or endoscopic treatment of plantar fasciitis include nerve injury, flattening of the longitudinal arch with resulting midtarsal pain, and persistent or recurrent pain.

Historically, FBLPN entrapment has been treated with nerve decompression without plantar fascia release.[7] However, a more recent study reported difficulty differentiating pain from plantar fascia and FBLPN entrapment and recommended partial plantar fascia release with FBLPN neurolysis. Decompression of the FBLPN is performed through a medial approach when the superficial and deep fascia of the abductor hallucis muscle is divided. The partial plantar fascia release is then performed through the distal aspect of the same incision. An extensive release of the tarsal tunnel can be performed with a plantar fascia release.[43]

Summary

Plantar heel pain remains a common disorder, most often caused by plantar fasciitis. Many safe, nonsurgical treatments are available; however, few data show that these modalities are more effective than sham treatment. The natural history of plantar fasciitis results in resolution of symptoms in less than 1 year in most patients. ESWT may be helpful in patients with chronic plantar fasciitis whose symptoms have not improved with other nonsurgical treatments. Surgical treatment of plantar fasciitis should be considered only after nonsurgical modalities have failed. If surgery is required, no more than 50% of the fascia should be released to avoid structural complications. If entrapment of the FBPLN is present, concurrent decompression of this nerve also should be performed. Heel pad atrophy is treated nonsurgically with shock-absorbing footwear.

Annotated References

1. McCarthy DJ, Gorecki GE: The anatomical basis of inferior calcaneal lesions: A cryomicrotomy study. *J Am Podiatry Assoc* 1979;69:527-536.

2. Pfeffer G, Bacchetti P, Deland J, et al: Comparison of custom and prefabricated orthoses in the initial treatment of proximal plantar fasciitis. *Foot Ankle Int* 1999; 20:214-221.

3. Davis PF, Severud E, Baxter DE: Painful heel syndrome: Results of nonoperative treatment. *Foot Ankle Int* 1994;15:531-535.

4. Lapidus PW, Guidotti FP: Painful heel: Report of 323 patients with 364 painful heels. *Clin Orthop Relat Res* 1965;39:178-186.

5. Martin RL, Irrgang JJ, Conti SF: Outcome study of subjects with insertional plantar fasciitis. *Foot Ankle Int* 1998;19:803-811.

6. Wolgin M, Cook C, Graham C, Mauldin D: Conservative treatment of plantar heel pain: Long-term follow-up. *Foot Ankle Int* 1994;15:97-102.

7. Baxter DE, Thigpen CM: Heel pain: Operative results. *Foot Ankle* 1984;5:16-25.

8. Jarde O, Diebold P, Havet E, Boulu G, Vernois J: Degenerative lesions of the plantar fascia: Surgical treatment by fasciectomy and excision of the heel spur. A report on 38 cases. *Acta Orthop Belg* 2003;69:267-274.

   The authors present a review of MRI, histologic, and surgical results of 38 patients treated with plantar fascia release and calcaneal spur resection. Level of evidence: IV.

9. Leach RE, Seavey MS, Salter DK: Results of surgery in athletes with plantar fasciitis. *Foot Ankle* 1986;7: 156-161.

10. Lemont H, Ammirati KM, Usen N: Plantar fasciitis: A degenerative process (fasciosis) without inflammation. *J Am Podiatr Med Assoc* 2003;93:234-237.

    The authors review histologic findings from 50 cases of heel spur surgery for chronic plantar fasciitis. Findings include myxoid degeneration with fragmentation and degeneration of the plantar fascia and bone marrow vascular ectasia. Histologic findings support the hypothesis that plantar fasciitis is a degenerative fasciosis without inflammation, not a fasciitis.

11. Kaya BK: Plantar fasciitis in athletes. *J Sport Rehabil* 1996;5:305-320.

12. Warren BL: Plantar fasciitis in runners: Treatment and prevention. *Sports Med* 1990;10:338-345.

13. Grasel RP, Schweitzer ME, Kovalovich AM, et al: MR imaging of plantar fasciitis: Edema, tears, and occult marrow abnormalities correlated with outcome. *AJR Am J Roentgenol* 1999;173:699-701.

14. LeMelle DP, Kisilewicz P, Janis LR: Chronic plantar fascial inflammation and fibrosis. *Clin Podiatr Med Surg* 1990;7:385-389.

15. Schepsis AA, Leach RE, Gorzyca J: Plantar fasciitis: Etiology, treatment, surgical results, and review of the literature. *Clin Orthop Relat Res* 1991;266:185-196.

16. Snider MP, Clancy WG, McBeath AA: Plantar fascia release for chronic plantar fasciitis in runners. *Am J Sports Med* 1983;11:215-219.

6: Special Problems of the Foot and Ankle

17. Sammarco GJ, Helfrey RB: Surgical treatment of recalcitrant plantar fasciitis. *Foot Ankle Int* 1996;17: 520-526.

18. Groshar D, Alperson M, Toubi A, Gorenberg A, Liberson A, Bar-Meir E: Plantar fasciitis: Detection with ultrasonography versus bone scintigraphy. *Foot* 2000;10: 164-168.

19. Berkowitz JF, Kier R, Rudicel S: Plantar fasciitis: MR imaging. *Radiology* 1991;179:665-667.

20. Gibbon WW, Long G: Ultrasound of the plantar aponeurosis (fascia). *Skeletal Radiol* 1999;28:21-26.

21. Carlson RE, Fleming LL, Hutton WC: The biomechanical relationship between the tendoachilles, plantar fascia and metatarsophalangeal joint dorsiflexion angle. *Foot Ankle Int* 2000;21:18-25.

22. Erdemir A, Hamel AJ, Fauth AR, et al: Dynamic loading of the plantar aponeurosis in walking. *J Bone Joint Surg Am* 2004;86:546-552.

   Simulated walking with measurements of foot motion and the ground reaction forces during the stance phase were studied using cadaver feet. Plantar aponeurosis forces gradually increased during stance and peaked in late stance.

23. Riddle DL, Pulisic M, Pidcoe P, Johnson RE: Risk factors for plantar fasciitis: A matched case-control study. *J Bone Joint Surg Am* 2003;85:872-877.

   In a matched, case-controlled study with two controls for each patient, decreased ankle dorsiflexion, increased body mass index, and standing for most of the workday were reported to be independent risk factors for the development of plantar fasciitis. Level of evidence: II.

24. Singh D, Angel J, Bentley G, Trevino SG: Plantar fasciitis. *BMJ* 1997;315:172-175.

25. Young CC, Rutherford DS, Niedfeldt MW: Treatment of plantar fasciitis. *Am Fam Physician* 2001;63: 467-478.

26. DiGiovanni BF, Nawoczenski DA, Lintal ME, et al: Tissue-specific plantar fascia-stretching exercise enhances outcomes in patients with chronic heel pain: A prospective, randomized study. *J Bone Joint Surg Am* 2003;85:1270-1277.

   Plantar fascia stretching exercises produced more improvement in pain scores than Achilles tendon stretching after 8 weeks of treatment in patients with chronic plantar fasciitis. Level of evidence: I.

27. DiGiovanni BF, Nawoczenski DA, Malay DP, et al: Plantar fascia-specific stretching exercise improves outcomes in patients with chronic plantar fasciitis: A prospective clinical trial with two-year follow-up. *J Bone Joint Surg Am* 2006;88:1775-1781.

   The long-term results of plantar fascia-specific stretching exercises for patients with plantar fasciitis were evaluated. In comparison with a group treated with Achilles tendon stretching in another study, long-term follow-up showed that the significant difference between the groups was no longer present. Level of evidence: II.

28. Radford JA, Burns J, Buchbinder R, Landorf KB, Cook C: Does stretching increase ankle dorsiflexion range of motion? A systematic review. *Br J Sports Med* 2006;40:870-875.

   Ninety-two patients with plantar fasciitis were treated with calf stretching with sham ultrasound or sham ultrasound alone. No significant differences were reported between the groups after 2 weeks of treatment. Level of evidence: I.

29. Powell M, Post WR, Keener J, Wearden S: Effective treatment of chronic plantar fasciitis with dorsiflexion night splints: A crossover prospective randomized outcome study. *Foot Ankle Int* 1998;19:10-18.

30. Probe RA, Baca M, Adams R, Preece C: Night splint treatment for plantar fasciitis: A prospective randomized study. *Clin Orthop Relat Res* 1999;368:190-195.

31. Landorf KB, Keenan AM, Herbert RD: Effectiveness of foot orthoses to treat plantar fasciitis: A randomized trial. *Arch Intern Med* 2006;166:1305-1310.

   In this study, 135 patients were randomized to treatment with a sham orthosis, prefabricated orthosis, or customized orthosis. A short-term functional benefit was reported for patients using an orthosis; however, they did not have long-term beneficial effects when compared with the use of a sham device.

32. Donley BG, Moore T, Sferra J, et al: The efficacy of oral nonsteroidal anti-inflammatory medication (NSAID) in the treatment of plantar fasciitis: A randomized, prospective, placebo-controlled study. *Foot Ankle Int* 2007; 28:20-23.

   Twenty-nine patients were randomly assigned to receive either celecoxib or a placebo as part of a treatment regimen for plantar fasciitis. No significant differences between the groups were reported at 1-, 2-, and 6-month follow-up. Level of evidence: II.

33. Crawford F, Atkins D, Young P, Edwards J: Steroid injection for heel pain: Evidence of short-term effectiveness: A randomized controlled trial. *Rheumatology (Oxford)* 1999;38:974-977.

34. Sellman JR: Plantar fascia rupture associated with corticosteroid injection. *Foot Ankle Int* 1994;15:376-381.

35. Acevedo JI, Beskin JL: Complications of plantar fascia rupture associated with corticosteroid injection. *Foot Ankle Int* 1998;19:91-97.

36. Gudeman SD, Eisele SA, Heidt RS Jr, et al: Treatment of plantar fasciitis by iontophoresis of 0.4% dexamethasone: A randomized, double-blind, placebo-controlled study. *Am J Sports Med* 1997;25:312-316.

37. Buchbinder R, Ptasznik R, Gordon J, et al: Ultrasound-

guided extracorporeal shock wave therapy for plantar fasciitis: A randomized controlled trial. *JAMA* 2002; 288:1364-1372.

38. Ogden JA, Alvarez RG, Levitt RL, Johnson JE, Marlow ME: Electrohydraulic high-energy shock-wave treatment for chronic plantar fasciitis. *J Bone Joint Surg Am* 2004;86:2216-2228.

    This randomized, placebo-controlled, blinded, multicenter study evaluated 293 patients treated with high-energy ESWT or sham treatment for chronic plantar fasciitis. At 3 months, significant improvement was reported in the ESWT treatment group. Level of evidence: I.

39. Rompe JD, Schoellner C, Nafe B: Evaluation of low-energy extracorporeal shock-wave application for treatment of chronic plantar fasciitis. *J Bone Joint Surg Am* 2002;84:335-341.

40. Thomson CE, Crawford F, Murray GD: The effectiveness of extra corporeal shock wave therapy for plantar heel pain: A systematic review and meta-analysis. *BMC Musculoskelet Disord* 2005;6:19.

    This meta-analysis on the use of ESWT for treating plantar fasciitis reported a small but statistically significant improvement in pain with ESWT. Level of evidence: I.

41. Bazaz R, Ferkel RD: Results of endoscopic plantar fascia release. *Foot Ankle Int* 2007;28:549-556.

    The authors reviewed the results of 20 patients with chronic plantar fasciitis who underwent endoscopic release of the plantar fascia. Patients with the greatest improvement included women, nonworkers' compensation patients, and those who had symptoms for less than 2 years. Level of evidence: IV.

42. Conflitti JM, Tarquinio TA: Operative outcome of partial plantar fasciectomy and neurolysis to the nerve of the abductor digiti minimi muscle for recalcitrant plantar fasciitis. *Foot Ankle Int* 2004;25:482-487.

    Twenty-three patients had improvement in visual analog scale scores from 9.2 to 1.7 at 2 years following plantar fascia release and FBLPN neurolysis. Level of evidence: IV.

43. Gould JS: Chronic plantar fasciitis with neuritic symptoms. American Academy of Orthopaedic Surgeons Website. Orthopaedic Knowledge Online. http://www5.aaos.org/oko/description.cfm?topic=FOO008& referringPage=http://www5.aaos.org/oko/menus/foot.cfm. Accessed April 2, 2008.

    A review of the literature is provided, and a video demonstration of a posterior medial release for recalcitrant plantar fasciitis is shown.

44. Tomczak RL, Haverstock BD: A retrospective comparison of endoscopic plantar fasciotomy to open fasciotomy with heel spur resection for chronic plantar fasciitis/heel spur syndrome. *J Foot Ankle Surg* 1995;34: 305-311.

6: Special Problems of the Foot and Ankle

Chapter 27

Bone and Soft-Tissue Tumors of the Foot and Ankle

Henry DeGroot III, MD

Introduction

A tumor is any type of mass or swelling of bone or soft tissue. Tumors can arise from hamartomas (an overgrowth of normal tissues), reactive or posttraumatic processes, inflammatory lesions, or true neoplasms, which can be benign or malignant. Because the foot is composed of numerous, tightly defined, and well-vascularized anatomic compartments, it is predisposed to local and distant spread of disease. An informed and systematic approach is necessary when treating a patient with a tumor of the foot or ankle.

Recent Developments

Recent developments in treating foot and ankle tumors include a new approach to diagnosing soft-tissue masses and a newly described tumor (acral myxoinflammatory fibroblastic sarcoma) that is often misdiagnosed and has a predilection for the foot. New material on managing physician-patient communication and practical methods of avoiding medical and legal problems unique to musculoskeletal cancer care are presented.

Incidence and Pathogenesis

Tumors of the foot and ankle represent a unique subset of all bone and soft-tissue tumors, and vary from other tumors of the musculoskeletal system in type, location, age of affected patients, prognosis, and treatment. Bone tumors in the foot and ankle occur more often in males than in females by a ratio of 4:3. Most tumors are cartilaginous or cystic; a smaller number are osteoblastic. Approximately 5% of tumors are malignant, whereas 20% of mass-forming lesions are malignant.[1,2] Malignancies make up a larger proportion of tumors in the foot and ankle than elsewhere in the body; however, survival rates are significantly better in patients with distal lower extremity tumors than for those with sarcomas at other musculoskeletal sites.[3]

Chondrosarcoma and osteosarcoma are the most common bone sarcomas in the foot and ankle.[1] The American Cancer Society estimates that 10,390 soft-tissue sarcomas will be diagnosed in the United States in 2008; approximately 10% of these sarcomas will occur in the distal lower extremity.[3,4] Synovial sarcoma, clear cell sarcoma, and Ewing sarcoma are the most common soft-tissue sarcomas in the foot and ankle. Soft-tissue sarcomas have no predilection for race or sex. Bone and soft-tissue sarcomas are believed to be caused by a series of alterations in the structure or expression of the genetic material of the mesenchymal cell of origin. A few sarcomas are caused by exposure to radiation or by an underlying genetic abnormality such as the *RB-1* gene in hereditary retinoblastoma or the *p53* gene in Li-Fraumeni syndrome.

The treatment of sarcomas requires resection with a wide margin, plus adjuvant chemotherapy and/or radiotherapy depending on the tumor type. In the foot and ankle, adequate resection with a wide margin may require partial or complete amputation of the affected part. Limb salvage following the removal of tumors in the foot and ankle is complicated by the loads on the skeletal elements and the generally limited soft-tissue coverage. The ultimate goal of treatment is elimination of the tumor and restoration of long-term mobility and function.

Initial Patient Assessment and Examination

A complete history and physical examination is needed for the patient presenting with a mass in the foot or ankle. It is important to precisely determine the onset of pain, the rate of progression, and the precise location of the lesion. This information allows the clinician to determine if the pain is actually originating from the tumor or from a nearby abnormality. In patients with bone tumors, the examination only occasionally provides useful information for diagnosing the lesion. The palpable size, local extent, and presence of a soft-tissue mass should be documented in the patient's chart. For soft-tissue tumors, physical examination findings are helpful in assessing the potential for malignancy. Malignant tumors tend to be large, deep, progressively growing, firm, and detectable as a definite soft-tissue mass.

Benign tumors tend to be small, superficial, soft, and not growing or intermittently increasing and decreasing in size; they are more difficult to detect as a definite soft-tissue mass. Certain findings of the physical examination can indicate a specific diagnosis. For example, hemangiomas have a characteristic blue-purple color that may be visible at the skin level and typically elicit pain when palpated.

Laboratory Testing

Because laboratory testing is not particularly helpful in diagnosing or managing tumors in the foot and ankle, ordering a large battery of nonspecific laboratory tests is not recommended. If infection is suspected, an erythrocyte sedimentation rate, C-reactive protein level, and blood cultures are useful. In patients with known or suspected prostate cancer or multiple myeloma, a prostate-specific antigen test or protein immunoelectrophoresis may help confirm the diagnosis.

Imaging Studies

For bone and soft-tissue lesions, two orthogonal, high-quality, plain radiographs are recommended. The characteristics of the tumor, its location, and the findings from the history and physical examination may indicate the need for additional cross-sectional imaging. Both fine-cut CT scans and high-field strength MRI scans are essential for determining the local extent, anatomic relationships, and possible origins of bone tumors. All soft-tissue masses larger than 2 cm should be evaluated with MRI. Information from CT can be valuable for determining the location and extent of bony invasion of soft-tissue masses. When a metastatic bone lesion in the foot or ankle area is suspected and the primary site is unknown, CT of the chest, abdomen, and pelvis with oral and intravenous contrast is recommended. Bone scans are useful in identifying multiple and occult bone lesions in patients with metastasis. Bone scan findings are nonspecific in patients with solitary bone tumors (if metastasis is not suspected) and in those with soft-tissue tumors.

Assessing the Potential for Malignancy

Bone Lesions
The malignancy potential of bone tumors can be estimated by carefully analyzing their appearance on plain radiographs. Bone tumors are described as latent, active, or aggressive based on an analysis of the tumor margins, the zone of transition, and any permeation or extension into nearby structures. Latent lesions exhibit little or no growth and often have a well-developed sclerotic rim at their margins. Active lesions exhibit gradual growth with progressive local destruction of

bone, no sclerotic rim, a zone of transition of 1 mm to a few millimeters wide, and no tendency to permeate the bone or expand into the soft tissues.[5] Aggressive lesions exhibit rapid growth with complete destruction of nearby bone, a wide zone of transition of several millimeters or more, permeation through adjacent bone and soft tissues, and sometimes a soft-tissue mass. Lesions that are latent may require no treatment, and biopsy is often unnecessary. Active lesions typically require complete local removal based on the results of a preliminary biopsy. Aggressive lesions are best managed with prompt referral to an orthopaedic oncologist for a complete systemic cancer workup and biopsy.

Soft-Tissue Tumors
The malignant potential of soft-tissue tumors is more difficult to determine; the patient history and physical examination findings may be unhelpful or even misleading. MRI provides valuable information about soft-tissue masses. In some instances, MRI signal characteristics may be adequate to identify the exact nature of the lesion or may allow narrowing of the differential diagnosis. In other instances, MRI findings are nonspecific and inadequate to rule out malignancy. A new approach to assessing potential malignancy divides soft-tissue tumors into two groups, determinate and indeterminate, with the subsequent management plan based on this initial assessment. If a specific diagnosis is possible based on a combination of the history, physical examination, and analysis of the MRI findings, the tumor is considered a determinate lesion.[6] Lesions that are determinate include lipomas, hemangiomas, ganglion cysts, pigmented villonodular synovitis (PVNS), and aneurysms. If these lesions can be diagnosed with sufficient confidence, biopsy is not necessary. Lesions that cannot be identified based on the MRI findings are called indeterminate lesions. These lesions are typically isointense with muscle on T1-weighted images and hyperintense on T2-weighted images. This group of tumors includes various soft-tissue sarcomas, such as synovial sarcoma, Ewing sarcoma, clear cell sarcoma, and leiomyosarcoma, as well as several benign tumors. Patients with indeterminate lesions should be referred to an orthopaedic oncologist. A complete workup followed by a carefully planned and executed biopsy is necessary. In most instances, definitive local surgical removal of the lesion must await the final pathologic diagnosis and should be performed as a separate procedure.

Biopsy Techniques

Most orthopaedic surgeons refer patients with bone and soft-tissue tumors to an orthopaedic oncologist for definitive treatment, but some surgeons perform the diagnostic biopsy. Improper timing, technique, or management of the biopsy process can impair outcomes. Complications of poorly planned biopsies include errors in diagnosis, obtaining nondiagnostic biopsy material, infection, hematoma, and uncontrolled spread of the tumor. A poorly planned biopsy can lead to an otherwise avoidable amputation. It is essential to understand proper biopsy techniques and to appreciate the potential morbidity associated with this seemingly simple procedure. For bone lesions, the pathologic diagnosis can be difficult to determine based on small samples. Because of this, open biopsy techniques are more likely to yield diagnostic material than needle biopsy or aspiration techniques. During the procedure, the pathologist should examine a frozen section of the biopsy material to ensure that diagnostic material has been obtained. The biopsy should be performed as the last stage in the tumor workup. All diagnostic scans should precede the biopsy because the biopsy will alter the appearance of the tumor on the scans.

The biopsy should be performed through adequate longitudinal incisions that approach the lesion most directly. Because the compartments of the foot are numerous, small, and have incomplete boundaries, it may be difficult to approach a lesion surgically without contaminating nearby normal tissues. It is essential to prevent unintentional spread of the tumor caused by postbiopsy bleeding. The tourniquet should be released after the tumor is sampled, and measures should be taken to ensure that meticulous hemostasis has been achieved. Bleeding bone may require packing with a small amount of methylmethacrylate cement or bone wax. A moderate compressive dressing should be applied, the patient should not bear weight, and the extremity should be elevated for 3 or 4 days to prevent formation of a hematoma that can carry tumor cells and track under subcutaneous tissues or through intramuscular spaces, causing a wide zone of contaminated tissues.

Excisional biopsy is rarely preferable for bone tumors in the foot or ankle, with the exception of osteochondromas and unicameral bone cysts (UBCs) in which there is a reliable diagnosis based on the examination and imaging studies. Completely superficial soft-tissue masses that are smaller than 2 cm in their greatest dimension can be treated with excisional biopsy. During excisional biopsy, care should be taken that the tumor is not exposed or entered. The entire tumor, the surrounding capsule, and a small amount of surrounding normal soft tissue is removed en bloc. Excisional biopsy is never appropriate for large or deep soft-tissue tumors.

Needle biopsy should be performed in medical centers with dedicated teams of surgeons and pathologists experienced with the technique. If there is little doubt concerning the diagnosis, needle biopsy can be used for confirmation. Core needle biopsy is a good technique for patients with a biopsy-proven cancer diagnosis with a suspected recurrence or a metastatic lesion in the foot or ankle. In these instances, the histopathologic characteristics of the cells aspirated from the new lesion can be matched against the tissue from the original biopsy.

Factors in Treating Musculoskeletal Tumors

Patient Management After an Unplanned Excision of a Malignant Tumor
Studies of patients following unplanned or inadequate excision of a soft-tissue tumor suggest that favorable outcomes can still be achieved if additional surgical treatment is initiated without delay, although overall outcomes may not be optimal. It is necessary to achieve a wide margin by complete excision of the entire tumor bed and any surgically contaminated tissues. Following repeat excision in patients without a clinically palpable residual tumor, one study showed that 50% of patients had a microscopic residual tumor.[7] Following repeat excision, 85% of the patients were alive and disease free at 5 years. However, unplanned removal of a soft-tissue sarcoma is associated with a higher risk of positive margins and local recurrence, both of which are associated with poor outcomes.

Delayed Diagnosis
Despite advances in detection methods and treatment, tumors of the musculoskeletal system are sometimes missed, misdiagnosed, or mismanaged.[8] This delay in diagnosing tumors may be caused by the overlap in presentation between tumors and more common orthopaedic conditions, the rarity and confusing variety of tumors, or other factors.[9] Diagnostic delay is linked to both patient sociodemographic and physician-associated factors. Females, younger patients, single or divorced patients, and those of a lower socioeconomic status are more likely to have a delayed tumor diagnosis.[10] A delayed cancer diagnosis is the most common reason for malpractice litigation in the United States and is the most costly for physicians. Medicolegal claims analysis has shown that several physician factors are associated with a delayed diagnosis.[11] The physician may ignore or fail to follow up on the patient's reported symptoms or may believe that the patient is too young or too healthy to have cancer. The physician may not provide follow-up or referral, may rely on an apparently negative imaging study, or may not document salient facts. The duration of the delay seems to have an impact on the ultimate legal outcome in medical malpractice claims. In an analysis of 338 closed malpractice claims in which a delayed diagnosis was alleged, there was a finding in favor of the physician in 65% of cases in which the delay was 1 to 3 months and in 33% of cases in which the delay was longer than 6 months.[12]

Treatment of Malignant Tumors
The goals of surgical treatment of tumors in the distal lower extremity do not differ from those for any other part of the body; however, the unique anatomic and functional characteristics of the area require special consideration. The surgical goal is resection with a wide margin, while maintaining a sensate, plantigrade foot. Wide margins reduce the risks for local recurrence,

which has a strong negative impact on survival. Because of the anatomy of the foot and ankle, it may be difficult to achieve a wide margin without at least a partial amputation. Limb-sparing surgery is preferable to amputation only if a durable, functional, and pain-free extremity can be achieved. The soft-tissue coverage of areas of the distal lower extremities is often scant and subjected to high loads and repetitive shear stresses. The bony and articular elements must provide durable support and flexibility and still be capable of withstanding the stresses of weight bearing. For these reasons, limb-sparing surgery, although considered the treatment of choice for sarcomas in most anatomic locations, must be carefully weighed against other options for tumors of the foot and ankle. In a review of 175 patients with sarcoma in the distal lower extremity, 23% of patients required amputation, whereas the amputation rate for tumors in other body parts was 3%.[3]

A recent study showed that following resection of one or more rays in patients with malignant sarcoma, reconstruction with an osteomyocutaneous flap resulted in an encouraging rate of overall limb salvage and function; however, multiple procedures were required in all patients because of complications.[13] Efforts to preserve the limb may result in significant functional impairment. In one study, fewer than 50% of patients regained normal functional status.[14] Because of poor soft-tissue coverage of the area and the need to replace the resected bony part, local island flaps, reverse pedicle myocutaneous flaps, split-thickness skin grafts, free vascularized latissimus dorsi flaps, free vascularized fibular or iliac crest grafts, and fresh frozen allografts have been used with varying degrees of success.[13-15] For pediatric sarcomas in the foot, such as Ewing sarcoma and rhabdomyosarcoma, limb-sparing surgery combined with adjuvant radiation may provide better overall function than amputation. These tumors more often recur at a distant site rather than locally.[16]

Management of Patient Expectations and Anxiety

The patient with a tumor in the foot or ankle requires systematic and knowledgeable orthopaedic care delivered in a caring and supportive manner. The treating physician should focus on providing an accurate diagnosis, a comprehensive treatment plan, and information regarding the prospects for recovery. Radiologists, pathologists, and other physicians should be part of the treatment team. Information should be shared with the patient and the patient's family and presented in an understandable and emotionally sensitive manner to lessen the patient's anxiety.

Primary Benign Bone Tumors

Giant Cell Tumor

Giant cell tumor is a benign but locally aggressive tumor that can occur in any bone but is uncommon in the foot. The peak age at diagnosis is the second or third decade of life. The typical patient has a history of gradually increasing pain but no mass. Pathologic fracture or microfracture may cause the patient to seek treatment. The lesion originates in the metaphyseal segment of the bone adjacent to the physeal scar and expands proximally and distally into the diaphysis and epiphysis. The tumor grows until it reaches the subchondral surface of the joint, which forms a partial barrier against further tumor extension. The adjacent cortex may be expanded, thin, or destroyed, and the tumor can extend into the nearby soft tissues. There may be numerous septae or longitudinal striations in the involved bone. The zone of transition is 1 to 4 mm wide, with no permeation and no matrix mineralization. If the lesion has been present long enough, the involved bone can balloon to many times its original volume. CT can be used to define the local extent of the tumor and help confirm the absence of matrix mineralization. MRI findings are nondiagnostic, although the lesions tend to be highly heterogeneous if they are large enough. There may be cystic loculated blood-filled internal spaces. Bone scan findings are nonspecific.

Treatment consists of curettage followed by extension of the zone of curettage with application of a motorized burr, phenol, or liquid nitrogen to the tumor cavity. Filling of the cavity with morcellized autogenous or allogenous bone graft allows more complete remodeling and normalization of the bone. However, filling of the cavity with polymethylmethacrylate bone cement appears to be associated with a lower rate of local recurrence, perhaps because of the heat of polymerization released by the cement. Lesser bones may be excised completely or reconstructed with structural allograft. Large lesions of the phalanges of the lesser toes should be amputated. Treatment is followed by recurrence in approximately 10% of patients. Recurrent tumors should be treated by repeat curettage, or, if adequate local control is impossible, by wide resection and reconstruction.

Osteochondroma

Osteochondromas occur in the distal fibula and the distal tibia, where they can cause recurrent sprains, ankle stiffness, or a palpable mass. Distal fibular lesions often impinge on the tibia and require removal. Large or multiple lesions in the distal leg result in differential longitudinal growth of the tibia and fibula, leading to valgus deformity of the ankle. The valgus deformity will remodel if these lesions are removed early. Patients with osteochondromatosis present in early adulthood with valgus overload of the ankle. Severe ankle deformities will not remodel, and supramalleolar osteotomy may be required to correct symptomatic valgus (Figure 1).

Osteochondroma is relatively rare in the bones of the foot. It usually occurs in the forefoot on a metatarsal. This lesion occurs in teenagers and young adults and is characterized by mild pain, a palpable mass, and a typical radiographic appearance as a pedunculated or

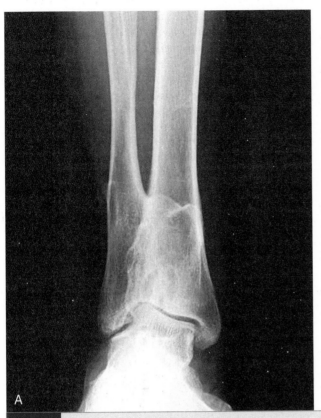
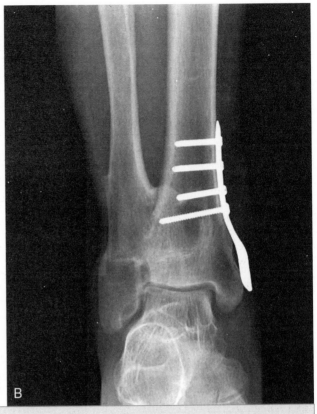

Figure 1 Ankle deformity caused by osteochondromatosis. **A,** Preoperative AP view shows valgus deformity. **B,** Postoperative AP view shows the results of a closing wedge osteotomy of the distal tibia and fibula.

sessile mature bony mass on the surface of the metaphyseal portion of the bone. The cortex of the lesion is continuous with the nearby normal cortex. CT can be helpful in verifying the pathognomonic appearance of the lesion. The CT scan should show that the cortex and medullary cavity of the underlying bone are continuous with the cortex and medullary cavity of the lesion. MRI is helpful in evaluating the thickness of the cartilage cap. Growth of the cartilage cap or growth of the lesion after skeletal maturity is a worrisome finding and should be investigated as a potential sign of malignant degeneration. These lesions may be treated with simple excision by osteotomy through the base of the lesion. It is not necessary to remove every vestige of the lesion to achieve symptom resolution. Treatment should be delayed until skeletal maturity (if possible) when the lesions are better defined and easier to remove and when the active cartilaginous portion of the lesion is located farther from the underlying bone. If the entire active cartilaginous portion of the lesion is not removed, recurrence is possible (**Figure 2**).

Enchondroma

Approximately 8% of enchondromas occur in the bones of the foot. The peak age at diagnosis is approximately the middle of the fourth decade of life, but the tumor may occur at any age.[17] Enchondromas usually occur in the metatarsals or phalanges of the lesser toes.

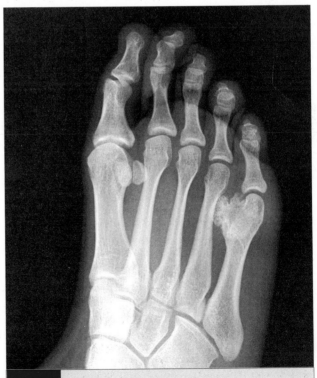

Figure 2 Osteochondroma of the metatarsal in a 17-year-old girl. The patient had an injury to the area at age 12 years.

The hindfoot is rarely involved. The lesion is typically a solitary, slightly expansile, lucent lesion with minimal matrix calcification; it can be thin and expanding, or can fracture the nearby cortex. Patients present with pain during activities or after an injury, but there is rarely any palpable mass on physical examination. Occasionally, pathologic fracture through the lesion will cause the patient to seek medical care. Small, peripheral cartilage tumors tend to be benign, whereas large central cartilage lesions are more likely to be malignant. Reliable differentiation of benign from malignant cartilage tumors is difficult. Larger tumors, tumors located in the hindfoot or midfoot, or new tumors occurring in a patient with a known history of enchondromatosis (Ollier disease) have an increased risk of malignancy. Other radiologic findings, such as the presence or absence of matrix mineralization, amount and extent of cortical thinning or expansion, and findings on technetium bone scans are not well correlated with the presence or absence of malignancy. Asymptomatic, latent lesions that are not causing bone fragility may be observed without biopsy. Painful or problematic enchondromas can be treated with simple curettage and packing with bone graft. Recurrence is rare. Extremely expansile lesions may require complete excision and substitution of a structural allograft. Partial amputation of the toe should be considered for large lesions in the distal phalanges because the functional and cosmetic result of curettage and bone grafting may be unacceptable.

Chondromyxoid Fibroma

Chondromyxoid fibroma is a rare benign tumor that has a striking predilection for the bones of the tibia and foot. Most affected patients are younger than 30 years, and the tumor occurs more often in males, typically in the second or third decade of life. Approximately 25% of all chondromyxoid fibromas involve the foot, with the metatarsals the most common location. Patients present with pain and a slowly growing mass. Plain radiographs show an expansile, lobulated, lytic lesion in the metaphysis, with partial cortical erosion and local extension into the soft tissues. There may be a sclerotic margin, with the long axis typically parallel to the bone. The matrix lacks detectable calcification. CT can help identify the local extent of the lesion and can confirm the absence of matrix mineralization. MRI findings are similar to those reported for other cartilage tumors, with low-signal intensity on T1-weighted images and high-signal intensity on T2-weighted images. MRI is helpful in identifying the soft-tissue mass and for preoperative planning. Careful biopsy and evaluation by an experienced pathologist are necessary to distinguish this tumor from similar aggressive or malignant lesions. Curettage may be adequate but may result in local recurrence in up to 25% of patients. Unlike giant cell tumor, this tumor has a propensity to recur because of seeding of the soft tissues during curettage. Local recurrence can be treated with meticulous repeat curettage

and excision of the entire soft-tissue mass. Marginal or wide excision and substitution of the involved bone with a structural bone graft is usually curative.

Osteoid Osteoma

Osteoid osteomas are painful, benign tumors; approximately 11% occur in the bones of the foot, with the neck of the talus as the most common location. The peak age of incidence is the second decade of life. Patients present with persistent pain and swelling that is unrelated to activity. The pain may be more intense at night. In most patients, nonsteroidal anti-inflammatory drugs (NSAIDs) provide substantial pain relief. If NSAIDs do not relieve pain, the diagnosis of osteoid osteoma is less likely. Lesions adjacent to a joint may cause ankylosis or mimic a pauciarticular inflammatory arthritis, such as Reiter disease. The local swelling, erythema, and tenderness can mimic infection. Pain relief from NSAIDs can be less dramatic when there is significant involvement of a nearby joint. On plain radiographs and CT scans, a central nidus smaller than 1 cm is identified within a larger zone of sclerotic reactive bone. If the nidus is larger than 2 cm, the diagnosis of osteoid osteoma is excluded. The sclerotic bone surrounding the nidus can be minimal when the tumor involves a small bone. Bone scans show a small, very intense focus of increased uptake. Characteristic findings on plain radiographs, CT scans, and bone scans are sufficient to diagnosis this tumor. MRI findings are nonspecific.

Patients who respond well to NSAIDs and aspirin may be successfully treated with these medications until the lesion disappears. The average time to resolution is 22 months. Many patients are unable to tolerate the pain for such an extended period and prefer surgical removal of the lesion. The goal of surgery is complete removal of the lesion by the least invasive means possible. For lesions in the hindfoot and midfoot, radiofrequency ablation with a CT-guided needle is the recommended technique. With the patient under general anesthesia, the tip of a radiofrequency generator electrode is placed into the center of the lesion using CT guidance. A radiofrequency generator produces an alternating high-frequency radio wave that passes from the electrode tip into the surrounding tissue, where energy is dissipated as heat. The tissue itself is heated, not the radiofrequency probe. A sphere with a diameter of up to 1 cm can be effectively treated in this manner, making this treatment ideal for osteoid osteoma. Before treatment with radiofrequency ablation, there should be a high degree of confidence in the diagnosis, which has been confirmed with imaging studies. There should be sufficient distance between the lesion and any major neurovascular structure, and the lesion should have a clearly deformed nidus smaller than 1 cm in its largest dimension. Although radiofrequency ablation was previously available only in tertiary medical centers, it is now more widely available. A high success rate and an extremely low rate of complications strongly favor this technique. Radiofrequency ablation can be more challenging to use in smaller bones because of difficulties with targeting the lesion in the CT scanner and with the increased risk of damaging nearby tendons or neurovascular structures. For superficial lesions in the forefoot, open surgery is still the preferred treatment. The surgeon must be able to locate the nidus using radiographs, anatomic landmarks, and direct observation. Other techniques for locating the nidus have been described. The surrounding reactive bone can be extremely dense and may also be hypervascular and somewhat porous. It is essential to remove the entire nidus to prevent recurrence. Surgical removal of the lesion often leads to weakening of the affected bone, which may necessitate bone grafting, plating, a prolonged period of not bearing weight, and other activity restrictions.

Osteoblastoma

Osteoblastoma is an osteoid-producing, benign bone lesion that can demonstrate aggressive clinical behavior. The foot is the third most common location of osteoblastoma after the spine and the femur, with 12.5% of osteoblastomas occurring in the bones of the foot.[18] Most lesions occur in the hindfoot, and the talus is the most commonly affected bone. The mean age of patients affected with osteoblastomas is 22 years. In one study of 41 osteoblastomas in the foot, 2 evolved into malignant sarcomas.[18] Careful correlation of clinical, radiologic, and histologic information is required to determine the proper treatment. There is no consensus on which histologic characteristics are associated with the aggressive behavior of osteoblastomas.

Chondroblastoma

About 12% of all chondroblastomas occur in the bones of the foot. Males are affected six times as often as females. The average patient age at presentation is 25 years, which is significantly older than the average age of patients with chondroblastomas in other parts of the skeleton.[19] Patients report pain (that can be severe) and swelling or a mass near the joint. The nearby joint may be locally inflamed. Radiographically, the lesion is located exclusively in the epiphysis, although in the small bones of the foot the location within the epiphysis may not be obvious. The lesions appear well defined, expansile, and lucent, and there may be stippled calcification or no matrix mineralization. The tumor is adjacent to an articular surface or an apophysis. Chondroblastoma in the foot most commonly occurs in subchondral areas of the talus and calcaneus as well as the calcaneal apophysis. CT is useful for defining the relationship of the tumor to the joint, defining the integrity of the underlying bone, and identifying intralesional calcifications. Chondroblastoma can behave aggressively and invade soft tissue. Benign pulmonary metastases have been observed. Treatment of the primary lesion consists of complete curettage and bone grafting. To reduce the risk of recurrence, it has been recom-

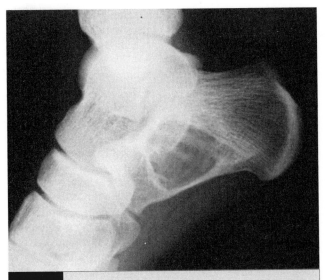

Figure 3 Lateral radiograph showing UBC in the calcaneus.

mended that the zone of curettage be extended by removing an additional 2 or 3 mm of bone using a mechanical burr or by using phenol or liquid nitrogen placed in the tumor cavity. Recurrence is common; recurrent lesions should be treated with repeat curettage. If a recurrent lesion is located in a readily reconstructible location, marginal resection with structural allograft or autograft reconstruction is preferable. Patients with recurrent lesions should have follow-up CT scans of the chest to detect pulmonary nodules. Pulmonary nodules should be excised.[19]

Unicameral Bone Cyst

A UBC is a benign lesion of uncertain origin. Several etiologies have been proposed, including expansion of synovial tissue trapped in the bone during development, local failure of ossification, or obstruction of the venous outflow of the bone. In the foot, UBCs occur almost exclusively in the calcaneus and are detected in teenagers or young adults as an incidental finding or during evaluation for mild aching pain caused by sports participation or running. The location and appearance is characteristic, and biopsy may not be needed to confirm the diagnosis. UBCs occur in the lateral portion of the calcaneus subadjacent to the middle facet (**Figure 3**). The apex of the lesion is toward the forefoot. There is no matrix mineralization. Displaced fractures through UBCs in the calcaneus are uncommon. Asymptomatic patients are treated with observation and follow-up radiographs to ensure the lesion is not expanding or changing. Painful cysts can be treated with a wide variety of techniques; there is no consensus regarding the optimal treatment method. Minimally invasive techniques include aspiration and injection with methylprednisolone, bone marrow, autogenous or allogenous bone graft, bone graft substitutes, or a combination of these materials. UBCs also can be treated with curettage without grafting, creating multiple drill holes, or percutaneous screw decompression. Open

6: Special Problems of the Foot and Ankle

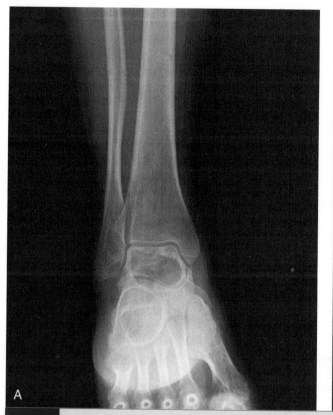
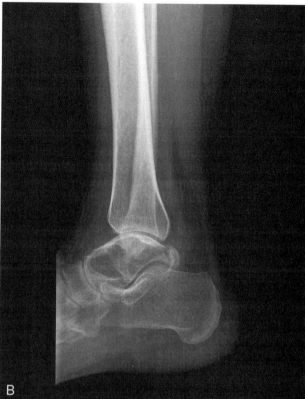

Figure 4   AP **(A)** and lateral **(B)** radiographs showing mesenchymal chondrosarcoma of the talus. The location of a cartilage lesion in the hindfoot is associated with malignancy. (*Courtesy of F. Zhao, Zhejiang, China.*)

curettage and bone grafting may have a higher rate of success, but invasive treatments should be reserved for large or troublesome lesions.

Aneurysmal Bone Cyst

Aneurysmal bone cysts usually occur in the second and third decades of life. Some patients have a history of trauma to the area of the lesion. Patients report pain and a slowly growing mass. The lesion may be located on the surface of the bone or in the metaphysis or epiphysis. Plain radiographs show an expansile lesion with internal septations or longitudinal striations. The lesion may be highly expansile, causing the bone to balloon to many times its original diameter. Even in highly expansile lesions, an overlying eggshell thin layer of bone remains. The radiographic appearance of aneurysmal bone cysts can be variable; these lesions may appear to be highly aggressive. CT scans will show the local extent of the tumor. MRI scans may show fluid levels within the lesion, a finding that is suggestive but not diagnostic. Treatment of most lesions can be accomplished by curettage and using a high-speed burr to remove an additional 2 mm of bone. During surgical treatment, aneurysmal bone cysts bleed profusely until removal is complete. Recurrence is more common in younger patients with open growth plates and can be as high as 20%. Where appropriate, the lesions may be resected with a wide margin, such as in the fibula.

Primary Malignant Bone Tumors

Chondrosarcoma

Chondrosarcomas are relatively rare in the bones of the foot, with this location accounting for approximately 2% of all such tumors.[20] The tumors may be primary or develop as a secondary malignancy in an enchondroma or osteochondroma. Because enchondromas often occur in the foot, it is essential to properly differentiate between benign and malignant cartilage tumors (Figure 4). In the foot, the radiographic appearance of chondrosarcoma may considerably overlap with the appearance of enchondroma. Both types of tumors are lytic and may extend into the soft tissues around the bone. Matrix mineralization, in the form of rings and arcs, occurs in approximately two thirds of both benign and malignant lesions. The presence of scalloping and cortical and periosteal destruction is not a reliable method for distinguishing benign from malignant lesions. In a recent study, lesions larger than 5 cm and location in the hindfoot were associated with the potential for malignancy.[20] Management of these lesions includes close follow-up and biopsy when indicated. Chondrosarcoma is treated by surgical resection with a wide margin. Chemotherapy and radiation therapy are used if surgical control is inadequate or impossible. Innovative limb-salvage procedures, such as total calcaneus allograft implantation, have been reported. Treatment consists of wide excision of the tumor and maximal restoration of mobility, preferably with conservation of a durable, minimally painful, plantigrade foot.

Osteosarcoma

Osteosarcoma can occur in any bone of the foot, but the calcaneus is the most commonly involved bone. The peak age of incidence is approximately 20 years, but very young and very old patients also are affected. The patient presents with insidious pain; eventually, a mass is detectable. Because the pain may be initially intermittent and related to a minor injury or exercise activity, the condition may be misdiagnosed as a common sprain or strain. The pain will become persistent with time and will begin to occur at night. Initial radiographs will show a lesion with subtle mixed lysis and sclerosis, followed by increasing sclerosis, permeation, destruction, and expansion into the adjacent soft-tissues, with bone formation in the soft-tissue mass.

The differential diagnoses include other sarcomas, such as Ewing sarcoma and synovial sarcoma, and metastatic lesions. Plain radiographs, CT, MRI, technetium Tc99m bone scans, and a CT scan of the chest are required to determine the local extent and stage of the tumor. Most osteosarcomas present in stage IIB, which is defined as a tumor that has broken out of its compartment of origin but is not yet metastatic. The prognosis for patients with osteosarcoma depends on the tumor grade and stage at presentation. Low-grade tumors are associated with long-term survival rates of approximately 90%, whereas high-grade tumors have an overall survival rate of approximately 60%. Survival in patients with metastasis is poor.[21]

Ewing Sarcoma

Ewing sarcoma is relatively rare in the bones of the foot. The calcaneus is the most commonly involved site, but this tumor can occur in any bone or as a mass in the soft tissues. Delayed diagnosis is common in patients with Ewing sarcoma in the foot. The mean age at presentation for lesions in the foot is 17 years, with an average duration of symptoms of 14 months.[22] Patients with forefoot tumors have an average of 7 months of symptoms before diagnosis, whereas patients with hindfoot tumors have an average of 22 months of symptoms before diagnosis.[22] Many patients are treated for osteomyelitis before the correct diagnosis is made. The lesion causes pain, which initially follows a sports activity or minor injury. The patient appears entirely healthy other than the foot and ankle symptoms. The initial radiographs will show minor, unimpressive changes, with focal lysis and permeation of the involved bone. If the diagnosis is delayed, extensive permeation, bony destruction, and a soft-tissue mass will develop. The characteristic "onion skinning" or lamellar periosteal reaction is not usually seen because of the anatomy of the foot.

Initial evaluation should include plain radiographs

of the foot, CT and MRI scans of the primary tumor, a whole-body bone scan, and a CT scan of the chest. Biopsy should be delayed until all of the imaging studies are completed. In one study, patients with Ewing sarcoma in the forefoot had an overall survival rate of 70%, whereas patients with Ewing sarcoma in the hindfoot had an overall survival rate of 33%.[22] The survival rate for patients with metastasis at the time of presentation was 0%. Treatment depends on the stage and local extent of the tumor. Localized tumors are treated with chemotherapy and wide surgical excision with or without radiation. Radiation can be avoided if adequate margins can be achieved at the time of surgery. Because radiation carries the risk of development of secondary sarcomas in the radiated field, amputation may be the procedure of choice for treating Ewing sarcoma of the foot.

Metastatic Tumors of the Foot

Metastases to the foot from neoplasms elsewhere in the body are relatively rare. However, the rate of metastasis has been underestimated in some reports in the literature because of inadequate imaging of the distal extremities. When a careful survey of the entire skeleton is performed, there is an increase in the number of metastatic lesions that are identified in the foot. For patients with lung, prostate, kidney, and other cancers, metastatic lesions in the bones of the foot account for 2.8% to 3.7% of all skeletal lesions (**Figure 5**). The authors of one study reported that in patients with breast cancer, metastatic lesions in the foot accounted for 9.4% of all lesions.[23] Patients with metastasis to the foot are usually older than 60 years, present with pain and swelling, and have a bone lesion that is visible on plain radiographs. The radiographic changes may be subtle at first, leading to a missed diagnosis. In 25% of patients presenting with a painful bony metastasis, there is no previous history of cancer. The tarsal bones are most commonly affected (50%), with most lesions located in the calcaneus, followed by the metatarsals (23%) and phalanges (17%).[23] Radiographically, the lesions are lytic or blastic and destructive; they can be expansile but only occasionally transgress the cortex or invade a nearby joint. Multiple lesions may develop. Technetium Tc 99m bone scanning has a 98% yield for skeletal lesions and is an excellent screening and detection tool. The level of serum alkaline phosphatase shows a good correlation with the number of metastatic lesions overall, but the level may be normal in the early stages. Because patients tend to have widespread cancer when a metastatic lesion is detected in the foot, reconstructive surgery is rarely feasible or advisable. Most patients are palliated with bisphosphonates, radiation, casts or braces, and walking aids. For patients with good functional and survival prospects, treatment by curettage and packing with methylmethacrylate or amputation has been advocated.

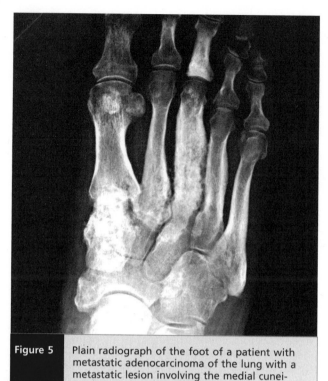

Figure 5 Plain radiograph of the foot of a patient with metastatic adenocarcinoma of the lung with a metastatic lesion involving the medial cuneiform and portions of the third ray.

Benign Soft-Tissue Tumors

A large number of benign soft-tissue tumors and tumorlike conditions occur in the foot and ankle, including ganglion cyst, runner's bump, plantar fibromatosis, schwannoma, and neurofibroma. The correct treatment for benign soft-tissue tumors primarily involves definitively ruling out the potential for malignancy. Once the clinician is certain that the lesion is benign, appropriate nonsurgical or surgical management can begin. Typically, the lesion is removed with a minimal or marginal resection with maximal preservation of nearby bone and soft-tissue structures.

Ganglion Cysts

The origin of ganglion cysts is unclear, but they are commonly associated with degenerative conditions of soft-tissue or bone. Ganglion cysts arise from a synovial-lined space such as a joint, fascia, or tendon sheath. These cysts can occur adjacent to joints, tendons, and fascial planes and within bone. Most ganglion cysts can be definitively diagnosed based on a careful physical examination. A ganglion cyst typically has a superficial location and a tendency to both increase and decrease in size over time. The mass is often soft when the nearby joint is relaxed and becomes firm when the nearby joint or muscle is tensed. A penlight or a small laser pointer may transilluminate the cyst.

Aspiration with a large bore needle should yield characteristic clear viscous material from the mass to confirm the diagnosis (**Figure 6**). If the characteristic fluid is not obtained, further attempts at aspiration should not be made. MRI should be used to further delineate the mass. Ganglion cysts have a characteristic MRI appearance. The lesion is well defined, lobular, homogeneous, and has low signal intensity on T1-weighted sequences and high signal intensity on T2-weighted sequences, which is typical of water or fluid. After the diagnosis of a ganglion cyst is confirmed, the cyst can be treated with aspiration and injection with cortisone, which should lead to resolution in 50% of patients. Surgical removal is indicated for persistent, large, or troublesome cysts. The mass should be explored and the origin of the cyst and the stalk identified, if possible. A portion of the joint capsule and the stalk should be excised in continuity with the mass. Loupe magnification and tourniquet hemostasis will assist in visualizing the stalk and may decrease the risk of recurrence. Approximately 10% of these cysts recur following surgery.

Plantar Fibromatosis

Plantar fibromatosis is a nonencapsulated thickening and proliferation of the central and medial bands of the plantar fascia. This lesion is histologically similar to Dupuytren contracture. Plantar fibromatosis usually occurs in the second to fourth decades of life. Most patients are asymptomatic, but some report activity-related pain. Bilateral nodules occur in approximately 33% to 50% of patients. MRI signal characteristics of the lesion are characteristic and allow differentiation of this lesion from more worrisome conditions. The lesion appears as a poorly defined area of thickening of the plantar fascia with low-signal intensity on T1-weighted and T2-weighted images. Initial treatment includes shoe modifications and pain medication. Surgical removal is reserved for large lesions causing significant disability. Aggressive resection with a wide margin is necessary to avoid recurrence but may be associated with significant complications, including scar sensitivity, pain, and nerve injury.

Synovial Chondromatosis

Synovial chondromatosis originates from cartilaginous metaplasia of synovial tissue near joints, tendon sheaths, or bursae and occasionally occurs around the ankle but is rare in the foot. The lesions can grow to a significant size and may present a diagnostic dilemma. The lesion characteristically is adjacent to a joint or contained within the tendon sheath and has MRI features that are characteristic of partially calcified cartilage. It is lobular, well-defined, and has low-signal intensity on T1-weighted images and high-signal intensity on T2-weighted images. Treatment consists of arthroscopic or open surgical removal.

Pigmented Villonodular Synovitis

PVNS and giant cell tumor of the tendon sheath are benign tumors that are characterized by invasive and destructive proliferation of synovial tissue within a joint

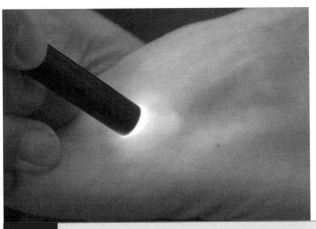 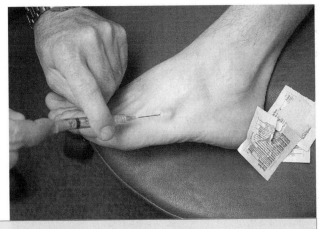

Figure 6   Diagnosis of a ganglion cyst can be confirmed by transillumination and aspiration.

or tendon sheath. The lesion most commonly occurs as a localized, nodular mass in or adjacent to a joint or tendon sheath. The nodular form occurs around the joints and tendons of the hands and feet. The diffuse form usually involves larger joints and may involve several adjacent joints. The ankle is the third most common location for diffuse intra-articular PVNS. A diagnosis of PVNS usually occurs in the second decade of life, with men and women equally affected. The ankle and hindfoot are affected approximately twice as often as the forefoot.

The tumor can present as a soft-tissue mass or a periarticular mass with or without pain. Patients with PVNS of the ankle have a monarticular swelling and aching pain with activity. A significant effusion is characteristic. Although mild inflammation is usually present, findings are less impressive than those that are seen in patients with gout or rheumatoid arthritis. In early or mild PVNS, the only finding is soft-tissue swelling with no changes to bone. The joint space is preserved, and the periarticular bone density is not affected. More advanced PVNS can cause focal destruction of the bone, juxta-articular osteoporosis, and joint-space narrowing. Long-standing nodular lesions can mildly invade or erode adjacent bone. In larger joints and in patients with more extensive PVNS, severe lytic subchondral bone lesions may occur on both sides of the joint, which is a characteristic unique to this tumor. On MRI scans, the nodular lesions appear solitary and well circumscribed. Severe PVNS can mimic the MRI appearance of a malignancy; however, PVNS has a characteristic MRI finding that often allows the diagnosis to be made based on the imaging studies. When the tumor contains sufficient amounts of iron-rich hemosiderin, a paramagnetic "blooming" effect can be seen on T2-weighted, gradient echo sequences. This finding is diagnostic of PVNS.

The treatment of PVNS depends on the location, extent, and the damage to nearby structures that has occurred at the time of diagnosis. Solitary nodular lesions can be easily excised, and recurrence is uncommon. In diffuse PVNS involving larger joints with mild symptoms and no joint damage, nonsurgical treatment consisting of prolonged (4 to 6 months) activity restrictions, protected weight bearing, and the use of NSAIDs should be considered. Mild or moderate PVNS of the ankle can be treated with open or arthroscopic synovectomy and curettage of the cystic lesions. The prognosis for patients is fair because of frequent recurrences. To reduce the chance of recurrence after surgical treatment, prolonged activity restrictions and protected weight bearing are helpful. Adjuvant therapies, such as radiation and synoviorthesis (radionuclide synovectomy) using phosphorus-32 chromic phosphate can be used to treat patients with difficult, recurrent PVNS. Lesions that cause severe damage require aggressive synovectomy combined with fusion or replacement of the involved joint. For permeative and destructive lesions involving the distal lesser toes, amputation is recommended.

Malignant Soft-Tissue Tumors

Acral Myxoinflammatory Fibroblastic Sarcoma
First identified in 1998, acral myxoinflammatory fibroblastic sarcoma is a rare, low-grade sarcoma. The tumor presents as a painless subcutaneous mass of months or years duration. Approximately 30% of these tumors occur in the foot and ankle, 65% in the hand and wrist, and the rest at other sites.[24] This sarcoma usually occurs in the middle adult years (median age, 53 years) but can occur in the third to ninth decades of life; males and females are equally affected. The lesions average 3 cm in size. The mass is poorly circumscribed and subcutaneous and is often misdiagnosed as a ganglion cyst or tenosynovitis. Because of the innocuous presentation, the initial surgical margins are frequently inadequate. Recurrence is reported in 60% to 70% of patients.[24] Approximately 25% of patients require amputation because of repeated local recurrence of the tumor. Metastasis is uncommon, but tumor spread to re-

gional lymph nodes and the lung have been reported. Appropriate management begins with the recognition of the malignant potential of this sarcoma. MRI scans will show the extent of the tumor. A complete workup includes assessing the regional lymph nodes and lungs for potential metastasis. Excision with a wide margin and long-term follow-up is required. Outcomes are similar to those of other low-grade sarcomas, with two thirds of patients alive without disease and the remainder alive with disease at 5-year follow-up.[24]

Aggressive Digital Capillary Adenoma/Adenocarcinoma

Aggressive digital capillary adenocarcinoma is a rare cutaneous tumor of eccrine sweat gland origin that occurs on the plantar surfaces of the digits in the hand and foot. Because it can have an indolent clinical course without symptoms or change for years, it may be misdiagnosed as a benign entity. Excisional biopsy is recommended for indolent soft-tissue masses on the plantar surfaces of the digits. Metastasis has been reported in 14% of patients, with both widespread metastasis and frequent metastasis to the lungs.[25] The usefulness of lymph node sampling has not been defined. No effective treatment is available for metastatic disease. Aggressive surgical resection or amputation is necessary to avoid local recurrence. Aggressive surgical treatment is associated with a decrease in the rate of local recurrence from 50% to 5%.[25]

Both a benign and a malignant variant of this tumor have been described, but a more recent review has cast doubt on the reliability of the histologic diagnosis. It appears that the histologic characteristics of this lesion do not allow reliable differentiation between the benign and malignant forms or provide a distinction between aggressive tumors that metastasize from tumors that have a benign course. Both digital capillary adenoma and digital capillary adenocarcinoma should be treated in a similar manner and can be designated as aggressive digital capillary adenocarcinoma.[25]

Synovial Sarcoma

Synovial sarcoma is the most common malignant soft-tissue sarcoma in the foot and accounts for 18% to 22% of all such tumors. It has been reported to be the single most common sarcoma of any type in the distal lower extremity.[26] This tumor deserves special attention and study because of its potential for slow, painless growth, its peak incidence in young patients, and the serious consequences of delayed diagnosis. Synovial sarcoma occurs in the second through fifth decades of life (mean age, 28 years). The most common location of this tumor is the leg, ankle, or foot. The presentation of synovial sarcoma is variable and can mimic a benign process, such as a ganglion cyst. The patient may have a mass that has been present for months, years, or even decades, with slow growth and few or no symptoms. There may be recent rapid growth of a lesion that has been present for years without apparent change. Con-

versely, some of these sarcomas can cause pain from their outset. The average duration of symptoms before diagnosis is 21 months.[26] The lesion is usually deeply seated, firm, and painless; however, small superficial lesions also occur. The tumor is firm on examination and does not transilluminate. Because metastasis to regional lymph nodes can occur, these nodes should be included in the physical examination.

Imaging studies are not adequate to distinguish this tumor from a benign soft-tissue mass. Plain radiographs are useful and may show the invasiveness and the stippled calcification characteristic of some synovial sarcomas. MRI findings are indeterminate, with intermediate or low signal intensity on T1-weighted images and high signal intensity on T2-weighted images. Axial imaging may show the lesion's potential to invade and destroy adjacent bones or soft tissues, but the tumor may appear well circumscribed. Most lesions present in stage II, which indicates it has spread beyond the compartment of origin. Imaging of regional lymph nodes should be included in the MRI examination.

The overall prognosis of patients with synovial sarcoma is fair. Approximately 50% to 60% of patients will be free of disease at 5-year follow-up.[26] There is an inverse correlation between prognosis and age at presentation. Location of the tumor in the distal lower extremity may be a positive prognostic factor. Negative prognostic factors include large tumor size, high histologic grade, and metastasis at presentation.

Recent data have shown that synovial sarcoma displays two distinct types of chromosomal translocations t(X;18)(p11;q11), named fusion types *SYT-SSX1* and *SYT-SSX2*.[27] The fusion type seems to have a significant impact on the disease course and patient survival. In one study, median and 5-year overall survival rates for the *SYT-SSX1* and *SYT-SSX2* groups were 6.1 years and 53%, and 13.7 years and 73%, respectively.[27] Surgical resection with a wide margin remains the cornerstone of treatment. Both chemotherapy and radiotherapy have a positive effect on patient survival. In one study, 10 of 12 patients who had surgical treatment of synovial sarcoma in the foot required either a below-knee or a Chopart amputation.[26]

Epithelioid Sarcoma

Epithelioid sarcoma is a challenging tumor to treat. Although this sarcoma is generally rare, the most common location is the distal upper and lower extremities. Most patients are young adults, but children are occasionally affected. Men are affected three times as often as women. The tumor can present as a small, firm, superficial or deep nodule or a focal cluster of nodules. Regional multifocal presentation is an unusual characteristic displayed by this tumor. Epithelioid sarcoma is frequently misdiagnosed as a skin condition, warts, or corns. Delay in providing a correct diagnosis may cause serious medical consequences for the patient and legal consequences for the treating physician. Approximately 50% of the tumors are not painful. The tumor grows and spreads along lymph and vascular channels and tendon sheaths, leading to more generalized swelling and a permeative mass.

Contrast-enhanced MRI and positron emission tomography of the entire limb is essential for detecting the complete extent of the disease and locating the frequently occurring local and regional metastases. For surgically controllable disease, surgical removal of the tumor with a wide margin is mandatory. Local and regional metastasis may necessitate amputation. The local recurrence rate is approximately 35% and the rate of distant metastasis is 40%, with the lungs being the most common metastatic site. Metastasis to regional lymph nodes occurs in 25% of patients. Five- and 10-year survival rates are 70% and 42%, respectively.[28]

Malignant Melanoma

Primary cutaneous melanoma is the most common malignant tumor of any type in the foot. The term acral lentiginous melanoma is applied to melanoma affecting the hand or foot. Despite years of research, outcomes for patients with malignant melanoma are poor. Not only does malignant melanoma in the foot have a significantly worse prognosis then melanoma in other body sites, but the prevalence of melanoma is increasing faster than any other type of cancer.

Most patients are young adults; the most frequent age at presentation is the fourth decade of life. Women are often affected, with this cancer presenting a particular risk for young women.[29] This tumor is the most common malignancy in women in the latter part of the second decade of life and is the second most common type of cancer (breast cancer is the most common) in women in the third decade of life. The most common sites of presentation are the plantar surface and subungual regions, but the tumor may occur anywhere on the foot. These lesions are frequently misdiagnosed as benign nevus, subungual hematoma, blisters, pyogenic granuloma, and other dermatologic lesions. The foot and ankle surgeon should be suspicious of pigmented lesions anywhere on the foot or ankle. Patients with suspicious lesions should be promptly referred for appropriate management. Careful documentation and follow-up on all patients referred for potential cancers can increase the chance of early diagnosis and reduce the risk of litigation related to a delayed diagnosis. Melanoma of the foot tends to present at a more advanced stage and at a greater depth than lesions elsewhere in the body. These factors may be related to frequent delays in diagnosing this lesion. Delayed diagnosis of malignant melanoma is associated with a significant negative impact on patient survival.

Based on the staging system of the American Joint Committee on Cancer, stage I and stage II melanoma are localized diseases, stage III indicates lymph node involvement or in-transit or regional metastasis, and stage IV indicates visceral metastasis. Thin lesions are less than 1 mm in thickness, intermediate lesions are up to 4 mm, and thick lesions are more than 4 mm.[29] The thickness of the tumor is the single most important prognostic factor. Surgical removal with a surgical margin of up to 3 cm is recommended based on the thickness of the tumor. Thin lesions are excised with a 1-cm margin, intermediate lesions with a 2-cm margin, and thick lesions with a 3-cm margin. Lesions in the toes are generally treated with amputation. Wide resection with split-thickness skin graft coverage or locoregional flap coverage is necessary for all lesions. Depending on the location and available soft-tissue coverage, amputation may be required. Elective regional lymph node dissection can be combined with surgical removal of the primary tumor. Lymph node dissection is used to stage the disease in thick and intermediate tumors, but its use is controversial in thin tumors and is no longer considered mandatory. Overall patient survival at 5 years is 63% and at 10 years is 51%.[29]

Summary

The distal lower extremity is affected by a unique subset of bone and soft-tissue tumors. A systematic approach to the patient history, physical examination, and imaging studies will allow the orthopaedic surgeon to make the proper choices for managing these tumors. The differentiation of lesions that are probably benign from those that are probably malignant relies mainly on the patient history and plain radiographs for bone tumors and on the examination and the MRI findings for soft-tissue tumors. For benign tumors and nonmetastatic malignant tumors of the foot and ankle, most patients can be restored to full health and mobility following surgical treatment.

Annotated References

1. Pollandt K, Werner M, Delling G: Tumors of the footbones: A report from the Hamburg Bone Tumor Registry. *Z Orthop Ihre Grenzgeb* 2003;141:445-451.

   The authors reviewed 367 tumors and tumorlike lesions in the foot and ankle and reported that 20% of the mass-forming lesions were malignant. In the calcaneus, a solitary bone cyst was the most common lesion. Slightly less than 50% of all lesions were cartilaginous.

2. Jiang ZM, Zhang HZ, Chen JQ, Liu L: Clinicopathologic analysis of 154 cases of tumors and tumor-like lesions in the bones of hands and feet. *Zhonghua Bing Li Xue Za Zhi* 2003;32:417-421.

   Clinical, pathologic, and radiographic features of 154 cases of tumors and tumorlike lesions in the bones of the hands and feet were reviewed. Cartilage lesions accounted for 60% of the lesions. Benign tumors were more prevalent than malignant tumors by a ratio of 20 to 1. The authors reported significant differences between the frequency of tumors occurring in the foot and in other parts of the skeleton.

3. Zeytoonjian T, Mankin HJ, Gebhardt MC, Hornicek FJ: Distal lower extremity sarcomas: Frequency of occurrence and patient survival rate. *Foot Ankle Int* 2004;25:325-330.

   The authors report on 175 sarcomas in the distal lower extremity compared with 2,367 lesions in other parts of the body. Survival rates for patients with sarcoma in the distal lower extremity were significantly better than for sarcoma in other body parts.

4. American Cancer Society Website: What Are the Key Statistics About Soft Tissue Sarcoma? http://www.cancer.org/docroot/CRI/content/CRI_2_4_1X_What_are_the_key_statistics_for_sarcoma_38.asp?sitearea=. Accessed September 2008.

   The American Cancer Society provides a detailed guide to adult soft-tissue cancer.

5. Lodwick GS: A systematic approach to the roentgen diagnosis of bone tumors, in *Tumors of the Bone and Soft Tissue*. Chicago, IL, Year Book Medical Publishers, 1965, pp 49-68.

6. Papp DF, Khanna AJ, McCarthy EF, Carrino JA, Farber AJ, Frassica FJ: Magnetic resonance imaging of soft-tissue tumors: Determinate and indeterminate lesions. *J Bone Joint Surg Am* 2007;89(suppl 3):103-115.

   The authors review the use of MRI for diagnosing soft-tissue tumors. An algorithm is proposed for dividing tumors into determinate and indeterminate lesions based on their appearance on T1-weighted, T2-weighted, and fat-suppressed T2-weighted images. If a diagnosis cannot be determined based on the patient history, the physical examination, and advanced imaging studies, the lesion is considered indeterminate and possibly malignant. A tissue sample must be obtained for diagnosis prior to planning treatment.

7. Gibbs CP, Peabody TD, Mundt AJ, Montag AG, Simon MA: Oncological outcomes of operative treatment of subcutaneous soft-tissue sarcomas of the extremities. *J Bone Joint Surg Am* 1997;79:888-897.

8. Mankin HJ, Mankin CJ, Simon MA: The hazards of the biopsy, revisited: Members of the Musculoskeletal Tumor Society. *J Bone Joint Surg Am* 1996;78:656-663.

9. Wurtz LD, Peabody TD, Simon MA: Delay in the diagnosis and treatment of primary bone sarcoma of the pelvis. *J Bone Joint Surg Am* 1999;81:317-325.

10. Neal RD, Allgar VL: Sociodemographic factors and delays in the diagnosis of six cancers: Analysis of data from the "National Survey of NHS Patients: Cancer." *Br J Cancer* 2005;92:1971-1975.

    Factors associated with diagnostic delays were analyzed for six types of cancer. Female sex; younger age; single, separated, or divorced marital status; lower social class; and minority status were associated with diagnostic delays.

11. Strunk AL, Kenyon S: Medicolegal considerations in the diagnosis of breast cancer. *Obstet Gynecol Clin North Am* 2002;29:43-49.

12. Kern KA: Medicolegal analysis of the delayed diagnosis of cancer in 338 cases in the United States. *Arch Surg* 1994;129:397-403.

13. Ozger H, Eralp L, Türker M, Basaran M: Surgical treatment of malignant tumors of the foot and ankle. *Int J Clin Oncol* 2005;10:127-132.

    Outcomes of surgical treatment for 16 patients with malignancies in the foot are reported. Of 14 patients treated with limb-sparing surgery, fewer than 50% had normal function. In most patients, soft-tissue defects required local and free tissue flaps for coverage.

14. Toma CD, Dominkus M, Pfeiffer M, Giovanoli P, Assadian O, Kotz R: Metatarsal reconstruction with use of free vascularized osteomyocutaneous fibular grafts following resection of malignant tumors of the midfoot: A series of six cases. *J Bone Joint Surg Am* 2007;89:1553-1564.

    The authors report on six patients with primary malignant tumors of the foot who had reconstruction with free vascularized fibula grafts. Five patients had successful limb salvage; all patients required revision surgery.

15. Luna JT, DeGroot H III: Five-year follow-up of structural allograft reconstruction for epithelioid hemangioma of the talus and navicular: A case report and review of the literature. *Foot Ankle Int* 2007;28:379-384.

    The authors review the outcome of a patient with an aggressive benign tumor of the talus that was reconstructed with an allograft and multiple fusions.

16. Johnstone PA, Wexler LH, Venzon DJ, et al: Sarcomas of the hand and foot: Analysis of local control and functional result with combined modality therapy in extremity preservation. *Int J Radiat Oncol Biol Phys* 1994;29:735-745.

17. Mirra JM (ed): *Bone Tumors: Clinical, Radiologic, and Pathologic Correlation*. Philadelphia, PA, Lea & Febiger, 1989, p 482.

18. Temple HT, Mizel MS, Murphey MD, Sweet DE: Osteoblastoma of the foot and ankle. *Foot Ankle Int* 1998;19:698-704.

19. Fink BR, Temple HT, Chiricosta FM, Mizel MS, Murphey MD: Chondroblastoma of the foot. *Foot Ankle Int* 1997;18:236-242.

20. Gajewski DA, Burnette JB, Murphey MD, Temple HT: Differentiating clinical and radiographic features of enchondroma and secondary chondrosarcoma in the foot. *Foot Ankle Int* 2006;27:240-244.

    The authors examined the medical records and radiographs of 48 patients with enchondroma and chondrosarcoma of the foot to identify clinical or radiographic findings that could be helpful in differentiating these two types of tumors. There was a considerable overlap between the two groups, which illustrated the difficulty in reliably diagnosing these tumors without biopsy confirmation.

21. Simon MA, Springfield DS (eds): *Surgery for Bone and Soft-Tissue Tumors*. Philadelphia, PA, Lippincott-Raven Press, 1998, pp 48-53.

22. Adkins CD, Kitaoka HB, Seidl RK, Pritchard DJ: Ewing's sarcoma of the foot. *Clin Orthop Relat Res* 1997; 343:173-182.

23. Krishnamurthy GT, Tubis M, Hiss J, Blahd WH: Distribution pattern of metastatic bone disease: A need for total body skeletal image. *JAMA* 1977;237:2504-2506.

24. Meis-Kindblom JM, Kindblom LG: Acral myxoinflammatory fibroblastic sarcoma: A low-grade tumor of the hands and feet. *Am J Surg Pathol* 1998;22:911-924.

25. Duke WH, Sherrod TT, Lupton GP: Aggressive digital papillary adenocarcinoma (aggressive digital papillary adenoma and adenocarcinoma revisited). *Am J Surg Pathol* 2000;24:775-784.

26. Scully SP, Temple HT, Harrelson JM: Synovial sarcoma of the foot and ankle. *Clin Orthop Relat Res* 1999;364: 220-226.

27. Ladanyi M, Antonescu CR, Leung DH, et al: Impact of SYT-SSX fusion type on the clinical behavior of synovial sarcoma: A multi-institutional retrospective study of 243 patients. *Cancer Res* 2002;62:135-140.

28. Spillane AJ, Thomas JM, Fischer C: Epithelioid sarcoma: The clinicopathological complexities of this rare soft tissue sarcoma. *Ann Surg Oncol* 2000;7:218-225.

29. National Cancer Institute Website. Surveillance epidemiology and end results: Melanoma of the skin. http://seer.cancer.gov/statfacts/html/melan.html. Accessed August 2008.

This Website provides a brief synopsis of cancer facts on melanoma of the skin. An overview of the incidence, mortality, trends in rates of occurrence, survival by stage, lifetime risk, and prevalence data from one of the largest available data sets is presented.

6: Special Problems of the Foot and Ankle

Chapter 28

Nail and Skin Disorders of the Foot and Ankle

Steven B. Weinfeld, MD

Nail Disorders

The nail unit consists of the nail plate, which arises from beneath the proximal nail fold. The eponychium is the skin in the ventral surface of the proximal nail fold. The floor of the proximal nail groove is called the nail matrix. Between the ventral surface of the eponychium and the nail matrix is the nail plate. The lunula is the area where the nail matrix extends beyond the proximal nail fold; the nail bed begins where the nail matrix or lunula ends. The distal phalanx of the toe lies immediately beneath the nail unit. The blood supply to the nail unit arises from the two digital arteries of the toe.

Subungual Hematomas

Subungual hematomas occur between the nail and the nail bed and usually occur secondary to trauma. Laceration to the nail bed and concomitant fracture of the distal phalanx is common. In patients with no traumatic injury to the nail, subungual melanoma should be considered in the differential diagnosis. A melanoma usually forms a band of pigmentation (known as the Hutchinson sign) as the toenail grows. It is often necessary to evacuate the subungual hematoma with a heat cautery. If the nail bed is lacerated, the nail can be elevated from the nail bed, and the laceration can be repaired with 5-0 absorbable suture. A nail bed laceration with an underlying phalangeal fracture should be treated as an open fracture with irrigation and débridement along with the administration of intravenous antibiotics.[1]

Subungual Exostosis

A subungual exostosis is an outgrowth of normal bone beneath the nail bed. Histologically similar to osteochondroma, two distinct types of subungual exostosis have been described. Type I subungual exostosis, which occurs in women ages 20 to 40 years, is an outgrowth on the dorsomedial aspect of the phalanx and tends to disrupt the entire nail plate, causing pain and difficulty with shoe wear. Type II subungual exostosis occurs more frequently in women who are older than those affected by type I exostosis.

On examination, pain with palpation of the distal nail plate is usually present. The diagnosis is confirmed with radiography. Type II lesions often occur on the distal aspect of the hallux and elevate the tip of the nail. Resection of the exostosis can be performed either through an incision in the nail bed or at the tip of the toe. Resection through the nail bed often leads to a nail deformity that may remain painful. Attempting to remove the exostosis through elevation of the nail bed can lead to inadequate resection of the exostosis or perforation of the nail bed, with subsequent recurrence of the exostosis.

Paronychia

Paronychia occurs when the nail plate grows into the surrounding soft tissues, resulting in pain and often infection with the development of a pyogenic granuloma. This condition is most common in men who are ages 20 to 30 years; the hallux is most often affected. Initially, paronychia was believed to be caused by improper nail cutting or shoe wear; however, more recent studies have shown that paronychia is likely caused by congenital abnormalities of the nail plate.[2,3] Nail fold width, medial rotation of the hallux, and nail thickness are associated risk factors for paronychia.

Examination findings include pain with palpation of the nail fold, erythema, edema, and, if persistent, hypertrophy of the nail fold. Purulent discharge may be present with obvious infection. Radiographs may be necessary to rule out osteomyelitis. Untreated paronychial infections can lead to cellulitis of the foot and leg, osteomyelitis of the distal phalanx, or gangrene in patients with peripheral vascular disease. Patients with peripheral neuropathy or vascular disease have an increased risk for complications with paronychial infection.

Partial or total nail avulsion is the preferred treatment for paronychia. The nail avulsion can be accompanied by a partial or total matricectomy, which can be surgical or chemical. A local anesthetic is used when treating an acute paronychial infection; the offending portion of the nail plate is removed using an English nail splitter. The infected material, including a pyogenic granuloma, is débrided. The patient is instructed to soak the toe in warm water several times per day for 3

6: Special Problems of the Foot and Ankle

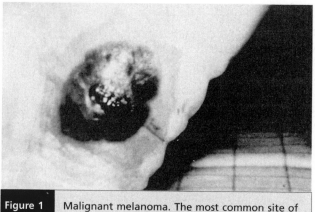

Figure 1   Malignant melanoma. The most common site of foot involvement is on the plantar surface. (Reproduced from Chou LB: Skin and nail disorders, in Mizel MS, Miller RA, Scioli MW (eds): Orthopaedic Knowledge Update: Foot and Ankle 2. Rosemont, IL, American Academy of Orthopaedic Surgeons, 1998, pp 27-38.)

to 5 days. Oral antibiotics are often administered to treat the local cellulitis. A first generation cephalosporin is an excellent antibiotic choice and is taken for 7 to 10 days. For recurrent paronychial infections, a partial or complete matricectomy can be used to prevent future toe infections. With the Winograd method, either the medial or lateral nail plate is removed with subsequent surgical excision of the corresponding nail matrix and nail fold. The skin edges are sutured to the remaining nail plate. This method prevents regrowth of the offending portion of the nail plate.

Other authors have recommended matricectomy using a phenol alcohol combination.[4] The affected portion of the nail plate is removed, an 88% liquid phenol solution is applied to the nail matrix, and the matrix then is curetted. The toe is immediately soaked in saline solution to neutralize the strong phenol solution. This process may be repeated to ensure complete removal of the nail matrix.

Total matricectomy may be performed by either of two methods. In the Zadik method, the entire nail matrix is removed without phalangeal resection. In the terminal Symes method, the distal phalanx is amputated with removal of the nail matrix, nail bed, and medial and lateral nail folds. The most common complications of paronychial surgery are infection, recurrence, delayed healing, incomplete nail matrix removal, nail deformity, and tissue necrosis.[5]

Traumatic Injury

Repeated trauma to the toenails may lead to thickening and deformity of the nail and yellowish discoloration. Subungual hyperkeratosis can develop from nail trauma caused by ill-fitting shoes or repeated striking of the toes against the end of the shoe. Yellow discoloration of the nail with subungual hyperkeratosis is more likely caused by trauma than by fungal infection.

Onychomycosis

Fungal infections of the toenail are extremely common, with up to 20% of the population affected. *Trichophyton rubrum* is the most common fungus to affect the nails, followed by *Trichophyton mentagrophytes*. The yeast, *Candida*, also may affect the toenail. It initially infests the nail folds before attacking the nail plate. Yellowish streaks in the nail plate are seen, usually beginning at the distal end of the plate. With chronic infection, the nail plate thickens and may elevate from the nail bed. *Candida* infection is more common in patients with diabetes. The diagnosis of onychomycosis is made using light microscopy to examine nail scrapings treated with sodium hydroxide. Topical treatments usually do not eradicate the fungus but will soften the nail and facilitate trimming. More recently, systemic treatment, with antifungal agents such as ketoconazole and terbinafine, has proven effective but has produced significant adverse side effects, including liver toxicity and cardiovascular effects.[6,7] Successful treatment of onychomycosis with photodynamic therapy has been reported.[8]

Malignant Melanoma

Malignant melanoma is a tumor of the melanocytes and usually occurs on areas of the body not normally exposed to the sun. The plantar aspect of the foot is the most common site on the foot for malignant melanoma (Figure 1). This tumor also may occur in the nail. The appearance of melanonychia striata is an important criterion for diagnosis; however, up to 20% of subungual melanomas have been reported as amelanotic.[9] Malignant melanoma of the nail is significantly more common in the African American and Asian populations (median patient age, 50 to 60 years at presentation). Several studies have shown that a delayed diagnosis is an important factor in the poor prognosis associated with this lesion.[10] A poor prognosis also is associated with advanced clinical stage, deep invasion, ulceration, and active cell division. Simple nail biopsy is not adequate to confirm the diagnosis; nail matrix tissue also must be sampled.[11] The nail is removed, and the nail bed is biopsied. Surgical treatment of subungual melanoma is controversial, with recommended treatment ranging from wide excision to ray resection. Lymph node dissection also is controversial. Estimated 5-year survival rates have been reported as 26% to 80%; limited resection and preservation of the digit has not affected the survival rates.[12]

Glomus Tumor

This benign lesion usually occurs in the subungual area and presents as a purple nodule measuring only a few millimeters. These lesions are tender to palpation and exhibit hypersensitivity to cold. Treatment is similar to glomus tumor in the finger, with surgical treatment usually providing a cure. The differential diagnoses include hemangioma, neuroma, hemangiopericytoma, and granuloma telangiectaticum.

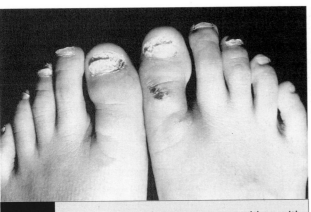

Figure 2 | Psoriasis. Nail involvement can occur with or without skin lesions. This patient shows abnormality of the nail plate with severe thickening. *(Reproduced from Chou LB: Skin and nail disorders, in Mizel MS, Miller RA, Scioli MW (eds): Orthopaedic Knowledge Update: Foot and Ankle 2. Rosemont, IL, American Academy of Orthopaedic Surgeons, 1998, pp 27-38.)*

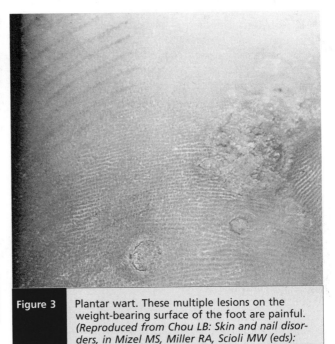

Figure 3 | Plantar wart. These multiple lesions on the weight-bearing surface of the foot are painful. *(Reproduced from Chou LB: Skin and nail disorders, in Mizel MS, Miller RA, Scioli MW (eds): Orthopaedic Knowledge Update: Foot and Ankle 2. Rosemont, IL, American Academy of Orthopaedic Surgeons, 1998, pp 27-38.)*

Psoriasis

Psoriasis is a common skin disease with nail involvement in up to 50% of patients (**Figure 2**). Psoriasis can cause multiple deformities of the toenail, with the most severe form of nail involvement seen in those with psoriatic arthritis. Psoriasis can cause pitting of the nail, onycholysis (separation of the nail plate), crumbling of the nail plate, and subungual keratosis. Multiple forms of treatment have been described, including excision of the nail plate and the use of topical and injected steroids, cyclosporine A, and radiation therapy. Currently there is no standardized therapeutic regimen available for the treatment of psoriasis of the nails.[13]

Contact Dermatitis and Eczema

Contact dermatitis and eczema frequently affect the proximal and lateral nail folds, ultimately causing abnormalities of the nail plate. Transverse ridges and discoloration of the nail plate may develop. Serous fluid may accumulate beneath the nail plate, causing onycholysis. Initial treatment includes identifying the cause of the acute inflammatory process and removing the offending allergen. Effective treatment leads to eventual resolution of the toenail abnormality. Topical steroids may be used.

Infectious Diseases of the Skin

Plantar Warts

Plantar warts are viral tumors caused by a papillomavirus and commonly occur in children and young adults. Multiple plantar warts often appear on the weight-bearing surface of the foot (**Figure 3**). Pinpoint bleeding of the wart when the callus is pared with a knife helps to differentiate these tumors from corns and calluses. There are many treatment options for plantar

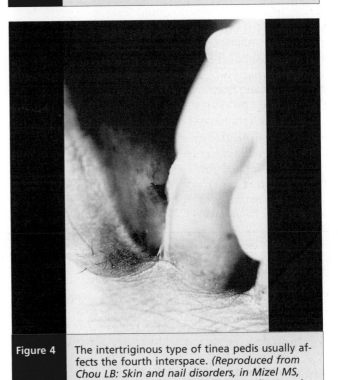

Figure 4 | The intertriginous type of tinea pedis usually affects the fourth interspace. *(Reproduced from Chou LB: Skin and nail disorders, in Mizel MS, Miller RA, Scioli MW (eds): Orthopaedic Knowledge Update: Foot and Ankle 2. Rosemont, IL, American Academy of Orthopaedic Surgeons, 1998, pp 27-38.)*

warts. Nonsurgical treatment includes salicylic acid applied in either liquid form or on a pad in concentrations up to 40%. Acetic acid, lactic acid, cantharidin, and liquid nitrogen also may be used. Orthotics, padding,

6: Special Problems of the Foot and Ankle

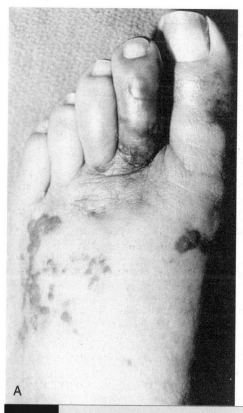 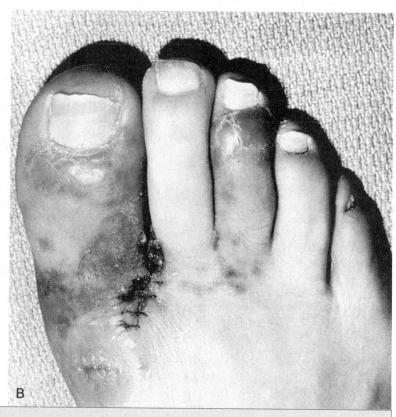

Figure 5 Although Kaposi sarcoma lesions usually occur on the plantar aspect of the foot, they can also involve the dorsum. **A,** The typical appearance of multiple, small, red lesions. **B,** These lesions are purplish, flat, and more diffuse than those in part A. *(Reproduced from Chou LB: Skin and nail disorders, in Mizel MS, Miller RA, Scioli MW (eds): Orthopaedic Knowledge Update: Foot and Ankle 2. Rosemont, IL, American Academy of Orthopaedic Surgeons, 1998, pp 27-38.)*

and shoe wear modification may be helpful in off-loading pressure on the affected areas. Surgical excision is used for painful warts or in those patients in whom nonsurgical treatment was unsuccessful. After infiltration of the area with a local anesthetic, the wart is excised using sharp dissection. A curette may be used to detach the wart from its base. Excision with a laser is an effective method for treating plantar warts.[14]

Fungal Infections
Fungal infections of the foot are commonly referred to as athlete's foot or tinea pedis (**Figure 4**). The most common infecting fungi are *T rubrum* and *T mentagrophytes*. Superinfection may occur with gram-negative bacteria such as *Pseudomonas aeruginosa*. A fungal infection is confirmed by placing scrapings from the foot onto a glass slide with 10% potassium hydroxide and examining the sample with a microscope for the presence of fungi. Fungal cultures also can be grown, with results often taking several weeks. Treatment with topical antifungal creams is usually effective.

Kaposi Sarcoma
Kaposi sarcoma, most often seen in patients with human immunodeficiency virus (HIV) and acquired immunodeficiency syndrome, may present as violaceous patches, plaques, or nodules. These lesions may appear as purplish discolorations of the skin (Figure 5). Kaposi sarcoma may be treated with liquid nitrogen, radiation, and an intralesional injection with vinblastine.[15] Changes in the toenails may occur in patients with HIV. Some medications used to treat HIV can cause discoloration of the nail; onychomycosis is more frequent in the HIV population.

Atopic Dermatitis
Atopic dermatitis presents as scaly, dry, and often pruritic skin on the feet. In children, the soles of the feet are often affected, with the toes specifically affected. These children have a form of atopic dermatitis aggravated by cold, dry weather. Atopic dermatitis should be differentiated from a fungal infection by performing fungal cultures. Steroid creams are often effective in treating this disorder.

Contact Dermatitis
Contact dermatitis of the foot is an inflammation of the skin of the foot in response to contact with an irritant or an allergen. There is a primary irritant dermatitis and allergic dermatitis. Usually, more itching occurs with allergic dermatitis. Both forms of contact dermatitis are treated with wet compresses and topical steroids.

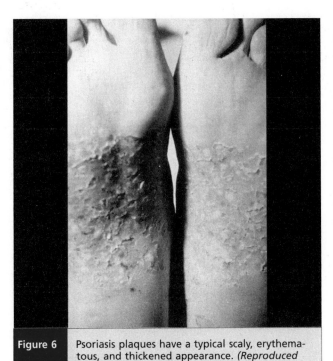

| Figure 6 | Psoriasis plaques have a typical scaly, erythematous, and thickened appearance. *(Reproduced from Chou LB: Skin and nail disorders, in Mizel MS, Miller RA, Scioli MW (eds):* Orthopaedic Knowledge Update: Foot and Ankle 2. *Rosemont, IL, American Academy of Orthopaedic Surgeons, 1998, pp 27-38.)* |

Patients may exhibit allergic contact dermatitis to material in shoe wear. Avoidance of these allergens usually resolves the condition.

Psoriasis

Psoriasis is a common skin disorder that presents with scaly reddish plaques typically seen on the elbows, knees, scalp, and feet (**Figure 6**). Psoriasis can affect any area of the foot, with whitish scales that bleed when stripped off. Psoriasis of the sole of the foot may present as pustular psoriasis or keratoderma climacterium. Pustular psoriasis exhibits sharply outlined areas of redness on the soles of the feet with yellowish pustules. These can be distinguished from a fungal infection with appropriate cultures. Psoriatic arthritis is a disfiguring form of erosive arthritis with a predilection for the distal interphalangeal joints of the foot, although any joint in the foot may be affected. The treatment for pustular psoriasis is incision and drainage of the pustules and application of topical steroids. Ultraviolet light may also be an effective treatment.

Summary

The nails of the foot are affected by many diseases, including paronychial infections, onychomycosis, psoriasis, subungual hematoma, exostoses, and melanoma. Skin disorders of the foot and ankle include fungal infections, psoriasis, dermatitis, plantar warts, and Ka-

posi sarcoma. It is important for the physician to be familiar with these conditions to ensure accurate diagnosis and timely treatment.

Paronychial infections most often require surgical débridement of the nail plate, whereas onychomycosis is effectively treated with oral medication. Patients with malignant melanoma have an excellent survival rate if the diagnosis is made early; surgical treatment is most effective. Kaposi sarcoma may be treated with surgical excision or chemotherapy. Topical antifungals are effective in treating fungal infections of the skin. Psoriasis can be treated with topical steroids and ultraviolet light therapy. Plantar warts require surgical excision. Early diagnosis and treatment of these disorders most often leads to a successful outcome.

Annotated References

1. Kensinger DR, Guille JT, Horn BD, Herman MJ: The stubbed toe: Importance of early recognition and treatment of open fractures of the distal phalanx. *J Pediatr Orthop* 2001;21:31-34.

2. Langford DT, Burke C, Robertson K: Risk factors in onychocryptosis. *Br J Surg* 1989;76:45-48.

3. Heifetz CJ: Ingrown toenail: A clinical study. *Am J Surg* 1937;38:298-315.

4. Gallocher J: The phenol alcohol method of nail matrix sterilization. *N Z Med J* 1977;86:140-141.

5. Boll OF: Surgical correction of ingrowing nails. *J Natl Assoc Chiropodists* 1945;35:7-8.

6. Sigurgeirsson B, Olafsson JH, Stinsson JB, et al: Long-term effectiveness of treatment with terbinafine vs itraconazole in onychomycosis: A 5-year blinded prospective follow-up study. *Arch Dermatol* 2002;138: 353-357.

7. Finch JJ, Warshaw EM: Toenail onychomycosis: Current and future treatment options. *Dermatol Ther* 2007; 20:31-46.
   Treatment of onychomycosis is challenging, with low cure rates and relatively high recurrence rates. The authors review the efficacy of oral, topical, and surgical treatment options. The current treatment of choice for toenail onychomycosis is oral terbinafine because of its high efficacy rate, low relapse rate, and cost effectiveness. Oral itraconazole or fluconazole can be considered for infections caused by *Candida*. Topical therapies may be a useful adjunct to these systemic therapies but are less effective when used alone. More research is needed to determine effective measures to prevent reinfection.

8. Watanabe D, Kawamura C, Masuda Y, et al: Successful treatment of toenail onychomycosis with photodynamic therapy. *Arch Dermatol* 2008;144:19-21.
   The authors describe the use of photodynamic therapy

6: Special Problems of the Foot and Ankle

for treating onychomycosis. This therapy has proven useful in treating a variety of malignant skin tumors and inflammatory diseases. An occlusive dressing with urea ointment was applied to the nail prior to the initiation of the therapy. An irradiation dose of 100 J/cm² was used. Two patients with chronic onychomycosis were successfully treated.

9. Norton LA: Tumors, in Scher R, Daniels CR (eds): *Nails: Therapy, Diagnosis, Surgery*. Philadelphia, PA, WB Saunders, 1990.

10. Dawber RP, Colver GB: The spectrum of malignant melanoma of the nail apparatus. *Semin Dermatol* 1991; 10:82-87.

11. Jellinek N: Nail matrix biopsy of longitudinal melanonychia: Diagnostic algorithm including the matrix shave biopsy. *J Am Acad Dermatol* 2007;56:803-810.

The author describes longitudinal melanonychia, which may represent nail matrix melanocyte activation, benign hyperplasia, or melanoma. An algorithm is provided for treating longitudinal melanonychia that includes a careful patient history, physical examination, dermoscopy, and sampling of the nail matrix using three biopsy techniques. The use of all three techniques allows appropriate sampling of the nail matrix for accurate diagnosis.

12. Moehrle M, Metzger S, Schippert W, et al: Functional surgery in subungual melanoma. *Dermatol Surg* 2003; 29:366-374.

A retrospective review of 62 patients who were surgically treated for stage I and II subungual melanoma is presented. Functional surgery with preservation of the distal phalanx was performed in 31 patients, and traditional surgery with amputation of the distal phalanx was used in 31 patients. No statistically significant differences in disease-free, 5-year survival were reported between the two groups.

13. Jiaravuthisan MM, Sasseville D, Vender RB, et al: Psoriasis of the nail: Anatomy, pathology, clinical presentation, and a review of the literature on therapy. *J Am Acad Dermatol* 2007;57:1-27.

The authors discuss the normal anatomy of the nail unit and the current understanding of psoriasis. An extensive review of the literature on psoriatic nail therapy is presented. There are many treatment options available, but there is an absence of clear evidence favoring one treatment over another. Treatment includes topical, intralesional, radiation, systemic, and combination therapies. The authors conclude that better documented studies are needed to provide a successful approach to treating psoriatic nail disease.

14. Serour F, Somekh E: Successful treatment of recalcitrant warts in pediatric patients with carbon dioxide laser. *Eur J Pediatr Surg* 2003;13:219-223.

The efficacy of the carbon dioxide laser treatment for recalcitrant warts in pediatric patients is evaluated in this study of 40 patients (54 warts). Laser treatment was used with local anesthetic. No curettage was used. Healing time was 4 to 5 weeks. No recurrence of the warts was reported at 12 month follow-up. Hyperpigmentation occurred in 27% of cases.

15. Levi MJ: Classic Kaposi's sarcoma. *J Am Podiatr Med Assoc* 2005;95:586-588.

Kaposi sarcoma usually occurs on the skin of the lower extremity. Lesions increase in size, number, and color over time. Early diagnosis is critical to prevent metastasis to the lungs, liver, and kidneys. Kaposi sarcoma is confirmed by skin biopsy and is treated with local radiation. Successful outcomes have been reported in 73% of patients treated with vinblastine.

Chapter 29

Transtibial Amputation: Traumatic and Dysvascular

CDR John J. Keeling, MD, MC, USN   LTC Scott B. Shawen, MD, MC, USA
LTC Romney C. Andersen, MD, MC, USA

Introduction

Amputation surgery should be viewed by the patient and surgeon as the next step toward reconstructive surgery and recovery. The ultimate goal of amputation is to surgically remove diseased and nonfunctional distal extremity tissues and to fashion a competent and painless residual limb for ambulation. The transtibial (below-knee) amputation level provides acceptable outcomes for patients with a wide range of morbidities.

According to the National Center for Health Statistics, more than 300,000 amputees currently reside in the United States. Peripheral vascular disease has been implicated in at least two thirds of these amputations.[1] The current incidence of more than 100,000 amputations per year will likely increase as obesity and diabetes reach epidemic proportions in the US population, which has a higher number of lower extremity amputations than other developed countries.[2] The effectiveness of prevention strategies for obesity and diabetes should be reevaluated and new strategies explored.[3] The number of wounded personnel surviving current military conflicts also is contributing to the growing number of amputees in the United States.

Historical Perspective

Improvements in prosthetic design were spurred by knowledge gained in treating World War II veterans who required amputation. Those improvements and advancements in surgical amputation techniques have resulted in better care and treatment for current amputees.[4]

In the 1920s, the Ertl technique was introduced as a new approach to transtibial and transfemoral amputation to treat injured Hungarian soldiers.[5] Flexible bone graft and osteomyoplastic flaps were used to enhance the prosthetic endbearing capability of the residual limb. The surgical procedure consisted of using flexible corticoperiosteal flaps harvested after subcorticoperiosteal resection of the osseous stumps to create a bridge of mature bone between the tibia and fibula. It was be-

lieved that this procedure resulted in an improved endbearing residual limb that was likened to the heel of the foot. The approximation of antagonistic muscles and sealing of the intramedullary canal also afforded a more normal physiologic state of the limb and helped prevent muscle atrophy. Although not supported by evidence, there is growing interest in the Ertl bone-bridging technique.

Indications

There are four main categories of morbidity for which lower extremity amputation is widely described. Peripheral vascular disease with or without associated diabetes that leads to dysvascular or infected gangrenous distal extremity tissue is the most common cause of amputation in the United States.[2] Patients with acute, unreconstructable, lower extremity and foot trauma or failed limb-salvage surgeries also should be considered for transtibial amputation. Chronic, unremitting, lower extremity nerve pain following trauma has been successfully treated with transtibial amputation.[6] Congenital deformity and invasive soft-tissue and bone tumors also have been traditionally treated with amputation; however, with newer and more successful limb-sparing procedures, the number of amputations performed for these diagnoses has significantly declined in recent years.[7] Bridge synostosis can be considered as an alternative to traditional amputation techniques in all four types of morbidities and is often necessary in a chronically painful transtibial amputation when there is injury to the intraosseous structures and associated fibular instability.

Contraindications

Regardless of etiology, a dysvascular limb that will not support closure of the transtibial wound should be considered for amputation at a higher level. Wound failure or persistent wound infection also requires revision to a more proximal amputation level. If bridge synostosis will require nonvascularized free osseous transfer to

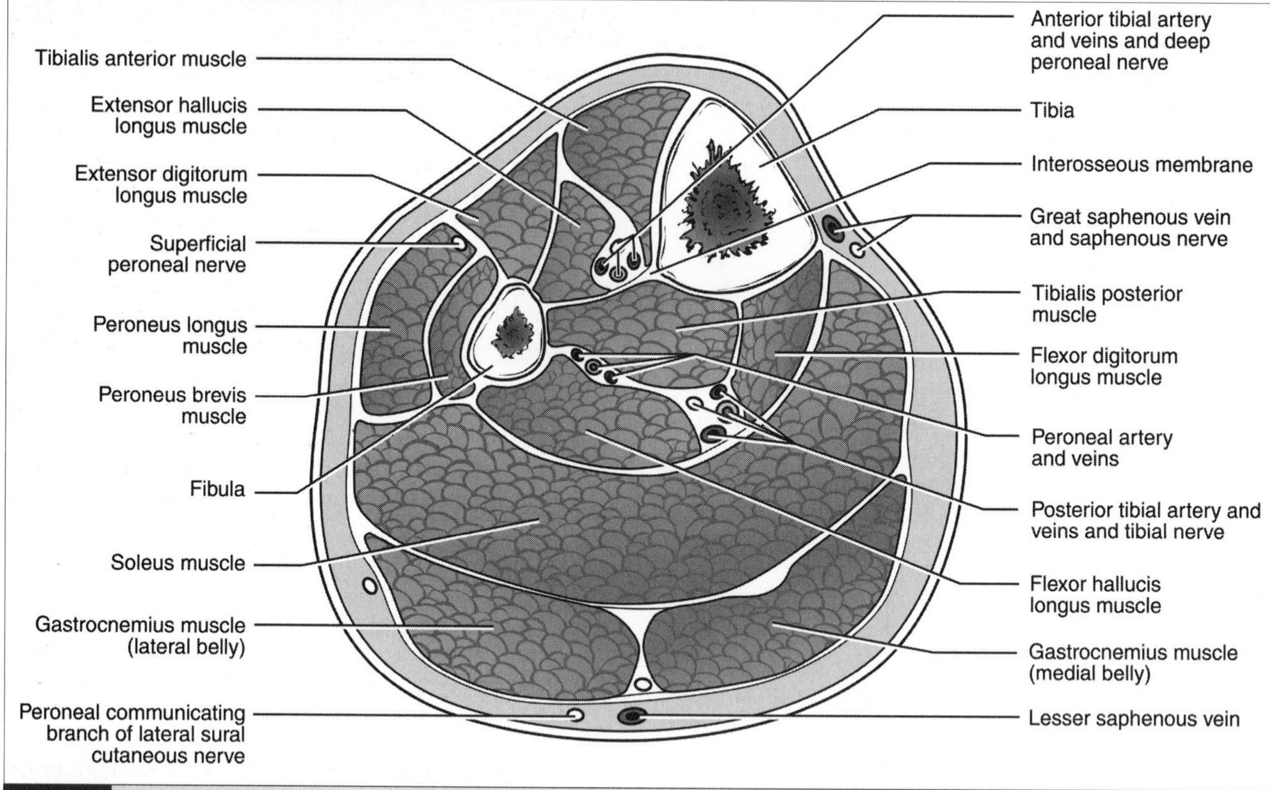
Tibialis anterior muscle
Extensor hallucis longus muscle
Extensor digitorum longus muscle
Superficial peroneal nerve
Peroneus longus muscle
Peroneus brevis muscle
Fibula
Soleus muscle
Gastrocnemius muscle (lateral belly)
Peroneal communicating branch of lateral sural cutaneous nerve
Anterior tibial artery and veins and deep peroneal nerve
Tibia
Interosseous membrane
Great saphenous vein and saphenous nerve
Tibialis posterior muscle
Flexor digitorum longus muscle
Peroneal artery and veins
Posterior tibial artery and veins and tibial nerve
Flexor hallucis longus muscle
Gastrocnemius muscle (medial belly)
Lesser saphenous vein

Figure 1 A cross section of the middle of the leg.

complete the bridge in a potentially contaminated soft-tissue environment, traditional surgery should be performed.

Cross-Sectional Anatomy

It is essential that the surgeon have a firm grasp of the cross-sectional anatomy when performing a transtibial amputation. Anatomic relationships of critical structures in the middle leg should be fully understood and key soft-tissue structures identified for successful surgery (Figure 1). The leg contains four compartments: anterior, lateral, superficial posterior, and deep posterior, each with its own associated muscle groups and neurovascular anatomy.

Because most transtibial amputations are currently performed using a long posterior myocutaneous flap, the gastrocnemius muscle must be identified and protected in the superficial posterior compartment. A recent meta-analysis showed that the choice of amputation skin flap, including skew and sagittal flaps, has not resulted in outcome improvements when compared with posterior myocutaneous flaps.[8] Because the blood supply to the anterolateral and anterior leg is relatively less abundant in ischemic legs, there is reason to use a long posterior myocutaneous flap. The long posterior skin flap is supplied with anastomotic vascularity from perforating vessels originating from the gastrocnemius muscle and runoff from the more proximal genicular branches. The soleus muscle need not be preserved because it usually adds unwanted bulk and supplies no blood to the posterior skin flap. The sural nerve and lesser saphenous vein are located within the posterior adipocutaneous flap. The saphenous nerve and vein also should be isolated along the posteromedial border of the tibia in the adipocutaneous layer.

The deep posterior muscle compartment contains the major vasculature and large tibial nerve. The deep musculature is typically transected at the level of the tibial osteotomy; the posterior tibial artery and veins are located in the intermuscular plane adjacent to the tibialis posterior in the neurovascular sheath. The peroneal artery and veins should be dissected free approximately 2 cm lateral to the tibial nerve.

The anterior compartment musculature also is usually transected at the level of the tibial osteotomy, allowing the creation of an adequate soft-tissue envelope. The anterior tibial artery and associated veins are usually located along the posterolateral border of the tibia at this level, adjacent to the tibialis anterior muscle. The deep peroneal nerve can usually be found in the intermuscular plane or adjacent to the anterior tibial artery, depending on how distally the amputation is performed. Similarly, the superficial peroneal nerve is most often located in the intermuscular plane of the lateral compartment. It typically becomes extrafascial approximately 12 cm proximal to the ankle joint and occasionally can be located outside the muscle compartment.[9] The lateral compartment musculature can be transected at the level of the fibula osteotomy for traditional transtibial amputation; however, if a fibula strut graft is used for a bone-bridging procedure, the peroneus longus and peroneus brevis muscle origins should remain attached to the fibula.

The osseous anatomy is relatively simple to understand; however, it is important to realize that the tibia is a triangular bone in cross section. When considering a distal tibiofibular bone-bridging procedure, it is essential to recognize that the fibula is a posterior structure relative to the tibia. This alignment should be taken into consideration when preparing a fibula osteotomy and tibial bone troughs for seating the fibula strut in the posterolateral tibia.

Preoperative Evaluation

A multidisciplinary team, including the surgeon, internist, prosthetist, physiatrist, psychiatrist, occupational therapist, and physical therapist should work together to counsel the patient on the role of amputation surgery, eventual postoperative rehabilitation, and long-term recovery goals. A team approach has consistently been shown to improve both short- and long-term outcomes.[10] Incorporating peer support groups, job retraining courses, community reintegration programs, and recreational activities improves the patient's quality of life and ability to adjust to the amputation. These concepts have been implemented by the US military and include the creation of amputee Centers of Excellence, which provide a model of interdisciplinary cooperation that effectively maximizes functional improvement for each amputee. **Figure 2** is a flowchart that can be used to guide the treatment of amputees to ensure optimal functional recovery.

The goal of amputation is to provide a more functional and less painful extremity. Emphasis must be placed on the fact that the amputation is a step toward recovery and not a failure of previous interventions.[11] The patient may have difficulty in dealing with the issue of limb loss or may believe that the exhaustive and lengthy attempt at limb salvage was a waste of time (**Figure 3**). To ensure that the patient's decision is informed and accepting, it is often helpful to encourage the patient to discuss the prospect of amputation versus continued attempts at limb salvage with other patients who have confronted these difficult options. Family support and understanding also are paramount in achieving a successful transition to amputation. Psychological counseling for both the patient and family members should be considered during the preoperative and postoperative periods of adjustment.

Dysvascular Amputations

In patients with diabetes, peripheral vascular disease, or both, who are being considered for amputation, a preoperative internal medicine consultation is usually required for optimal treatment. Routine laboratory tests should be performed. Ideally, a serum albumin level greater than 3.5 g/dL and absolute lymphocyte cell count greater than 1.5×10^9/L should be achieved preoperatively to ensure that the patient's nutritional status is adequate for wound healing.[12] Risk factors for mortality associated with lower extremity amputation in patients with peripheral vascular disease include the lack of a previous coronary artery bypass graft, advancing age, transfemoral amputation, and low albumin levels. Factors that increased the 90-day wound complication rate were transtibial amputation, community living (rather than living in a care facility), hematocrit levels greater than 30 mg/dL, and not using a general anesthetic (for example, using spinal or regional anesthesia).[13] Although counterintuitive, an increased hematocrit level is believed to result in vascular congestion because of increased blood viscosity. Dysvascular patients with limited preoperative ambulatory ability; those age 70 years or older; or those with dementia, end-stage renal disease, and advanced coronary artery disease had poor perioperative performance and rarely regained ambulatory ability. These patients are probably best treated in a manner similar to bedridden patients, who traditionally have been managed with a palliative knee disarticulation or transfemoral amputation.[14]

In patients with a preoperative pulse discrepancy, a vascular surgery consultation is necessary to ensure that the limb is adequately vascularized for postoperative recovery. Consideration must be given to a preoperative arteriogram to assess the need for revascularization or angioplasty before surgery. Preoperative pain in the calf (when at rest) and loss of soft tissue from the foot, along with perioperative wound infection, are variables that predict the failure of a transtibial amputation and subsequent transfemoral amputation. These factors should be assessed preoperatively, and the patient should be informed of the risks.[15]

Several studies have attempted to objectively quantify wound healing potential at a particular amputation level. Pressures greater than 70 mm Hg on Doppler ultrasonography are necessary to promote healing.[16] Transcutaneous oxygen pressures also can be measured to predict wound healing potential. This minimally invasive test is inexpensive, can be performed bedside, and is probably the best objective measure of wound healing. Values of 40 mm Hg or greater imply adequate wound-healing potential. A rise in oxygen pressure after oxygen inhalation also is a positive sign of good local tissue perfusion.[17]

Clinically, there is no substitute for a thorough preoperative assessment by a trained surgeon familiar with amputation. Capillary refill, hair growth, and overall

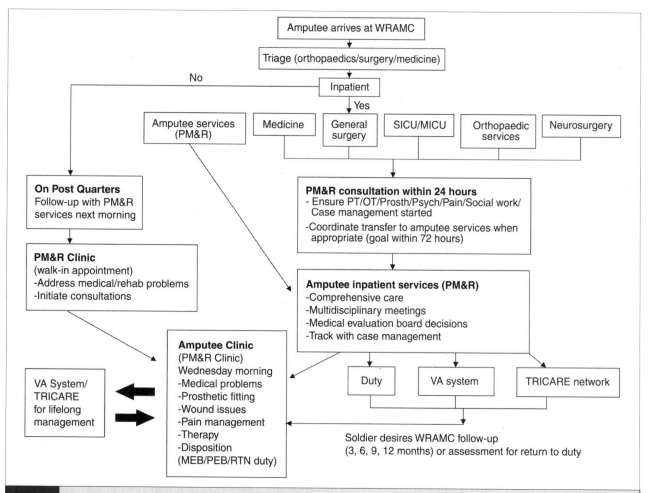

Figure 2   Flowchart of an amputee management protocol used by the US military. WRAMC = Walter Reed Army Medical Center, PM&R = preventive medicine and rehabilitation, PT = physical therapy, OT = occupational therapy, Prosth = prosthetic, Psych = psychological, SICU/MICU = surgical intensive care unit/medical intensive care unit, MEB/PEB/RTN duty = medical evaluation board/physical evaluation board/return to duty. (Adapted with permission from Pasquina PF, Bryant PR, Huang ME, Roberts TL, Nelson VS, Flood KM: Advances in amputee care. Arch Phys Med Rehabil 2006; 87(3 suppl 1):S34-S43.)

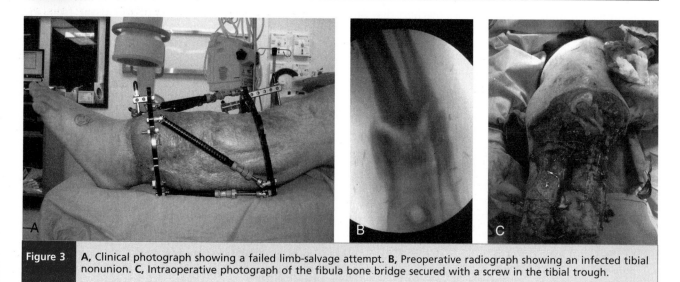

Figure 3   A, Clinical photograph showing a failed limb-salvage attempt. B, Preoperative radiograph showing an infected tibial nonunion. C, Intraoperative photograph of the fibula bone bridge secured with a screw in the tibial trough.

skin hygiene and warmth should be observed and documented. An intraoperative assessment by visualization of healthy bleeding tissue should be the final determinant of the appropriate amputation level.

AP, lateral, and lateral oblique radiographs of the involved extremity should be obtained preoperatively. The lateral oblique radiograph allows assessment of preoperative tibiofibular distance to ensure that this distance remains constant if a bone-bridging procedure is chosen. For suspected infection, supplemental MRI and bone scanning should be performed to ensure that the pathology is well outside the area of amputation reconstruction. In infected or gangrenous distal extremities, a staged procedure should be considered because guillotine ankle amputation followed by delayed definitive closure for the nonsalvageable, infected lower extremity is associated with a significantly lower transtibial amputation failure rate than primary definitive amputation.[18]

Trauma-Related Amputations

Indications

The decision to perform a lower extremity amputation following acute trauma can be extremely challenging because there is typically only a brief period of time to critically assess the extent of injury and make a life-changing decision. For blast-injured military personnel, multiple extremity injuries and associated traumatic brain injury complicate the decision-making process. Absolute indications for amputation of a lower extremity limb after significant trauma include either a crush injury with major arterial injury and warm ischemia for more than 6 hours (which remains the only absolute indication) or complete transection of the sciatic or posterior tibial nerve. Two of three relative indications, including severe associated multiple-trauma, severe ipsilateral foot injury, or a predicted prolonged course to full recovery also suggest that amputation should be considered.[19]

Scoring Systems

Several scoring systems have been developed to assist in determining the potential survivability of a limb after major trauma. Injury severity scoring systems for the lower extremity include the Limb Salvage Index, the Predictive Salvage Index, the NISSSA index (acronym for Nerve injury, Ischemia, Soft-tissue contamination, Skeletal damage, Shock, and Age), the Hannover Fracture Scale-97, and the Mangled Extremity Severity Score (MESS). The most widely accepted scoring system used by orthopaedic surgeons is MESS, which evaluates the bone and soft-tissue injury, warm ischemia time, shock, and the patient's age. Points are assigned in each category depending on the magnitude of the injury. A higher score indicates a worse prognosis for limb salvage. A MESS of 7 to 8 is a relative indication for amputation. Limb reconstruction with a MESS of 9 or more is contraindicated.[20]

More recently, the Lower Extremity Assessment Project (LEAP) study group prospectively evaluated the usefulness of these five scoring systems in predicting which traumatized limbs should be salvaged and which should be amputated.[21] Analysis did not validate the clinical utility of any of the lower extremity injury severity scoring systems. The high specificity of the scores in all of the patient subgroups confirmed that low scores could be used to help predict the potential for limb salvage. However, lower extremity injury severity scores at or above the amputation threshold should be used with caution to decide if amputation is necessary in a patient with a high-energy, lower extremity injury. Based on the LEAP study data, the most important factor affecting a surgeon's decision to amputate rather than to attempt limb salvage was the extent of soft-tissue injury, most notably severe muscle injury and lack of plantar sensation.[22] Subsequently, however, the LEAP study group reported that more than 50% of patients who initially presented with an insensate foot and were treated with limb salvage regained full plantar sensation within 2 years. The group concluded that the lack of plantar sensation at initial presentation should not be a factor in the decision to salvage or amputate an extremity after trauma.[23]

If the clinical situation permits, a preoperative counseling session with the patient and family, information from the scoring systems, and an intraoperative assessment of the osseous and soft-tissue injury performed by one or more surgeons experienced with both limb salvage and amputation should be used to determine the most appropriate treatment for the patient.

Anesthesia and Pain Control

Numerous types of postamputation sensations have been reported; the three main categories include painless phantom limb sensations, phantom limb pain, and stump pain. Phantom limb sensations are defined as painless sensations that are referred to the missing limb; these sensations are estimated to be present in 4% to 20% of congenitally absent limbs and 53% to 100% of traumatically or surgically removed limbs. Sensations of tingling, itching, pins and needles, and numbness can occur that are referred to the missing limb. "Super-added" phenomena, such as the sensation of wearing a ring or sock, may be present. The phantom limb sensations can over time "telescope" in size, leaving a relatively small area of foot and/or digits perceived on the stump. These sensations usually stabilize within the first year following amputation.[24]

Phantom limb pain is nociceptive afferent pain from the amputated limb. The quality of phantom limb pain varies but is generally either a burning or throbbing sensation or an abnormal ischemic discomfort that can range from a mild sensation to excruciating, intolerable pain.[25] Phantom limb pain occurs in 50% to 80% of patients with trauma-related amputations.

Stump pain has a characteristically more dull character and is localized to the amputation site. It has been reported in 6% to 76% of amputees and is not believed to be related to the central neuraxis.[24]

The associations between preamputation pain, acute postamputation pain, and chronic amputation-related pain have been recognized and studied. Patients who have the most intense preamputation pain are most likely to have chronic phantom limb pain 24 months after surgery. Patients who report the most intense acute phantom limb pain are likely to have phantom limb pain at 6 and 12 months after surgery.[26]

These associations have led to an attempt to prevent or reduce the rate and intensity of amputation-related phantom limb pain using preemptive epidural treatments, early regional nerve blocks, and stimulatory techniques. A recent meta-analysis examined 12 clinical trials that included 375 patients with follow-ups ranging from 1 week to 2 years.[27] Three trials showed a positive impact of intervention on phantom limb pain, but the remainder showed no difference between the treated groups and control groups. Although not fully supported by controlled trials, many centers continue to use preemptive epidural and early regional nerve block techniques.

Current anesthesia guidelines continue to focus on methods to prevent central neuroplastic changes from occurring by using preventive, multimodal, analgesic techniques. The rationale for this strategy is the achievement of sufficient analgesia based on the additive and synergistic effects of different analgesics. Effective multimodal analgesic techniques include the use of nonsteroidal anti-inflammatory drugs, local anesthetics (nerve sheath injections), alpha-2 agonists, ketamine, alpha(2)-delta ligands, and opioids.[28] Several other centrally acting agents, including gabapentin, pregabalin, amitriptyline, and tramadol, all have shown a positive effect on reducing amputation-related phantom limb pain in the short term.[29,30] Future improvements in pain control may include mirror feedback therapy and perineural injections of substances to prevent local cytokine-induced sensory excitation.[31,32]

Surgical Techniques

A pneumatic tourniquet reduces blood loss and transfusion requirements during transtibial amputation and may have the added benefit of reducing the revision rate by providing better hemostasis and easier visualization, even in patients with dysvascular disease.[33,34] An assessment of perfusion should be performed without the tourniquet inflated at least once before definitive closure to ensure adequate bleeding tissue and hemostasis. An increase in tourniquet time of approximately 43 minutes is associated with use of the bone-bridging amputation technique; however, the additional surgical time has not been predictive of increased perioperative complications when compared with non–bone-bridging techniques.[35]

Preoperative prophylactic antibiotics should be administered. Antibiotic selection should include standard perioperative prophylaxis for patients who do not have an infection. For amputations associated with infection, the use of culture-specific antibiotics is warranted, and consultation with an infectious-disease specialist should be considered. Recent evidence shows a significantly lower risk of wound complications and infection in dysvascular patients treated with 5 days of prophylactic postoperative antibiotic therapy compared with standard perioperative dosing regimens.[36]

In patients with a traumatic injury, a preoperative plan for expected soft-tissue closure should be formulated that uses well-vascularized and noncontaminated muscle and skin flaps extending beyond the level of bony amputation, known as "flaps of opportunity." Because preservation of knee joint function is paramount, an attempt to salvage the limb at the transtibial level is warranted, with the use of skin grafts for local soft-tissue coverage. Skin grafts do not withstand shear forces after prosthetic fitting; therefore, a plan for later tissue expansion and eventual coverage with native skin is usually necessary.[37,38] Additional challenges in closing traumatic wounds have been reported by military centers that treat blast victims. A wound complication rate of almost 67% has been reported for amputation closure within the zone of injury.[35] Approximately 63% of blast-related amputations are complicated by heterotopic ossification, which most closely correlates with closure through the zone of injury.[39] For amputations with adequate uninjured distal soft tissue, a long posterior myocutaneous flap will off-load the suture line anteriorly and is beneficial for fitting the prosthesis.[40]

For determining the appropriate residual limb length for the patient's stature, a guideline of 2.5 cm for each 30 cm of height is useful. Typically, the final tibia length for nonischemic limbs is 12.5 to 17.5 cm below the tibiofemoral joint line. In a patient with dysvascular disease, a shorter stump to aid wound healing may be considered and weighed against the benefits of a longer more functional residual limb.[11] Preserving limb length improves energy expenditure[41,42] (Table 1). The maximum length of the residual limb after a transtibial amputation is limited by the length necessary for fitting the pylon and prosthesis. Most amputees adjust their self-selected walking speed to offset the increased energy expenditure.

For a non–bone-bridging amputation, the fibula is usually osteotomized no more than 1 cm proximal to the tibia. The anterior third of the tibia should be beveled at 30° to prevent a bony prominence postoperatively.[2] For bone-bridging procedures, several modifications of the original Ertl technique can be performed to create a bone bridge between the tibia and fibula with either a fibula strut graft or periosteal sleeve.[5,43-45]

A systematic anatomic dissection is performed to isolate each named peripheral nerve. It is crucial to identify each nerve to prevent the formation of a painful postoperative neuroma. Each nerve is gently grasped but not clamped, pulled distally, transected as proximally as possible with a sharp scalpel, and allowed to retract into the deep soft-tissue cushion.[46] Local perineural injection of lidocaine may provide additional multimodal anesthetic at this point in the procedure.[28] Current research is attempting to verify the effectiveness of targeted reinnervation. This process involves rerouting the peripheral nerves to a functional muscle motor end plate to prevent postoperative neuroma formation. The large named arteries and their associated veins also should be individually identified and clamped proximal to the wound. Each should be separately double-suture ligated.

The long posterior flap can then be brought anteriorly and fashioned with sharp transection of muscle and skin to the desired length for a tension-free closure without excessive redundancy (**Figure 4**). Care should be taken to provide adequate muscle bulk overlying the anterior distal tibia to allow cushioning for weight bearing. The posterior gastrocnemius muscle fascia should be securely attached to the tibia (via drill holes) or the anterior periosteum and anterior compartment fascia to provide adequate soft tissue for cushioning the terminal amputation stump and preventing soft-tissue retraction. Other factors that can influence the choice of closure techniques include the surgeon's previous experience with a particular technique, the extent of nonviable tissue, and the location of preexisting surgical scars.[8] Myodesis of the muscle through bone holes in the tibia prevents retraction and muscle atrophy.[40]

Postoperative Recovery

Care of the Residual Limb

Compression of the residual limb is important in the postoperative period because it helps to control swelling, which minimizes postoperative pain and promotes a stable limb volume. Support of tissues also is impor-

tant because the muscle and skin flaps need a tension-free environment for optimal healing. Sutures are removed when the wounds are healed (usually 2 to 3 weeks). The incision should be kept dry until all signs of eschar along the incision have healed. Wound care is dependent on the condition of the tissues at the level of the amputation.[47] If infection is a concern at the level of the amputation, more frequent dressing changes may be necessary.

A rigid dressing in the form of a splint or cast is the gold standard after transtibial amputation.[48] Theoretically, injured tissues heal more consistently and with less pain when at rest. Rigid immobilization also has the added benefit of preventing knee flexion contractures.[2] Extra padding should be placed over the patella when placing a rigid dressing for a transtibial amputation to prevent skin irritation and pressure. The distal

Table 1

Energy Expenditure in Amputees

Amputation Level	Energy Above Baseline, %	Speed, m/min	Oxygen Cost, mL/kg/m
Long transtibial	10	70	0.17
Average transtibial	25	60	0.20
Short transtibial	40	50	0.20
Bilateral transtibial	41	50	0.20
Transfemoral	65	40	0.28
Wheelchair	0-8	70	0.16

(Reproduced with permission from Ertl JP, Ertl W, Pritchett JW: Amputations of the lower extremity. http://www.emedicine.com/orthoped/topic9.htm. Accessed May 2007.)

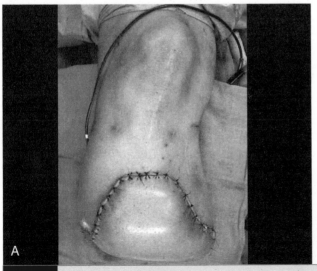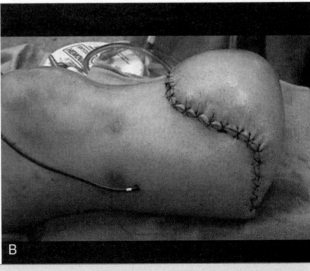

| **Figure 4** | AP **(A)** and lateral **(B)** views of an extended long posterior myocutaneous flap. *(Reproduced with permission from Pinzur MS, Gottschalk FA, Pinto MA, Smith DG: Controversies in lower extremity amputation. Instr Course Lect 2008;57:663-672.)* |

6: Special Problems of the Foot and Ankle

end should be well padded to maintain distal pressure using closed-cell foam or a similar material. A supracondylar mold helps to maintain the dressing in place, avoiding distal migration. With loss of distal pressure, terminal edema can occur, possibly leading to severe wound complications.

The most common dressing, but not necessarily most effective, is a soft dressing.[49] Often first applied in the operating room, it provides a sterile dressing and is covered by an elastic bandage. The elastic bandage is classically applied in the figure-of-8 pattern. This type of dressing, with modifications, can be applied to any residual limb. Careful application is necessary to avoid overcompression or possibly the creation of a tourniquet effect above the amputation as the patient flexes and extends the joint.

A prefabricated, immediate postoperative prosthesis (IPOP) and early weight bearing is an advantageous postoperative management strategy. In one study, 31 transtibial amputees treated with a prefabricated IPOP and early weight bearing were prospectively evaluated and compared with a matched control group of 23 transtibial amputees treated with soft dressings and no weight bearing on the residual limb.[50] Patients in the IPOP group had significantly fewer postoperative complications, required fewer revisions, and had a shorter time interval to their first custom prosthetic fitting than did those in the control group.

A shrinker sock provides transition to the fitting of the prosthesis. The timing of its application varies between surgeons from as early as 5 days following surgery (if the incision and wounds allow) to weeks later if a rigid dressing or IPOP is used. The sock should be worn at all times except during bathing and dressing changes because the sock helps to reduce the volume of the residual limb, shape it, and prepare it for the prosthetic fitting.

Prosthetic Fitting

The prosthetic fitting is initiated after the incisions and wounds have healed and the volume of the residual limb has stabilized. A thorough evaluation is necessary to determine the type of liner, socket, and prosthetic components that will be used. The patient's expected activity level (not necessarily dependent on age), geographic location, time since amputation (state of soft tissues), medical condition, employment, condition of the residual limb, and range of motion and condition of the knee joint should be considered. Each factor plays a role in deciding what type of liner, socket, and prosthesis will best suit the patient.[51]

The basic types of socket designs are total surface-bearing and hydrostatic socket designs. Each type should place some pressure on all areas of the residual limb to prevent distal edema. If all of the weight is supported proximally with the distal portion open, as was the situation with older socket designs, distal edema results.

The selection of foot and linkage designs has continued to expand. The type of pylon, the alignment and length of the toe lever arm, flexibility of the heel, softness of the heel cushion, and fit within the shoe should be considered. Alignment of the prosthesis and foot can have a significant effect on the overall outcome of the amputation. One of the most important aspects of rehabilitation is the patient's ability to consult with a prosthetist for modifications needed to ensure proper fit and pressure relief. Standing, weight-bearing radiographs taken with the patient wearing the prosthesis and gait analysis can help in evaluating and resolving issues related to the fit of the prosthesis. A prosthesis that causes pain will not be used by the patient.[51]

Outcomes and Complications

Dysvascular Amputation

Although technical advances in prosthetic design and rehabilitation protocols have improved outcomes, there is concern regarding several aspects of amputee care and recovery. The authors of a 2006 study retrospectively assessed the survival rates of dysvascular lower limb amputees and reported that significant mortality accompanies dysvascular amputation in the short term (median survival, 4 years), which was similar to outcomes in previously published studies.[52] Diabetic patients had a poorer survival prognosis and a 46% complication rate for stump wound healing.

Another study confirmed the high rate of morbidity and mortality associated with transfemoral and transtibial amputation in diabetic patients.[53] Median survival was significantly less after transfemoral amputation (20 months) than after transtibial amputation (52 months). Diabetes was a significant predictor of 10-year mortality. A history of renal insufficiency also portends a poor outcome. Transfemoral amputation should be considered high-risk surgery, whereas transtibial amputation is intermediate-risk surgery because patients selected for transtibial amputation generally have better preoperative health. Patients with transtibial amputations infrequently require revision or conversion to a transfemoral amputation. It is estimated that approximately 90% of transtibial amputees will eventually obtain adequate ambulatory function, whereas approximately 25% of transfemoral amputees become ambulatory.[54]

An analysis of prognostic factors for locomotion in patients after transtibial amputation showed that early prosthesis fitting and rehabilitation results in a more than fourfold increase in achieving very good or good locomotion and shortens the time needed to reach this goal by twofold.[55]

Trauma-Related Amputation

The LEAP study group examined functional outcomes following trauma-related lower extremity amputations and compared outcomes based on the amputation level.[56] The Sickness Impact Profile showed no significant difference in scores between patients treated with transfemoral amputation and those treated with transtibial amputation. Patients with a transtibial amputation performed better than patients with a transfemoral amputation on the timed test for walking speed. Severe disability often accompanies above-the-ankle lower extremity amputations following trauma, regardless of the amputation level. The LEAP study group subsequently reported on longer term follow-up of patients managed with amputation compared with patients who had undergone limb-salvage surgery. They found that reconstruction for below-knee injuries resulted in functional outcomes equivalent to those of amputation. Regardless of the treatment option, long-term functional outcomes were poor. Patient characteristics significantly associated with poorer outcomes included older age, female gender, nonwhite race, lower educational level, living in a poor household, current or previous smoking, low self-efficacy, poor self-reported health status before the injury, and involvement with the legal system in an effort to obtain disability payments.[57]

High-functioning posttraumatic amputees also have perceived physical limitations and pain. A retrospective review of patients treated with transtibial amputation during a 7-year period at one institution found that Medical Outcomes Study 36-Item Short Form health status scores were significantly lower than published scores for a normal age-matched group in the categories of physical function and role limitations caused by physical health problems and pain.[58] Similarly, another study reported that the largest differences were found in scales sensitive to physical health when comparing war-injured soldiers with unilateral transtibial amputations and a group of uninjured age-matched controls.[59] Higher levels of amputation and complications involving the stump and sound leg had a significant association with poor physical and mental health scores.

One retrospective study evaluated patients with posttraumatic lower extremity injuries with unremitting nerve pain who were treated with transtibial amputation.[6] Twenty patients met the inclusion criteria, which included intractable foot or ankle pain, continued pain after maximal medical therapy, failure of prior surgical reconstruction, and a minimum follow-up period of 24 months after the transtibial amputation. Results showed that 10 patients discontinued the use of narcotics, and 7 decreased the level and/or dosage of pain medicine after the amputation. Three patients worked before the amputation, and eight worked after the amputation. Transtibial amputation can be considered a salvage procedure for intractable foot and ankle pain that is unresponsive to medical and local surgical reconstructive techniques.

Bridge Synostosis

In a 28-year follow-up study of 72 Vietnam War veterans with trauma-related amputations, isolated transtibial amputees and transtibial amputees with other injuries were assessed to ascertain overall well-being and family situation; patients completed the Medical Outcomes Study 36-Item Short Form.[60] An increased need for psychological care and more significant long-term consequences for patients with additional injuries was reported. In a comparison of 42 amputees treated with bone-bridge synostosis compared with 30 patients with traditional transtibial amputations, no significant differences were found between the two groups.

Another study reported on the results at 5-year follow-up of 155 soldiers treated with bone-bridge synostosis.[61] Most patients required stump revision after open guillotine amputation. Autologous bone graft was used for 38 patients. Postoperative infection occurred in 15 patients but compromised the formation of the terminal synostosis in 4 patients. All amputees achieved prosthetic usage.

Researchers reported on 143 patients with 150 symptomatic transtibial amputations that required revision.[42] More than 92% of patients reported good or excellent outcomes. Primary amputations in the group were trauma related in 63% of patients, related to vascular disease in 28%, infection in 7%, and tumor in 2%. Poor results were reported in dysvascular amputees who had persistent postoperative residual extremity pain.

In a study of 15 amputees treated with transtibial amputations with a fibular segment in place of tibial osteoperiosteal flaps, 5 patients required revision amputations.[45] Four patients had diabetes. All patients produced a solid synostosis clinically within 8 to 10 weeks and were rehabilitated with the use of prostheses. Complications included a fibula bone bridge dislocation caused by a fall 2 days after surgery, which required revision, and wound dehiscence in a diabetic patient requiring 6 months of local wound care to close.

Thirty-two patients of varying ages with multiple diagnoses who had bone bridging of the distal tibia and fibula at the time of transtibial amputation were compared with a selected group of 17 highly functioning amputees who had been treated with a traditional transtibial amputation.[62] The group treated with the bone-bridging technique had better or comparable scores on the Prosthetics Evaluation Questionnaire than the amputees treated with a traditional transtibial amputation. This study suggests that bone bridging at the time of transtibial amputation may enhance the patient's perceived functional outcome.

Summary

Transtibial amputation continues to provide adequate outcomes for a wide range of morbidities. Although recent advances in technique and prosthetic design have improved outcomes and comfort, even high-functioning amputees may have significant, persistent pain and health-related complications. These issues are compounded when associated with contralateral limb deficiencies or medical comorbidities. An interdisciplinary

6: Special Problems of the Foot and Ankle

team approach to amputee management is important for successful outcomes and should include job retraining, social reintegration, and establishing a social network for amputees.

Bone-bridge synostosis seems to offer benefits that optimize functional prosthetic use. Research is needed to achieve better pain control and prevent chronic pain in residual limbs. Randomized, controlled, prospective outcomes studies are needed to identify optimal surgical techniques, prosthetic designs, and functional rehabilitation strategies for amputees.

The views expressed in this article are those of the authors and do not reflect the official policy or position of the Department of the Navy, Department of the Army, Department of Defense, or the US government.

Annotated References

1. Russell JN, Hendershot GE, LeClaire F, Howie J, Adler M: Trends and differential use of assistive technology devices: United States, 1994. http://www.cdc.gov/nchs/data/ad/ad292.pdf. Accessed July 23, 2008.

2. Smith DG, Fergason JR: Transtibial amputations. *Clin Orthop Relat Res* 1999;361:108-115.

3. Renzi R, Unwin N, Jubelirer R, Haag L: An international comparison of lower extremity amputations. *Ann Vasc Surg* 2006;20:346-350.

   Amputation rates in 12 US counties distributed throughout the country was compared with the amputation rate in counties in other countries. Results showed that the United States has a higher number of amputations. Level of evidence: IV.

4. Hoaglund FT, Jergensen HE, Wilson L, Lamoreux LW, Roberts R: Evaluation of problems and needs of veteran lower-extremity amputees in the San Francisco Bay area during the period 1977-1980. *J Rehabil R D* 1983;20:57-71.

5. Ertl J: Uber amputationsstumpfe. *Chirurg* 1949;20:218-224.

6. Honkamp N, Amendola A, Hurwitz S, et al: Retrospective review of eighteen patients who underwent transtibial amputation for intractable pain. *J Bone Joint Surg Am* 2001;83:1479-1483.

7. Dillingham TR, Pezzin LE, MacKenzie EJ: Limb amputation and limb deficiency: Epidemiology and recent trends in the United States. *South Med J* 2002;95:875-883.

8. Tisi PV, Callum MJ: Type of incision for below knee amputation. *Cochrane Database Syst Rev* 2004;1:CD003749.

9. Blair JM, Botte MJ: Surgical anatomy of the superficial peroneal nerve in the ankle and foot. *Clin Orthop Relat Res* 1994;305:229-238.

10. Pasquina PF, Bryant PR, Huang ME, Roberts TL, Nelson VS, Flood KM: Advances in amputee care. *Arch Phys Med Rehabil* 2006;87(suppl 1):S34-S43.

    This focused review article describes the key elements of a successful comprehensive amputee program. Level of evidence: V.

11. Burgess EM, Matsen FA III: Determining amputation levels in peripheral vascular disease. *J Bone Joint Surg Am* 1981;63:1493-1497.

12. Dickhaut SC, DeLee JC, Page CP: Nutritional status: Importance in predicting wound-healing after amputation. *J Bone Joint Surg Am* 1984;66:71-75.

13. Stone PA, Flaherty SK, Aburahma AF, et al: Factors affecting perioperative mortality and wound-related complications following major lower extremity amputations. *Ann Vasc Surg* 2006;20:209-216.

    A retrospective review was conducted of all adult patients who underwent nontraumatic major lower extremity amputations over a 5-year period at a single tertiary-care center in southern West Virginia to determine factors that affect mortality and wound-related complications. Level of evidence: IV.

14. Taylor SM, Kalbaugh CA, Blackhurst DW, et al: Preoperative clinical factors predict postoperative functional outcomes after major lower limb amputation: An analysis of 553 consecutive patients. *J Vasc Surg* 2005;42:227-235.

    An investigation of the relationship between a variety of preoperative clinical characteristics and postoperative functional outcomes was performed to formulate treatment recommendations for patients requiring major dysvascular lower limb amputation. Level of evidence: IV.

15. Yip VS, Teo NB, Johnstone R, et al: An analysis of risk factors associated with failure of below knee amputations. *World J Surg* 2006;30:1081-1087.

    The authors present the results of a retrospective review of 47 patients to identify risk factors associated with failure of transtibial amputations. Level of evidence: IV.

16. Barnes RW, Shanik GD, Slaymaker EE: An index of healing in below-knee amputation: Leg blood pressure by Doppler ultrasound. *Surgery* 1976;79:13-20.

17. Burgess EM, Matsen FA III, Wyss CR, et al: Segmental transcutaneous measurements of PO_2 in patients requiring below-the-knee amputation for peripheral vascular insufficiency. *J Bone Joint Surg Am* 1982;64:378-382.

Evidence suggests that the choice of amputation technique has no effect on outcome. The surgeon's previous experience with a particular technique, the extent of nonviable tissue, and the location of preexisting surgical scars may influence the choice of technique. Level of evidence: II.

18. McIntyre KE Jr, Bailey SA, Malone JM, Goldstone J: Guillotine amputation in the treatment of nonsalvageable lower-extremity infections. *Arch Surg* 1984;119: 450-453.

19. Lange RH, Bach AW, Hansen ST Jr, Johansen KH: Open tibial fractures with associated vascular injuries: Prognosis for limb salvage. *J Trauma* 1985;25:203-208.

20. Helfet DL, Howey T, Sanders R, Johansen K: Limb salvage versus amputation: Preliminary results of the Mangled Extremity Severity Score. *Clin Orthop Relat Res* 1990;256:80-86.

21. Bosse MJ, MacKenzie EJ, Kellam JF, et al: A prospective evaluation of the clinical utility of the lower-extremity injury-severity scores. *J Bone Joint Surg Am* 2001;83-A:3-14.

22. MacKenzie EJ, Bosse MJ, Kellam JF, et al: Factors influencing the decision to amputate or reconstruct after high-energy lower extremity trauma. *J Trauma* 2002;52: 641-649.

23. Bosse MJ, McCarthy ML, Jones AL, et al: The insensate foot following severe lower extremity trauma: An indication for amputation? *J Bone Joint Surg Am* 2005;87: 2601-2608.

   The authors present a retrospective review of the outcomes of a subset of 55 patients with an insensate extremity at the time of presentation for treatment. Level of evidence: IV.

24. Richardson C, Glenn S, Nurmikko T, Horgan M: Incidence of phantom phenomena including phantom limb pain 6 months after major lower limb amputation in patients with peripheral vascular disease. *Clin J Pain* 2006;22:353-358.

   Fifty-two patients treated with amputation of a lower limb because of peripheral vascular disease were evaluated at 6-month follow-up to determine the incidence of phantom limb pain and other associated postamputation phenomena. Pain and coping style were the primary outcome measures. Level of evidence: IV.

25. Danshaw CB: An anesthetic approach to amputation and pain syndromes. *Phys Med Rehabil Clin N Am* 2000;11:553-557.

26. Hanley MA, Jensen MP, Smith DG, Ehde DM, Edwards WT, Robinson LR: Preamputation pain and acute pain predict chronic pain after lower extremity amputation. *J Pain* 2007;8:102-109.

   This prospective study examined the associations of preamputation pain and acute postamputation pain with chronic amputation-related pain. Level of evidence: IV.

27. Halbert J, Crotty M, Cameron ID: Evidence for the optimal management of acute and chronic phantom pain: A systematic review. *Clin J Pain* 2002;18:84-92.

28. Reuben SS, Buvanendran A: Preventing the development of chronic pain after orthopaedic surgery with preventive multimodal analgesic techniques. *J Bone Joint Surg Am* 2007;89:1343-1358.

   The results of this study provide a rational approach to using preventive multimodal analgesic techniques after orthopaedic surgery. Level of evidence: V.

29. Wilder-Smith CH, Hill LT, Laurent S: Postamputation pain and sensory changes in treatment-naive patients: Characteristics and responses to treatment with tramadol, amitriptyline, and placebo. *Anesthesiology* 2005; 103:619-628.

   Ninety-four treatment-naive posttraumatic limb amputees with phantom pain were randomly assigned to receive individually titrated doses of tramadol, placebo, or amitriptyline for 1 month. Amitriptyline and tramadol provided excellent control for phantom limb and stump pain with no major adverse events. Level of evidence: I.

30. Bone M, Critchley P, Buggy DJ: Gabapentin in postamputation phantom limb pain: A randomized, double-blind, placebo-controlled, cross-over study. *Reg Anesth Pain Med* 2002;27:481-486.

31. Chan BL, Witt R, Charrow AP, et al: Mirror therapy for phantom limb pain. *N Engl J Med* 2007;357:2206-2207.

   The authors present the results of a comparative analysis investigating the use of mirror feedback therapy to control postoperative phantom limb pain.

32. Dahl E, Cohen SP: Perineural injection of etanercept as a treatment for postamputation pain. *Clin J Pain* 2008; 24:172-175.

   The authors report on use of perineural etanercept in six traumatic amputees with postamputation pain. Level of evidence: IV.

33. Choksy SA, Lee Chong P, Smith C, Ireland M, Beard J: A randomised controlled trial of the use of a tourniquet to reduce blood loss during transtibial amputation for peripheral arterial disease. *Eur J Vasc Endovasc Surg* 2006;31:646-650.

   Sixty-four patients undergoing transtibial amputation for nonreconstructible peripheral artery disease were randomized to either tourniquet or no tourniquet use during surgery. The use of a tourniquet reduced blood loss and the need for transfusion. Level of evidence: I.

34. Wolthuis AM, Whitehead E, Ridler BM, Cowan AR, Campbell WB, Thompson JF: Use of a pneumatic tourniquet improves outcome following trans-tibial amputation. *Eur J Vasc Endovasc Surg* 2006;31:642-645.

   The authors of a prospective, nonrandomized study of 89 adult patients who underwent transtibial amputation with or without the use of a tourniquet reported that pneumatic tourniquet use was safe and significantly reduced blood loss and the need for transfusion during transtibial amputation. Level of evidence: II.

35. Gwinn DE, Keeling JJ, Froehner JA, McGuigan FX, Andersen RC: Perioperative differences between bone-bridging and non-bone-bridging transtibial amputations for wartime lower extremity trauma. *Foot Ankle Int* 2008;29:787-793.

6: Special Problems of the Foot and Ankle

36. Sadat U, Chaudhuri A, Hayes PD, Gaunt ME, Boyle JR, Varty K: Five day antibiotic prophylaxis for major lower limb amputation reduces wound infection rates and the length of in-hospital stay. *Eur J Vasc Endovasc Surg* 2008;35:75-78.

The outcomes of a consecutive series of 40 major lower limb amputations in patients receiving a short (24-hour) course of combined prophylactic antibiotics were retrospectively analyzed and compared with a consecutive group of 40 major lower limb amputations treated with a 5-day course of combined antibiotic therapy. The 5-day regimen appeared to reduce stump infection rates, leading to shorter in-hospital stays. Level of evidence: III.

37. Anderson WD, Stewart KJ, Wilson Y, Quaba AA: Skin grafts for the salvage of degloved below-knee amputation stumps. *Br J Plast Surg* 2002;55:320-323.

38. Watier E, Georgieu N, Manise O, Husson JL, Pailheret JP: Use of tissue expansion in revision of unhealed below-knee amputation stumps. *Scand J Plast Reconstr Surg Hand Surg* 2001;35:193-196.

39. Potter BK, Burns TC, Lacap AP, Granville RR, Gajewski DA: Heterotopic ossification following traumatic and combat-related amputations: Prevalence, risk factors, and preliminary results of excision. *J Bone Joint Surg Am* 2007;89:476-486.

The authors evaluated 330 patients with 373 traumatic and combat-related amputations. Patients were reviewed for complications associated with heterotopic bone formation. Level of evidence: IV.

40. Pinzur MS, Gottschalk FA, Pinto MA, Smith DG, American Academy of Orthopaedic Surgeons: Controversies in lower-extremity amputation. *J Bone Joint Surg Am* 2007;89:1118-1127.

The American Academy of Orthopaedic Surgeons current concepts review of amputation controversies is presented. Level of evidence: IV.

41. Waters RL, Perry J, Antonelli D, Hislop H: Energy cost of walking of amputees: The influence of level of amputation. *J Bone Joint Surg Am* 1976;58:42-46.

42. Ertl JP, Ertl W, Pritchett JW: Amputations of the lower extremity. eMedicine Website. http://www.emedicine.com/orthoped/topic9.htm. Accessed July 23, 2008.

This article provides an overview of important factors in lower extremity amputations and includes a discussion of anatomy, indications, treatment, and outcomes.

43. Keeling JJ, Schon LC: Tibiofibular bridge synostosis in below knee amputation. *Tech Foot Ankle Surg* 2007;6:156-161.

The authors review and describe surgical techniques for bone-bridging distal tibiofibular synostosis transtibial amputation. Level of evidence: V.

44. Stewart JD, Anderson CD, Unger DV: The Portsmouth modification of the Ertl bone-bridge transtibial amputa-tion: The challenge of returning amputees back to active duty. *Oper Tech Sports Med* 2006;13:222-226.

The authors present a review and description of the Portsmouth modification to the Ertl techniques for bone-bridging transtibial distal tibiofibular synostosis. Level of evidence: V.

45. Pinto MA, Harris WW: Fibular segment bone bridging in trans-tibial amputation. *Prosthet Orthot Int* 2004;28:220-224.

The authors present a retrospective review of a unique bone-bridging technique used to treat 15 patients. Results were compared with a cohort of high functioning patients treated with traditional transtibial amputation. The patients treated with the bone-bridging technique had more capacity for distal weight bearing on the stump. Level of evidence: IV.

46. Burgess EM, Romano RL, Zettl JH, et al: Amputations of the leg for peripheral vascular insufficiency. *J Bone Joint Surg Am* 1971;53:874-890.

47. Smith DG, Berke GM: Postoperative management of the lower extremity amputee. *J Prosthetic Orthotic* 2004;16(suppl):3.

Descriptive postoperative management techniques for lower extremity amputees are provided by the authors.

48. Smith DG, McFarland LV, Sangeorzan BJ, Reiber GE, Czerniecki JM: Postoperative dressing and management strategies for transtibial amputations: A critical review. *J Rehabil Res Dev* 2003;40:213-224.

The authors review the current literature and compare the safety, efficacy, and outcomes of various postoperative management strategies. Level of evidence: V.

49. Choudhury SR, Reiber GE, Pecoraro JA, Czerniecki JM, Smith DG, Sangeorzan BJ: Postoperative management of transtibial amputations in VA hospitals. *J Rehabil Res Dev* 2001;38:293-298.

50. Schon LC, Short KW, Soupiou O, Noll K, Rheinstein J: Benefits of early prosthetic management of transtibial amputees: A prospective clinical study of a prefabricated prosthesis. *Foot Ankle Int* 2002;23:509-514.

51. Fergason J, Smith DG: Socket considerations for the patient with a transtibial amputation. *Clin Orthop Relat Res* 1999;361:76-84.

52. Kulkarni J, Pande S, Morris J: Survival rates in dysvascular lower limb amputees. *Int J Surg* 2006;4:217-221.

Five- and 10-year survival rates of major dysvascular lower limb amputees attending a center specializing in amputee rehabilitation are presented. Median survival remained at 4 years, which was similar to outcomes in previously published studies. Level of evidence: IV.

53. Subramaniam B, Pomposelli F, Talmor D, Park KW: Perioperative and long-term morbidity and mortality after above-knee and below-knee amputations in diabetics and nondiabetics. *Anesth Analg* 2005;100:1241-1247.

6: Special Problems of the Foot and Ankle

A retrospective review of a vascular surgery quality assurance database was performed to evaluate the perioperative and long-term morbidity and mortality of transtibial ($n = 720$) and transfemoral ($n = 234$) amputations. The effects of diabetes mellitus were also examined. Level of evidence: IV.

54. Aulivola B, Hile CN, Hamdan AD, et al: Major lower extremity amputation: Outcome of a modern series. *Arch Surg* 2004;139:395-399.

    The authors present a retrospective review of major lower extremity amputations performed in an academic center. It was concluded that long-term survival prospects for patients with diabetes and renal failure are poor. Level of evidence: IV.

55. Wasiak K: Analysis of prognostic factors for locomotion in patients after amputation of the tibia performed due to atherosclerotic critical limb ischemia. *Ortop Traumatol Rehabil* 2005;7:411-417.

    The authors report on a retrospective analysis of locomotion performance in patients following transtibial amputation for atherosclerotic critical limb ischemia to determine factors that influence final outcomes. Level of evidence: IV.

56. MacKenzie EJ, Bosse MJ, Castillo RC, et al: Functional outcomes following trauma-related lower-extremity amputation. *J Bone Joint Surg Am* 2004;86-A:1636-1645.

    The authors provide an analysis of functional outcomes based on data gathered during the LEAP project to compare outcomes based on the level of amputation. Significant disability is reported for patients with above-ankle traumatic amputations. Level of evidence: III.

57. MacKenzie EJ, Bosse MJ, Pollak AN, et al: Long-term persistence of disability following severe lower-limb trauma: Results of a seven-year follow-up. *J Bone Joint Surg Am* 2005;87:1801-1809.

    The authors report on 397 patients treated with amputation or reconstruction of the lower extremity. Patients were evaluated an average of 48 months after injury. Functional outcomes were assessed with the Sickness Impact Profile. Reconstruction for injuries below the distal part of the femur usually have functional outcomes equivalent to those of amputation. Regardless of treatment, long-term functional outcomes are poor. Level of evidence: III.

58. Smith DG, Horn P, Malchow D, Boone DA, Reiber GE, Hansen ST Jr: Prosthetic history, prosthetic charges, and functional outcome of the isolated, traumatic below-knee amputee. *J Trauma* 1995;38:44-47.

59. Gunawardena NS, Seneviratne Rde A, Athauda T: Functional outcomes of unilateral lower limb amputee soldiers in two districts of Sri Lanka. *Mil Med* 2006; 171:283-287.

    Functional outcomes of unilateral, lower-limb, amputee soldiers was compared with function in male nonamputees to identify factors affecting functional outcomes. Level of evidence: III.

60. Dougherty PJ: Transtibial amputees from the Vietnam War: Twenty-eight-year follow-up. *J Bone Joint Surg Am* 2001;83:383-389.

61. Deffer PA, Moll JH, LaNoue AM: The Ertl osteoplastic below knee amputation. *J Bone Joint Surg Am* 1971;53: 1028.

62. Pinzur MS, Pinto MA, Saltzman M, Batista F, Gottschalk F, Juknelis D: Health-related quality of life in patients with transtibial amputation and reconstruction with bone bridging of the distal tibia and fibula. *Foot Ankle Int* 2006;27:907-912.

    Thirty-two patients of varying ages with multiple diagnoses who had bone bridging of the distal tibia and fibula at the time of transtibial amputation were retrospectively compared with a selected group of 17 high functioning patients who were treated with traditional transtibial amputation. The group treated with the bone-bridging technique had better or comparable scores on the Prosthetics Evaluation Questionnaire compared with the amputees treated with traditional transtibial amputation. Level of evidence: III.

6: Special Problems of the Foot and Ankle

Index

V

Vacuum-assisted closure (VAC), 168
  in healing ulcers, 278
Valgus deviation, 208
Vancomycin for methicillin-resistant
  Staphylococcus aureus (MRSA), 337
Varus malalignment, 196

Varus malunion, 91
V-Y advancement for Achilles tendon
  injury, 123

W

Waddling gait, 6–7
Walking velocity, 6

Warts, plantar, 369–370, 369*f*
Weil osteotomy, 9, 9*f*
Wilson procedure, 264, 265

Z

Zadik method, for total matricectomy, 368